Chemoinformatics in Drug Design and Discovery

Chemoinformatics in Drug Design and Discovery

Editor: Tosha McCallum

AMERICAN
MEDICAL PUBLISHERS
www.americanmedicalpublishers.com

AMERICAN
MEDICAL PUBLISHERS
www.americanmedicalpublishers.com

Cataloging-in-Publication Data

Chemoinformatics in drug design and discovery / edited by Tosha McCallum.
p. cm.
Includes bibliographical references and index.
ISBN 978-1-63927-976-0
1. Cheminformatics. 2. Drugs--Design. 3. Drug development. 4. Chemistry--Data processing.
5. Computational chemistry. 6. Chemistry--Information services. I. McCallum, Tosha.
RS418 .C44 2023
615.19--dc23

American Medical Publishers,
41 Flatbush Avenue,
1st Floor, New York,
NY 11217, USA

ISBN 978-1-63927-976-0 (Hardback)

Contents

Preface

The world is advancing at a fast pace like never before. Therefore, the need is to keep up with the latest developments. This book was an idea that came to fruition when the specialists in the area realized the need to coordinate together and document essential themes in the subject. That's when I was requested to be the editor. Editing this book has been an honour as it brings together diverse authors researching on different streams of the field. The book collates essential materials contributed by veterans in the area which can be utilized by students and researchers alike.

Chemoinformatics is a relatively recent approach to chemistry based on computational analysis to analyze data about chemical and molecular structures. An examination of data helps in determining the relationship among chemical structures, chemical characteristics, and molecular activity of new drugs. Chemoinformatics is an in-silico technique, which implies that it is a type of scientific investigation that is done with the help of computers and simulations. A typical drug development process begins by selecting a disease to target, followed by the search for potential compounds and molecules that can be used to cure or reduce the severity of the disease. This is accomplished by screening the different procedures for examining the efficacy of various compounds and molecules in stopping a biochemical mechanism. It leads to significant improvement in terms of cost, time, and difficulty in discovery of new drugs. The different techniques used in chemoinformatics are virtual screening, high throughput screening (HTS), and in silico ADMET. This book is a valuable compilation of topics, ranging from the basic to the most complex advancements in the field of chemoinformatics. It aims to serve as a resource guide for students and experts alike.

Each chapter is a sole-standing publication that reflects each author´s interpretation. Thus, the book displays a multi-facetted picture of our current understanding of application, resources and aspects of the field. I would like to thank the contributors of this book and my family for their endless support.

Editor

1

Scaffold Diversity of Fungal Metabolites

*Mariana González-Medina [1], John R. Owen [2], Tamam El-Elimat [3], Cedric J. Pearce [4], Nicholas H. Oberlies [5], Mario Figueroa [1] and José L. Medina-Franco [1]**

[1] Departamento de Farmacia, Facultad de Química, Universidad Nacional Autónoma de México, Mexico, Mexico, [2] High-Performance Computing Research Group, ECIT Institute, Northern Ireland Science Park, Belfast, UK, [3] Department of Medicinal Chemistry and Pharmacognosy, Faculty of Pharmacy, Jordan University of Science and Technology, Irbid, Jordan, [4] Mycosynthetix, Inc., Hillsborough, NC, USA, [5] Department of Chemistry and Biochemistry, University of North Carolina at Greensboro, Greensboro, NC, USA

***Correspondence:**
José L. Medina-Franco
medinajl@unam.mx;
jose.medina.franco@gmail.com

Many drug discovery projects rely on commercial compounds to discover active leads. However, current commercial libraries, with mostly synthetic compounds, access a small fraction of the possible chemical diversity. Natural products, in contrast, possess a vast structural diversity and have proven to be an outstanding source of new drugs. Several chemoinformatic analyses of natural products have demonstrated their diversity and structural complexity. However, to our knowledge, the scaffold content and structural diversity of fungal secondary metabolites have never been studied. Herein, the scaffold diversity of 223 fungal metabolites was measured and compared to the diversity of approved drugs and commercial libraries for HTS containing natural, synthetic, and semi-synthetic compounds. In addition, the global diversity of the fungal isolates was assessed and compared to other reference data sets using Consensus Diversity Plots, a chemoinformatic tool recently developed. It was concluded that fungal secondary metabolites are cyclic systems with few ramifications and more diverse than the commercial libraries with natural products and semi-synthetic compounds. The fungal metabolites data set was one of the most structurally diverse, containing a large proportion of different and unique scaffolds not found in the other compound data sets including ChEMBL. Therefore, fungal metabolites offer a rich source of molecules suited for identifying diverse candidates for drug discovery.

Keywords: chemical space, cheminformatics, consensus diversity plots, generative topographic mapping, molecular diversity, natural products, fungal metabolites

INTRODUCTION

With a dramatic increase in commercially available compounds and the accessibility to high throughput screening (HTS), many current drug discovery projects rely on commercial libraries to uncover novel active compounds against different molecular targets (Roy et al., 2010). However, numerous analyses have revealed that libraries with poor diversity undermine HTS productivity, thus reducing the probability to find active compounds. Many research groups are investing in enhancing their collections by adding compounds with different chemotypes rather than simply increasing the size of their compound libraries (Macarron et al., 2011). Although, a highly diverse compound library would be considered the most profitable starting point to find new leads, the term diversity generates constant debate since the optimum composition of a library depends on the research objectives. Nonetheless, it has been shown that a diverse compound library is directly linked to a higher hit discovery rate than a similar sized combinatorial library with limited structural variation (Harper et al., 2004).

Natural products have a vast diversity and are rich sources of bioactive compounds (Hong, 2011). Several studies have shown that natural products and drugs approved by the United States Food and Drug Administration (FDA) share regions of chemical space and have similar molecular properties (Gu et al., 2013). Moreover, natural products have novel and complex chemotypes (Yongye et al., 2012) and new chemical structures from natural origin are constantly being discovered (Rosen et al., 2009). Therefore, natural products offer an excellent opportunity to enrich chemical libraries (Gu et al., 2013).

Specifically, natural products derived from fungi have been the source of many important approved drugs with diverse mechanisms of action (Pearce, 1997; Pearce et al., 2009). Fungi are widely found in nature and are able to generate novel structures with chemical diversity from simple starting materials including organic acids, sugars, amino acids, terpenes, and bases such as purines and pyrimidines. Gene sequencing has demonstrated there are multiple "silent" biosynthetic pathways, meaning there is genetic information that encodes for the synthesis of new products that have not been studied. Taken together with the vast number of unstudied fungal species in the world (Hawksworth and Rossman, 1997), fungi are a highly promising source for new medicines.

The number of *in silico* analyses of fungal metabolites is still limited but the interest in this area is increasing. El-Elimat et al. (2012) studied the chemical space of 105 compounds isolated from filamentous fungi using nine molecular descriptors, and compared them to other natural products and FDA-approved anticancer drugs. In that work it was concluded that fungal metabolites had a high overlap with the chemical space of anticancer drugs, which was an encouraging finding for the ongoing efforts to discover active anticancer compounds of fungal origin (Kinghorn et al., 2016). Gonzalez-Medina et al. (2016) analyzed a larger data set with 207 fungal isolates, adding more information on structural complexity and diversity of the fungal metabolites. In that work fungal metabolites were demonstrated to be more complex than approved drugs and commercial libraries, and as complex as compounds used in the food industry, Generally Recognized as Safe (GRAS). Those results suggested that fungal metabolites could be selective and have an appropriate toxicity profile. Furthermore, fungal metabolites had drug-like properties and covered similar chemical space of approved drugs as well as unexplored areas. However, the scaffold composition and diversity of fungal metabolites has not been studied in a systematic and quantitative manner.

The goal of this work was to measure the scaffold content and diversity of an in-house library with 223 fungal metabolites. Five data sets were used as reference: non-anticancer drugs approved by the FDA, anticancer drugs approved by the FDA, compounds based on the Flavor and Extract Manufacturers Association of the United States (FEMA), and two commercial libraries containing natural products and semi-synthetic compounds. Additional criteria, including molecular properties and fingerprints were used to obtain a complete scaffold analysis and to compare datasets of different size containing cyclic and acyclic compounds. Consensus Diversity Plot (CDP) (González-Medina et al., 2016), a novel chemoinformatic tool developed to analyze the global diversity of compound data sets, was employed to compare the total diversity of fungal metabolites with other reference collections.

METHODS

Data Sets

The chemotype diversity was analyzed for a unique in-house library of 223 fungal metabolites (El-Elimat et al., 2012; Gonzalez-Medina et al., 2016). For reference, five data sets containing between 76 and 2,500 compounds were included in the analysis: compounds based on the FEMA GRAS list (hereafter referred to as GRAS; Burdock et al., 2006; Medina-Franco et al., 2012); FDA approved drugs obtained from DrugBank, version 4.0 (Wishart et al., 2006; Law et al., 2014) subdivided into: anticancer and non-anticancer drugs; and two datasets from a commercial vendor (http://www.ac-discovery.com) containing mostly natural products derived from plants (MEGx) and semi-synthetic compounds (NATx). **Table 1** summarizes all data sets used, including source and number of unique compounds after data curation. Duplicates in each data set were removed using Molecular Operating Environment (MOE), version 2014.0 (MOE, 2016). The complete data set of fungal metabolites is available upon request, the other data sets

TABLE 1 | Compound data sets analyzed in this work.

Data set	Unique compounds	Sources
Fungal metabolites	223	El-Elimat et al., 2012
Natural products screening compounds (MEGx)	2,500	http://www.ac-discovery.com
Semi-synthetic screening compounds (NATx)	2,500	http://www.ac-discovery.com
Generally Recognized as Safe (GRAS)	2,249	Burdock et al., 2006; Medina-Franco et al., 2012
Anticancer drugs from DrugBank	76	Wishart et al., 2006; Law et al., 2014
Non-anticancer drugs from DrugBank	1,399	Wishart et al., 2006; Law et al., 2014

Abbreviations: AUC, area under the curve; CDP, Consensus Diversity Plot; CSR curves, cyclic system retrieval curves; FDA, Food and Drug Administration; FEMA, Flavor and Extract Manufacturers Association; GRAS, Generally Recognized as Safe; GTM, Generative Topographic Mapping; HBA, hydrogen bond acceptors; HBD, hydrogen bond donors; HTS, high throughput screening; Log P, the octanol/water partition coefficient; MACCS, Molecular ACCess System; MEQI, Molecular Equivalent Indices; MOE, Molecular Operating Environment; MW, molecular weight; N, number of chemotypes: N_{sing}, number of singletons; PCA, Principal Component Analysis; RBF, Radial Basis Function; RTB, number of rotatable bonds; SE, Shannon entropy; SSE, scaled Shannon Entropy; TPSA, topological polar surface area.

and the compounds information can be downloaded from the supporting information (Data Sheet 2).

Scaffold Definition and Acyclic Molecules

The term scaffold is now used extensively to describe the core structure of a molecule. Different ways to obtain the scaffold of a molecule have been reviewed elsewhere (Brown and Jacoby, 2006; Yan et al., 2009). In this work the scaffolds were derived with the methodology previously described by Johnson and Xu (Xu and Johnson, 2002). Chemotypes were calculated with the program Molecular Equivalent Indices (MEQI; Xu and Johnson, 2001, 2002) resulting in a code of five characters assigned to each chemotype using a unique naming algorithm (**Figure 1**). For this work, both acyclic and cyclic systems (hereafter referred to as chemotypes) were used to compare the structural diversity.

Chemotype Diversity

For each data set the number of unique chemotypes was recorded as well as the number of chemotypes containing only one compound. The fraction of chemotypes and singletons relative to the number of molecules in the data set were analyzed.

Cyclic system retrieval (CSR) curves were computed for each data set to analyze the distribution of chemotypes (Lipkus et al., 2008). To generate the CSR curves, the fraction of chemotypes was plotted on the X-axis and the fraction of compounds that contain those chemotypes was plotted on the Y-axis. Information such as the fraction of chemotypes required to retrieve a certain percentage of the molecules in the database and the area under the curve (AUC) can be obtained from these curves. For this work CSR curves were characterized calculating the AUC and the fraction of chemotypes required to retrieve 50% of the molecules (F50). The F50 metric has been used as a measure of scaffold diversity (Krier et al., 2006; Lipkus et al., 2008; Medina-Franco et al., 2009; Yongye et al., 2012).

As previously reported, the concept of Shannon entropy (SE) (Godden and Bajorath, 2007) was used to determine the distribution of compounds in the n most populated chemotypes based on histogram representations (Medina-Franco et al., 2009). The SE of a population of P compounds in n systems is defined as:

$$SE = -\sum\nolimits_{i=1}^{n} p_i log_2 p_i \tag{1}$$

$$p_i = \frac{c_i}{P} \tag{2}$$

where p_i is the estimated probability, or frequency, of the occurrence of a specific chemotype i in a population of P compounds containing a total of n chemotypes and c_i is the number of molecules containing a particular chemotype. The value of SE ranges from 0, when all the compounds have the same chemotype, and it takes its maximum value when SE equals to $log_2\ n$, meaning that all the compounds are evenly distributed among the n chemotypes representing a highly diverse data set.

To normalize SE by the different most populated chemotypes n, the scaled Shannon entropy (SSE) is defined as:

$$SSE = \frac{SE}{log_2 n} \tag{3}$$

SSE values range from 0, when all the molecules in the data set contain only one chemotype, to 1 indicating high diversity within the n chemotypes. Here, different numbers of n (from 5 to 70) were analyzed.

Fingerprints and Molecular Properties

The inter- and intra-molecular properties diversity for each data set was analyzed based on structural fingerprints and molecular properties. Molecular ACCess System (MACCS) keys (166-bits) fingerprints were computed with MayaChem Tools (Sud, 2016) and R Studio scripts (Team, 2015). To compare the data sets, six properties of pharmaceutical relevance were calculated

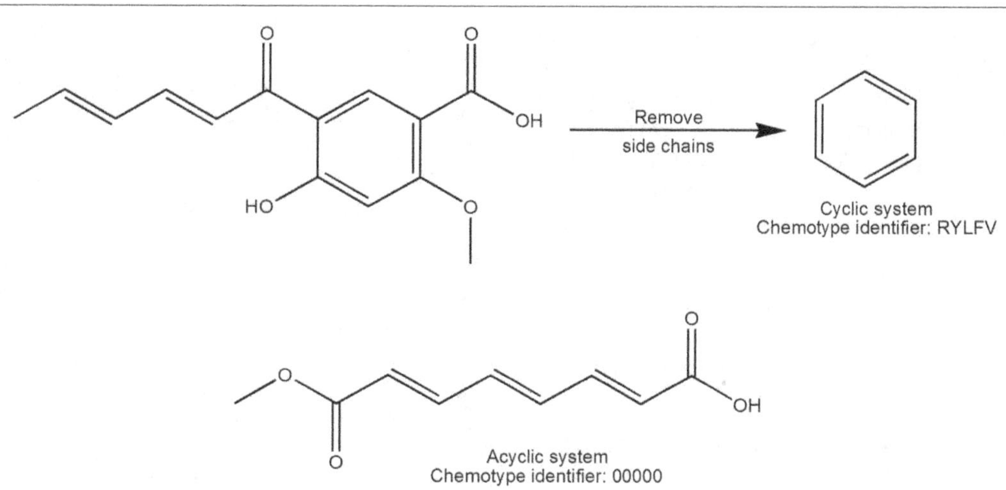

FIGURE 1 | Definition of scaffold used in this work. The cyclic system was obtained after iteratively removing the side chains of the entire molecule. Acyclic and cyclic systems were considered for this work and were defined by a code of five characters.

with MOE software: hydrogen bond donors (HBD), hydrogen bond acceptors (HBA), the octanol/water partition coefficient (LogP), molecular weight (MW), topological polar surface area (TPSA), and number of rotatable bonds (RTB). These molecular descriptors have been used previously to measure molecular properties diversity (Gonzalez-Medina et al., 2016).

Similarity Coefficients

There are many ways in which the similarities between pairs of molecules can be calculated. Here, we used two well-known measures to compare discrete and continuous variables. The Soergel distance function is a complement of Tanimoto similarity coefficient (Owen et al., 2011), widely used for binary fingerprints.

$$\text{Tanimoto}\,(\mathrm{x},\mathrm{y}) = \left(\frac{x.y^T}{x.x^T + y.y^T - x.y^T}\right) \quad (4)$$

$$\text{Soergel}\,(\mathrm{x},\mathrm{y}) = 1 - \text{tanimoto}\,(\mathrm{x},\mathrm{y}) \quad (5)$$

The similarity coefficient between data sets (d_{uv}) was calculated with a Soergel-based inter-data set distance function, previously described by Owen et al. (2011).

$$\mathrm{d_{uv}} = \frac{1}{N_u N_v} \sum\nolimits_{i=1}^{N_u} \sum\nolimits_{j=1}^{Nv} soergel\,(x_i^u, x_j^v) \quad (6)$$

where N_u and N_v are the number of molecules in data sets D_u and D_v, and x_i^u and x_j^v are the fingerprint vectors from the compounds i or j of the fingerprint array for the data sets D_u or D_v, respectively. The diversity of the molecules within a single data set (d_u) was calculated rearranging the Equation 6:

$$\mathrm{d_u} = \frac{2}{N_u^2} \sum\nolimits_{i=1}^{Nu-1} \sum\nolimits_{j=i+1}^{Nu} soergel\,(x_i^u, x_j^u) \quad (7)$$

The distance (or dissimilarity) between any two data sets, D_u and D_v, was computed using the Euclidean distance (Perez, 2005; Karthikeyan and Vyas, 2014), Equation (8), as follows. Let x_i be the N-dimensional vector of molecular properties for molecule i in data set D_u; similarly, let y_i be the N-dimensional vector of molecular properties for molecule j in data set D_v. (For the analyses in this article, 6 molecular properties where used, so $N = 6$). Let the number of molecules in data sets D_u and D_v be U and V, respectively. Then the inter-data set distance between data sets D_u and D_v, was computed as introduced in Equation (9):

$$\text{Euclidean}\,(X_i, Y_j) = \sqrt{\sum\nolimits_{k=1}^{N} (X_{ik} - Y_{jk})^2} \quad (8)$$

$$I_{uv} = \frac{1}{UV} \sum\nolimits_{i=1}^{U} \sum\nolimits_{j=1}^{V} euclidean\,(X_i, Y_j) \quad (9)$$

Global Diversity Analysis with Consensus Diversity Plots (CDPs)

CDPs have been designed to compare the diversity of compound data sets analyzing, in two dimensions, four criteria of diversity (González-Medina et al., 2016). Herein, we employed two metrics to quantify structural diversity: MACCs keys/Soergel-based distance, plotted on the X axis, and AUC, on the Y axis. The third property analyzed in the CDPs was the molecular properties intra-data set distance, calculated with Euclidean distance. This property is represented in the plot by the color of each data point: data sets in red had the highest Euclidean distances, i.e., are the most diverse, data sets in orange/brown have intermediate diversity values and data sets in green are the least diverse. The fourth property represented on this plot was the size of the data sets. This property is represented by the relative size of the data point representing each set; bigger data points correspond to data sets with more compounds. Four regions, in different colors, can be distinguished on the plot: the region in red contains the most diverse data sets, i.e., this data sets are diverse either by their scaffold content or if features of the entire molecule are analyzed and compared using fingerprints; the white region shows the least diverse data sets, i.e., these data sets were the least diverse by scaffold content and fingerprints/similarity; blue, all data sets in this region contain either acyclic compounds which are diverse if the entire molecule is compared (i.e., using fingerprints) or data sets containing cyclic systems for which side chains contribute significantly to their diversity; yellow, this fourth region contains data sets diverse by the number of different scaffolds with few ramifications. To set the four regions on the plots we chose a threshold for each axis: a value of 0.75 was chosen as the threshold for the y axis, considering that the lowest AUC value a data set could have is 0.5, if it is highly diverse by scaffolds, and the highest AUC value it could have is 1; the threshold for the x axis was the median of the Soergel intra-data set distance obtained from MACCS keys fingerprints for each set, therefore this threshold is specifically for the data sets analyzed in this work. As previously discussed, other thresholds can be set up to define the quadrants of the CDPs (González-Medina et al., 2016).

Visual Representation of the Chemical Space

Two approaches were used to cluster and visualize the molecules in the data sets based on their molecular properties and structural features: Principal Component Analysis (PCA) (Jolliffe, 2002) and Generative Topographic Mapping (GTM) (Osolodkin et al., 2015). PCA is a technique often used to emphasize variation and find patterns in a data set. The main disadvantage of PCA is that it is a linear mapping technique and is unable to map non-linear data. GTM is a nonlinear method that trains a Radial Basis Function (RBF) neuronal network to produce a mapping from an n-dimensional data space to a two dimensional latent space (Owen et al., 2011; Gaspar et al., 2013). For further explanation on each model, the reader is referred to the cited papers (Gaspar et al., 2013, 2015). To represent the chemical space using molecular fingerprints, a fingerprint array was assembled from the MACCS key fingerprint results, consisting of 166 bits in which each element is either 0 or 1 to indicate the absence or presence, respectively, of structural elements in the corresponding molecular structure. The six molecular properties of pharmaceutical relevance (HBD, HBA, LogP, MW, TPSA, and RTB) were arranged in a similar way and were used as the data set for the models. GTM and PCA were used as dimensionality reduction techniques to encode all the molecular properties and fingerprints into two-dimensional spaces that could be visualized easily. All the models and visualizations were implemented using the Matlab toolbox Netlab (Nabney, 2002).

RESULTS AND DISCUSSION

The scaffold diversity of the fungal metabolites was compared to data sets with biological relevance like approved drugs and commercial libraries available for HTS. In this work the chemotypes were calculated with the program MEQI (Xu and Johnson, 2001, 2002), as described in the Section Materials and Methods. Table S1 shows the most frequent chemotypes found in the fungal metabolites data set, along with their chemotype identifier. Interestingly, it was found that this library has several unique scaffolds not found in the reference data sets. To further explore the uniqueness of the scaffolds of the fungal metabolites, we compared the scaffolds from this data set with the scaffolds of all the compounds found in ChEMBL, version 22 (Bento et al., 2014; Davies et al., 2015). An exceptional finding was that out of the 130 different scaffolds in the fungal metabolites set, 26 were not found in ChEMBL or any other data set studied in this work. **Figure 2** shows representative scaffolds in the fungal metabolites data set not found in other data sets. Most of these compounds have been shown to have cytotoxicity against a variety of human tumor cell lines. For example, the chemotype TBEMM corresponds to the cytotoxic compounds Acremonidin C and Acremonidin A, reported by Ayers et al. (2012). The scaffolds with the chemotype V7D6X and YVGCT correspond to Palmarumycin CP3 and Palmarumycin CP4, whose cytotoxic activity has not been reported. However, their structural similarity with Palmarumycin CP1 could indicate that the compounds in the fungal metabolites data set with these scaffolds could have antibacterial, antifungal and antitumoral activities (Kornienko et al., 2015). The scaffolds with the codes 8MY2X and ROFC5 belong to new secondary metabolites isolated from *Eupenicillium brefeldianum* and *Aspergillus fumigatus,* respectively, and their biological activity has not been reported. **Figure 2** exemplifies the considerable structural variation among substances that have been isolated and characterized from filamentous fungi.

Counts

Table 2 summarizes the number of chemotypes (N) in each database, the fraction of chemotypes relative to the number of molecules in each data set (N/M), and the number and fraction of singletons (N_{sing}). Based on N/M values, the set of fungal

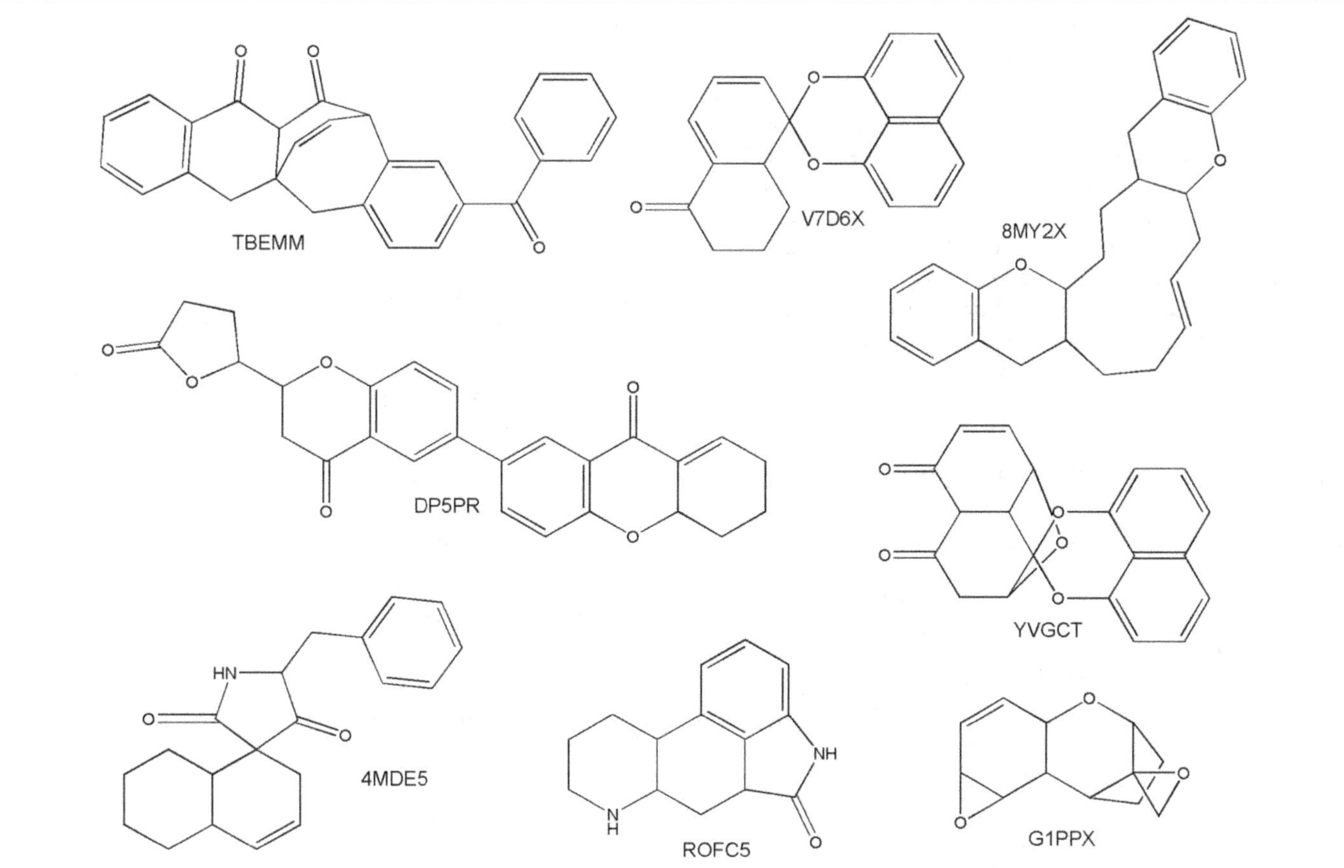

FIGURE 2 | Unique scaffolds of fungal origin.

metabolites, containing 223 compounds, has an intermediate chemotype diversity (N/M = 0.587), similar to the proportion of chemotypes in the non-anticancer drugs library, containing 1,399 compounds (N/M = 0.572). The set of anticancer drugs has fewer compounds but the largest proportion of chemotypes relative to the number of molecules (N/M = 0.921) and the largest proportion of singletons relative to the number of molecules (N_{sing}/M = 0.855). In contrast, GRAS, NATx, and MEGx data sets with more compounds (**Table 1**) have the lowest scaffold diversity with a smaller proportion of chemotypes and singletons.

CSR Curves

CSR curves represent the fraction of compounds in the data set (y-axis) contained in a fraction of chemotypes (x-axis). A data set with maximum diversity would contain a different chemotype for each molecule in the library and the CSR curve would be a diagonal with an AUC of 0.5. **Figure 3** shows the CSR curves calculated using the chemotypes of all the data sets analyzed in this study.

The CSR curve for the fungal metabolites indicates this data set contains more different scaffolds than MEGx, NATx, GRAS, and the non-anticancer drugs. All these data sets contain at least six times more compounds than the set with fungal metabolites (**Table 1**). The CSR curve for the anticancer drugs is closer to a diagonal indicating large diversity, while the curves for GRAS undergoes a sudden increase on its slope indicating this data set has the lowest chemotype diversity. AUC and the fraction of chemotypes that contains 50% of the molecules in the data set (F_{50}) were used to compare the curves for each set quantitatively (**Table 2**). An AUC value closer to one indicates low chemotype diversity and higher F_{50} values indicate higher diversity. Based on these metrics, the fungal metabolites are more diverse than MEGx and NATx, commercial data sets with 2,500 natural products and semi-synthetic compounds and approved non-anticancer drugs, with an AUC of 0.644 and a F_{50} = 0.244. As expected, anticancer drugs showed the lowest AUC and the largest F_{50} values (0.537 and 0.457, respectively). In agreement with other metrics of scaffold diversity (i.e., N/M), the GRAS and MEGx libraries had the highest AUC and lowest F_{50} values, respectively, indicating low diversity.

TABLE 2 | Results of different chemotypes diversity analyses on the data sets.

Database	*N*	*N/M*	N_{sing}	N_{sing}/N	N_{sing}/M	AUC	F_{50}
Fungal metabolites	131	0.587	87	0.664	0.390	0.664	0.244
MEGx	935	0.374	642	0.687	0.257	0.781	0.072
NATx	799	0.320	400	0.501	0.160	0.768	0.116
GRAS	238	0.106	150	0.630	0.067	0.926	0.004
Anticancer drugs	70	0.921	65	0.929	0.855	0.537	0.457
Non-anticancer drugs	844	0.572	686	0.813	0.465	0.699	0.157

N, number of chemotypes; M, number of molecules; N_{sing}, number of singletons; AUC, area under the curve; F_{50}, fraction of chemotypes that contains 50% of the data set.

Scaled Shannon Entropy (SSE)

SSE was computed to get an idea of the compound distribution in the most populated chemotypes. For this approach, a SSE value closer to 1 indicates that compounds are evenly distributed in the different chemotypes and a low SSE value (i.e., closer to 0) means all the compounds share the same chemotype. SSE will have its maximum value only when all chemotypes contain the same number of compounds, or when each chemotype contains only one compound. **Table 3** summarizes the SSE for the first 70 most populated chemotypes in each library. The chemotype diversity of the fungal metabolites is higher (SSE values ranging from 0.942 to 0.967) compared to the non-anticancer drugs and the

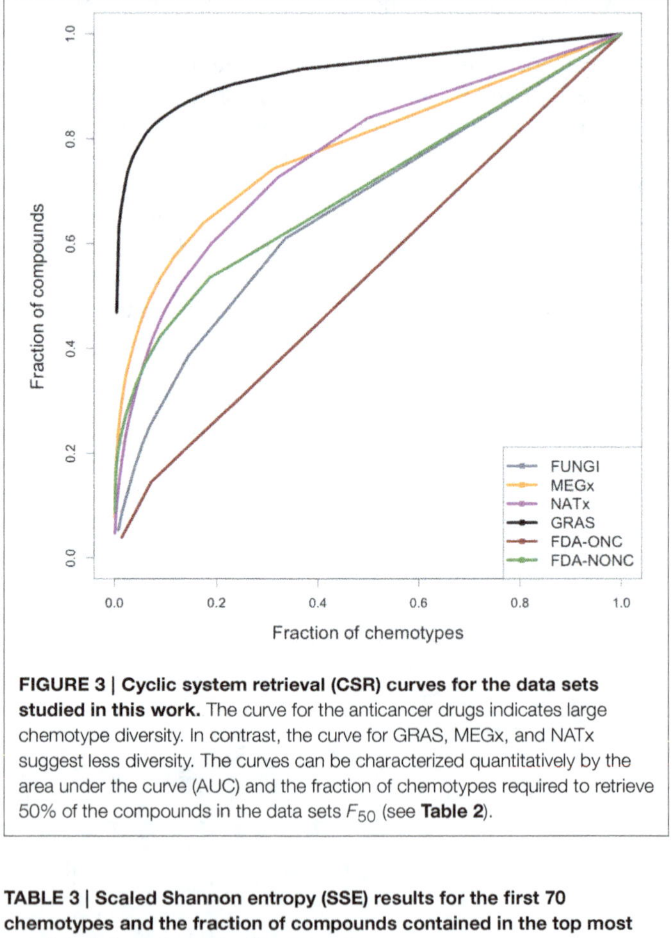

FIGURE 3 | Cyclic system retrieval (CSR) curves for the data sets studied in this work. The curve for the anticancer drugs indicates large chemotype diversity. In contrast, the curve for GRAS, MEGx, and NATx suggest less diversity. The curves can be characterized quantitatively by the area under the curve (AUC) and the fraction of chemotypes required to retrieve 50% of the compounds in the data sets F_{50} (see **Table 2**).

TABLE 3 | Scaled Shannon entropy (SSE) results for the first 70 chemotypes and the fraction of compounds contained in the top most populated chemotypes for the data sets.

Database	SSE5	SSE10	SSE20	SSE30	SSE40	SSE50	SSE60	SSE70
Fungal metabolites	0.967	0.959	0.954	0.954	0.956	0.947	0.943	0.942
MEGx	0.883	0.873	0.869	0.858	0.858	0.858	0.857	0.856
NATx	0.916	0.931	0.938	0.939	0.939	0.938	0.938	0.936
GRAS	0.617	0.57	0.541	0.526	0.517	0.512	0.507	0.501
Anticancer drugs	0.991	0.964	0.974	0.981	0.986	0.989	0.991	0.992
Non-anticancer drugs	0.769	0.750	0.762	0.777	0.789	0.799	0.803	0.809

commercial libraries NATx and MEGx, which represent larger data sets containing natural products. Compounds in the library with anticancer drugs are more evenly distributed among the chemotypes studied (SSE values higher than 0.960). The least diverse set is GRAS (SSE values ranging from 0.502 to 0.617). Of note, the most diverse data sets, the fungal metabolites and the anticancer drugs, are also the smallest data sets containing only 223 and 76 compounds, respectively (**Table 1**). Overall, the SSE values vary for the rest of the libraries, indicating that that scaffold diversity decreases in this order: anticancer drugs, fungal metabolites, NATx, MEGx, non-anticancer drugs, and GRAS. Interestingly, if the most populated chemotypes in NATx and MEGx are analyzed, these sets are more diverse than that of the non-anticancer drugs.

Figure 4 shows the distribution and SSE values of compounds in the top 70 most populated chemotypes of representative data sets. Data sets with higher SSE are colored dark red and data sets with lower SSE are light red. The chemotypes for the fungal metabolites, **Figure 4B**, are more evenly distributed after the top 10 most populated chemotypes and is the second most diverse data set. **Figure 4A** shows that anticancer drugs take its maximum SSE value when all the chemotypes are considered, indicating there is almost one different chemotype for each molecule in this data set. MEGx (**Figure 4C**) has SSE values

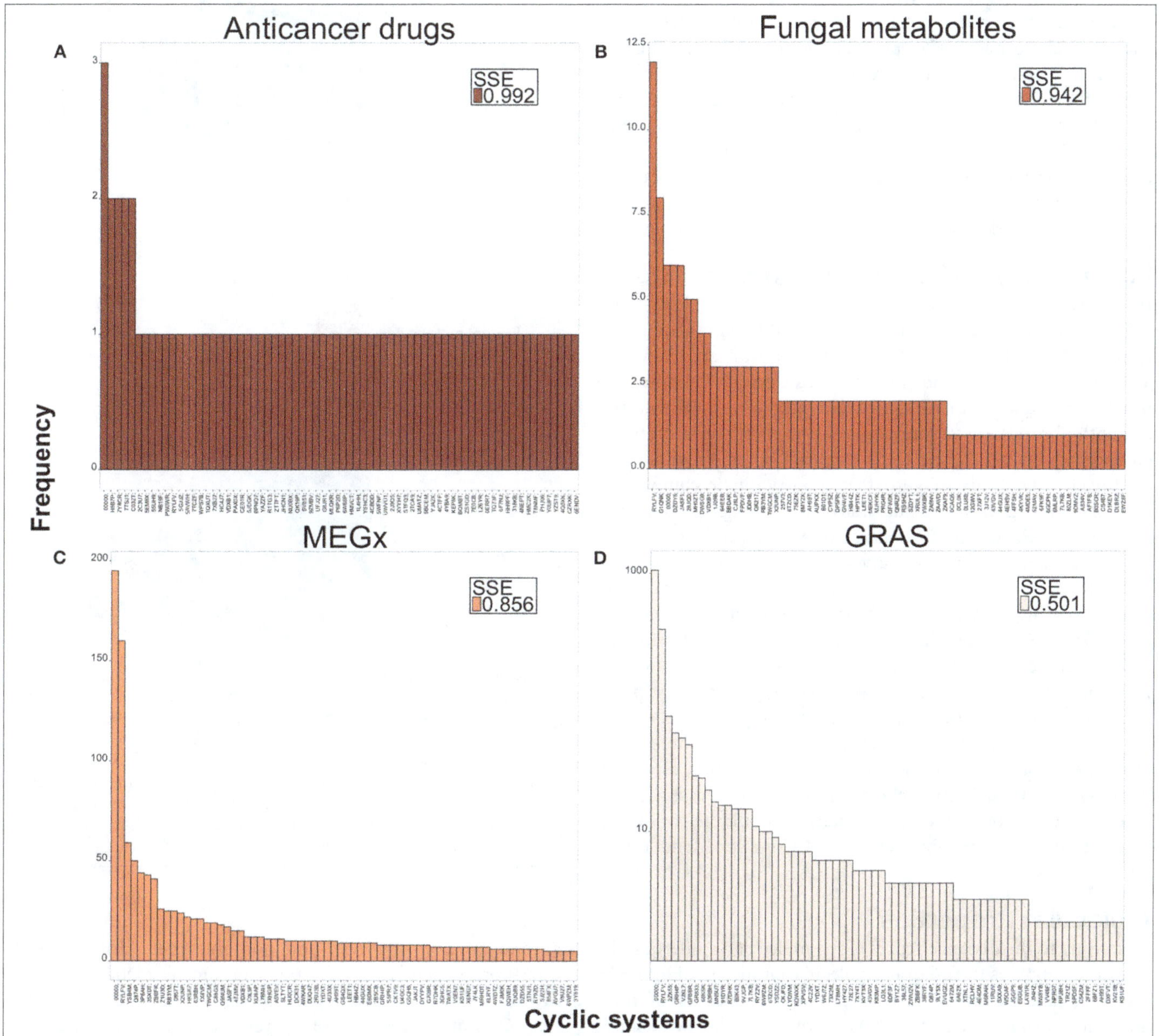

FIGURE 4 | Distribution of compounds in the top 70 most populated chemotypes. Values of SSE70 close to 1.0 are dark red and indicate large chemotype diversity, smaller SSE values are in light red indicating less diversity. **(A)** Anticancer drugs, **(B)** fungal metabolites, **(C)** MEGx, **(D)** GRAS.

between 0.883 and 0.856; for this library the first most populated chemotype contains 195 compounds and the scaffolds are more evenly distributed after the first 20 most populated chemotypes. This is also the case with GRAS (**Figure 4D**), the least diverse set, measured with SSE, for which the most populated chemotype contains 1,055 compounds, nearly half of the data set. The distribution of the compounds in each chemotype and the SSE70 value for the other data sets are shown in Figure S1.

Inter- and Intra-Library Similarities Using MACCS Keys and Molecular Properties

As stated in the Methods, the inter- and intra- library similarity was computed using MACCS keys/Soergel-based distance and molecular properties/Euclidean distance. **Figures 5A,B** show the corresponding distance matrices computed with MACCS keys and molecular properties, respectively. Values along the diagonal in red represent the intra-library diversity, i.e., the diversity within the compounds contained in a data set: the least diverse libraries are in light red while the most diverse libraries are in dark red. The values in blue represent the inter-library diversity, i.e., the diversity between the compounds in all the data sets: the least diverse libraries are in light blue while the most diverse libraries are in dark blue.

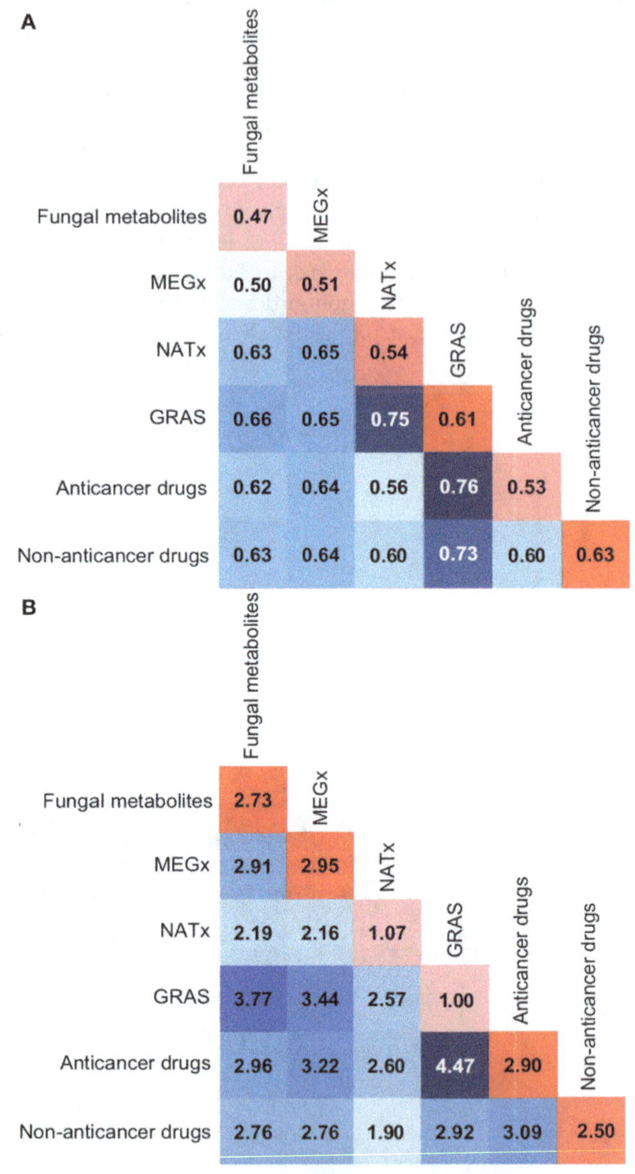

FIGURE 5 | Intra and inter-library similarity. The diagonal in red depicts intra-library comparisons, i.e., the similarity between the compounds in a data set. Dark red scores indicate large distance or low similarity, while light red colors indicate small distance or high similarity. The matrix in blue depicts inter-library similarity comparisons, i.e., the similarity between the compounds in the data sets. Dark blue scores indicate large distance or low similarity, while white or light blue colors indicate small distance or high similarity. **(A)** Soergel distance using MACCS keys (166-bit) fingerprints. **(B)** Euclidean distance function using molecular properties.

MACCS Keys—Structural Features

In **Figure 5A** the inter-library similarity matrix, in blue, shows that the fungal metabolites are structurally different to approved drugs, with a distance of 0.62 to the anticancer drugs and a distance of 0.63 to the non-anticancer drugs. Of note, the fungal metabolites and MEGx have similar structural features, but both libraries are structurally different to the semi-synthetic compounds in NATx. NATx is the data set most similar to approved drugs. This suggests that semi-synthetic compounds have been modified to be structurally similar to approved drugs, decreasing their structural similarity to natural products.

In **Figure 5A** the intra-library similarity in the red diagonal shows that GRAS and non-anticancer drugs are the most diverse data sets using MACCs keys (with intra-set distance of 0.61 and 0.63, respectively). In contrast, GRAS is the set with the lowest scaffold diversity. The reason for this is that 65% of GRAS molecules are classified into two chemotypes, namely, non-cyclic structure (49%; 00000), and benzene ring (16.3%; RYLFV). Nonetheless, having the same chemotype does not imply that molecules should present the same chemical features, especially with very common/simple chemotypes as in this case. This is a good example of how diversity analysis should be conducted using multiple metrics (Singh et al., 2009; Gonzalez-Medina et al., 2016).

Molecular Properties

According to the distance scores of the molecular properties, the fungal metabolites intra-library molecular properties, **Figure 5B** red diagonal, are more diverse than the properties of non-anticancer drugs, GRAS and NATx, with a Euclidian distance equal to 2.73. Comparing the fungal metabolites inter-library distances to the lowest inter and intra-library distances obtained for other data sets, e.g., GRAS intra-library similarity with a value of 1.00 or NATx and non-anticancer drugs with an inter-library similarity of 1.90, the fungal metabolites have diverse molecular properties compared to the other data sets. Of note, the inter-library results, in a blue scale, show that the fungal metabolites have the largest dissimilarity with GRAS, which has been previously demonstrated to contain smaller compounds with less HBD, HBA, MW, and TPSA than the fungal metabolites (Gonzalez-Medina et al., 2016). Table S2 contains the statistics of each property for all the data sets. **Figure 5B** also shows that NATx has the lowest inter-data set distance (more similar) to the rest of the data sets studied and GRAS is the least similar (i.e., the most distant) to the other libraries. Interestingly, approved anticancer drugs and GRAS present the largest distance to the other data sets, with an added distance of 28.72 and 27.37, respectively. As previously discussed (Gonzalez-Medina et al., 2016), compounds in the data set containing approved anticancer drugs show the largest distance (dissimilarity) to the non-anticancer drugs.

Global Diversity Analysis with Consensus Diversity Plots (CDPs)

Figure 6 shows a CDP, which compares the global structural diversity of all data sets, by plotting MACCs keys/Soergel-based distance in the x axis and AUC in the y axis. The size of the data points represents the relative size of each data set (**Table 1**) and the color of each data point represents the molecular properties diversity (**Figure 5B**). Remarkably, the fungal metabolites, a data set with 223 compounds, had more different scaffolds than data sets with 2,500 compounds, such as MEGx and NATx; the fungal metabolite dataset is on average, more structurally diverse than MEGx and more diverse than NATx when considering molecular properties. The fungal metabolites and the anticancer drugs are located in the yellow quadrant, indicating high scaffold diversity but low structure (fingerprint-based) diversity. Furthermore, the data point in red, representing the fungal metabolites, indicates this data has diverse molecular properties. Overall, non-anticancer drugs, in the red quadrant, are the most structurally diverse (with a Soergel-based distance of 0.63 and an AUC of 0.699). However, non-anticancer drugs in orange/brown are less diverse by molecular properties than the fungal isolates. GRAS, in the blue quadrant, is the most diverse library when structural features are taken into account, but the compounds in this data set have low molecular properties diversity. Compared to the other data sets, MEGx, in the white quadrant, is the least structural diverse. The molecular properties diversity is independent of the structural diversity or the size of the libraries, that is, small data sets can be both structurally diverse and diverse by their molecular properties, or structurally diverse but with low molecular properties diversity.

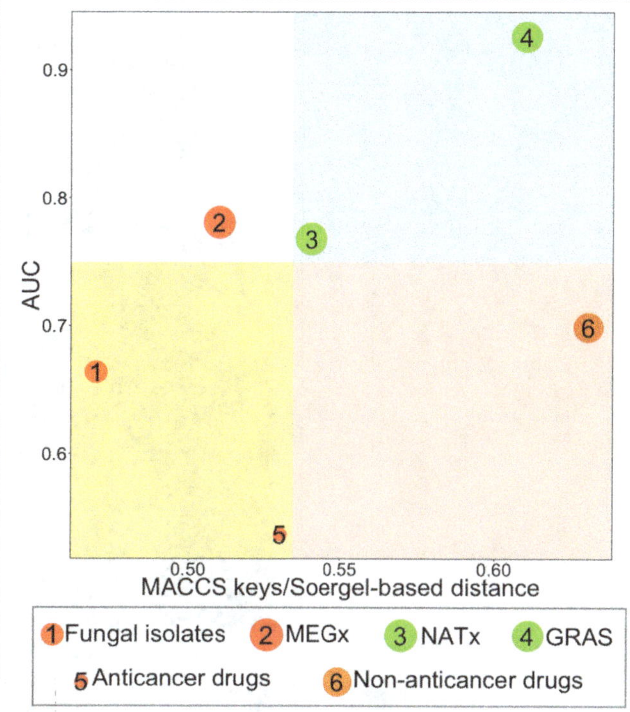

FIGURE 6 | Consensus Diversity Plot comparing the diversity of six data sets. The structural diversity was defined with MACCs keys fingerprints/Soergel-based distance and area under curve (AUC). The quadrants color codes are as follows: red, indicates the library is diverse considering its scaffolds and/or side chains; white, the library is not diverse; blue, the library is diverse if the chemical features of the entire molecule are considered and/or side chains contribute significantly to the diversity; yellow, the scaffolds of the molecules are the main factor contributing to the diversity and/or this set contains mostly rings with few side chains. Data points are colored by the diversity of the physicochemical properties of the data set as measured by the Euclidean distance of six properties of pharmaceutical relevance. The distance is represented with a continuous color scale from red (more diverse), to orange/brown (intermediate diversity) to green (less diverse). The relative size of the data set is represented with the size of the data point: smaller data points indicate compound data sets with fewer molecules. A value of 0.75 for AUC and the median value of the MACCs keys fingerprints/Soergel-based distance were used to set the quadrants.

Visual Representation of the Chemical Space

Figure 7 depicts the visual representation of the six data sets generated with GTM using the structural features MACCS keys. The fungal metabolites occupy similar areas of the structural space of MEGx, which is in agreement with the results observed on **Figure 5A**. The clusters of compounds in the structural space of the fungal metabolites are in different areas of the space of most of the approved drugs, and particularly, from the approved anticancer drugs. This is also in line with the results on **Figure 5A** and could give the notion that different structural features found in the fungal metabolites are not found in the approved drugs. Interestingly, semi-synthetic compounds (NATx) are in different areas of the structural space of natural products, compared with the fungal metabolites and MEGx. Approved non-anticancer drugs and MEGx are the most dispersed, whereas GRAS seems to be more clustered in a high-density region that contains some compounds from MEGx.

Figure S2 depicts the visual representation of the chemical space generated with GTM using physicochemical properties. The fungal metabolites form small clusters and occupy similar areas of the physicochemical space of MEGx, NATx, and the non-anticancer drugs, with a few exceptions found on the bottom left of the fungal metabolites plot, but occupy different areas than the anticancer drugs. NATx and GRAS are less distributed in the chemical space. This result is in agreement with **Figure 5B**.

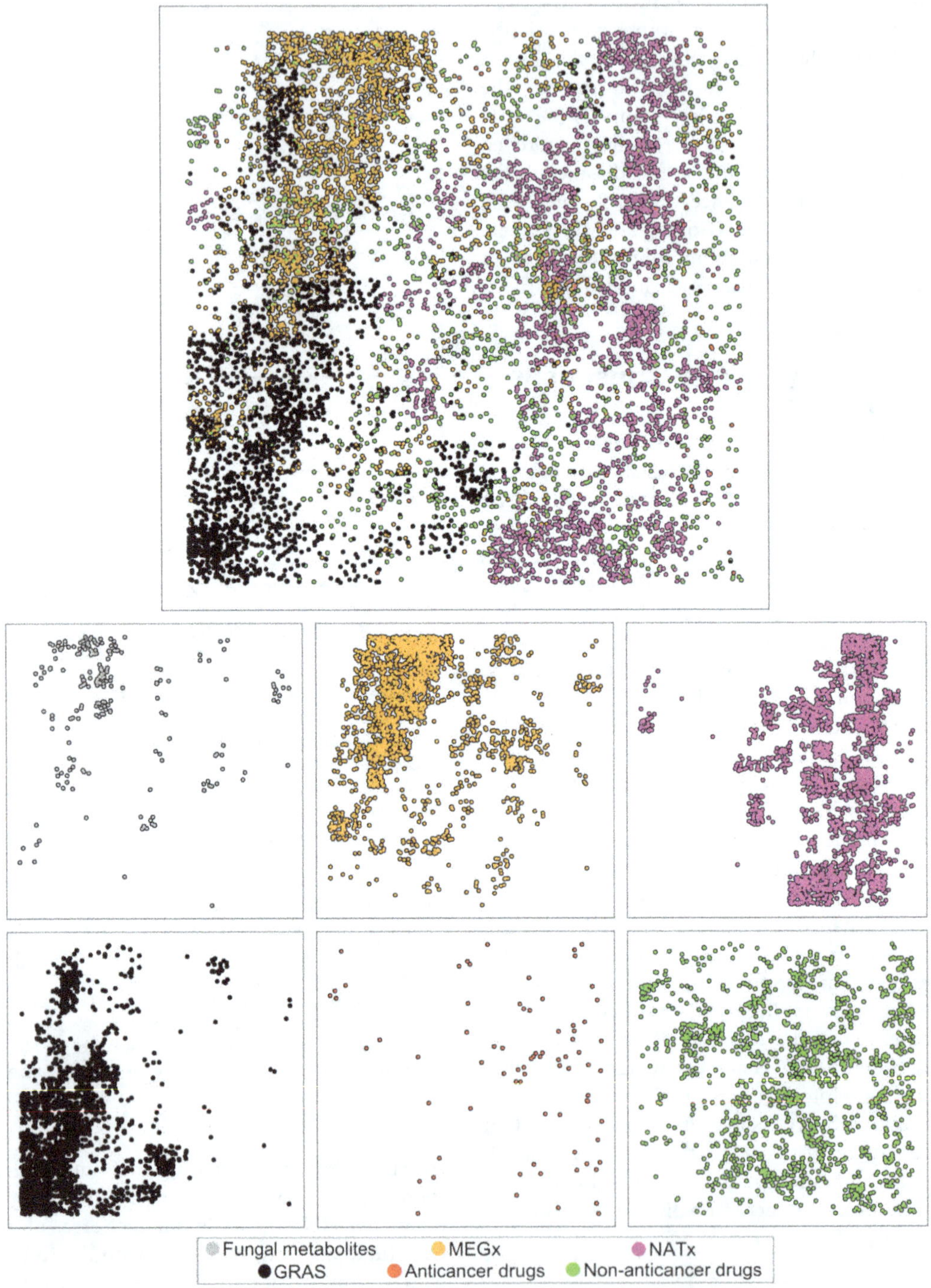

FIGURE 7 | Visual representation of the chemical space of the six data sets generated with Generative Topographic Mapping (GTM) using MACCS keys fingerprints.

The visualization generated with PCA using MACCS keys fingerprints (Figure S3) generated clusters of molecules easier to interpret. The results obtained with this representation were in line with the results obtained with GTM. Based on the structural features encoded by MACCS keys, some fungal metabolites are in the same region as the approved anticancer and non-anticancer drugs. However, most of the molecules in the data sets containing natural products, MEGx and the fungal metabolites, are clustered together in a region separated from the other data sets. Figure S4 depicts the visualization of the six molecular properties (described in the Materials and Methods Section) using PCA: the fungal metabolites are in similar regions as the non-anticancer drugs, with a few compounds dispersed similarly to MEGx. Anticancer drugs are the most spread (more diverse), while GRAS is more constrained in to specific areas of the chemical space. These results are also in agreement with results derived from **Figure 5B**.

CONCLUSIONS

Using computational-driven approaches, this work reports the structural diversity and scaffold content of a set of 223 fungal metabolites isolated and characterized in discovery projects funded by the USA National Cancer Institute and the Mexican National Research Council of Science and Technology. Generally speaking, most of these compounds were isolated while pursuing new anticancer drug leads. The structural diversity of the fungal metabolites was quantified using three complementary approaches: Cyclic Systems Retrieval curves, Shannon entropy, and molecular fingerprints. The dataset of fungal metabolites was compared to datasets that represent synthetic, semi-synthetic, and natural products commercially available for HTS and approved drugs. It was concluded that most of the chemical structures of the fungal metabolites are cyclic compounds with few side chains. The diversity analysis showed that the set of fungal secondary metabolites herein studied is more diverse than commercial libraries with natural products and semi-synthetic compounds despite the fact that the reference collections are expected to be diverse and contain more compounds. Moreover, the fungal dataset was developed mostly via pursuing leads that were cytotoxic to cancer cell lines; if the diversity of the targets were to be expanded, the resultant chemical diversity may expand as well. Moreover, the fungal metabolites have a large proportion of different and unique scaffolds not found in the other reference sets, including ChEMBL. Additionally, visualizations of the chemical space, based both on molecular fingerprints and molecular properties, revealed that the fungal metabolites cover different areas of chemical space when compared to that of approved drugs, offering the possibility to expand the medicinally-relevant chemical space. For example, this diverse data set could be used for HTS to find new hits with new scaffolds and diverse properties. The high and unique scaffold diversity of fungal metabolites revealed in this work, in addition to the high structural complexity and balanced molecular properties revealed in previous studies (Greve et al., 2010; El-Elimat et al., 2012; Cragg and Newman, 2013; Gonzalez-Medina et al., 2016), further supports fungal metabolites as a promising sources of novel compounds for drug discovery.

AUTHOR CONTRIBUTIONS

MG and JO performed the calculations. MG and JM designed the study. TE, CP, NO, and MF participate in interpreting the calculations. All authors participate in analyzing data and writing the manuscript.

ACKNOWLEDGMENTS

We thank the Universidad Nacional Autónoma de México (UNAM) for grant PAPIME PE200116 and the Consejo Nacional de Ciencia y Tecnología (CONACyT) for grant 236564. The isolation of fungal metabolites from the Mycosynthetix library via researchers at the University of North Carolina at Greensboro was funded in part by grant P01 CA125066 from the National Institutes of Health/National Cancer Institute. We thank Fernando Prieto-Martinez and Oscar Méndez-Lucio for helpful discussions.

REFERENCES

Ayers, S., Graf, T. N., Adcock, A. F., Kroll, D. J., Shen, Q., Swanson, S. M., et al. (2012). Cytotoxic xanthone-anthraquinone heterodimers from an unidentified fungus of the order Hypocreales (MSX 17022). *J. Antibiot.* 65, 3–8. doi: 10.1038/ja.2011.95

Bento, A. P., Gaulton, A., Hersey, A., Bellis, L. J., Chambers, J., Davies, M., et al. (2014). The ChEMBL bioactivity database: an update. *Nucleic Acids Res.* 42, D1083–D1090. doi: 10.1093/nar/gkt1031

Brown, N., and Jacoby, E. (2006). On scaffolds and hopping in medicinal chemistry. *Mini Rev. Med. Chem.* 6, 1217–1229. doi: 10.2174/138955706778742768

Burdock, G. A., Carabin, I. G., and Griffiths, J. C. (2006). The importance of GRAS to the functional food and nutraceutical industries. *Toxicology* 221, 17–27. doi: 10.1016/j.tox.2006.01.012

Cragg, G. M., and Newman, D. J. (2013). Natural products: a continuing source of novel drug leads. *Biochim. Biophys. Acta* 1830, 3670–3695. doi: 10.1016/j.bbagen.2013.02.008

Davies, M., Nowotka, M., Papadatos, G., Dedman, N., Gaulton, A., Atkinson, F., et al. (2015). ChEMBL web services: streamlining access to drug discovery data and utilities. *Nucleic Acids Res.* 43, W612–W620. doi: 10.1093/nar/gkv352

El-Elimat, T., Zhang, X., Jarjoura, D., Moy, F. J., Orjala, J., Kinghorn, A. D., et al. (2012). Chemical diversity of metabolites from fungi, cyanobacteria, and plants relative to FDA-approved anticancer agents. *ACS Med. Chem. Lett.* 3, 645–649. doi: 10.1021/ml300105s

Gaspar, H. A., Baskin, I. I., Marcou, G., Horvath, D., and Varnek, A. (2015). Chemical data visualization and analysis with incremental generative topographic mapping: big data challenge. *J. Chem. Inf. Model.* 55, 84–94. doi: 10.1021/ci500575y

Gaspar, H. A., Marcou, G., Horvath, D., Arault, A., Lozano, S., Vayer, P., et al. (2013). Generative topographic mapping-based classification models and their applicability domain: application to the Biopharmaceutics Drug Disposition Classification System (BDDCS). *J. Chem. Inf. Model.* 53, 3318–3325. doi: 10.1021/ci400423c

Godden, J. W., and Bajorath, J. (2007). "Analysis of chemical information content using shannon entropy," in *Reviews in Computational Chemistry*, eds K. B. Lipkowitz and T. R. Cundari (Hoboken, NJ: John Wiley & Sons, Inc.), 263–289.

Gonzalez-Medina, M., Prieto-Martinez, F. D., Naveja, J. J., Mendez-Lucio, O., El-Elimat, T., Pearce, C. J., et al. (2016). Chemoinformatic expedition of the chemical space of fungal products. *Future Med. Chem.* 8, 1399–1412. doi: 10.4155/fmc-2016-0079

González-Medina, M., Prieto-Martínez, F. D., Owen, J. R., and Medina-Franco, J. L. (2016). Consensus diversity plots: a global diversity analysis of chemical libraries. *J. Cheminform.* 8:63. doi: 10.1186/s13321-016-0176-9

Greve, H., Mohamed, I. E., Pontius, A., Kehraus, S., Gross, H., and König, G. M. (2010). Fungal metabolites: structural diversity as incentive for anticancer drug development. *Phytochem. Rev.* 9, 537–545. doi: 10.1007/s11101-010-9198-5

Gu, J., Gui, Y., Chen, L., Yuan, G., Lu, H.-Z., and Xu, X. (2013). Use of natural products as chemical library for drug discovery and network pharmacology. *PLoS ONE* 8:e62839. doi: 10.1371/journal.pone.0062839

Harper, G., Pickett, S. D., and Green, D. V. (2004). Design of a compound screening collection for use in high throughput screening. *Comb. Chem. High Throughput Screen.* 7, 63–70. doi: 10.2174/138620704772884832

Hawksworth, D. L., and Rossman, A. Y. (1997). Where are all the undescribed fungi? *Phytopathology* 87, 888–891. doi: 10.1094/PHYTO.1997.87.9.888

Hong, J. (2011). Role of natural product diversity in chemical biology. *Curr. Opin. Chem. Biol.* 15, 350–354. doi: 10.1016/j.cbpa.2011.03.004

Jolliffe, I. T. (2002). *Principal Component Analysis*. New York, NY: Springer.

Karthikeyan, M., and Vyas, R. (2014). *Practical Chemoinformatics*. New York, NY: Springer.

Kinghorn, A. D., DE Blanco, E. J., Lucas, D. M., Rakotondraibe, H. L., Orjala, J., Soejarto, D. D., et al. (2016). Discovery of anticancer agents of diverse natural origin. *Anticancer Res.* 36, 5623–5637. doi: 10.21873/anticanres.11146

Kornienko, A., Evidente, A., Vurro, M., Mathieu, V., Cimmino, A., Evidente, M., et al. (2015). Towards a cancer drug of fungal origin. *Med. Res. Rev.* 35, 937–967. doi: 10.1002/med.21348

Krier, M., Bret, G., and Rognan, D. (2006). Assessing the scaffold diversity of screening libraries. *J. Chem. Inf. Model.* 46, 512–524. doi: 10.1021/ci050352v

Law, V., Knox, C., Djoumbou, Y., Jewison, T., Guo, A. C., Liu, Y., et al. (2014). DrugBank 4.0: shedding new light on drug metabolism. *Nucleic Acids Res.* 42, D1091–D1097. doi: 10.1093/nar/gkt1068

Lipkus, A. H., Yuan, Q., Lucas, K. A., Funk, S. A., Bartelt, W. F. III, Schenck, R. J., et al. (2008). Structural diversity of organic chemistry. A scaffold analysis of the CAS Registry. *J. Org. Chem.* 73, 4443–4451. doi: 10.1021/jo8001276

Macarron, R., Banks, M. N., Bojanic, D., Burns, D. J., Cirovic, D. A., Garyantes, T., et al. (2011). Impact of high-throughput screening in biomedical research. *Nat. Rev. Drug Discov.* 10, 188–195. doi: 10.1038/nrd3368

Medina-Franco, J. L., Martínez-Mayorga, K., Bender, A., and Scior, T. (2009). Scaffold diversity analysis of compound data sets using an entropy-based measure. *QSAR Comb. Sci.* 28, 1551–1560. doi: 10.1002/qsar.200960069

Medina-Franco, J. L., Martinez-Mayorga, K., Peppard, T. L., and Del Rio, A. (2012). Chemoinformatic analysis of GRAS (Generally Recognized as Safe) flavor chemicals and natural products. *PLoS ONE* 7:e50798. doi: 10.1371/journal.pone.0050798

MOE (2016). *Molecular Operating Environment (MOE)*. 2013.08 ed. Montreal, QC: Chemical Computing Group Inc.

Nabney, I. T. (2002). *NETLAB: Algorithms for Pattern Recognition*. London: Springer.

Osolodkin, D. I., Radchenko, E. V., Orlov, A. A., Voronkov, A. E., Palyulin, V. A., and Zefirov, N. S. (2015). Progress in visual representations of chemical space. *Expert Opin. Drug Discov.* 10, 959–973. doi: 10.1517/17460441.2015.1060216

Owen, J. R., Nabney, I. T., Medina-Franco, J. L., and Lopez-Vallejo, F. (2011). Visualization of molecular fingerprints. *J. Chem. Inf. Model.* 51, 1552–1563. doi: 10.1021/ci1004042

Pearce, C. (1997). Biologically active fungal metabolites. *Adv. Appl. Microbiol.* 44, 1–80. doi: 10.1016/S0065-2164(08)70459-3

Pearce, C., Eckard, P., Gruen-Wollny, I., and Hansske, F. G. (2009). "Chapter 7 microorganisms: their role in the discovery and development of medicines," in *Natural Product Chemistry for Drug Discovery*, eds A. D. Buss and M. S. Buttler (Cambridge: The Royal Society of Chemistry), 215–241.

Perez, J. J. (2005). Managing molecular diversity. *Chem. Soc. Rev.* 34, 143–152. doi: 10.1039/b209064n

Rosen, J., Gottfries, J., Muresan, S., Backlund, A., and Oprea, T. I. (2009). Novel chemical space exploration via natural products. *J. Med. Chem.* 52, 1953–1962. doi: 10.1021/jm801514w

Roy, A., McDonald, P. R., Sittampalam, S., and Chaguturu, R. (2010). Open access high throughput drug discovery in the public domain: a mount everest in the making. *Curr. Pharm. Biotechnol.* 11, 764–778. doi: 10.2174/138920110792927757

Singh, N., Guha, R., Giulianotti, M. A., Pinilla, C., Houghten, R. A., and Medina-Franco, J. L. (2009). Chemoinformatic analysis of combinatorial libraries, drugs, natural products, and molecular libraries small molecule repository. *J. Chem. Inf. Model.* 49, 1010–1024. doi: 10.1021/ci800426u

Sud, M. (2016). MayaChemTools: an open source package for computational drug discovery. *J. Chem. Inf. Model.* 56, 2292–2297. doi: 10.1021/acs.jcim.6b00505

Team, R. (2015). *RStudio: Integrated Development for R*. Boston, MA: RStudio, Inc.

Wishart, D. S., Knox, C., Guo, A. C., Shrivastava, S., Hassanali, M., Stothard, P., et al. (2006). DrugBank: a comprehensive resource for *in silico* drug discovery and exploration. *Nucleic Acids Res.* 34, D668–D672. doi: 10.1093/nar/gkj067

Xu, Y.-J., and Johnson, M. (2001). Algorithm for Naming Molecular Equivalence classes represented by labeled pseudographs. *J. Chem. Inf. Comp. Sci.* 41, 181–185. doi: 10.1021/ci0003911

Xu, Y.-J., and Johnson, M. (2002). Using molecular equivalence numbers to visually explore structural features that distinguish chemical libraries. *J. Chem. Inf. Comp. Sci.* 42, 912–926. doi: 10.1021/ci025535l

Yan, B., Xue, M., Xiong, B., Liu, K., Hu, D., and Shen, J. (2009). ScafBank: a public comprehensive Scaffold database to support molecular hopping. *Acta Pharmacol. Sin.* 30, 251–258. doi: 10.1038/aps.2008.22

Yongye, A. B., Waddell, J., and Medina-Franco, J. L. (2012). Molecular scaffold analysis of natural products databases in the public domain. *Chem. Biol. Drug Des.* 80, 717–724. doi: 10.1111/cbdd.12011

2

QSAR-Driven Design and Discovery of Novel Compounds with Antiplasmodial and Transmission Blocking Activities

Marilia N. N. Lima[1†], Cleber C. Melo-Filho[1†], Gustavo C. Cassiano[2], Bruno J. Neves[1,3], Vinicius M. Alves[1], Rodolpho C. Braga[1], Pedro V. L. Cravo[4], Eugene N. Muratov[5,6], Juliana Calit[7], Daniel Y. Bargieri[7], Fabio T. M. Costa[2] and Carolina H. Andrade[1,2]*

[1] LabMol – Laboratory for Molecular Modeling and Drug Design, Faculty of Pharmacy, Federal University of Goiás, Goiânia, Brazil, [2] Laboratory of Tropical Diseases – Prof. Dr. Luiz Jacintho da Silva, Department of Genetics, Evolution, Microbiology and Immunology, Institute of Biology, UNICAMP, Campinas, Brazil, [3] Laboratory of Cheminformatics, PPG-SOMA, University Center of Anápolis/UniEVANGELICA, Anápolis, Brazil, [4] Global Health and Tropical Medicine Centre, Unidade de Parasitologia Médica, Instituto de Higiene e Medicina Tropical, Universidade Nova de Lisboa, Lisbon, Portugal, [5] Laboratory for Molecular Modeling, Division of Chemical Biology and Medicinal Chemistry, Eshelman School of Pharmacy, University of North Carolina at Chapel Hill, Chapel Hill, NC, United States, [6] Department of Chemical Technology, Odessa National Polytechnic University, Odessa, Ukraine, [7] Department of Parasitology, Institute of Biomedical Sciences, University of São Paulo, São Paulo, Brazil

***Correspondence:**
Carolina H. Andrade
carolina@ufg.br

† These authors have contributed equally to this work.

Malaria is a life-threatening infectious disease caused by parasites of the genus *Plasmodium*, affecting more than 200 million people worldwide every year and leading to about a half million deaths. Malaria parasites of humans have evolved resistance to all current antimalarial drugs, urging for the discovery of new effective compounds. Given that the inhibition of deoxyuridine triphosphatase of *Plasmodium falciparum* (*Pf*dUTPase) induces wrong insertions in plasmodial DNA and consequently leading the parasite to death, this enzyme is considered an attractive antimalarial drug target. Using a combi-QSAR (quantitative structure-activity relationship) approach followed by virtual screening and *in vitro* experimental evaluation, we report herein the discovery of novel chemical scaffolds with *in vitro* potency against asexual blood stages of both *P. falciparum* multidrug-resistant and sensitive strains and against sporogonic development of *P. berghei*. We developed 2D- and 3D-QSAR models using a series of nucleosides reported in the literature as *Pf*dUTPase inhibitors. The best models were combined in a consensus approach and used for virtual screening of the ChemBridge database, leading to the identification of five new virtual *Pf*dUTPase inhibitors. Further *in vitro* testing on *P. falciparum* multidrug-resistant (W2) and sensitive (3D7) parasites showed that compounds LabMol-144 and LabMol-146 demonstrated fair activity against both strains and presented good selectivity versus mammalian cells. In addition, LabMol-144 showed good *in vitro* inhibition of *P. berghei* ookinete formation, demonstrating that hit-to-lead optimization based on this compound may also lead to new antimalarials with transmission blocking activity.

Keywords: malaria, virtual screening, QSAR, *Plasmodium falciparum*, dUTPase, transmission blocker

INTRODUCTION

Malaria is an infectious disease caused by protozoans of the genus *Plasmodium* and transmitted through the bite of insect vectors of the genus *Anopheles. Plasmodium falciparum* is the most prevalent and lethal species infecting humans in the African continent, being responsible for 99% of all malaria-attributed deaths (World Health Organization [WHO], 2016). Despite the fact that integrated control interventions have achieved significant progress in the reducing malaria cases and related mortality in recent years, malaria still causes 429,000 deaths every year, being endemic in 91 countries and territories of sub-Saharan Africa, South-East Asia, Latin America, and the Middle East (World Health Organization [WHO], 2016).

When compared to viruses and bacteria, these eukaryotic protozoans present a larger genome, have multiple stages in their life cycle, and a complex biology, which hinder the development of vaccines (Hoffman et al., 2015). Consequently, malaria control strategies largely rely on drug-dependent case management. Currently, artemisinin-based combination therapy (ACT) is the recommended official treatment for malaria. However, resistance to artemisinins has been detected in five countries in the Greater Mekong sub region of South-east Asia, endangering the future of *P. falciparum* elimination (Vogel, 2014; World Health Organization [WHO], 2016; Thu et al., 2017). Therefore, there is an urgent need for the discovery and development of new antimalarial therapies.

The enzyme 2′-deoxyuridine 5′-triphosphate nucleotide hydrolase (dUTPase) has emerged as a promising biological target in *P. falciparum*, and it is responsible for the hydrolytic cleavage of dUTP (deoxyuridine triphosphate) in dUMP (deoxyuridine monophosphate) and pyrophosphate (Nyman, 2001). The inhibition of dUTPase may cause dUTP accumulation and erroneous incorporation of uracil into DNA, leading to parasite death. Although another enzyme, DNA glycosylase, could repair the erroneous insertions, the excessive number of repairs would result in a fatal break of DNA strand (Whittingham et al., 2005). Given that DNA replication in *Plasmodium* takes place in all distinct stages of the parasite life cycle and given the importance of the enzyme dUTPase in this process, this enzyme is expressed in both asexual and sexual stages of the parasite (ring, trophozoite, schizont, gametocyte, and ookinete), as demonstrated in previous studies on *P. falciparum* 3D7 and *P. berghei* (López-Barragán et al., 2011; Otto et al., 2014). Thus, dUTPase inhibitors might not only act against blood-stage parasites, but also could block parasite transmission/development in mosquitoes. Experimental findings categorize dUTPase as essential for various organisms, such as *Escherichia coli, Saccharomyces cerevisiae, and Mycobacterium smegmatis* (El-hajj et al., 1988; Gadsden et al., 1993; Pecsi et al., 2012). The dUTPase of *P. falciparum* (*Pf*dUTPase) is an attractive target for the development of selective inhibitors since it presents relatively low sequence similarity with its human ortholog *Hs*dUTPase (28.4% identity) (Whittingham et al., 2005).

Due to the importance of dUTPase in the parasite's DNA repair, we decided to use computer-aided drug design (CADD) approaches for discovering new dUTPase inhibitors. In the last several decades, CADD approaches have been widely applied in early stages of drug discovery, making the process faster and more financially viable (Leelananda and Lindert, 2016). Among these approaches, quantitative structure-activity relationships (QSARs) have been extensively used for lead optimization and virtual screening (Verma et al., 2010). Different QSAR approaches have been used by our group for identification of new promising hits for infectious diseases (Melo-Filho et al., 2016; Neves et al., 2016; Gomes et al., 2017).

In this work, we applied a combi-QSAR approach, combining 2D- and 3D-QSAR models, in a virtual screening campaign of the ChemBridge database for selection of new antimalarial virtual hits. Finally, we performed *in vitro* experimental evaluation of the potential *Pf*dUTPase inhibitors against chloroquine-sensitive and multidrug-resistant strains of *P. falciparum*, and in gametocyte to ookinete conversion of *P. berghei*, aiming to identify new potential and selective antimalarial hits.

MATERIALS AND METHODS

The steps of the modeling study are briefly presented in **Figure 1**. The workflow encompasses the following steps: (i) data compilation and integration; (ii) data curation; (iii) model generation; (iv) virtual screening and (v) experimental validation. Our workflow was built following the best practices of QSAR modeling and CADD (Tropsha, 2010; Cherkasov et al., 2014).

Dataset Preparation

2D and 3D QSAR models were built using a series of *Pf*dUTPase inhibitors reported in the literature (Supplementary Table S1) (Nguyen et al., 2005, 2006; Whittingham et al., 2005; McCarthy et al., 2009; Baragaña et al., 2011; Hampton et al., 2011; Ruda et al., 2011). The data set was prepared and curated according to the protocol described by Fourches et al. (2010, 2015, 2016). Counterions were removed as chemotypes, and specific and nitroaromatic groups were standardized using Standardizer (v. 6.1, ChemAxon, Budapest, Hungary[1]). Duplicates were identified using ISIDA Duplicates program (Varnek et al., 2008) and HiTQSAR (Kuz'min et al., 2008). If values of properties of identical compounds were equal, one of these compounds was kept in the data set. However, if properties were significantly different, all records were removed. After curation, 127 compounds (Supplementary Table S1) with activity against *Pf*dUTPase were kept for molecular modeling. The activity against both *Plasmodium* and human enzymes was available only for 45 compounds and used for calculation of selectivity (*S*) (Eq. 1). The activity was represented as K_i (inhibition constant) and converted to the corresponding pK_i ($-\log K_i$). In a similar approach, selectivity was converted to the logarithmic scale:

$$S = \log \frac{HsdUTPase\,Ki}{PfdUTPase\,Ki} \tag{1}$$

Values of *S* greater than zero indicate selective compounds while values below zero indicate compounds with poor selectivity.

[1] http://www.chemaxon.com

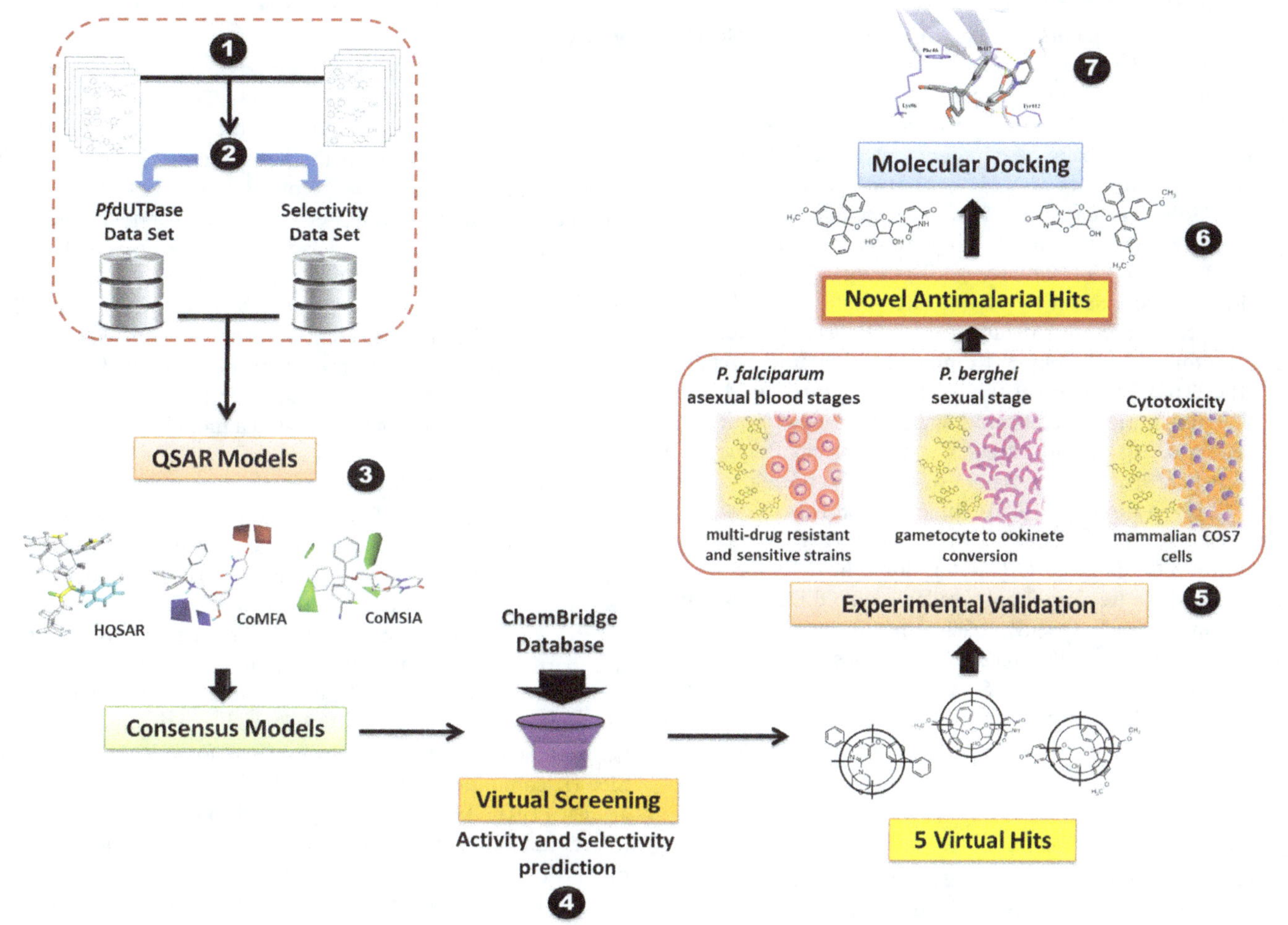

FIGURE 1 | General workflow of the computer-aided design and discovery of new antimalarial hits using Combi-QSAR models for virtual screening followed by experimental validation. Briefly, the following steps were performed: (1) data integration and compilation; (2) data curation; (3) QSAR models generation and validation; (4) virtual screening of the ChemBridge database and selection of the compounds with higher predicted potency and selectivity; (5) experimental validation against *P. falciparum* asexual blood stages, *P. berghei* sexual stage, and mammalian COS7 cells; (6) identification of novel antimalarial hits; (7) molecular docking of the most promising antimalarial hit in plasmodial and human dUTPase.

The data sets were divided into training and test sets using the Hierarchical Cluster Analysis method (HCA) available in the SYBYL v.1.2 (SYBYL-X 1.2, Tripos International, St. Louis, MO, United States). Molecules representing each cluster were manually selected for test set to maximize the coverage across the entire range of inhibition activity and selectivity. The final proportion between training and test set compounds was 3:1.

HQSAR

Hologram QSAR (HQSAR), available on SYBYL-X v.1.2 (SYBYL-X 1.2, Tripos International, St. Louis, MO, United States; TRIPOS, 2010a), was used to build 2D QSAR models. Holograms were generated using six distinct fragment sizes (2–5, 3–6, 4–7, 5–8, 6–9, 7–10 atoms) over a series of hologram lengths (53–997). Different combinations of fragment distinction were also considered, such as atoms (A), bonds (B), connectivity (C), hydrogen atoms (H), chirality (Ch), and hydrogen bond donor/acceptor (DA).

Conformer Generation and Atomic Charges Assignment

The structures were converted into 3D format, and initial conformations were generated using the OMEGA v.2.5.1.4 (Hawkins et al., 2010; OMEGA 2.5.1.4: OpenEye Scientific Software, Santa Fe, NM, United States[2]). Two different methods were used for the calculation of the partial atomic charges: the empirical method of Gasteiger-Hückel available on SYBYL-X v.1.2 (SYBYL-X 1.2, Tripos International, St. Louis, MO, United States) and the semi-empirical AM1-BCC (Jakalian et al., 1999, 2002) implemented in QUACPAC v.1.6.3.1 (QUACPAC 1.6.3.1: OpenEye Scientific Software, Santa Fe, NM, United States[2]). The protonation state of the molecules were performed at pH 7.4, using QUACPAC 1.6.3 (QUACPAC 1.6.3.1: OpenEye Scientific Software, Santa Fe, NM, United States[2]).

[2]http://www.eyesopen.com

Molecular Alignment

Compounds were submitted to three different molecular alignments: (i) alignment based on the morphological similarity function implemented in Surflex-Sim, accessible in SYBYL-X 1.2 (SYBYL-X 1.2, Tripos International, St. Louis, MO, United States); (ii) shape-based alignment from ROCS 3.2.1.4 software (Hawkins et al., 2007; ROCS 3.2.1.4: OpenEye Scientific Software, Santa Fe, NM, United States[2]); and (iii) alignment by molecular docking of molecules on *Pf*dUTPase, using OEDocking 3.0.1 software (OEDocking 3.2.0.2: OpenEye Scientific Software, Santa Fe, NM, United States[2]). For the last alignment, X-ray crystal structure of *Pf*dUTPase complexed with the inhibitor 2′,5′-dideoxy-5′-[(diphenylmethyl)amino]uridine (PDB ID: 3T64) (Hampton et al., 2011) was imported to Maestro v. 9.3 (Epik version 3.0, Schrödinger, LLC, New York, NY, United States, 2014.) and prepared using Protein Preparation Wizard, where hydrogen atoms were added according to Epik v. 2.7 (Epik version 3.0, Schrödinger, LLC, New York, NY, United States, 2014.; Shelley et al., 2007) (pH 7.4 ± 0.5), and minimized using the OPLS-2005 force field (Banks et al., 2005). On Make Receptor tool, available on OEDocking 3.0.1 (OEDocking 3.2.0.2: OpenEye Scientific Software, Santa Fe, NM, United States[2]), the receptor grid was generated with dimensions 22.34 Å × 19.65 Å × 25.24 Å and volume of 11,078 $Å^3$. All compounds of the data set were docked and the best pose for each molecule was selected for alignment.

3D-QSAR

Comparative Molecular Field Analysis (CoMFA) and Comparative Molecular Similarity Indices Analysis (CoMSIA), available in SYBYL-X v.1.2 (SYBYL-X 1.2, Tripos International, St. Louis, MO, United States; TRIPOS, 2010b), were used to build 3D QSAR models for *Pf*dUTPase inhibitors.

CoMFA

The aligned training set molecules were placed in a 3D lattice box with grid spacing of 2 Å. Then, CoMFA steric and electrostatic fields were calculated at each grid point with the Tripos force field using a carbon atom probe with sp^3 hybridization (Csp^3) and charge +1.0. The energy cutoff was set to 30 kcal/mol. The standard deviation coefficient method (SDC) was used for region focusing with values varying from 0.3 to 1.5.

CoMSIA

The models were generated using the same molecular alignments used for CoMFA. The aligned compounds were placed in the 3D lattice box with grid spacing of 2 Å. The steric, electrostatic, hydrophobic, hydrogen bond donor and acceptor descriptors were calculated at each grid point. A probe carbon atom with radius of 1.0 Å and charge +1.0, was used to obtain the similarity indices. A Gaussian function was used to describe the energy terms according to the distance between the probe atom and aligned molecules. The attenuation factor (α) was used on default value of 0.3.

Generation and Validation of QSAR Models

Partial least squares regression (PLS) was used for development of statistical models (Lindberg et al., 1983). The internal validation of QSAR models was performed using the full cross-validation r^2 (q^2) leave-one-out (LOO) method. The predictive ability of the models was assessed by Q^2_{ext} (Tropsha et al., 2003) estimated on external set compounds that were not used for model building or selection. The consensus models were obtained by combination of three QSAR models (HQSAR + CoMFA + CoMSIA). The models were built and used separately for predictions. The predicted activity of each compound by the consensus model was the result of the arithmetic mean of individual models predictions. The external validation of these models was done using the same metrics as for individual models.

Virtual Screening

The virtual screening of new potential *Pf*dUTPase inhibitors was performed on Hit2Lead library of the ChemBridge database (ChemBridge Online Chemical Store, 2017). All compounds were prepared using the same protocol and software used in the preparation of the modeling dataset. The methods of alignment and partial charges calculation were the same used in the best individual CoMFA and CoMSIA models. Then compounds had their activity and selectivity predicted by the consensus QSAR models. Two criteria were used for selection of virtual hits: (i) compounds should have the highest predicted potency against *Pf*dUTPase (predicted pK_i); (ii) the predicted selectivity (*S*) should be greater than zero. Furthermore, some ADMET properties were predicted for the best virtual hits, such as physicochemical properties (log*P* and logS)[3]), acute oral toxicity by GUSAR[4] (Filimonov et al., 2004; Lagunin et al., 2009, 2011), carcinogenicity using admetSAR[5] (Cheng et al., 2012), and hERG K+ channel blockage using Pred-hERG[6]) (Alves et al., 2014; Braga et al., 2014, 2015).

Molecular Docking

The selected virtual hits were submitted to molecular docking in Glide (Friesner et al., 2004), available on Maestro v. 9.3.5, to predict their binding mode in *Pf*dUTPase and human dUTPase (*Hs*dUTPase). Ligands were prepared on LigPrep module of Maestro software, the correct protonation states and energy minimization were performed on Epik v. 2.7 (pH 7.4 ± 2.0) using OPLS-2005 force field. The previously prepared structure of *Pf*dUTPase, used for docking-based alignment, was used here. The search space was defined as a box with 10 x 10 x 10 $Å^3$. The box was centered on the geometrical center of co-crystallized ligand (−7.7431 Å × 27.0662 Å × −3.9483 Å, *x*, *y* and *z* axes, respectively). The structure of *Hs*dUTPase (PDB ID: 3ARA, resolution of 1.7 Å) (Miyakoshi et al., 2012) was prepared using the same protocol described for plasmodial enzyme. The grid was defined with dimensions 10 × 10 × 10 $Å^3$ and was

[3]http://www.hit2lead.com/

[4]http://cactus.nci.nih.gov/chemical/apps/cap

[5]https://omictools.com/admetsar-tool

[6]http://labmol.com.br/predherg/

centered on the co-crystallized ligand at 6.3901 Å × 11.1138 Å × −17.3607 Å, *x*, *y* and *z* coordinates. After docking, the poses of each virtual hit were submitted to rescoring using the Molecular Mechanics/Generalized Born Surface Area (MM-GBSA) approach, available on Prime v.3.1 (Prime version 3.1, Schrödinger, LLC, New York, NY, United States, 2014), using default conditions.

Experimental Evaluation

Plasmodium Culture

Chloroquine-sensitive (3D7) and multidrug-resistant (W2) strains were cultured in RPMI 1640 medium supplemented with 0.05 mg/mL gentamycin, 38.4 mM HEPES, 0.2% sodium bicarbonate, and 10% O^+ human serum, as previously described in a standardized protocol (Trager and Jensen, 1976). Then, erythrocytes were added to the culture to obtain a 5% hematocrit, and incubated at 37°C under 5% CO_2 atmosphere, with daily exchange of medium. The parasitemia was monitored daily in smears stained with Giemsa. Synchronic cultures in the ring stage were obtained by two consecutive treatments at 48 h intervals with a 5% solution of D-sorbitol (Lambros and Vanderberg, 1979).

Determination of Growth Inhibition by SYBR Green I

Parasites synchronized at the ring stage, with 0.5% parasitemia and 2% hematocrit were distributed in each well, separately. The compounds were tested in triplicates, using 12 point of concentration, prepared in two-fold dilution (40 μM – ∼0.019 μM) over 72 h. Chloroquine and pyrimethamine were used as control. Subsequently, the *in vitro* susceptibility of parasite to tested drugs was measured by SYBR Green according to Hartwig et al. (2013). Briefly, 100 μL of lysis buffer (20 mM Tris, 5 mM EDTA, 0.008% wt/vol saponin, 0.08% vol/vol Triton X-100, and 0.4 μL/mL of SYBR Green) were added in each well of a new black 96-well plate and 100 μL of parasite culture incubated with drugs were added. After homogenization, the plates were incubated for 1 h in the dark. Fluorescence was measured at 490 nm excitation and 540 nm emission (CLARIOstar, Labtech BMG). The IC_{50} was calculated by plotting the Log doses vs. Inhibition (expressed as a percentage relative to the control) in Prism 6 (GraphPad Software Inc.).

Cytotoxicity Assay

Cytotoxicity assays used COS7 cells (fibroblast-like cell lines derived from monkey kidney tissue), grown in DMEM medium supplemented with 10% fetal bovine serum and 0.05 mg/mL gentamicin in atmosphere containing 5% CO_2 at 37°C. Drug cytotoxicity in COS7 cells was determined in duplicate, using 12 point of concentration, prepared in two-fold dilution (200 μM – ∼ 0.097 μM). After the incubation period (72 h), the cell viability analysis were done by the MMT reduction method (3-[4,5-dimethyl-thiazol-2-yl]-2,5-diphenyltetrazolium chloride (Mosmann, 1983). The optical density was determined at 570 nm (CLARIOstar, Labtech BMG) and the 50% cytotoxicity concentrations (CC_{50}) was expressed as the percent viability relative to the control. The selectivity index of the compounds was determined by the following expression:

$$S = \frac{COS7\ CC_{50}}{Pf\ IC_{50}} \quad (2)$$

Where COS7 CC_{50} corresponds to the 50% cytotoxic concentration on COS7 cells and *Pf* IC_{50} is the 50 % inhibitory concentration on *P. falciparum* (3D7).

Ookinete Assay

All animal procedures were carried out in accordance to the Brazilian College of Animal Experimentation (COBEA). This research protocol was approved by the Ethics Committee of the Institute of Biomedical Sciences – University of Sao Paulo, protocol number 132/2014-CEUA. C57BL/6 mice received an intraperitoneal injection of *P. berghei* ANKA infected erythrocytes, and four days after infection, a mouse with parasitemia between 4 and 6% and gametocytemia > 0.4% was selected as blood donor for cardiac puncture. Four microliters of the infected blood was dispensed in 80 μl of ookinete medium (Blagborough et al., 2012) at 21°C with DMSO control or with 10 μM of the tested compounds. The assay was incubated at 21°C for 24 h and 2 μl of the blood at the bottom of the tubes was spread onto a glass slide, stained with Giemsa and analyzed under a direct light microscope. The total number of formed ookinetes were counted in each slide (triplicate for each condition), and inhibition was calculated in relation to the total ookinetes formed in the control condition.

RESULTS AND DISCUSSION

QSAR Modeling

Various combinations of hologram length, fragment size, and fragment distinction were tested with an aim to build robust and predictive HQSAR models. The original data set was divided into training and test sets in a ratio of approximately 3:1 using the HCA method. The three best HQSAR models for *Pf*dUTPase inhibition are shown in Supplementary Table S2. The models displayed very similar statistical features, but the model with fragment distinction A/C (Supplementary Table S2) performed slightly better than others in terms of robustness (q^2_{LOO} = 0.70) and external predictivity (Q^2_{ext} = 0.71). In addition, the best model presented a Durbin-Watson metric (Savin and White, 1977) (*d*) closest to the ideal value ($d = 1.99$), indicating that this model is less biased. The Durbin-Watson test is useful to evaluate the presence or absence of autocorrelation of residuals from regression analysis. The values range from 0 to 4. Values of *d* near or equal to 2 indicate no autocorrelation of residuals. Values of $d < 2$ or $d > 2$ indicate that residuals are positively or negatively auto correlated and predictions are more biased (Savin and White, 1977). The best HQSAR models for selectivity (using human dUTPase data) are also presented in Supplementary Table S2. The best model, with fragment distinction B/C (Supplementary Table S2), showed good external predictivity (Q^2_{ext} = 0.83), with *d*-value close to the reference value ($d = 2.02$). The plots comparing the experimental and predicted biological activity for the best HQSAR models are shown in Supplementary Figures S1A,D. These plots demonstrate a good agreement between experimental data and predictions from the models.

The HQSAR contribution maps are useful to highlight the relationships between specific structural fragments and the biological property/activity. Colors close to the red end (red, red orange, and orange) indicate fragments with negative contribution, while colors in the green region (yellow, green blue, and green) indicate fragments with positive contribution to biological activity. The common substructure is represented in cyan (**Figure 2**).

The contribution maps of the most potent (4) and least potent inhibitors (127) and of the most selective (20) and least selective inhibitor (87) are presented in **Figure 2**. As one can see, the trityl ring has a positive contribution for both inhibition and selectivity (compounds 4 and 20, **Figure 2**). Additionally, the absence of the trityl group results in drastic decrease in activity against *Pf*dUTPase, as observed in compounds 4 and 127 (**Figures 2A,B**, respectively), and a clear decrease in selectivity, when we compare compounds 20 and 87 (**Figures 2C,D**, respectively). These observations corroborate previous studies (Whittingham et al., 2005; McCarthy et al., 2009; Baragaña et al., 2011; Hampton et al., 2011; Recio et al., 2011; Ruda et al., 2011; Ojha and Roy, 2013), indicating that two of the three phenyl rings from the trityl group have significant interactions with the hydrophobic pocket formed by residues Phe46 and Ile117 from *Pf*dUTPase (Hampton et al., 2011). In contrast, in the human enzyme, such residues are replaced by hydrophilic residues Val42 and Gly87. Therefore, there is no corresponding hydrophobic pocket in *Hs*dUTPase (Whittingham et al., 2005; Hampton et al., 2011). In a previous study by Ojha and Roy (2013), some nucleoside inhibitors were used for QSAR studies and pharmacophore mapping of *Pf*dUTPase inhibitors. The results revealed that two phenyl rings from the trityl group are responsible for stablishing important hydrophobic interactions and one phenyl ring may form a π–π stacking interaction with the amino acid residue Phe46 from *Pf*dUTPase (Ojha and Roy, 2013).

Two steps are critical for the development of CoMFA and CoMSIA models: the partial atomic charge assignment and structural alignment (Doweyko, 2004; Melo-Filho et al., 2014). In this study, two different charges (Gasteiger-Hückel and AM1-BCC) and three different molecular alignment approaches (morphological similarity function on Surflex-Sim, shape-based superposition on ROCS and alignment accessed by molecular docking) were evaluated. The Surflex-Sim alignment was performed using the most potent inhibitors of the data set (compounds 1 and 2) as templates, which were used for the flexible alignment of the remaining compounds of the data set. The shape-based alignment was executed with previously generated conformers. These conformers were superimposed to compound 3, which is the co-crystallized inhibitor of *Pf*dUTPase, available at Protein Data Bank (PDB code: 3T64) (Hampton et al., 2011). The superposition was evaluated by the *TanimotoCombo* score (Hawkins et al., 2010). Based on this score, the best conformation of each compound was selected. In the docking-based alignment, the previously generated conformers were docked and classified using the Chemgauss4 score function (McGann, 2011). The best conformer for each compound was selected based on the Chemgauss4 score. Additionally, conformers were visually inspected for selection of those with better superposition to the co-crystallized inhibitor.

The results of the best CoMFA and CoMSIA models are available at Supplementary Tables S3 and S4, respectively. The plots comparing the experimental and predicted biological

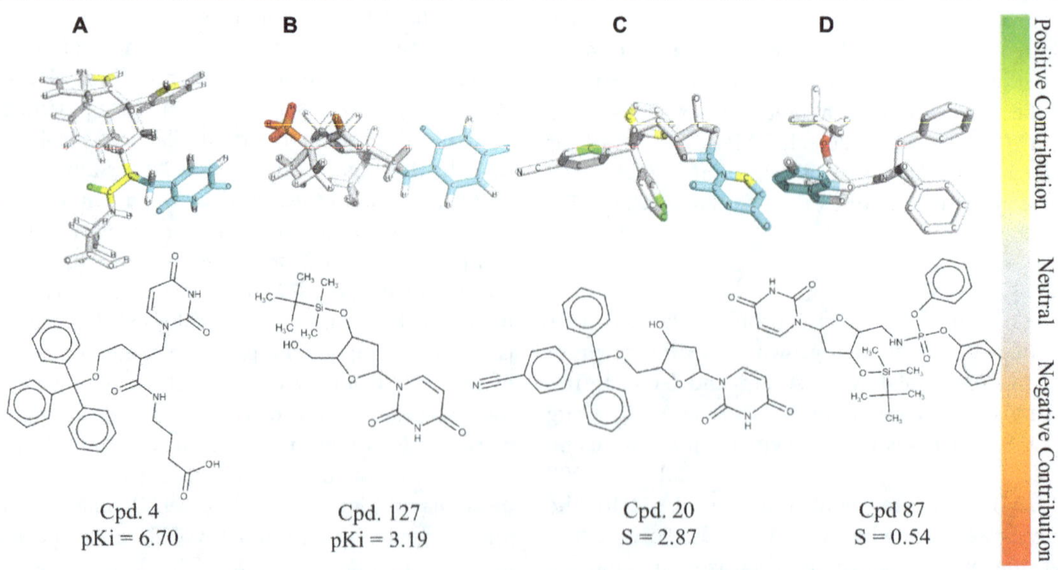

FIGURE 2 | HQSAR contribution maps for the most potent *Pf*dUTPase inhibitor of the dataset (**A**, Cpd. 4) and the less potent compound (**B**, Cpd. 127). The most selective (**C**, Cpd. 20) and less selective (**D**, Cpd. 87) compounds are also displayed. The uracil ring, which is the common substructure, is highlighted in cyan.

activity for the best COMFA and CoMSIA models are shown in Supplementary Figures S1B,C,E,F. The best CoMFA models for inhibition and selectivity presented good robustness (q^2_{LOO} = 0.63 and 0.86, respectively) and good external predictivity (Q^2_{ext} = 0.75 and 0.61). Furthermore, presented good *d* values, indicating a low probability of biased predictions (d = 1.86 and 1.99, respectively). In general, for CoMFA models, the shape-based and Surflex-Sim alignments performed better than the docking-based alignment (Supplementary Table S3). The best CoMSIA models were obtained using shape-based alignment and AM1-BCC charges (Supplementary Table S4). The best CoMSIA model for *Pf*dUTPase inhibition presented good robustness and external predictivity (q^2_{LOO} = 0.68; Q^2_{ext} = 0.78, Supplementary Table S4). The best CoMSIA model for selectivity, despite its lower internal consistence (q^2_{LOO} = 0.59), presented an acceptable external predictivity (Q^2_{ext} = 0.63), as demonstrated on Supplementary Table S4.

The best CoMFA and CoMSIA models were used to generate contour maps by using STDEV*COEFF field type and the function "contour by actual." These maps could be useful for designing new potent and selective *Pf*dUTPase inhibitors as they indicate regions in the molecules where certain types of interactions are favorable and unfavorable for biological activity. The contour maps from the best CoMFA and CoMSIA models, for both inhibition and selectivity, are presented in **Figures 3**, **4**, respectively.

The obtained contour maps show that bulky and hydrophobic groups in the trityl group region are favorable for both *Pf*dUTPase inhibition and selectivity (**Figures 3A,C**, **4A,C,D**). These results corroborate with the HQSAR contribution maps and other studies highlighting the importance of the trytil hydrophobic group for inhibition and selectivity. The trytil group interacts with the hydrophobic pocket formed by residues Phe46 and Ile117 which are missing in the human dUTPase (Hampton et al., 2011). Thus, structural modifications in trytil group should be further explored in order to improve the interactions with the hydrophobic pocket and, consequently, to help the design of novel potent and selective *Pf*dUTPase inhibitors. The CoMFA and CoMSIA electrostatic contour maps also show that electropositive groups in sugar moiety and uracil group are favorable for inhibition and selectivity (**Figures 3D**, **4B,E**). Additionally, these maps show that electronegative groups near the region of the oxygen atom of the pentose sugar are favorable for *Pf*dUTPase selectivity (**Figure 4B**), while electronegative groups near the linker between the trityl group and the sugar moiety (**Figures 3B,D**, **4E**) are unfavorable for both inhibition and selectivity.

The best individual HQSAR, CoMFA, and CoMSIA models were combined in a consensus approach (Supplementary Table S5). Thus, one consensus model for inhibition of *Pf*dUTPase and another for selectivity were built. The external validation of the consensus models was performed using the same external evaluation set and metrics used for individual QSAR models. The statistical characteristics of the consensus models are presented in **Table 1**. Both models showed good external predictivity (Q^2_{ext} = 0.85 and 0.75; RMSEP = 0.40).

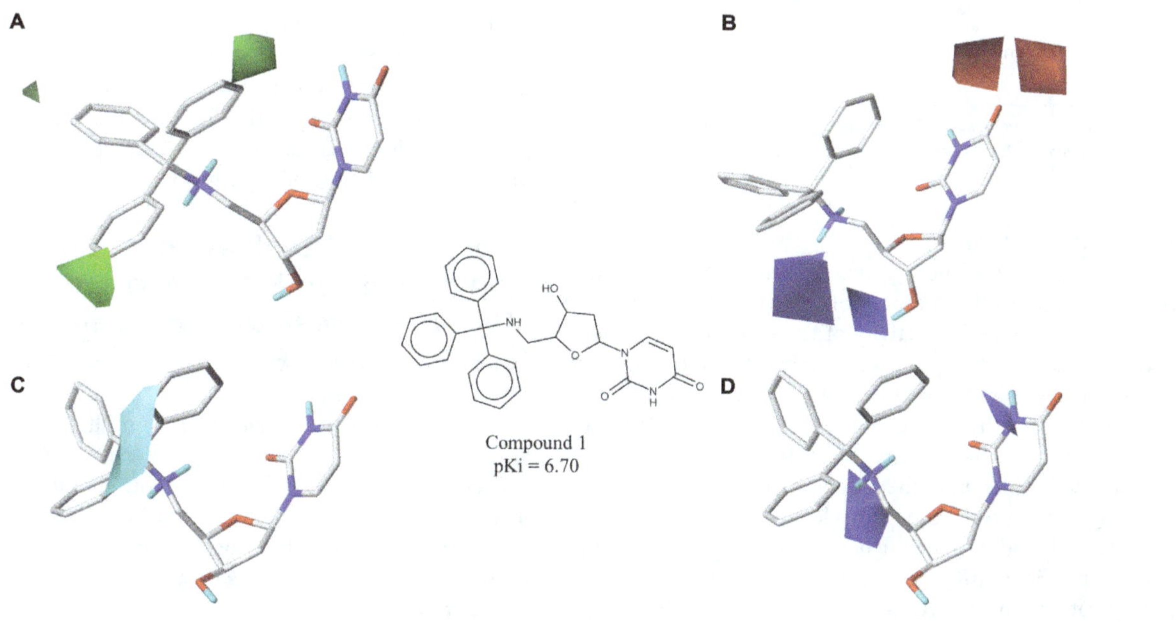

FIGURE 3 | Contour maps of the best CoMFA and CoMSIA models for *Pf*dUTPase inhibition surrounding the most potent inhibitor (cpd. 1); **(A,B)** CoMFA steric and electrostatic contour maps; **(C,D)** CoMSIA electrostatic and hydrophobic contour maps. Steric fields: green contours indicate regions where bulky groups are favorable to biological activity; electrostatic fields: red contours indicate regions where electronegative groups are favorable for biological activity, while blue contours indicate regions where electronegative groups are unfavorable; hydrophobic fields: cyan contours indicate regions where hydrophobic groups are favorable to biological activity.

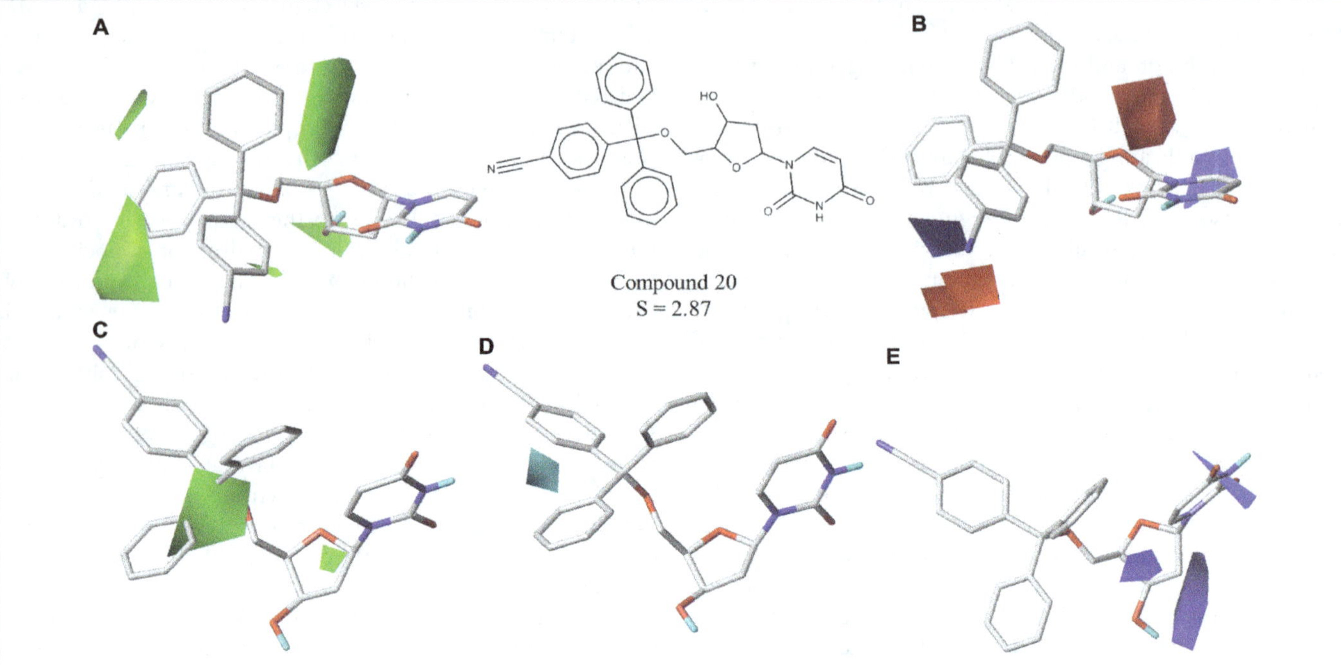

FIGURE 4 | Contour maps of the best CoMFA and CoMSIA models for selectivity surrounding one of the most selective inhibitors (cpd. 20); **(A,B)** CoMFA steric and electrostatic contour maps; **(C–E)** CoMSIA steric, hydrophobic and electrostatic contour maps. Steric fields: green contours indicate regions where bulky groups are favorable to selectivity; electrostatic fields: red contours indicate regions where electronegative groups are favorable to selectivity, while blue contours indicate regions where electronegative groups are unfavorable; hydrophobic fields: cyan contours indicate regions where hydrophobic groups are favorable to selectivity.

TABLE 1 | Statistical characteristics of consensus QSAR models for *Pf*dUTPase inhibition and selectivity.

Model	Q^2_{ext}	RMSEP
Consensus – *Pf*dUTPase Inhibition*	0.85	0.40
Consensus – Selectivity*	0.75	0.40

**Consensus of the best individual HQSAR, CoMFA and CoMSIA models; Q^2_{ext}: determination coefficient for external set; RMSEP, root mean-square error of prediction.*

Virtual Screening

The virtual screening of new potential *Pf*dUTPase inhibitors was performed on Hit2Lead library of ChemBridge database by prediction of activity and selectivity of the compounds through the developed and validated consensus QSAR models. Each consensus prediction was obtained by the arithmetic mean of the predictions from the best individual HQSAR, CoMFA, and CoMSIA models (Supplementary Table S6). All duplicates or compounds used to generate the models were excluded. Finally, the following criteria were used for selection of the virtual hits: (i) compounds should have the highest predicted potency against *Pf*dUTPase (predicted pK_i) and (ii) the predicted selectivity (*S*) should be greater than zero. At the end of this process, five virtual hits were chosen for experimental evaluation.

Inadequate ADMET properties contribute to high failure rates in late stages of drug development. The early prediction and optimization of such properties can help the reduction of late-stage failures and expenses (van de Waterbeemd and Gifford, 2003; Sanders et al., 2017). In this study, the five virtual hits were evaluated by predicting/analyzing a panel of properties including log*P* and log*S*, oral acute toxicity in rodents (Filimonov et al., 2004; Lagunin et al., 2009, 2011), carcinogenicity (Cheng et al., 2012), and binding affinity to hERG (Braga et al., 2015) (**Table 2**). All molecules were predicted as non-carcinogenic and non-blockers of hERG channel. Only LabMol-143 and LabMol-146 were predicted as positive for acute oral toxicity. LabMol-142 presented a high calculated logP (7.3), while the remaining hits presented log*P* below or slightly above 5.

Experimental Evaluation of Selected Compounds on *P. falciparum* Multi-Drug-Resistant and Sensitive Strains, and on *P. berghei* Sexual Stages

The five virtual hits selected were evaluated *in vitro* against asexual blood-stages of *P. falciparum* multi-drug-resistant (W2) and sensitive (3D7) strains. The half maximal inhibitory concentrations (IC_{50}) for each compound (**Table 3**) indicate that three compounds (LabMol-144, LabMol-145, and LabMol-146) were more potent at inhibiting parasite growth, showing activity in submicromolar range against both 3D7 and W2 strains. Furthermore, the cytotoxicity was measured in mammalian COS7 cells. LabMol-144 and LabMol-146 showed promising results in terms of selectivity (SI = 11.7 and 6.7, respectively; **Table 3**).

The five compounds were also tested against *P. berghei* sexual stages using *in vitro* gametocyte to ookinete conversion assays (**Table 3**). LabMol-144, a promising selected compound in terms

TABLE 2 | Chemical structures, predicted potency against *Pf*dUTPase, predicted selectivity, and some calculated ADMET properties of the virtual hits.

Cpd ID	Structure	*Pf*dUTPase inhibition (pK_i)[a]	Selectivity (S)[b]	clog*P*	log*S*	Acute oral toxicity[c]	Carcinogenicity[d]	hERG[e]
LabMol-142	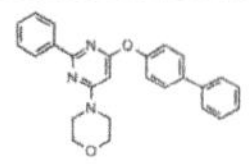	5.68	1.03	7.3	−8.42	No	No	Non-blocker
LabMol-143	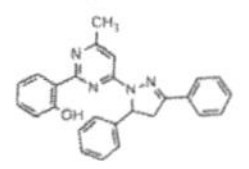	5.52	1.59	5.87	−6.6	Yes	No	Non-blocker
LabMol-144	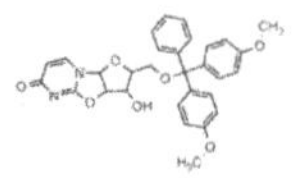	5.81	2.64	2.69	−5.36	No	No	Non-blocker
LabMol-145	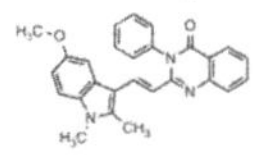	5.10	1.14	5.23	−6.74	No	No	Non-blocker
LabMol-146	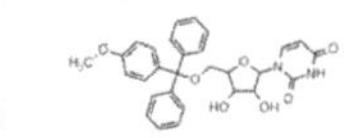	5.61	2.31	2.43	−5.04	Yes	No	Non-blocker

[a]Prediction based on consensus QSAR model for dUTPase inhibition; [b]Prediction based on consensus QSAR model for selectivity; logP and logS were extracted from Hit2Lead library; [c]Acute oral toxicity predicted using GUSAR; [d]Carcinogenicity predicted in admetSAR software (Cheng et al., 2012); [e]Prediction of hERG channel blockage in Pred-hERG web app (Alves et al., 2014; Braga et al., 2014, 2015).

of IC_{50} and SI against asexual stages and mammalian cells, showed inhibition of 44.6% of ookinete formation relative to control. Although the IC_{50} range of LabMol-144 and LabMol-146 are still far from that of chloroquine and pyrimethamine (**Table 3**), these compounds represent good starting points for further optimization studies and development of new antimalarial drugs. In addition, drug development based on LabMol-144 may also lead to new antimalarials with transmission blocking activity and new mechanism of action.

The two most promising compounds, LabMol-144 and LabMol-146, are similar to the most potent compound from the training set (cpd. 1) used for developing QSAR models (T_c of 0.72 and 0.84, respectively, Supplementary Table S6). However, LabMol-144 presents some differences in relation to compound 1. As demonstrated on **Figures 2–4**, and based on previous reports on literature, the presence of hydrophobic groups on trytil region is favorable for both activity and selectivity against *Pf*dUTPase (Whittingham et al., 2005; Hampton et al., 2011; Ojha and Roy, 2013). Thus, LabMol-144 can be a potent and selective inhibitor of *Pf*dUTPase due to the addition of two methoxy substituents on trytil group, which can contribute for improved affinity to the hydrophobic binding pocket of the enzyme. Other modifications in LabMol-144 in comparison to compound 1 are the presence of the oxazolidine ring between the sugar moiety and uracil ring, and the substitution of nitrogen by oxygen on the linker between the sugar moiety and the trytil group.

LabMol-144 has higher similarity to the most potent inhibitors of *Pf*dUTPase from the training set (compounds 1 to 6, **Figure 5**) $T_c = 0.58–0.72$, and it has a very low similarity to the currently used antimalarial drugs, $T_c = 0.23–0.54$ (**Figure 5**). Added to the fact that LabMol-144 showed similar activity against sensitive and multidrug resistant strains of *P. falciparum*, this further suggests that the mode of action of nucleosides and their derivatives is different from current antimalarials. This is particularly important considering parasite resistance in natural settings. Therefore, inhibitors of *Pf*dUTPase, a target different from the other test antimalarials, could overcome cross-resistance phenomena, and are very promising scaffolds to be explored as new antimalarial drugs. Certainly, the activity of compounds could be caused not only by *Pf*dUTPase inhibition but by different mechanisms of action. However, to explore this, further *in vitro* enzymatic studies should be performed. Exploring other mechanisms of action is out of the scope of this paper and should be considered in the next steps of the project.

Molecular Docking

The most promising compound (LabMol-144, $IC_{50} = 4.23\ \mu M$ against W2 strain, and highest predicted $pIC_{50} = 5.81$ against the parasite enzyme) was docked in *Pf*dUTPase and *Hs*dUTPase in order to compare the binding modes and to analyze how differences between the human and parasite enzymes can be explored for the design of selective inhibitors. The docking studies suggested a higher affinity of LabMol-144 to *Pf*dUTPase. The Glide Score on *Pf*dUTPase was −7.38 kcal/mol (**Figure 6A**) and −6.26 kcal/mol on *Hs*dUTPase (**Figure 6C**). After the docking, we performed MM-GBSA calculations to obtain the free energy of binding, in order to compare the affinities of the compounds. The results are available on Supplementary Table S7. These results suggested that LabMol-144 has a higher affinity to *Pf*dUTPase, with a twice higher affinity toward the parasitic enzyme in comparison to the human ortholog (estimated ΔG of binding of −107.8 and −52.8, respectively)."

As demonstrated on **Figures 6A,B**, the parasitic enzyme has the amino acid residues Phe46 and Ile117 in the hydrophobic region of the active site, while the human counterpart has Val65 and Gly110, respectively (**Figures 6C,D**). The presence of Phe46 in *Pf*dUTPase is responsible for an additional π–π stacking interaction with one ring from trytil group, while Ile117 can perform two hydrogen bonds with uracil and oxazolidine rings. These two hydrogen bonds contribute to the exposure of a hydroxyl group to Tyr112, allowing the molecule to stablish

TABLE 3 | *In vitro* evaluation of selected hits against asexual blood stage of *P. falciparum* 3D7 and W2 strains, cytotoxicity on mammalian cells (COS7), selectivity index, and inhibition of ookinete stage of *P. berghei*.

Cpd ID	IC_{50} 3D7 (μM)	IC_{50} W2 (μM)	CC_{50} COS7 (μM)	SI	% conversion inhibition (10 μM)
LabMol-142	>40	>40	>100	ND	10.2 ± 11.9
LabMol-143	>40	>40	>200	ND	0
LabMol-144	7.1 ± 2.53	4.23 ± 1.18	81.7 ± 25.7	11.7	44.6 ± 2.4
LabMol-145	17.1 ± 16.2	15.3 ± 3.29	46.0 ± 13.4	2.7	13.2 ± 24.0
LabMol-146	6.1 ± 1.95	3.20 ± 2.12	52.0 ± 16.4	6.7	7.3 ± 7.3
Chloroquine	0.011 ± 0.0006	0.181 ± 0.027	–	–	–
Pyrimethamine	0.044 ± 0.009	14.7 ± 3.94	–	–	–

IC_{50} 3D7: half maximal inhibitory concentration on 3D7 strain; IC_{50} W2: half maximal inhibitory concentration on W2 strain; CC_{50} COS7: half maximal cytotoxic concentration on COS7 cells; SI, selectivity index calculated between CC_{50} on COS7 and IC_{50} in 3D7 strain. The data are expressed as mean ± SD of three independent assays.

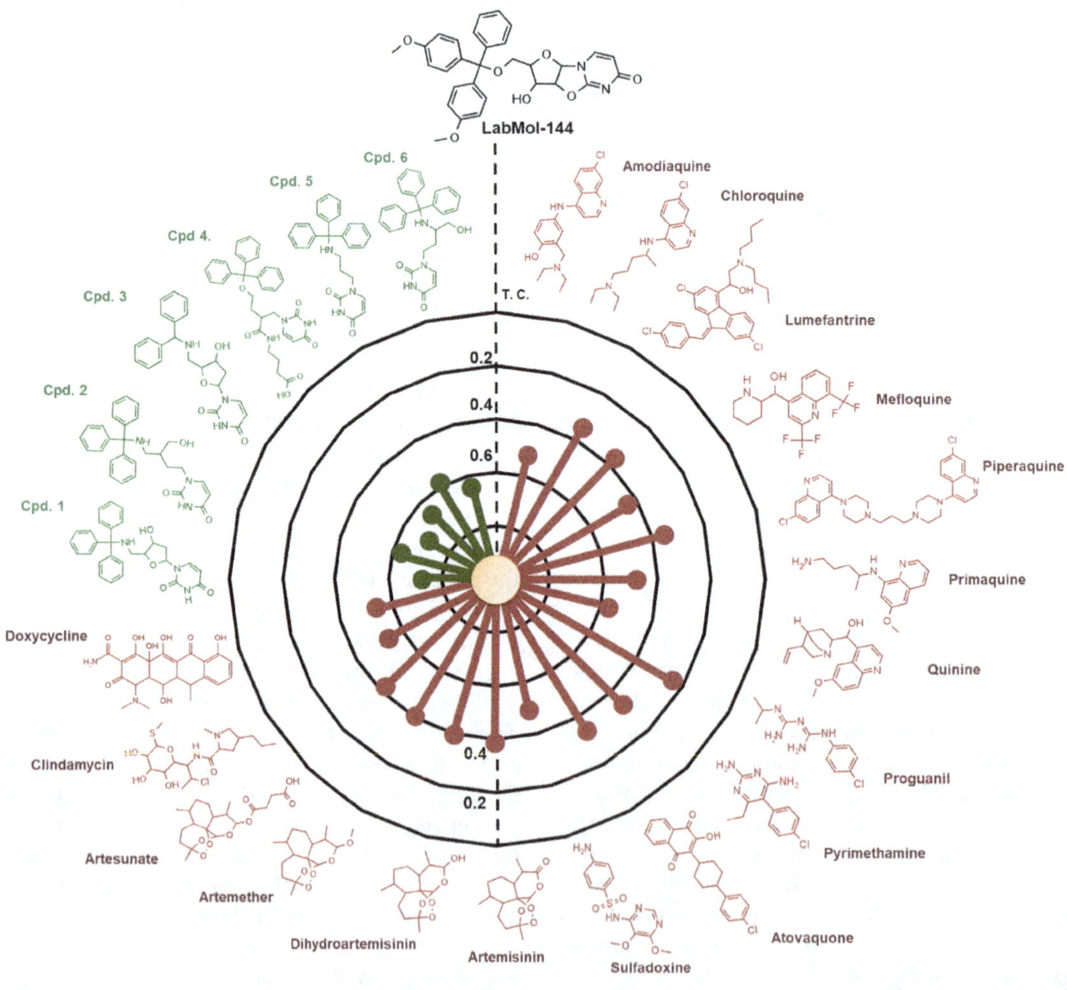

FIGURE 5 | Radial plot showing the similarity of the most promising compound discovered (LabMol-144) compared to known antimalarial drugs (red) and six of the most potent inhibitors of *Pf*dUTPase from the dataset used for QSAR modeling (green). The similarity was calculated using Tanimoto coefficient (T_c) and MACCS structural key fingerprints.

an additional hydrogen bond with this residue (**Figure 6A**). The absence of Phe46 and Ile117 on the human enzyme (**Figure 6C**) results in a weaker affinity for Labmol-144. In *Hs*dUTPase, there are no interactions with Val65 and Gly110, and consequently, no hydrogen bond with Tyr105. The main interactions with *Hs*dUTPase are the hydrogen bonds with Gly99 and two structural water molecules (**Figures 6C,D**).

These results corroborate with our QSAR contribution and contour maps and also with previous studies (Whittingham et al., 2005; Hampton et al., 2011; Ojha and Roy, 2013), highlighting

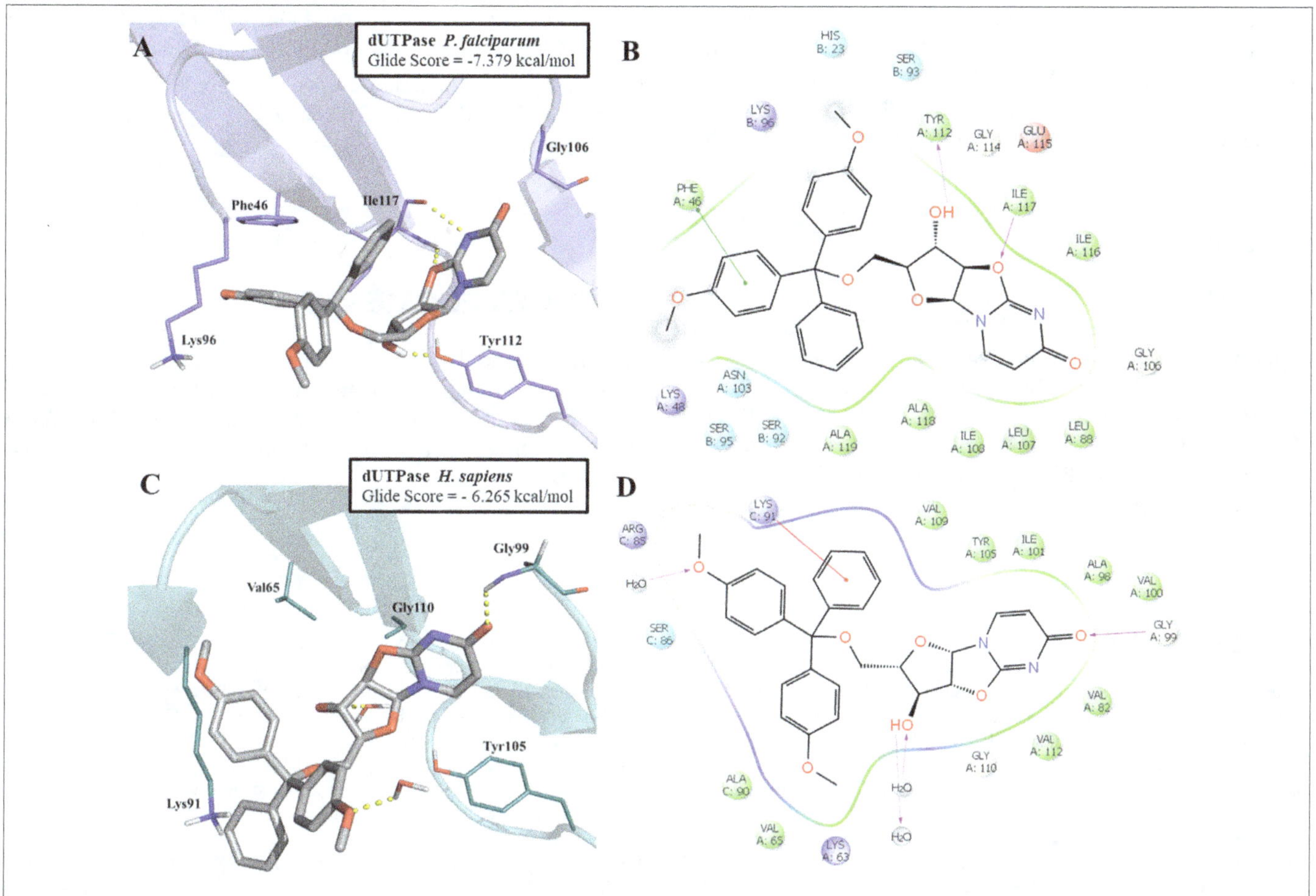

FIGURE 6 | Molecular docking of LabMol-144 in dUTPase of *P. falciparum* **(A,B)** and human **(C,D)**. In 3D representation **(A,C)**, hydrogen bonds are presented as yellow dashed lines. In 2D interaction diagrams **(B,C)**, hydrogen bonds are presented as magenta arrows and hydrophobic interactions as red lines.

the differences between human and parasite enzymes, and the importance of hydrophobic interactions with trytil group for increased potency and selectivity. In future studies, we aim to perform enzymatic assays against human and plasmodial enzymes aiming to confirm the findings observed here. Furthermore, the *in vitro* results against multi-drug and sensitive *P. falciparum* strains and inhibition of *P. berghei* ookinete formation are indicative that LabMol-144 is an attractive scaffold for further hit-to-lead optimization studies for the development of new antimalarials with transmission blocking activity.

CONCLUSION

In this work, we developed robust and externally predictive consensus QSAR models, merging 2D- (HQSAR) and 3D-QSAR (CoMFA and CoMSIA) models for prediction of inhibition and selectivity against *Pf*dUTPase. The QSAR models were applied for virtual screening of the ChemBridge database and allowed the selection of five new potential selective inhibitors of *Pf*dUTPase. The virtual hits were tested *in vitro* against sensitive (3D7) and multidrug-resistant (W2) strains of *P. falciparum*. Two compounds, LabMol-144 and LabMol-146, showed promising activity against both strains of *P. falciparum* and present chemical scaffolds very dissimilar from current antimalarial drugs. Thus, inhibitors of *Pf*dUTPase could be a good alternative for antimalarial drug combination. In addition, compound LabMol-144 showed potent *in vitro* inhibition of *P. berghei* ookinete formation, demonstrating that this compound is active against multiple parasite stages and, therefore, optimization based on this compound may also lead to new antimalarials with transmission blocking activity. In future studies, we aim to perform enzymatic assays against parasite and human enzymes. Furthermore, we aim to perform hit-to-lead optimization through structural modifications on the discovered scaffolds, based on the information gathered from the QSAR contribution and contour maps, aiming at designing new antimalarial drugs with transmission-blocking activity.

AUTHOR CONTRIBUTIONS

Each author has contributed significantly to this work. ML and CM-F contributed equally in the design, performing the computational experiments, and writing the paper. ML, CM-F, BN, VA, RB, PC, and CA conceived and designed the experiments. ML, CM-F, BN, VA, and RB performed the computational experiments. GC, FC, PC, JC, and DB performed the experimental assays. ML, CM-F, GC, FC, PC, EM, JC, and DB analyzed the data. ML, CM-F, GC, BN, EM, DB, and CA wrote the paper. All authors read, edited, and approved the final manuscript.

FUNDING

The authors would like to thank Brazilian funding agencies, CNPq, FAPEG, FAPESP, and CAPES for financial support and fellowships. FC, GC, and CA were supported by FAPESP (Grants #2012/16525-2, #2015/20774-6, and #2017/02353-9, respectively). DB was supported by FAPESP (Grant #2013/13119-6) and CNPq (Grant #405996/2016-0). JC was supported by FAPESP fellowship (#2016/16649-4). EM appreciates support from NIH (Grant 1U01CA207160 and GM5105946) and CNPq (Grant #400760/2014-2). CA, PC, and FC are CNPq research fellows. PC was partially supported by the Fundação Nacional de Desenvolvimento do Ensino Superior Particular - Funadesp, via UniEvangélica - Centro Universitário de Anápolis.

ACKNOWLEDGMENTS

We are thankful for Dr. Stephen Capuzzi for his kind help with editing the manuscript. We are also grateful to OpenEye Scientific Software Inc. and ChemAxon for providing us with academic licenses for their software.

REFERENCES

Alves, V. M., Braga, R. C., Silva, M. B., Muratov, E., Fourches, D., Tropsha, A., et al. (2014). "Pred-hERG: a novel web-accessible computational tool for predicting cardiac toxicity of drug candidates," in *Proceedings of the 248th ACS National Meeting & Exposition*, San Francisco, CA.

Banks, J. L., Beard, H. S., Cao, Y., Cho, A. E., Damm, W., Farid, R., et al. (2005). Integrated Modeling Program, Applied Chemical Theory (IMPACT). *J. Comput. Chem.* 26, 1752–1780. doi: 10.1002/jcc.20292

Baragaña, B., McCarthy, O., Sánchez, P., Bosch-Navarrete, C., Kaiser, M., Brun, R., et al. (2011). β-Branched acyclic nucleoside analogues as inhibitors of *Plasmodium falciparum* dUTPase. *Bioorg. Med. Chem.* 19, 2378–2391. doi: 10.1016/j.bmc.2011.02.012

Blagborough, A. M., Delves, M. J., Ramakrishnan, C., Lal, K., Butcher, G., and Sinden, R. E. (2012). "Assessing transmission blockade in Plasmodium spp," in *Malaria. Methods in Molecular Biology (Methods and Protocols)*, ed. R. Ménard (Totowa, NJ: Humana Press), 577–600.

Braga, R., Alves, V., Silva, M., Muratov, E., Fourches, D., Tropsha, A., et al. (2014). Tuning hERG Out: antitarget QSAR models for drug development. *Curr. Top. Med. Chem.* 14, 1399–1415. doi: 10.2174/1568026614666140506124442

Braga, R. C., Alves, V. M., Silva, M. F. B., Muratov, E., Fourches, D., Lião, L. M., et al. (2015). Pred-hERG: a novel web-accessible computational tool for predicting cardiac toxicity. *Mol. Inform.* 34, 698–701. doi: 10.1002/minf.201500040

ChemBridge Online Chemical Store (2017). Available at: http://www.hit2lead.com/ [accessed April 14, 2017].

Cheng, F., Li, W., Zhou, Y., Shen, J., Wu, Z., Liu, G., et al. (2012). admetSAR: a comprehensive source and free tool for assessment of chemical ADMET properties. *J. Chem. Inf. Model.* 52, 3099–3105. doi: 10.1021/ci300367a

Cherkasov, A., Muratov, E. N., Fourches, D., Varnek, A., Baskin, I. I., Cronin, M., et al. (2014). QSAR modeling: where have you been? Where are you going to? *J. Med. Chem.* 57, 4977–5010. doi: 10.1021/jm4004285

Doweyko, A. M. (2004). 3D-QSAR illusions. *J. Comput. Aided Mol. Des.* 18, 587–596. doi: 10.1007/s10822-004-4068-0

El-hajj, H. H., Zhang, H. U. I., and Weiss, B. (1988). Lethality of a dut (deoxyuridine triphosphatase) mutation in *Escherichia coli*. *J. Bacteriol.* 170, 1069–1075. doi: 10.1128/jb.170.3.1069-1075.1988

Filimonov, D. A., Akimov, D. V., and Poroikov, V. V. (2004). The method of self-consistent regression for the quantitative analysis of relationships between structure and properties of chemicals. *Pharm. Chem. J.* 38, 21–24. doi: 10.1023/B:PHAC.0000027639.17115.5d

Fourches, D., Muratov, E., and Tropsha, A. (2010). Trust, but verify: on the importance of chemical structure curation in cheminformatics and QSAR modeling research. *J. Chem. Inf. Model.* 50, 1189–1204. doi: 10.1021/ci100176x

Fourches, D., Muratov, E., and Tropsha, A. (2015). Curation of chemogenomics data. *Nat. Chem. Biol.* 11:535. doi: 10.1038/nchembio.1881

Fourches, D., Muratov, E. N., and Tropsha, A. (2016). Trust, but verify II: a practical guide to chemogenomics data curation. *J. Chem. Inf. Model.* 56, 1243–1252. doi: 10.1021/acs.jcim.6b00129

Friesner, R. A., Banks, J. L., Murphy, R. B., Halgren, T. A., Klicic, J. J., Mainz, D. T., et al. (2004). Glide: a new approach for rapid, accurate docking and scoring. 1. Method and assessment of docking accuracy. *J. Med. Chem.* 47, 1739–1749. doi: 10.1021/jm0306430

Gadsden, M. H., Mclntosh, E. M., Game, J. C., Wilson, P. J., and Haynes, R. H. (1993). dUTP pyrophosphatase is an essential enzyme in *Saccharomyces cerevisiae*. *EMBO J.* 12, 4425–4431.

Gomes, M. N., Braga, R. C., Grzelak, E. M., Neves, B. J., Muratov, E., Ma, R., et al. (2017). QSAR-driven design, synthesis and discovery of potent chalcone derivatives with antitubercular activity. *Eur. J. Med. Chem.* 137, 126–138. doi: 10.1016/j.ejmech.2017.05.026

Hampton, S. E., Baragaña, B., Schipani, A., Bosch-Navarrete, C., Musso-Buendía, J. A., Recio, E., et al. (2011). Design, synthesis, and evaluation of 5′-diphenyl nucleoside analogues as inhibitors of the *Plasmodium falciparum* dUTPase. *ChemMedChem* 6, 1816–1831. doi: 10.1002/cmdc.201100255

Hartwig, C. L., Ahmed, A. O. A., Cooper, R. A., and Stedman, T. T. (2013). "SYBR Green I®-based parasite growth inhibition assay for measurement of antimalarial drug susceptibility in *Plasmodium falciparum*," in *Methods in Malaria Research*, eds K. Moll, A. Kaneko, A. Scherf, and M. Wahlgren (Glasgow: European Virtual Institute for Malaria Research), 122–129.

Hawkins, P. C. D., Skillman, A. G., and Nicholls, A. (2007). Comparison of shape-matching and docking as virtual screening tools. *J. Med. Chem.* 50, 74–82. doi: 10.1021/jm0603365

Hawkins, P. C. D., Skillman, A. G., Warren, G. L., Ellingson, B. A., and Stahl, M. T. (2010). Conformer generation with OMEGA: algorithm and validation using high quality structures from the Protein Databank and Cambridge Structural Database. *J. Chem. Inf. Model.* 50, 572–584. doi: 10.1021/ci100031x

Hoffman, S. L., Vekemans, J., Richie, T. L., and Duffy, P. E. (2015). The march toward malaria vaccines. *Am. J. Prev. Med.* 49, S319–S333. doi: 10.1016/j.amepre.2015.09.011

Jakalian, A., Bush, B. L., Jack, D. B., and Bayly, C. I. (1999). Fast, efficient generation of high-quality atomic charges. AM1-BCC Model: I. Method. *J. Comput. Chem.* 21, 132–146. doi: 10.1002/(SICI)1096-987X(20000130)21:2<132::AID-JCC5>3.0.CO;2-P

Jakalian, A., Jack, D. B., and Bayly, C. I. (2002). Fast, efficient generation of high-quality atomic charges. AM1-BCC model: II. Parameterization and validation. *J. Comput. Chem.* 23, 1623–1641. doi: 10.1002/jcc.10128

Kuz'min, V. E., Artemenko, A. G., and Muratov, E. N. (2008). Hierarchical QSAR technology based on the Simplex representation of molecular structure. *J. Comput. Aided Mol. Des.* 22, 403–421. doi: 10.1007/s10822-008-9179-6

Lagunin, A., Zakharov, A., Filimonov, D., and Poroikov, V. (2009). In silico assessment of acute toxicity in rodents. *Toxicol. Lett.* 189:S264. doi: 10.1016/j.toxlet.2009.06.393

Lagunin, A., Zakharov, A., Filimonov, D., and Poroikov, V. (2011). QSAR modelling of rat acute toxicity on the basis of PASS prediction. *Mol. Inform.* 30, 241–250. doi: 10.1002/minf.201000151

Lambros, C., and Vanderberg, J. P. (1979). Synchronization of *Plasmodium falciparum* erythrocytic stages in culture. *J. Parasitol.* 65, 418–420. doi: 10.2307/3280287

Leelananda, S. P., and Lindert, S. (2016). Computational methods in drug discovery. *Beilstein J. Org. Chem.* 12, 2694–2718. doi: 10.3762/bjoc.12.267

Lindberg, W., Persson, J.-A., and Wold, S. (1983). Partial least-squares method for spectrofluorimetric analysis of mixtures of humic acid and lignin sulfonate. *Anal. Chem.* 55, 643–648. doi: 10.1021/ac00255a014

López-Barragán, M. J., Lemieux, J., Quiñones, M., Williamson, K. C., Molina-Cruz, A., Cui, K., et al. (2011). Directional gene expression and antisense transcripts in sexual and asexual stages of *Plasmodium falciparum*. *BMC Genomics* 12:587. doi: 10.1186/1471-2164-12-587

McCarthy, O., Musso-Buendia, A., Kaiser, M., Brun, R., Ruiz-Perez, L. M., Johansson, N. G., et al. (2009). Design, synthesis and evaluation of novel uracil acetamide derivatives as potential inhibitors of *Plasmodium falciparum* dUTP nucleotidohydrolase. *Eur. J. Med. Chem.* 44, 678–688. doi: 10.1016/j.ejmech.2008.05.018

McGann, M. (2011). FRED pose prediction and virtual screening accuracy. *J. Chem. Inf. Model.* 51, 578–596. doi: 10.1021/ci100436p

Melo-Filho, C. C., Braga, R. C., and Andrade, C. H. (2014). 3D-QSAR approaches in drug design: perspectives to generate reliable CoMFA models. *Curr. Comput. Aided Drug Des.* 10, 148–159. doi: 10.2174/1573409910666140410111043

Melo-Filho, C. C., Dantas, R. F., Braga, R. C., Neves, B. J., Senger, M. R., Valente, W. C. G. G., et al. (2016). QSAR-driven discovery of novel chemical scaffolds active against *Schistosoma mansoni*. *J. Chem. Inf. Model.* 56, 1357–1372. doi: 10.1021/acs.jcim.6b00055

Miyakoshi, H., Miyahara, S., Yokogawa, T., Chong, K. T., Taguchi, J., Endoh, K., et al. (2012). Synthesis and discovery of N-carbonylpyrrolidine- or N-sulfonylpyrrolidine-containing uracil derivatives as potent human deoxyuridine triphosphatase inhibitors. *J. Med. Chem.* 55, 2960–2969. doi: 10.1021/jm201627n

Mosmann, T. (1983). Rapid colorimetric assay for cellular growth and survival: application to proliferation and cytotoxicity assays. *J. Immunol. Methods* 65, 55–63. doi: 10.1016/0022-1759(83)90303-4

Neves, B. J., Dantas, R. F., Senger, M. R., Melo-Filho, C. C., Valente, W. C. G., De Almeida, A. C. M., et al. (2016). Discovery of new anti-schistosomal hits by integration of QSAR-based virtual screening and high content screening. *J. Med. Chem.* 59, 7075–7088. doi: 10.1021/acs.jmedchem.5b02038

Nguyen, C., Kasinathan, G., Leal-Cortijo, I., Musso-Buendia, A., Kaiser, M., Brun, R., et al. (2005). Deoxyuridine triphosphate nucleotidohydrolase as a potential antiparasitic drug target. *J. Med. Chem.* 48, 5942–5954. doi: 10.1021/jm050111e

Nguyen, C., Ruda, G. F., Schipani, A., Kasinathan, G., Leal, I., Musso-Buendia, A., et al. (2006). Acyclic nucleoside analogues as inhibitors of *Plasmodium falciparum* dUTPase. *J. Med. Chem.* 49, 4183–4195. doi: 10.1021/jm060126s

Nyman, P. O. (2001). Introduction. *Curr. Protein Pept. Sci.* 2, 277–285. doi: 10.2174/1389203013381071

Ojha, P. K., and Roy, K. (2013). Exploring structural requirements for a class of nucleoside inhibitors (PfdUTPase) as antimalarials: first report on QSAR, pharmacophore mapping and multiple docking studies. *Comb. Chem. High Throughput Screen.* 16, 739–757. doi: 10.2174/13862073113169990002

Otto, T. D., Böhme, U., Jackson, A. P., Hunt, M., Franke-Fayard, B., Hoeijmakers, W. A. M., et al. (2014). A comprehensive evaluation of rodent malaria parasite genomes and gene expression. *BMC Biol.* 12:86. doi: 10.1186/s12915-014-0086-0

Pecsi, I., Hirmondo, R., Brown, A. C., Lopata, A., Parish, T., Vertessy, B. G., et al. (2012). The dUTPase enzyme is essential in *Mycobacterium smegmatis*. *PLoS One* 7:e37461. doi: 10.1371/journal.pone.0037461

Recio, E., Musso-Buendía, A., Vidal, A. E., Ruda, G. F., Kasinathan, G., Nguyen, C., et al. (2011). Site-directed mutagenesis provides insights into the selective binding of trityl derivatives to *Plasmodium falciparum* dUTPase. *Eur. J. Med. Chem.* 46, 3309–3314. doi: 10.1016/j.ejmech.2011.04.052

Ruda, G. F., Nguyen, C., Ziemkowski, P., Felczak, K., Kasinathan, G., Musso-Buendia, A., et al. (2011). Modified 5'-trityl nucleosides as inhibitors of *Plasmodium falciparum* dUTPase. *ChemMedChem* 6, 309–320. doi: 10.1002/cmdc.201000445

Sanders, J. M., Beshore, D. C., Culberson, J. C., Fells, J. I., Imbriglio, J. E., Gunaydin, H., et al. (2017). Informing the selection of screening hit series with in Silico absorption, distribution, metabolism, excretion, and toxicity profiles. *J. Med. Chem.* 60, 6771–6780. doi: 10.1021/acs.jmedchem.6b01577

Savin, N. E., and White, K. J. (1977). The durbin-watson test for serial correlation with extreme sample sizes or many regressors. *Econometrica* 45, 1989–1996. doi: 10.2307/1914122

Shelley, J. C., Cholleti, A., Frye, L. L., Greenwood, J. R., Timlin, M. R., and Uchimaya, M. (2007). Epik: a software program for pK(a) prediction and protonation state generation for drug-like molecules. *J. Comput. Aided Mol. Des.* 21, 681–691. doi: 10.1007/s10822-007-9133-z

Thu, A. M., Phyo, A. P., Landier, J., Parker, D. M., and Nosten, F. H. (2017). Combating multidrug-resistant *Plasmodium falciparum* malaria. *FEBS J.* 284, 2569–2578. doi: 10.1111/febs.14127

Trager, W., and Jensen, J. (1976). Human malaria parasites in continuous culture. *Science* 193, 673–675. doi: 10.1126/science.781840

TRIPOS (2010a). *HQSAR TM Manual: SYBYL®-X 1.1* 2010. St. Louis, MO: TRIPOS.

TRIPOS (2010b). *QSAR and COMFA® Manual: SYBYL®-X 1.1* 2010. St. Louis, MO: TRIPOS.

Tropsha, A. (2010). Best practices for QSAR model development, validation, and exploitation. *Mol. Inform.* 29, 476–488. doi: 10.1002/minf.201000061

Tropsha, A., Gramatica, P., and Gombar, V. (2003). The importance of being earnest: validation is the absolute essential for successful application and interpretation of QSPR models. *QSAR Comb. Sci.* 22, 69–77. doi: 10.1002/qsar.200390007

van de Waterbeemd, H., and Gifford, E. (2003). ADMET in silico modelling: towards prediction paradise? *Nat. Rev. Drug Discov.* 2, 192–204. doi: 10.1038/nrd1032

Varnek, A., Fourches, D., Horvath, D., Klimchuk, O., Gaudin, C., Vayer, P., et al. (2008). ISIDA - platform for virtual screening based on fragment and pharmacophoric descriptors. *Curr. Comput. Aided Drug Des.* 4, 191–198. doi: 10.2174/157340908785747465

Verma, J., Khedkar, V. M., and Coutinho, E. C. (2010). 3D-QSAR in drug design–a review. *Curr. Top. Med. Chem.* 10, 95–115. doi: 10.2174/156802610790232260

Vogel, G. (2014). The genetics of resistant malaria. *Science* 346, 1276–1277. doi: 10.1126/science.346.6215.1276

Whittingham, J. L., Leal, I., Nguyen, C., Kasinathan, G., Bell, E., Jones, A. F., et al. (2005). dUTPase as a platform for antimalarial drug design: structural basis for the selectivity of a class of nucleoside inhibitors. *Structure* 13, 329–338. doi: 10.1016/j.str.2004.11.015

World Health Organization [WHO] (2016). *World Malaria Report 2016*. Geneva: World Health Organization.

3

Identification of a New Potent Inhibitor Targeting KRAS in Non-small Cell Lung Cancer Cells

Chun Xie[1†], Ying Li[1†], Lan-Lan Li[2], Xing-Xing Fan[1], Yu-Wei Wang[1], Chun-Li Wei[1], Liang Liu[1], Elaine Lai-Han Leung[1*] and Xiao-Jun Yao[1,2*]*

[1] *State Key Laboratory of Quality Research in Chinese Medicine, Macau Institute for Applied Research in Medicine and Health, Macau University of Science and Technology, Macau, China,* [2] *State Key Laboratory of Applied Organic Chemistry and Department of Chemistry, Lanzhou University, Lanzhou, China*

Correspondence:
Liang Liu
lliu@must.edu.mo
Elaine Lai-Han Leung
lhleung@must.edu.mo
Xiao-Jun Yao
xjyao@must.edu.mo

† These authors have contributed equally to this work.

KRAS (v-Ki-ras2 Kirsten rat sarcoma viral oncogene homolog) is an oncogenic driver with mutations in 30% of non-small cell lung cancer (NSCLC). However, there is no effective clinical drug even though it has been identified as an oncogene for 30 years. In this study, we identified a small molecule inhibitor compound 0375-0604 targeting KRAS by using molecular docking based virtual screening approach. Compound 0375-0604 had a good binding affinity to KRAS *in vitro* and exhibited cytotoxicity in oncogenic KRAS expressing NSCLC cell lines. Further mechanism study showed that compound 0375-0604 can block the formation of the complex of guanosine triphosphate (GTP) and KRAS *in vitro*. In addition, compound 0375-0604 inhibited KRAS downstream signaling pathway RAF/MEK/ERK and RAF/PI3K/AKT. Finally, we also found that this compound can inhibit the cell growth through G2/M cell cycle arrest and induce apoptosis on the NSCLC cell lines harboring KRAS mutation. Therefore, compound 0375-0604 may be considered as a potential KRAS inhibitor for treatment of NSCLC carrying KRAS oncogene.

Keywords: KRAS, NSCLC, small molecule inhibitor, molecular docking

INTRODUCTION

In lung cancer, NSCLC is the majority category and accounts for 85% (Ettinger et al., 2017). The overall survival of patients with advanced or metastatic NSCLC is still dismal (Shima et al., 2015; Lazo and Sharlow, 2016). With the development of modern sequencing technology, NSCLC was further classified into different subtypes according to the frequency of gene mutation, such as EGFR, ALK, MET, ROS-1, KRAS (Chen et al., 2014). Mutated KRAS genes are frequently found in human cancers, especially in approximately 30% of lung cancer. Ninety seven percent of mutated KRAS occurs in exon 2 and 3, including amino acid G12, G13, and Q61 (Karachaliou et al., 2013). Due to high morbidity and mortality, a great deal of attention has been paid to study NSCLC with KRAS mutations. However, there is still no direct and effective drug for clinical use (Jancik et al., 2010; Gysin et al., 2011; Vasan et al., 2014; Papke and Der, 2017).

KRAS plays an important role in normal cell development, such as proliferation and differentiation (Pylayeva-Gupta et al., 2011; Santarpia et al., 2012). As a small GTPase, KRAS normally cycles between inactive GDP-bound state and active GTP-bound state, which are tightly regulated by GTPase-activating proteins (GAPs) and Guanine nucleotide exchange factors (GEFs), respectively (Maurer et al., 2012; Burns et al., 2014; Leshchiner et al., 2015). However, mutant

KRAS impairs its GAPs activity, which locks KRAS at the active state (Smith et al., 2013; Clausen et al., 2015). Thereby mutant KRAS promotes its interaction with a variety of effector proteins and activates downstream signaling events, and finally results in tumor formation (Bos et al., 2007; Zimmermann et al., 2013; Lito et al., 2016). Therefore, it is urgently needed to find effective inhibitors to target and inhibit oncogenic KRAS in cancers.

To date, there are mainly three strategies for the discovery of potent KRAS inhibitors: (1) to inhibit KRAS membrane targeting (Laheru et al., 2012; Prakash and Gorfe, 2013; Chavan et al., 2015; Cox et al., 2015); (2) to directly target KRAS (Wang et al., 2012; Cromm et al., 2015; Leshchiner et al., 2015; Brock et al., 2016; Trinh et al., 2016); (3) to inhibit interaction between KRAS and its downstream effectors (Athuluri-Divakar et al., 2016; Upadhyaya et al., 2016; Keeton et al., 2017). However, there are multiple escape pathways by process of post-translation for inhibiting KRAS membrane targeting (Rowinsky et al., 1999; Van Cutsem et al., 2004). Inhibitor lonafarnib and tipifarnib showed effective inhibition to KRAS mutations through blocking prenylation of RAS, but failed in clinical trial, as the geranylgeranylation could be in replacement of prenylation when the farnesyltransferase was inhibited by these two inhibitors (Berndt et al., 2011). Additionally, it may be not a good choice to inhibit interaction between KRAS and its downstream effectors for developing KRAS inhibitors. Firstly, there are a lot of downstream effector proteins of KRAS involving in multiple signaling pathways, such as RAF (MAP kinase pathway), PI3K (AKT/mTOR pathway), and RalGDS (Ral pathway). Secondly, these effectors are not only highly complex but also regulating multiple pathways (Downward, 2003). Arguably, designing a small molecule inhibitor directly targeting KRAS may be one of the most effective ways. However, the biggest challenges to develop direct KRAS inhibitor are the high binding affinity between KRAS and GDP/GTP in the picomolar range and the relatively flat surface without deep hydrophobic pockets in KRAS protein (Ledford, 2015; Vo et al., 2016). Notably, in recent years, several reported works have shown the novel transient pockets on KRAS protein surfaces, which recover the hope in the development of KRAS inhibitors (Prakash and Gorfe, 2013; Wang et al., 2014).

In this study, we aimed to identify effective and potential KRAS inhibitors by directly targeting KRAS to prevent cell growth of NSCLC harboring KRAS mutation. We performed a molecular docking-based virtual screening from a small molecule database to screen KRAS inhibitors. A potential inhibitor compound 0375-0604 was found to bind to KRAS and exhibit the effective cytotoxicity to KRAS mutant NSCLC cell lines.

RESULTS

The Binding Mode between Compound 0375-0604 and KRAS

To discover potential small molecules targeting KRAS, virtual screening based on molecular docking was performed on Chemdiv library with about 1.36 million compounds. The most promising compound 0375-0604 (**Figure 1A**) was selected for further study. It was shown that the benzothiazole ring of 0375-0604 inserted into the binding pocket of KRAS with the linker sulfur atom exposed to solvent environment (**Figures 1B,C**). The amino group of compound 0375-0604 formed H-bond interactions with the backbone of Met67 and the side chain of Glu37, locating in switch I and II regions of $KRAS^{G12D}$, respectively. At the same time, 0375-0604 formed polar contacts and hydrophobic contacts with the surrounding residues. 0375-0604 bound to $KRAS^{G12C}$ with a similar manner (**Figure 1D**) as $KRAS^{G12D}$, except for the orientation of chlorobenzene rings. The orientation of benzothiazole ring and chlorobenzene rings of 0375-0604 switched in $KRAS^{Q61H}$ (**Figure 1E**). Docking score of 0375-0604 in various systems was shown in **Figure 1F**.

The Binding Affinity of Compound 0375-0604 with KRAS

To determine the binding affinity of this small molecule with KRAS, we used biolayer interferometry assay (BLI) (Rich and Myszka, 2007), a label-free technology, to measure biomolecular interactions. Different concentration of compound 0375-0604 was measured in real time by association with both-labeled KRAS protein, which was immobilized on the streptavidin (SA) biosensors. All the association/dissociation binding curves was shown in **Figure 2A**, and we further performed the steady-state analysis (**Figure 2B**) with ForteìBio data analysis software to obtain the binding affinity with K_D value of 92 μM (**Figure 2C**), which demonstrated their direct and reversible interaction with KRAS.

Compound 0375-0604 Decreased Cell Viability of NSCLC Cells with KRAS Mutations

Since compound 0375-0604 bound to KRAS *in vitro*, we further determined its cytotoxicity in NSCLC cell lines harboring mutant KRAS by using MTT assay, including H2122 ($KRAS^{G12C}$), H358 ($KRAS^{G12C}$) and H460 ($KRAS^{Q61H}$) cell lines. Cells were incubated with a range of compound 0375-0604 concentrations (0, 25, 50, 100 μM) for 24, 48, and 72 h. As shown in **Figure 3**, compound 0375-0604 inhibited three NSCLC cell lines in a dose- and time-dependent manner, but not in normal lung fibroblast cell line CCD-19Lu. Importantly, we found that the IC_{50} value of compound 0375-0604 in H2122, H358 and H460 cells were up to 6-fold less than that of CCD-19Lu cells, which suggested that compound 0375-0604 showed strong inhibition selectivity in NSCLC cells.

Compound 0375-0604 Blocked GTP-KRAS Formation in NSCLC Cells

Actually, mutant KRAS would interfere the balance between GEFs and GAPs, resulting in locking in the active GTP-bound KRAS state and aberrant stimulation of its downstream signaling. Hence, KRAS inhibitors should reduce the formation of GTP-KRAS to disrupt the mutant KRAS function.

In order to know whether compound 0375-0604 could inhibit activation of KRAS, we performed RAS activation assay to

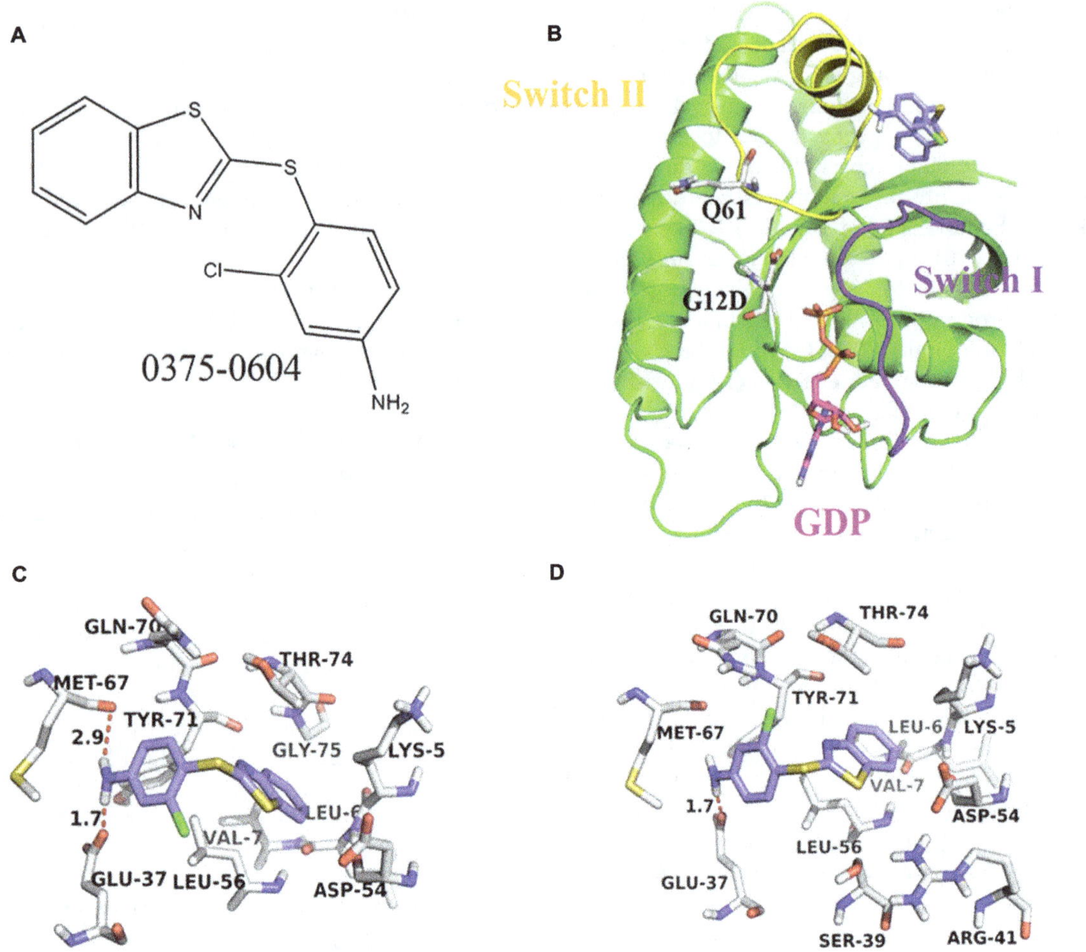

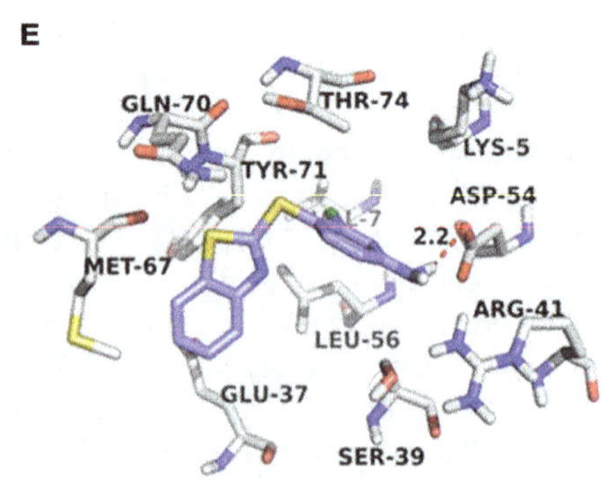

F

System	Docking score (kcal/mol)
$KRAS^{G12D}$	-5.38
$KRAS^{G12C}$	-5.41
$KRAS^{Q61H}$	-3.97

FIGURE 1 | The structural analysis between KRAS protein and 0375-0604. **(A)** The chemical structure of 0375-0604. **(B)** Structure of 0375-0604 binds to GDP-$KRAS^{G12D}$. The switch I and II region are colored in yellow and purple, respectively, while 0375-0604 and GDP are colored in blue and magenta, respectively. **(C–E)** Binding mode of 0375-0604 with $KRAS^{G12D}$, $KRAS^{G12C}$ and $KRAS^{Q61H}$, respectively. **(F)** Docking score of 0375-0604 in various systems.

examine the formation of GTP-bound KRAS after treatment with a range of concentrations of compound 0375-0604 in H2122, H358 and H460 cells at 24 h. As shown in **Figure 4**, the formation of GTP-KRAS was inhibited in KRAS mutant NSCLC by compound 0375-0604 treatment, compared to total amount of KRAS, suggesting this small molecule could partially rescue this unbalance resulted from mutant KRAS.

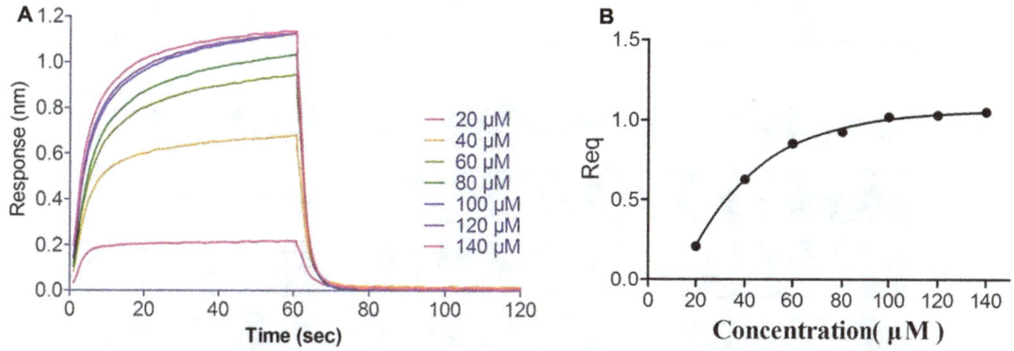

C

Kinetics of the interaction between KRAS and 0375-0604 by BLI

K_D (μM)	k_{on} (1/Ms)	k_{dis} (1/s)
92	$2.9\times10^{+03}$	2.6×10^{-01}

FIGURE 2 | The binding affinity of compound 0375-0604 with KRAS was determined by interferometry studies. **(A)** Binding curves of varying concentrations of compound 0375-0604 to the immobilized KRAS protein. **(B)** Steady-state analysis of the binding curves. **(C)** The binding affinity (K_D) of KRAS for compound 0375-0604 was determined. Experimental data for association and dissociation are represented as shown.

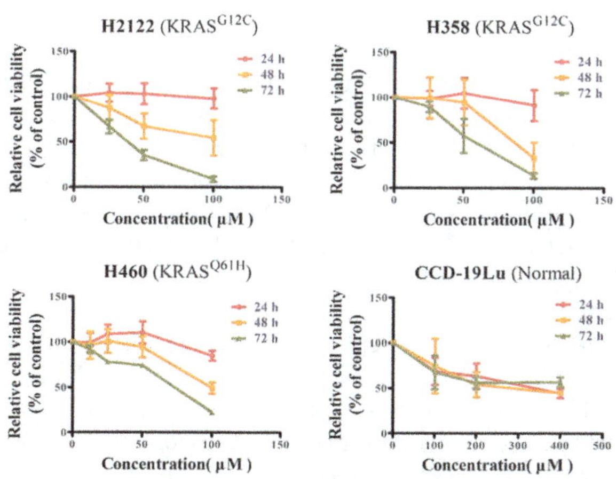

The IC_{50} values of 0375-0604

Cell lines	IC_{50} values (μM)		
	24 h	48 h	72 h
H2122	>100	>100	39.56±3.09
H358	>100	>100	63.83±3.89
H460	>100	100.30±13.30	66.02±11.82
CCD-19Lu	>400	>400	>400

FIGURE 3 | The cytotoxic effects of compound 0375-0604 on NSCLC cell lines were determined by MTT assay.

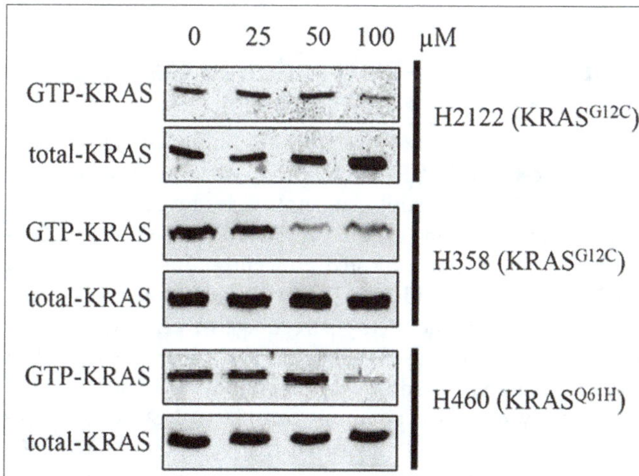

FIGURE 4 | The inhibition of compound 0375-0604 on active KRAS. KRAS mutant cells (H2122, H358 and H460) were treated with compound 0375-0604 for 24 h. The level of active KRAS (GTP-KRAS) was determined by a RAS activation assay and immunoblotted with a KRAS-specific antibody.

Compound 0375-0604 Inhibited the Activation of KRAS Downstream Signaling Pathway

Active KRAS stimulates downstream signaling pathways, especially for RAF/MEK/ERK and RAF/PI3K/AKT pathway, and then induces cell proliferation. Therefore, to investigate the effect of compound 0375-0604, we examined the phosphorylation levels of CRAF, AKT and ERK in NSCLC cell lines to monitor the impact of KRAS signaling by treatment with this compound for 48 h. As expected, compound 0375-0604 reduced the levels of phosphorylation of CRAF and AKT in a dose-dependent manner in all three NSCLC cell lines (**Figure 5**), which indicated that compound 0375-0604 may block oncogenic KRAS function through inhibiting its downstream signaling pathways.

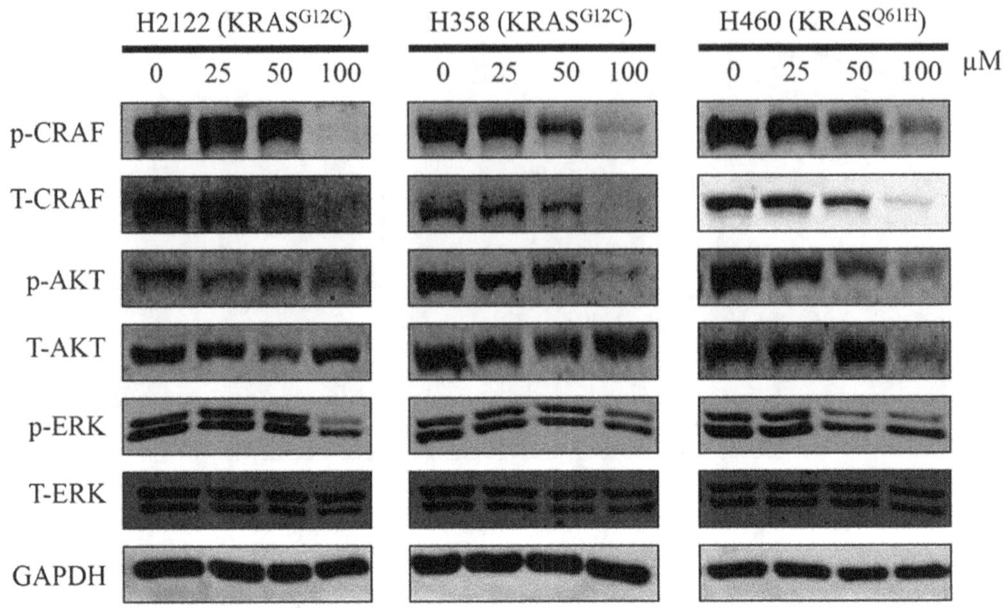

FIGURE 5 | The inhibitive effect of compound 0375-0604 on the KRAS signaling pathways in different NSCLC cell lines. Three NCSLC cell lines were treated with compound 0375-0604 for 48 h. The levels of phospho(p)-CRAF, p-ERK, p-AKT, CRAF, AKT, ERK and GAPDH were determined by western blot analysis. Untreated cells were used as a control. A representative of at least three independent experiments for each cell line is showed.

Compound 0375-0604 Induced Cell Cycle Arrest and Apoptosis in NSCLC

Since compound 0375-0604 significantly inhibited cell viability of NSCLC cells with KRAS mutation, we examined whether compound 0375-0604 exhibited cytotoxicity by cell cycle arrest or apoptotic effect in H2122, H358 and H460 cells. Cells were treated with the indicated concentrations of compound 0375-0604 for 24, 48, and 72 h. Flow cytometric analysis showed that after 24 h treatment, the percentage of cells significantly decreased in G0/G1 phase while remarkably increased in G2/M phase (**Figure 6A**). In addition, compound 0375-0604 induced a significantly increased apoptosis for 48h in NSCLC cell lines (**Figure 6B**). These result suggested that compound 0375-0604 may block cell proliferation and cause cell death via induction of G2/M cell cycle arrest or/and apoptosis in H2122, H358, and H460 cells.

DISCUSSION

In this study, we identified and characterized a small-molecule compound 0375-0604 as a new KRAS inhibitor. By using molecular docking approach, we found that compound 0375-0604 bound to the switch regions (switch I and II) of KRAS. KRAS conformation changes and its downstream signals are activated when its switch regions, either switch I or switch II, interact with GTP. A remarkable feature of compound 0375-0604 is that it formed two hydrogen bonds interaction with the backbone of Met67 and the side chain of Glu37, which are located in switch I and switch II, respectively. These two key hydrogen bonds could partially stabilize the interaction of KRAS and 0375-0604. The docking calculation indicated compound 0375-0604 exhibited potent binding affinity with KRAS. In addition, the chemical structure of this inhibitor has more potential to be modified and achieve more potent and effective inhibition to oncogenic KRAS NSCLC. Based on the docking result, the binding affinity of compound 0375-0604 with KRAS protein was further determined by using BLI and K_D value was 92 μM, which suggested that 0375-0604 could bind to KRAS with good performance.

There are two most extensively RAS-mediated pathways: PI3K/AKT/mTOR and RAF/MEK/ERK pathway (Papke and Der, 2017). The PI3K/AKT/mTOR pathway represents an important intracellular signaling pathway, which involved in transition of cell cycle. It is directly related to cell proliferation, cancer progress and longevity (Bryant et al., 2014). The RAF/MEK/ERK pathway is a chain of proteins in cell that communicates a signal from a receptor on the surface of cell to the DNA in the nucleus of cell. The RAF serine/threonine kinases (ARAF, BRAF and CRAF) are arguably the most important effectors of mutant RAS-dependent cancer growth, as they have a key driver role in RAS-mediated oncogenesis. In our study, we found that compound 0375-0604 could reduce the activation levels of AKT, CRAF and ERK and block the activation of KRAS downstream signaling pathways in NSCLC.

KRAS binds to GTP in its active state and then influences the expression of downstream genes involved in crucial pathways on regulating cell growth, differentiation and apoptosis (Lu et al., 2016). Compound 0375-0604 showed a strong anti-cancer activity by inhibiting the activation of KRAS proteins, and caused G2/M cell cycle arrest at the early stage and induced apoptosis

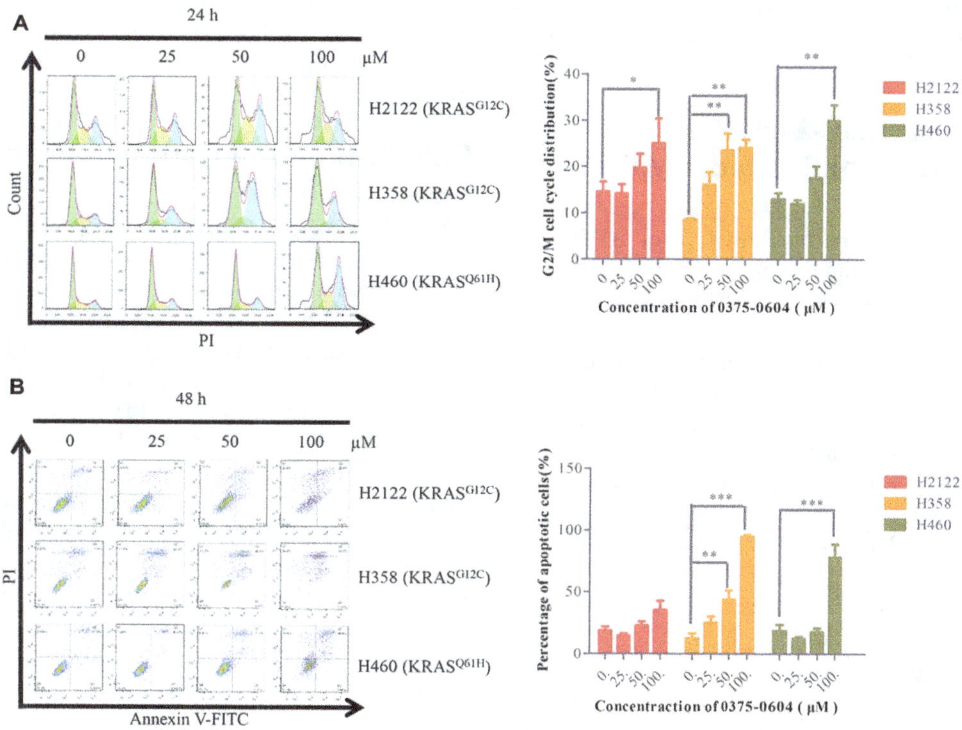

FIGURE 6 | Cell cycle arrest and apoptosis were induced by compound 0375-0604 in three NSCLC cell lines (H2122, H358 and H460). **(A)** Flow cytometric analysis of cell cycle arrest with compound 0375-0604 at different concentrations (0, 25, 50, 100 μM) was examined for 24 h. **(B)** Flow cytometric analysis of cell apoptosis with different concentrations (0, 25, 50, 100 μM) of compound 0375-0604 for 48 h was determined.

at the later stage in H2122, H358 and H460 cell lines harboring KRAS oncogene.

In summary, we identified a new small molecule compound 0375-0604 that bound to $KRAS^{G12D}$, $KRAS^{G12C}$ and $KRAS^{Q61H}$ protein with a moderate binding affinity of −5.38, −5.41, and −3.97 kcal/mol, respectively. In addition, 0375-0604 selectively inhibited the proliferation of NSCLC cells with KRAS mutation but not normal lung cells. Compound 0375-0604 also blocked the formation of GTP-KRAS and downstream activation of KRAS *in vivo*. Besides, compound 0375-0604 inhibited the growth of cancer cells by causing G2/M cell cycle arrest and inducing apoptosis. Regardless, our study provides further evidence for targeting to KRAS protein, which may contribute to the future study for lung cancer therapy.

MATERIALS AND METHODS

Molecular Docking

The $KRAS^{G12D}$ structure (PDB code: 4DSU) complexed with GDP and a compound benzimidazole (BZIM) was used for the modeling of possible binding modes between KRAS and 0375-0604. The crystal structure with GDP was prepared in the Prep Wiz module of Maestro (Version 9.1, Schrodinger) and water molecules within 5 Å of het groups were kept. Subsequently, the residues of D12 and Q61 were mutated into C12 and H61 using the BioLuminate module of Maestro, respectively. A grid file was generated based on the position of compound BZIM in the Grid Generation wizard. Then, 0375-0604 was prepared to assign atomic charges and generate alternative conformations chemical rings. Finally, the docking process was employed in the Glide Docking module based on the previous obtained grid file using an extra precision (XP) protocol followed by a post-docking minimization using MM-GBSA method.

Biotinylation

KRAS (Abcam, ab96817; 200 μg/ml) was biotinylated using the EZ-Link NHS-LC-LC-biotin (Thermo) in H_2O using a 3:1 molar ratio of biotin reagent: protein for 30 min at room temperature following the FortéBio suggested protocol. Biotinylated KRAS was separated from the biotinylation reaction reagents by Zeba desalying spin columns (Thermo). Streptavidin biosensors (SA) tips (ForteìBio, Inc., Menlo Park, CA, United States) were prewetted with PBS to establish a baseline before immobilization.

Biolayer Interferometry Analysis

A FortéBio Octet Red instrument was used in this assay. All the assays were performed at 96-well plate (Greiner Bio-One, PN:655209) and all the final volume for all the solutions was 200 μl/well. Biotinylated KRAS was immobilized onto SA tips. The experiments comprised three steps: (1) baseline, (2) association, (3) dissociation. The association and dissociation plot and kinetic constants were obtained with ForteìBio data analysis software. For measurement the interaction between compound 0375-0604 and KRAS, seven concentrations of compound 0375-0604 (20, 40, 60, 80, 100, 120, 140, 160 μM) were used for association step.

3-(4, 5-Dimethylthiazol-2-yl)-2, 5-Diphenyltetrazolium Bromide (MTT) Assay

H2122, H460 and H358 were purchased from ATCC and cultivated with RPMI 1640 medium supplemented with 10% fetal bovine serum (FBS), 100 units/mL penicillin and 100 μg/mL streptomycin. All the cells were cultivated at 37°C with 5% CO_2 incubator. Cells were seeded on a 96-well microplate with 3000, 4000, or 5000 cells/well, and were cultured overnight for cell adhesion. After add a range of compound 0375-0604 the microplates put back into incubator and incubated for 24, 48, or 72 h. Each dosage was repeated as triplicate. 10 μL MTT (5 mg/mL) solutions were added to each well. After incubated 4 h 100 μL DMSO was added to each well. After 15 min shake absorbance of the plate was measured at 570 nm (absorbance) and 650 nm (reference) by a microplate reader (Tecan).

Pull Down Assay

RAS activity was determined using RAS activation assay kit (EMD Millipore, 17–218). Briefly, lysates were incubated with glutathione S-transferase fusion of the Ras binding domain (RBD) of Raf1 along with glutathione agarose for 1 h. Agarose beads were collected by centrifugation and washed three times with Mg^{2+} lysis buffer. Each sample were resuspended and boiled for 5 min. Finally, samples were subjected to western blotting as previously described and blots probed using anti-KRAS antibody (Santa, sc-30).

Western Blot Analysis

After 48 h treatment with compound 0375-0604, RIPA lysis buffer (150 mM NaCl, 50 mM Tris pH 7.4, 1 mM EDTA, 0.25% sodium deoxycholate, 1% NP-40) containing protease (Roche) and phosphatase (Roche) inhibitors was added to extract the total whole cell protein. Bio-Rad DC™ protein assay kit was used to quantify the concentration of extract protein. Thirty microgram protein lysate was loaded and separated by 10% SDS-polyacrylamide gel electrophoresis and transferred to a nitrocellulose (Millipore) membrane. The membrane was incubated with the primary antibody (1:2000) and then with a fluorescence-conjugated secondary antibody (1:10000). GAPDH was used as the loading control and for normalization. The signal of the membranes was scanned with a LI-COR Odyssey Scanner (Belfast).

Cell Cycle and Apoptosis Assay Using Flow Cytometry

H2122, H358 and H460 cells were plated on a 6-well plate with 1.5×10^5 cells/well and cultured overnight for attachment. After treatment with compound 0375-0604 at 0, 25, 50, 100 μM for 24, 48, and 72 h, all cells were harvested and collected. For cell cycle analysis, cells pellets were re-suspended in 70% ethanol and fixation at 4°C for 30 min. Each cell pellet was stained in 300 μL propodium iodide (PI) (50 μg/ml) staining solution at 37°C for 30 min in dark. Then, cells were washed twice with PBS. Finally, cells were re-suspended in 300 μL PBS and transferred to the flow cytometer (FACSCalibur, BD Biosciences). For apoptosis analysis, cells will re-suspended with 100 μL annexin-binding buffer, stained with annexin V and PI staining solution and incubated 15 min at room temperature protect from light. Finally, cells were diluted in 300 μL annexin-binding buffer and quantitatively measured using flow cytometer (FACSCalibur, BD Biosciences).

Statistical Analysis

Descriptive analytical data are presented as means ± SD. Statistical analysis was conducted using Graph Prim 5.0. Significant differences between datasets were assessed by one-way analysis of variance (ANOVA).

AUTHOR CONTRIBUTIONS

X-JY, EL-HL, and LL conceived the project. X-JY, EL-HL, and CX designed the experiments. CX, YL, L-LL, X-XF, Y-WW, and C-LW carried out the research and analysis of data. X-JY, EL-HL, LL, and CX wrote the paper.

ACKNOWLEDGMENT

This work was supported by Macao Science and Technology Development Fund (Project No: 082/2013/A3 & 086/2015/A3 & 005/2014/AMJ&046/2016/A2).

REFERENCES

Athuluri-Divakar, S. K., Vasquez-Del Carpio, R., Dutta, K., Baker, S. J., Cosenza, S. C., Basu, I., et al. (2016). A small molecule RAS-mimetic disrupts RAS association with effector proteins to block signaling. *Cell* 165, 643–655. doi: 10.1016/j.cell.2016.03.045

Berndt, N., Hamilton, A. D., and Sebti, S. M. (2011). Targeting protein prenylation for cancer therapy. *Nat. Rev. Cancer* 11, 775–791. doi: 10.1038/nrc3151

Bos, J. L., Rehmann, H., and Wittinghofer, A. (2007). GEFs and GAPs: critical elements in the control of small G proteins. *Cell* 129, 865–877. doi: 10.1016/j.cell.2007.05.018

Brock, E. J., Ji, K., Reiners, J. J., and Mattingly, R. R. (2016). How to target activated RAS proteins: direct inhibition *vs.* induced Mislocalization. *Mini. Rev. Med. Chem.* 16, 358–369. doi: 10.2174/1389557515666151001154002

Bryant, K. L., Mancias, J. D., Kimmelman, A. C., and Der, C. J. (2014). KRAS: feeding pancreatic cancer proliferation. *Trends Biochem. Sci.* 39, 91–100. doi: 10.1016/j.tibs.2013.12.004

Burns, M. C., Sun, Q., Daniels, R. N., Camper, D., Kennedy, J. P., Phan, J., et al. (2014). Approach for targeting Ras with small molecules that activate SOS-mediated nucleotide exchange. *Proc. Natl. Acad. Sci. U.S.A.* 111, 3401–3406. doi: 10.1073/pnas.1315798111

Chavan, T. S., Muratcioglu, S., Marszalek, R., Jang, H., Keskin, O., Gursoy, A., et al. (2015). Plasma membrane regulates Ras signaling networks. *Cell. Logist.* 5:e1136374. doi: 10.1080/21592799.2015.1136374

Chen, Z., Fillmore, C. M., Hammerman, P. S., Kim, C. F., and Wong, K. K. (2014). Non-small-cell lung cancers: a heterogeneous set of diseases. *Nat. Rev. Cancer* 14, 535–546. doi: 10.1038/nrc3775

Clausen, R., Ma, B., Nussinov, R., and Shehu, A. (2015). Mapping the conformation space of wildtype and mutant H-Ras with a memetic, cellular, and multiscale evolutionary algorithm. *PLOS Comput. Biol.* 11:e1004470. doi: 10.1371/journal.pcbi.1004470

Cox, A. D., Der, C. J., and Philips, M. R. (2015). Targeting RAS membrane association: back to the future for anti-RAS drug discovery? *Clin. Cancer Res.* 21, 1819–1827. doi: 10.1158/1078-0432.CCR-14-3214

Cromm, P. M., Spiegel, J., Grossmann, T. N., and Waldmann, H. (2015). Direct modulation of small GTPase activity and function. *Angew. Chem. Int. Ed. Engl.* 54, 13516–13537. doi: 10.1002/anie.201504357

Downward, J. (2003). Targeting RAS signalling pathways in cancer therapy. *Nat. Rev. Cancer* 3, 11–22. doi: 10.1038/nrc969

Ettinger, D. S., Wood, D. E., Aisner, D. L., Akerley, W., Bauman, J., Chirieac, L. R., et al. (2017). Non-small cell lung cancer, version 5.2017, NCCN clinical practice guidelines in oncology. *J. Natl. Compr. Canc. Netw.* 15, 504–535. doi: 10.6004/jnccn.2017.0050

Gysin, S., Salt, M., Young, A., and Mccormick, F. (2011). Therapeutic strategies for targeting ras proteins. *Genes Cancer* 2, 359–372. doi: 10.1177/1947601911412376

Jancik, S., Drabek, J., Radzioch, D., and Hajduch, M. (2010). Clinical relevance of KRAS in human cancers. *J. Biomed. Biotechnol.* 2010:150960. doi: 10.1155/2010/150960

Karachaliou, N., Mayo, C., Costa, C., Magrí, I., Gimenez-Capitan, A., Molina-Vila, M. A., et al. (2013). KRAS mutations in lung cancer. *Clin. Lung Cancer* 14, 205. doi: 10.1016/j.cllc.2012.09.007

Keeton, A. B., Salter, E. A., and Piazza, G. A. (2017). The RAS-effector interaction as a drug target. *Cancer Res.* 77, 221–226. doi: 10.1158/0008-5472.CAN-16-0938

Laheru, D., Shah, P., Rajeshkumar, N. V., Mcallister, F., Taylor, G., Goldsweig, H., et al. (2012). Integrated preclinical and clinical development of S-*trans, trans*-farnesylthiosalicylic Acid (FTS, Salirasib) in pancreatic cancer. *Invest. New Drugs* 30, 2391–2399. doi: 10.1007/s10637-012-9818-6

Lazo, J. S., and Sharlow, E. R. (2016). Drugging undruggable molecular cancer targets. *Annu. Rev. Pharmacol. Toxicol.* 56, 23–40. doi: 10.1146/annurev-pharmtox-010715-103440

Ledford, H. (2015). Cancer: the Ras renaissance. *Nature* 520, 278–280. doi: 10.1038/520278a

Leshchiner, E. S., Parkhitko, A., Bird, G. H., Luccarelli, J., Bellairs, J. A., Escudero, S., et al. (2015). Direct inhibition of oncogenic KRAS by hydrocarbon-stapled SOS1 helices. *Proc. Natl. Acad. Sci. U.S.A.* 112, 1761–1766. doi: 10.1073/pnas.1413185112

Lito, P., Solomon, M., Li, L.-S., Hansen, R., and Rosen, N. (2016). Allele-specific inhibitors inactivate mutant KRAS G12C by a trapping mechanism. *Science* 351, 604–608. doi: 10.1126/science.aad6204

Lu, S. Y., Jang, H., Gu, S., Zhang, J., and Nussinov, R. (2016). Drugging Ras GTPase: a comprehensive mechanistic and signaling structural view. *Chem. Soc. Rev.* 45, 4929–4952. doi: 10.1039/c5cs00911a

Maurer, T., Garrenton, L. S., Oh, A., Pitts, K., Anderson, D. J., Skelton, N. J., et al. (2012). Small-molecule ligands bind to a distinct pocket in Ras and inhibit SOS-mediated nucleotide exchange activity. *Proc. Natl. Acad. Sci. U.S.A.* 109, 5299–5304. doi: 10.1073/pnas.1116510109

Papke, B., and Der, C. J. (2017). Drugging RAS: know the enemy. *Science* 355, 1158–1163. doi: 10.1126/science.aam7622

Prakash, P., and Gorfe, A. A. (2013). Lessons from computer simulations of Ras proteins in solution and in membrane. *Biochim. Biophys. Acta* 1830, 5211–5218. doi: 10.1016/j.bbagen.2013.07.024

Pylayeva-Gupta, Y., Grabocka, E., and Bar-Sagi, D. (2011). RAS oncogenes: weaving a tumorigenic web. *Nat. Rev. Cancer* 11, 761–774. doi: 10.1038/nrc3106

Rich, R. L., and Myszka, D. G. (2007). Higher-throughput, label-free, real-time molecular interaction analysis. *Anal. Biochem.* 361, 1–6. doi: 10.1016/j.ab.2006.10.040

Rowinsky, E. K., Windle, J. J., and Von Hoff, D. D. (1999). Ras protein farnesyltransferase: a strategic target for anticancer therapeutic development. *J. Clin. Oncol.* 17, 3631–3652. doi: 10.1200/JCO.1999.17.11.3631

Santarpia, L., Lippman, S. M., and El-Naggar, A. K. (2012). Targeting the MAPK-RAS-RAF signaling pathway in cancer therapy. *Expert Opin. Ther. Targets* 16, 103–119. doi: 10.1517/14728222.2011.645805

Shima, F., Matsumoto, S., Yoshikawa, Y., Kawamura, T., Isa, M., and Kataoka, T. (2015). Current status of the development of Ras inhibitors. *J. Biochem.* 158, 91–99. doi: 10.1093/jb/mvv060

Smith, M. J., Neel, B. G., and Ikura, M. (2013). NMR-based functional profiling of RASopathies and oncogenic RAS mutations. *Proc. Natl. Acad. Sci. U.S.A.* 110, 4574–4579. doi: 10.1073/pnas.1218173110

Trinh, T. B., Upadhyaya, P., Qian, Z., and Pei, D. (2016). Discovery of a direct Ras inhibitor by screening a combinatorial library of cell-permeable bicyclic peptides. *ACS Comb. Sci.* 18, 75–85. doi: 10.1021/acscombsci.5b00164

Upadhyaya, P., Bedewy, W., and Pei, D. (2016). Direct inhibitors of Ras-effector protein interactions. *Mini Rev. Med. Chem.* 16, 376–382. doi: 10.2174/1389557515666151001141713

Van Cutsem, E., Van De Velde, H., Karasek, P., Oettle, H., Vervenne, W. L., Szawlowski, A., et al. (2004). Phase III trial of gemcitabine plus tipifarnib compared with gemcitabine plus placebo in advanced pancreatic cancer. *J. Clin. Oncol.* 22, 1430–1438. doi: 10.1200/JCO.2004.10.112

Vasan, N., Boyer, J. L., and Herbst, R. S. (2014). A RAS renaissance: emerging targeted therapies for KRAS-mutated non-small cell lung cancer. *Clin. Cancer Res.* 20, 3921–3930. doi: 10.1158/1078-0432.ccr-13-1762

Vo, U., Vajpai, N., Flavell, L., Bobby, R., Breeze, A. L., Embrey, K. J., et al. (2016). Monitoring Ras interactions with the nucleotide exchange factor son of Sevenless (Sos) using site-specific NMR reporter signals and intrinsic fluorescence. *J. Biol. Chem.* 291, 1703–1718. doi: 10.1074/jbc.M115.691238

Wang, Q., Qi, Y., Yin, N., and Lai, L. (2014). Discovery of novel allosteric effectors based on the predicted allosteric sites for *Escherichia coli* D-3-phosphoglycerate dehydrogenase. *PLOS ONE* 9:e94829. doi: 10.1371/journal.pone.0094829

Wang, W., Fang, G., and Rudolph, J. (2012). Ras inhibition via direct Ras binding–is there a path forward? *Bioorg. Med. Chem. Lett.* 22, 5766–5776. doi: 10.1016/j.bmcl.2012.07.082

Zimmermann, G., Papke, B., Ismail, S., Vartak, N., Chandra, A., Hoffmann, M., et al. (2013). Small molecule inhibition of the KRAS-PDEdelta interaction impairs oncogenic KRAS signalling. *Nature* 497, 638–642. doi: 10.1038/nature12205

4

Comparison of Quantitative and Qualitative (Q)SAR Models Created for the Prediction of K_i and IC_{50} Values of Antitarget Inhibitors

Alexey A. Lagunin[1,2], Maria A. Romanova[2], Anton D. Zadorozhny[2], Natalia S. Kurilenko[2], Boris V. Shilov[2], Pavel V. Pogodin[1], Sergey M. Ivanov[1,2], Dmitry A. Filimonov[1] and Vladimir V. Poroikov[1]**

[1] Department of Bioinformatics, Institute of Biomedical Chemistry, Moscow, Russia, [2] Department of Bioinformatics, Pirogov Russian National Research Medical University, Moscow, Russia

***Correspondence:**
Alexey A. Lagunin
alexey.lagunin@ibmc.msk.ru
Vladimir V. Poroikov
vladimir.poroikov@ibmc.msk.ru

Estimation of interaction of drug-like compounds with antitargets is important for the assessment of possible toxic effects during drug development. Publicly available online databases provide data on the experimental results of chemical interactions with antitargets, which can be used for the creation of (Q)SAR models. The structures and experimental K_i and IC_{50} values for compounds tested on the inhibition of 30 antitargets from the ChEMBL 20 database were used. Data sets with K_i and IC_{50} values including more than 100 compounds were created for each antitarget. The (Q)SAR models were created by GUSAR software using quantitative neighborhoods of atoms (QNA), multilevel neighborhoods of atoms (MNA) descriptors, and self-consistent regression. The accuracy of (Q)SAR models was validated by the fivefold cross-validation procedure. The balanced accuracy was higher for qualitative SAR models (0.80 and 0.81 for K_i and IC_{50} values, respectively) than for quantitative QSAR models (0.73 and 0.76 for K_i and IC_{50} values, respectively). In most cases, sensitivity was higher for SAR models than for QSAR models, but specificity was higher for QSAR models. The mean R^2 and RMSE were 0.64 and 0.77 for K_i values and 0.59 and 0.73 for IC_{50} values, respectively. The number of compounds falling within the applicability domain was higher for SAR models than for the test sets.

Keywords: QSAR, antitarget, inhibition, adverse drug reactions, K_i, IC_{50}, GUSAR, ChEMBL

INTRODUCTION

Adverse drug reactions (ADRs) are one of the main problems in drug discovery and clinical practice (Böhm and Cascorbi, 2016). According to some estimates, ADR is one of the leading causes of hospitalization and death in developed countries (Starfield, 2000; Kochanek et al., 2016), the second most common cause of drug attrition in later stages of clinical trials and the major reason for drug withdrawal from the market (Hornberg et al., 2014). This situation is largely due to disadvantages of traditional animal toxicological experiments and clinical trials that cannot detect all serious ADRs because of inter-species differences and their idiosyncratic nature. Therefore, additional methods including *in vitro* and *in silico* approaches are currently being developed. *In silico* approaches are usually based on machine learning techniques and network analyses to link several chemical and biological features of approved and withdrawn drugs to ADRs, which include molecular descriptors, known or predicted drug targets, drug-induced gene expression profiles and cell phenotypic features (Ivanov et al., 2016). These approaches allow predict dangerous ADRs in the early stages of drug development and provide insights into potential toxic mechanisms of drug candidates. It is currently accepted that the most ADRs are the consequence of unintended interactions of drugs with human protein targets and are not related to a therapeutic mechanism of action. For example, blocking HERG potassium channels in the heart causes life-threatening arrhythmias (Siramshetty et al., 2016). There are dozens of human proteins that have known relationships to ADRs, and corresponding information has accumulated in public databases (Ji et al., 2003; Zhang et al., 2007) and been described in some publications (Whitebread et al., 2005; Bowes et al., 2012). These proteins are called "antitargets" because to avoid dangerous ADRs, they should not interact with drugs. Many pharmaceutical companies use *in vitro* assays to measure interactions of lead compounds with "antitargets" and select the least promiscuous ones for further development. To avoid performing hundreds of experiments, such interactions can also be predicted using ligand-based structure-activity relationship analysis or docking (Ivanov et al., 2016; Simões et al., 2018). Due to accumulation of data on chemical-protein interactions and three-dimensional protein structures in public databases such as ChEMBL (Gaulton et al., 2017), PubChem (Wang et al., 2017), and PDB (Berman et al., 2000), it has become possible to predict interactions with many hundreds of human proteins, including "antitargets." There are plenty of published (Q)SAR models (Poroikov et al., 2007; Filz et al., 2008; García-Sosa and Maran, 2014; Ivanov et al., 2016) and free available web-services (Zakharov et al., 2012; Braga et al., 2015) that may perform such predictions; however, no study was found with a comparison between the accuracy of classification (SAR) and quantitative (QSAR) models created based on the same data, descriptors and mathematical algorithm. The aim of this work is the creation, validation, and accuracy estimation of SAR and QSAR models for the prediction of the inhibition of 30 antitargets using GUSAR software and data on structures and K_i and IC_{50} values of tested compounds from the ChEMBL 20 database. Earlier, we published a study on the creation of reasonable QSAR models by GUSAR software and the appropriate web service[1] for the prediction of interaction between drug-like compounds and 18 antitargets (Zakharov et al., 2012). In this paper, we have significantly expanded the list of covered "antitargets" and significantly increased the volumes and diversity of training samples, which allowed us to expand the range of applicability of models and to obtain valuable results.

MATERIALS AND METHODS

Data Sets

Structures and experimental K_i and IC_{50} values of compounds tested on the inhibition of 30 antitargets were extracted from the ChEMBL 20 database. The data sets with K_i and IC_{50} values including more than 100 compounds were created for each antitarget (**Table 1**). Only the records with K_i or IC_{50} values in nM and symbol " = " in the field "Relation" were extracted from ChEMBL database. During the creation of data sets of compounds interacting with receptors, we included records with compounds studied as truly antagonists and records with compounds studied on biding affinity because of we could not divided them. In spite of Ki and IC50 values indicate the affinity of a compound by a given receptor, and they do not necessarily provide functional information related with agonism or antagonism of a compound to such target we decided to include such data because antagonism of receptors may be related with Ki and IC50 values, whereas agonism to receptors are usually represented by EC50 values. K_i or IC_{50} values were transformed in $pIC_{50} = -\log10(IC_{50}(M))$ and $pK_i = -\log10(K_i(M))$ values. **Table 1** also shows the known relations between the inhibition of antitargets and ADRs. The number of compounds with K_i values was approximately 1.5 times higher than that for IC_{50} values (46830 and 29678, respectively). The sets included structures of single electroneutral small (molecular weight in range from 50 to 1250 Da) organic molecules. In general, such representation of structure corresponds to the best QSAR practice (Fourches et al., 2016) implemented in the GUSAR software, which was used in our study (see below). If a compound had several experimental values for the parameter, then a median value was used. Such median values were calculated because the reference compounds usually had several experimental values, since they were tested in many experiments. Deleting such compounds reduces an important part of chemical space and significantly restricts the applicability domain of the global QSAR models. In several publications related to the creation of global QSAR models based on heterogeneous data, authors used average values (Politi et al., 2014; Cortes-Ciriano and Bender, 2015). The median value was used because it better characterizes the set of values for strongly skewed distributions. Zip file including SD files related with the appropriate target (the gene name of targets is used in a file name), and endpoint is provided in **Supplementary Materials**. Each SD file includes structures, ChEMBL_ID, and experimental values. For classification models and comparison of prediction results between the SAR and QSAR models, 1 μM was used as a threshold between active and inactive compounds. The sets were sorted by the ascending mode of the appropriate values. Then, successively, a number from 1 to 5 was assigned for each structure from a set. After that, the sets were divided into five unique parts according to the assigned number of structures. These parts were used for the fivefold cross-validation (fivefold CV) procedure, when

[1] http://www.way2drug.com/gusar/antitargets.html

TABLE 1 | Data related with antitargets and the number of compounds with Ki and IC50 values in data sets.

Target	UniProt ID	Chembl Target ID	K_i	IC_{50}	Effects at antagonism or inhibition
Acetylcholinesterase	P22303	CHEMBL220	272	2573	↓ BP; ↓ HR; ↑ GI motility (↓ at high doses); bronchoconstriction; ↑ respiratory secretions; anaphylaxis; anorexiant; arrhythmogenic; asystole; colic; diarrhea; emetic; gastrointestinal hemorrhage; headache; hypotension; muscle weakness; nausea; neurotoxic; nightmare; respiratory failure; sialorrhea; sweating; ulcer, gastric; urticaria
Adenosine receptor A2a	P29274	CHEMBL251	3258	213	Platelet aggregation; ↑ BP; nervousness (tremors, agitation); arousal; insomnia
Alpha-1A adrenergic receptor	P35348	CHEMBL229	942	100	↓ smooth muscle tone; orthostatic hypotension and ↑ HR; dizziness; impact on various aspects of sexual function; flushing; hypotension; impotence; nasal congestion; postural (orthostatic) hypotension; tachycardia; weakness
Alpha-2A adrenergic receptor	P08913	CHEMBL1867	557	201	↑ GI motility; ↑ insulin secretion; hypertension exacerbates heart failure; anxiety; depression
Beta-1 adrenergic receptor	P08588	CHEMBL213	278	512	↓ BP; ↓ HR; ↓ cardiac output; cardiotoxicity; heart failure
Beta-2 adrenergic receptor	P07550	CHEMBL210	352	472	↓ BP; increased bronchospasm
Androgen receptor	P10275	CHEMBL1871	631	1054	↓ spermatogenesis; impotence; gynecomastia, mastodynia; ↑ in breast carcinoma
Muscarinic acetylcholine receptor M1	P11229	CHEMBL216	635	544	↓ cognitive function; ↓ gastric acid secretion; blurred vision
Muscarinic acetylcholine receptor M2	P08172	CHEMBL211	799	422	Tachycardia; bronchoconstriction; tremors
Muscarinic acetylcholine receptor M3	P20309	CHEMBL245	644	606	Constipation; blurred vision; pupil dilation; dry mouth
Cannabinoid receptor 1	P21554	CHEMBL218	1998	904	↑ weight loss; emesis; depression
Cannabinoid receptor 2	P34972	CHEMBL253	2375	592	↑ inflammation; ↓ bone mass
D(1A) dopamine receptor	P21728	CHEMBL2056	681	106	Dyskinesia; parkinsonian symptoms (tremors); anti-emetic effects; depression; anxiety; suicidal intent
D(2) dopamine receptor	P14416	CHEMBL217	3946	431	Orthostatic hypotension; drowsiness; ↑ GI motility; dyskinesia; extrapyramidal effect; sedative
Endothelin-1 receptor	P25101	CHEMBL252	155	894	Teratogenicity
Histamine H1 receptor	P35367	CHEMBL231	753	264	Sedation; ↓ allergic responses; ↑ body weight; dizziness; extrapyramidal effect; hypnotic; hypotension; lassitude; tinnitus; xerostomia
5-hydroxytryptamine receptor 1A	P08908	CHEMBL214	2505	432	Anxiogenic
5-hydroxytryptamine receptor 1B	P28222	CHEMBL1898	662	266	↑ aggression
5-hydroxytryptamine receptor 2A	P28223	CHEMBL224	1768	659	hypnotic; sedative
5-hydroxytryptamine receptor 2B	P41595	CHEMBL1833	705	248	Possible cardiac effects, especially during embryonic development
Potassium voltage-gated channel subfamily H member 2	Q12809	CHEMBL240	935	4078	Prolongation of QT interval of ECG
Tyrosine-protein kinase Lck	P06239	CHEMBL258	364	1322	T cell inhibition; SCID-like immunodeficiency
Amine oxidase [flavin-containing] A	P21397	CHEMBL1951	342	1031	↑ BP when combined with amines such as tyramine; drug–drug interaction potential; dizziness; sleep disturbances; nausea
Neuropeptide Y receptor type 1	P25929	CHEMBL4777	321	304	Anxiogenic
Glucocorticoid receptor	P04150	CHEMBL2034	632	1086	Hypoglycemia
Delta-type opioid receptor	P41143	CHEMBL236	1603	534	↑ BP; ↑ cardiac contractility
Mu-type opioid receptor	P35372	CHEMBL233	1816	663	↑ GI motility; dyspepsia; flatulence
Sodium-dependent noradrenaline transporter	P23975	CHEMBL222	1346	1371	↑ HR; ↑ BP; ↑ locomotor activity; constipation; abuse potential
Sodium-dependent dopamine transporter	Q01959	SLC6A3	1195	1183	Addictive psychostimulation; dopaminergic hyperactivity; depression; parkinsonism; attention deficit–hyperactivity disorder; psychotic disorders; seizures; dystonia; dyskinesia; acne
Sodium-dependent serotonin transporter	P31645	CHEMBL228	1868	1938	↑ GI motility; ↓ upper GI transit; ↓ plasma renin; ↑ other serotonin-mediated effects; insomnia; anxiety; nausea; sexual dysfunction

BP, blood pressure; ECG, electrocardiogram; GI, gastrointestinal; HR, heart rate; SCID, severe-combined immunodeficiency.

each unique part was used as an external test set, and the remaining parts were used as a training set. As a result, different five training and five external test sets for K_i data and five training and five external test sets for IC_{50} data, including both quantitative and qualitative descriptions, were created for each antitarget.

GUSAR Software

The (Q)SAR models were created by GUSAR software[2], which used quantitative neighbourhoods of atoms (QNA), multilevel neighbourhoods of atom (MNA), and whole-molecule descriptors with self-consistent regression (Lagunin et al., 2007; Filimonov et al., 2009; Lagunin et al., 2011). QNA descriptors are calculated by two functions, P and Q. The values for P and Q for each atom *i* are calculated as:

$$P_i = B_i \sum_k (Exp(-\frac{1}{2}C))_{ik} B_k,$$

$$Q_i = B_i \sum_k (Exp(-\frac{1}{2}C))_{ik} B_k A_k,$$

where *k* is all other atoms in the molecule and

$$A_k = \tfrac{1}{2}(IP_k + EA_k),\ B_k = (IP_k - EA_k)^{-\frac{1}{2}}$$

Here, IP is the ionization potential, EA is the electron affinity for each atom, and C is the connectivity matrix for the molecule. QNA descriptors describe each particular atom of a molecule; at the same time, each *P* or *Q* value depends on the total molecule composition and structure. Two-dimensional Chebyshev polynomials are used for approximating the functions P and Q over all atoms of the molecule. A detailed description of QNA descriptors is represented in the publication of Filimonov et al. (2009).

MNA descriptors (Filimonov et al., 1999) are based on the molecular structure representation, which includes hydrogens according to the valences and partial charges of other atoms and does not specify the types of bonds. MNA descriptors are generated as a recursively defined sequence:

- zero-level MNA descriptor for each atom is the mark *A* of the atom itself;
- any next-level MNA descriptor for the atom is the substructure notation $A\ (D_1 D_2 ... D_i ...)$,

where D_i is the previous-level MNA descriptor for *i*–th immediate neighbor of the atom *A*.

The mark of the atom may include not only the atomic type but also any additional information about the atom. In particular, if the atom is not included in the ring, it is marked by "–". The neighbor descriptors $D_1 D_2 ... D_i ...$ are arranged in a unique manner, for example, in lexicographic order. The iterative process of MNA descriptors generation can be continued covering first, second, and so on, neighborhoods of each atom.

For regression analysis, this molecule structure representation was transformed using the original PASS (Prediction of Activity Spectra for Substances) algorithm (Lagunin et al., 2011). This algorithm estimates the biological activity profiles for chemical compounds using MNA descriptors as input parameters. Therefore, we used the results of PASS prediction as independent variables for regression analysis. The results of PASS prediction are given as a list of biological activities, for which the difference between probabilities of being active (Pa) and inactive (Pi) was calculated. The activities from the list of predicted biological activities were randomly selected as input independent variables for regression analysis. This allows obtaining different QSAR models. GUSAR incorporates a PASS version that predicts 4130 types of biological activity. This version of PASS has a mean prediction accuracy of approximately 95% calculated by leave-one-out cross-validation procedure (Filimonov et al., 2014). The list of predictable biological activities currently includes 501 pharmacotherapeutic effects (e.g., antihypertensive, hepatoprotectant, and nootropic), 3295 mechanisms of action (e.g., 5-hydroxytryptamine antagonist, acetylcholine M1 receptor agonist, and cyclooxygenase inhibitor), 57 adverse and toxic effects (e.g., carcinogenic, mutagenic, and hematotoxic), 199 metabolic terms (e.g., CYP1A inducer, CYP1A1 inhibitor, and CYP3A4 substrate), 49 transporter proteins (e.g., P-glycoprotein 3 inhibitor, nucleoside transporters inhibitors, and proline transporter inhibitor), and 29 activities related to gene expression (e.g., TH expression enhancer, TNF expression inhibitor, and VEGF expression inhibitor). Therefore, the maximum number of independent variables for the creation of MNA models is 4130. The detailed description of realization of PASS in GUSAR is represented in the publication of Lagunin et al. (2011).

QNA and MNA descriptors do not provide information on the shape and volume of a molecule, although this information may be important for determination of structure-activity relationships. Therefore, these parameters, which are called whole-molecule descriptors, are also used in GUSAR. The whole-molecule descriptors used in GUSAR are: topological length, topological volume, lipophilicity, number of positive charges, number of negative charges, number of hydrogen bond acceptors, number of aromatic atoms, molecular weight, and number of halogen atoms. GUSAR uses estimation of the applicability domain based on different types of structural similarity using calculation of QNA and MNA descriptors (Zakharov et al., 2016).

GUSAR may provide an equation of any single (Q)SAR model (Lagunin et al., 2011). But because we used consensus (Q)SAR models from dozens or even hundreds of single (Q)SAR models, it is not possible to provide a general equation describing all selected variables. By this reason, the created consensus (Q)SAR models could not provide information about positive and negatively influencing descriptors. Instead that GUSAR shows positive and negative impact of each atom of the structure in the predicted value (Khayrullina et al., 2015). Analysis of the influence of atoms on the predicted value and the search for general relationships between the structures of active compounds interacting with antitargets is a separate task (because of each structure in the set should be analyzed), and it is beyond the scope of this publication.

[2]http://www.way2drug.com/gusar/index.html

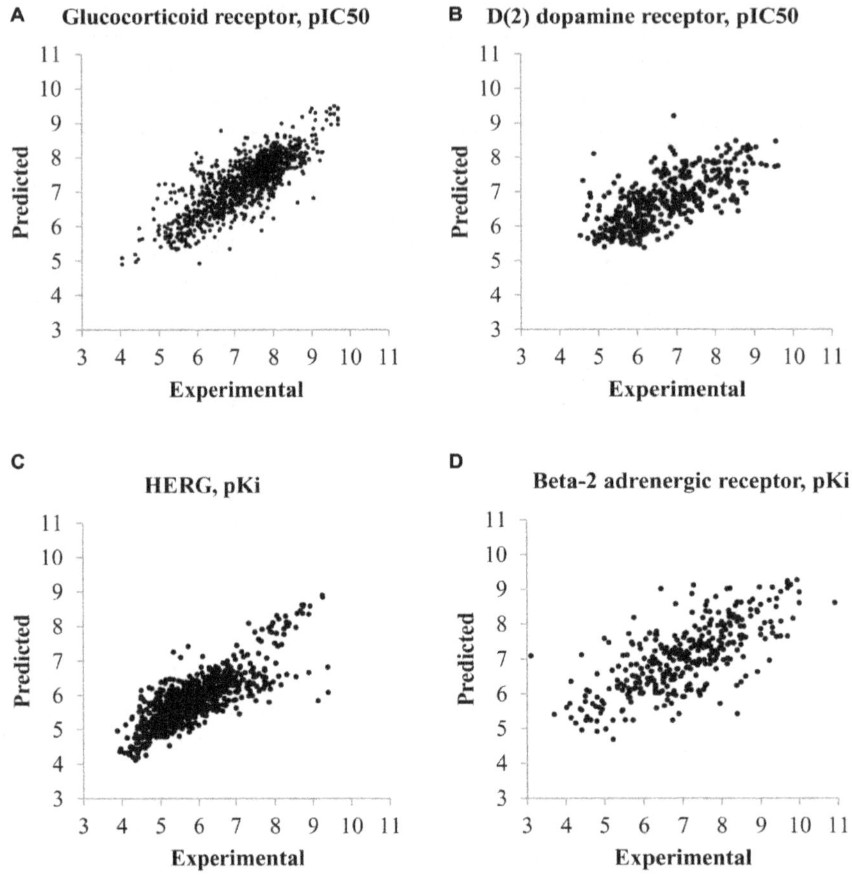

FIGURE 1 | Plots of predicted and experimental values for the best and worst QSAR models by RMSE values calculated during fivefold cross-validation procedure. **(A)** QSAR model for prediction of pIC_{50} values of compounds interacting with glucocorticoid receptor (the best QSAR model for IC_{50} values). **(B)** QSAR model for prediction of pIC_{50} values of compounds interacting with D(2) dopamine receptor (the worst QSAR model for IC_{50} values). **(C)** QSAR model for prediction of pK_i values of compounds interacting with HERG channel (Potassium voltage-gated channel subfamily H member 2) (the best QSAR model for K_i values). **(D)** QSAR model for prediction of pK_i values of compounds interacting with Beta-2 adrenergic receptor (the worst QSAR model for K_i values).

Evaluation of Prediction Accuracy

The following statistical parameters were calculated for estimating the accuracy of prediction:

(1) Sensitivity (Sens): $Sensitivity = \frac{TP}{FN+TP}$, where TP is true positive, and FN is false negative numbers.

(2) Specificity (Spec): $Specificity = \frac{TN}{TN+FP}$, where TN is true negative, and FP is false positive numbers.

(3) Accuracy:

$$Accuracy = \frac{TP + TN}{TP + TN + FP + FN}$$

(4) Balanced accuracy (BA): balance between sensitivity and specificity:

$$BA = \frac{Sensitivity + Specificity}{2}$$

(5) Root mean square error (RMSE):

$$RMSE = \sqrt{\frac{\sum(y_{exp} - y_{pred})^2}{n}}$$

(6) R-squared, coefficient of determination:

$$R^2 = 1 - \frac{\sum(y_{exp} - y_{pred})^2}{\sum(y_{exp} - y_{mean})^2},$$

where y_{exp} - experimental value, y_{pred} - predicted value, and y_{mean} - average value of experimental values in a training set.

Y-Randomization Procedure

Y-Randomization procedure is included in GUSAR software and allows to be ensuring that the developed continues QSAR models are robust and do not have the over fitting (Wold and Eriksson, 1995). In this procedure, the dependent-variable vector, Y vector (K_i or IC_{50} values in our case), is randomly shuffled and a new QSAR model is developed using the original independent variable matrix.

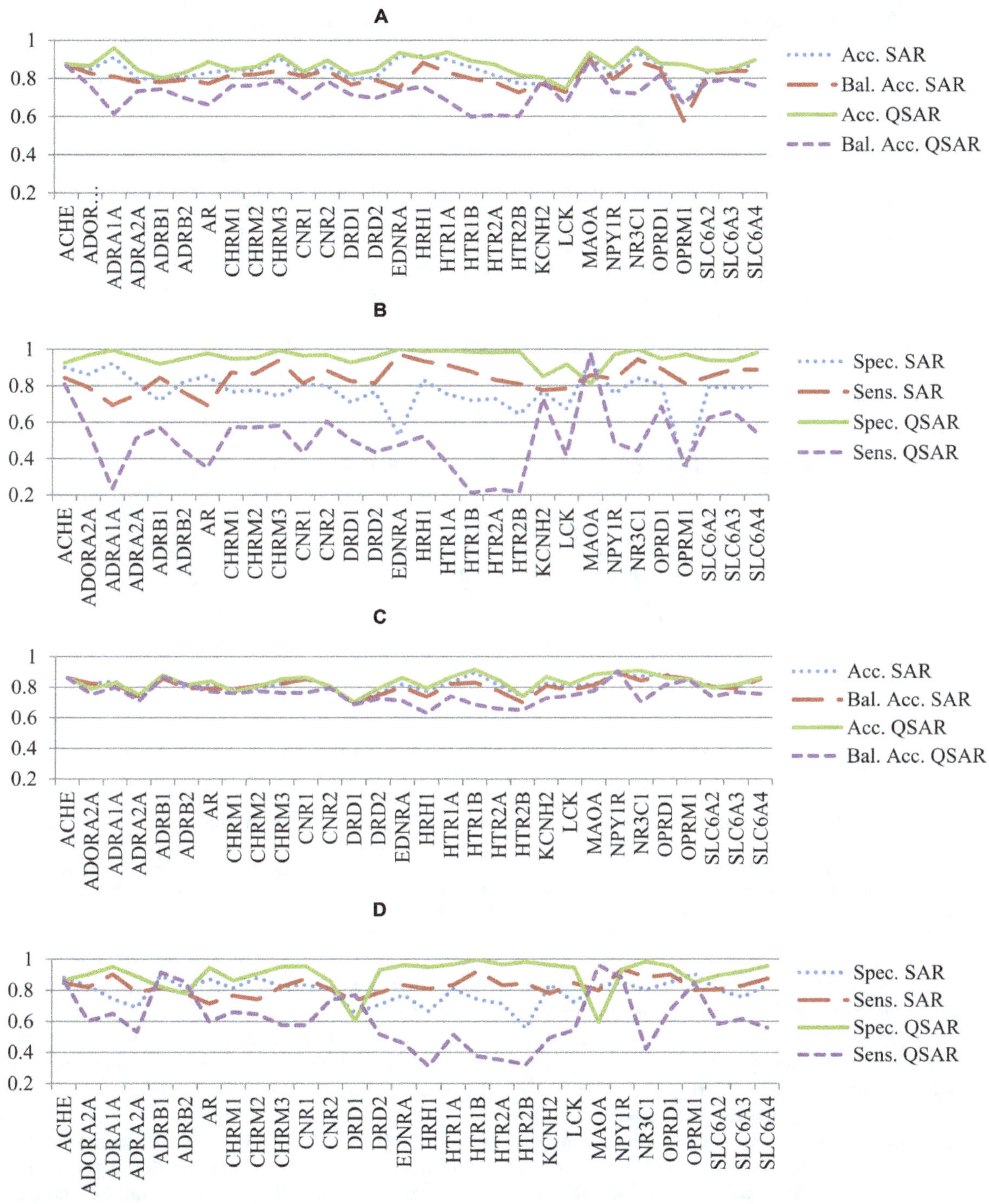

FIGURE 2 | Comparison of parameters of accuracy of prediction for SAR and QSAR models calculated by the fivefold cross-validation procedure for all antitargets. **(A)** Comparison of *Accuracy* (Acc.) and *Balanced Accuracy* (Bal. Acc.) between SAR and QSAR models for K_i data. **(B)** Comparison of *Sensitivity* (Sens.) and *Specificity* (Spec.) between SAR and QSAR models for K_i data. **(C)** Comparison of *Accuracy* (Acc.) and *Balanced Accuracy* (Bal. Acc.) between SAR and QSAR models for IC_{50} data. **(D)** Comparison of *Sensitivity* (Sens.) and *Specificity* (Spec.) between SAR and QSAR models for IC_{50} data.

It is expected that the resulting models should generally have low Q^2 values. This procedure was repeated five times for each model, and then the average Q^2 value was calculated.

RESULTS AND DISCUSSION

Three hundred twenty SAR and 320 QSAR models with modified calculation of descriptors and regression coefficients

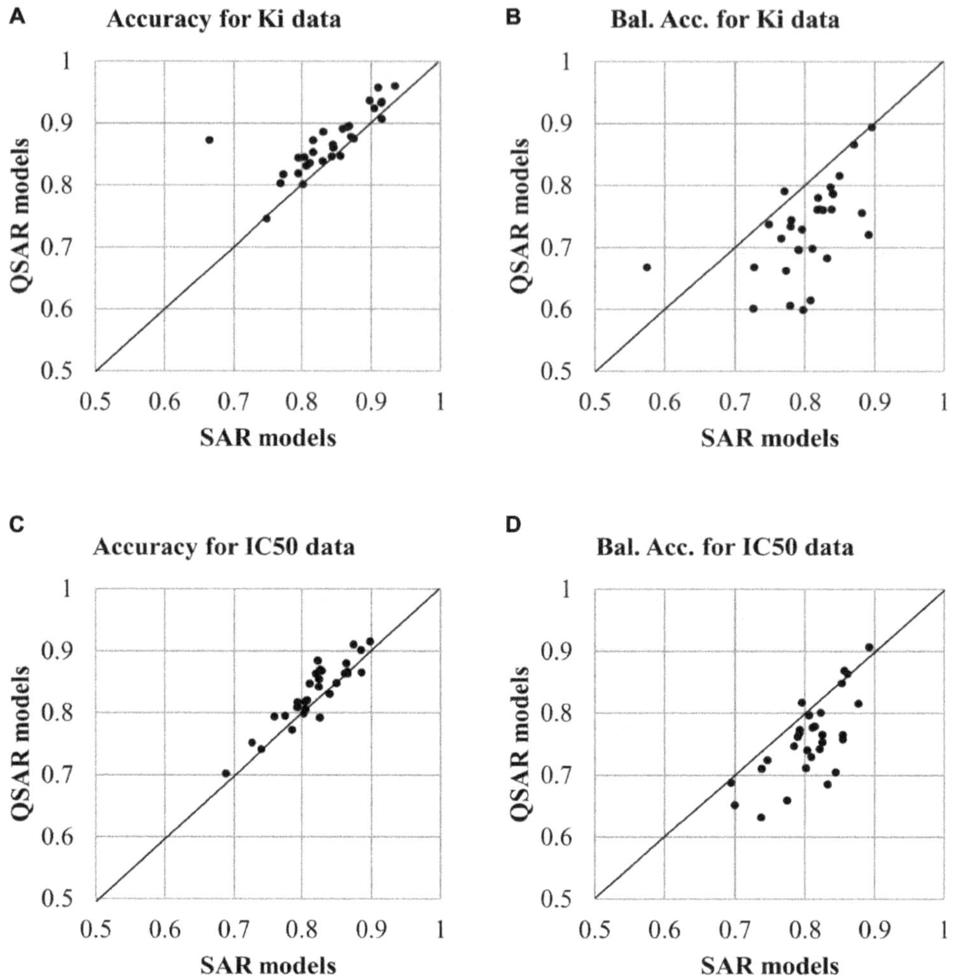

FIGURE 3 | Correlation of accuracy of prediction between SAR and QSAR models for all antitargets. **(A)** Correlation of *Accuracy* between SAR and QSAR models for K_i data. **(B)** Correlation of *Balanced Accuracy* (BA) between SAR and QSAR models for K_i data. **(C)** Correlation of *Accuracy* between SAR and QSAR models for IC_{50} data. **(D)** Correlation of *Balanced Accuracy* (BA) between SAR and QSAR models for IC_{50} data.

were created by GUSAR software for each from five training sets (five training sets with qualitative and quantitative data for K_i or IC_{50} values for each target) with internal validation (five times 20% from the training set was randomly used as an internal test set; this procedure is included into GUSAR). As a result, one consensus SAR model and one consensus QSAR model were created for each training set based on the appropriate single (Q)SAR model with R^2_{train} and Q^2_{train} and average R^2 calculated for internal validation sets more than 0.5. If R^2 of internal validation for (Q)SAR model was less than 0.5, then the model was excluded from the final consensus model [excluding QSAR models for D(1A) and D(2) dopamine receptors, histamine H1 and 5-hydroxytryptamine 2B receptors created on the basis of IC_{50} data]. The final predicted values for tested compounds were calculated using a weighted average of the predictions from the obtained (Q)SAR models. Each model is based on a different set of descriptors, and its predictions for each compound were weighted according to the similarity value that was calculated during the applicability domain assessment.

After SAR and QSAR consensus models were created based on a training set, they were used for prediction of inhibition of the antitarget by compounds from the appropriate external test set. It was repeated for five training sets with K_i values and five training sets with IC_{50} values for each antitarget (fivefold CV procedure). The average characteristics of the created (Q)SAR models including average results of Y-randomization procedure (Q^2_{Y-rand}) are represented in **Supplementary Tables S1, S2.** It was appeared that all Q^2_{Y-rand} values for all QSAR models were less 0.15. The average Q^2_{Y-rand} values were from 0.026 to 0.06 and from 0.026 to 0.078 for QSAR models created based on K_i and IC_{50} data, respectively. It is significant less in comparison with Q^2 values calculated based on original data of the training sets and displays robustness of the given models.

The plots between predicted and experimental values for the best and worst QSAR models by RMSE values

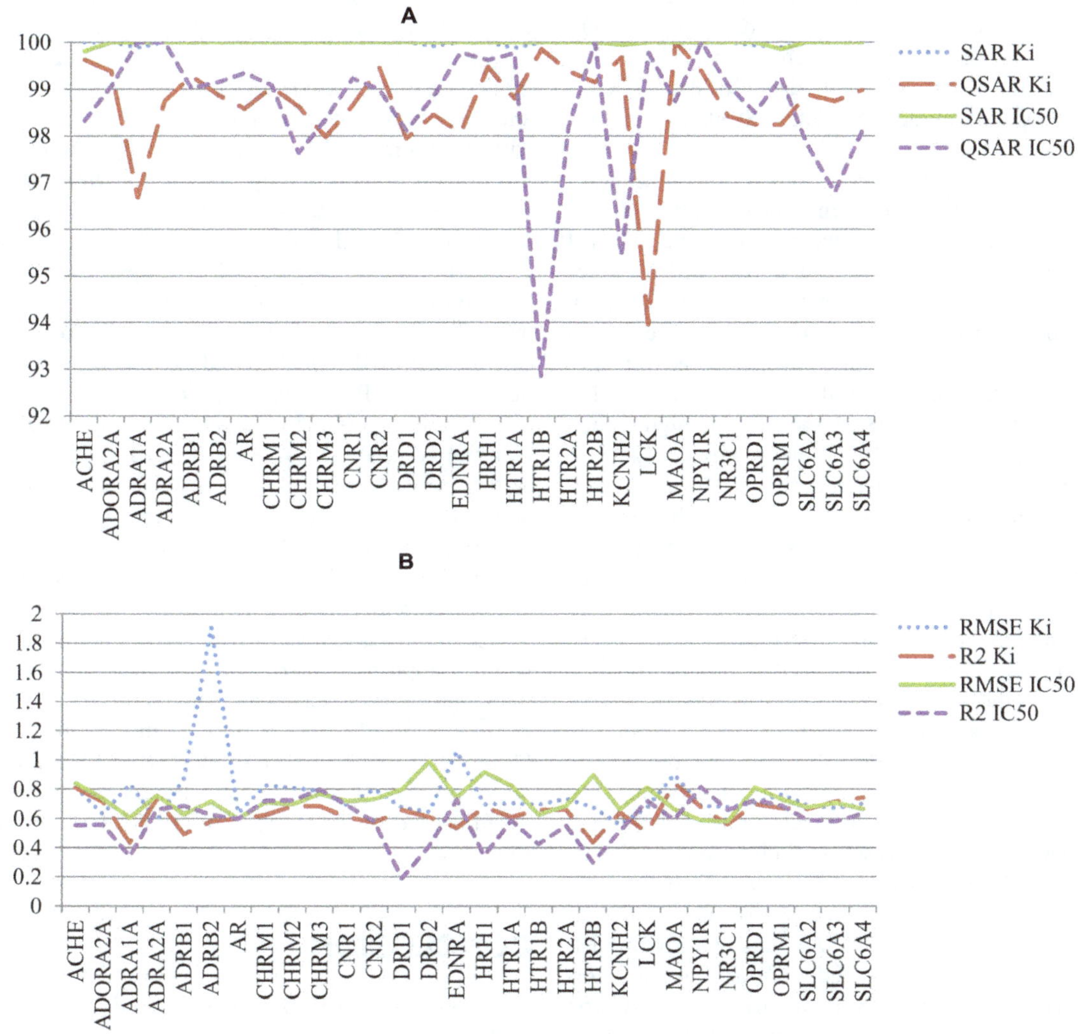

FIGURE 4 | Comparison of quality of (Q)SAR models for K_i and IC_{50} data for all antitargets. **(A)** Comparison of the percent of compounds in applicability domain (AD) for SAR and QSAR models; **(B)** Comparison of R^2 and RMSE values of QSAR models.

calculated by fivefold cross-validation are displayed in **Figure 1**. The relations between predicted and experimental values for others QSAR models are within these extreme cases.

The statistical parameters describing accuracy of prediction and mentioned in the section "Materials and Methods" were calculated based on the prediction results given during the fivefold CV procedure for both SAR and QSAR models. To compare the accuracy of prediction of QSAR and SAR models, the quantitative results of prediction were transformed into qualitative ones according to the threshold mentioned in the section "Materials and Methods." Statistical parameters of accuracy of prediction for SAR and QSAR models created based on K_i and IC_{50} data for all antitargets are represented in **Supplementary Tables S3, S4**, respectively. The graphical representation of statistical parameters of accuracy and their comparison are represented in **Figures 2–4**.

Figures 2A,B show a comparison of the accuracy between SAR and QSAR models created based on K_i values. **Figures 2C,D** show the results given based on IC_{50} values. The accuracy of the QSAR models was higher in most cases than the accuracy of SAR models for both K_i and IC_{50} values (**Figures 2A, 1C**). The mean accuracy of prediction for K_i values was 0.84 and 0.87 for SAR and QSAR models, respectively. This is statistically significant difference ($p < 0.05$). The mean accuracy of prediction for IC_{50} values was 0.82 and 0.83 for SAR and QSAR models, respectively. This is statistically insignificant difference ($p = 0.285$). The reverse result was observed for balanced accuracy (SAR models: K_i data – 0.80, IC_{50} data – 0.81; QSAR models: K_i data – 0.73, IC_{50} data – 0.76). The difference in balanced accuracy between SAR and QSAR models is statistically significant in both cases, for K_i and for IC_{50} values ($p < 0.05$). Specificity and sensitivity were similar for SAR and QSAR models (**Figures 2B, 1D**). The mean value of specificity was higher for QSAR models for both K_i and IC_{50} data (SAR models: K_i data – 0.76, IC_{50} data – 0.79; QSAR models: K_i data – 0.95, IC_{50} data – 0.90). The mean value of sensitivity was higher for SAR models for both K_i and IC_{50} data (SAR models: K_i data – 0.84, IC_{50} data – 0.82; QSAR models: K_i data – 0.50, IC_{50} data – 0.61).

The analysis of values of accuracy and balanced accuracy of SAR and QSAR models (**Supplementary Tables S1, S2**) shows that there is a correlation between them. **Figures 3A,B** show a correlation between accuracy and balanced accuracy for both SAR and QSAR models created based on K_i data. **Figures 3C,D** show a correlation between accuracy and balanced accuracy for SAR and QSAR models created based on IC_{50} data. One may see that in the both cases, the correlation between accuracy of SAR and QSAR models was higher than for balanced accuracy (**Figure 3**). If the values correlate, it means that there is no preference between SAR and QSAR models for the appropriate criterion of accuracy. But similar accuracy is achieved by different ways in the most cases (high sensitivity or high specificity, see **Figures 2B,D**). One can decide what is more important in the study: find as many as possible active compounds (the models with highest sensitivity should be selected) or reduce the number of false positive prediction (the models with highest specificity should be selected). The absence of correlation between the studied parameters shows that one of methods has preference. The values above the line show that QSAR models better than SAR ones. The values below the line show that SAR models better than QSAR ones. All cases excluding one which is displayed in **Figure 3C** (Correlation of *Accuracy* between SAR and QSAR models for IC_{50} data) had statistically significant difference between the values of SAR and QSAR models ($p < 0.05$). The values of balanced accuracy is the most important criterion for estimation of accuracy of prediction because of many used datasets were unbalanced (the number of active and inactive compounds is significant different). Therefore, the given results showed that SAR models are the more preferable for the use of prediction of drug adverse reactions.

The other parameters of SAR and QSAR models are represented in **Figure 4**. **Figure 4A** shows the percent of compounds in applicability domain (AD) of SAR and QSAR models. The number of compounds in AD was 100% approximately for all SAR models. At the same time, the number of compounds in AD approximately for all QSAR models was less 100%. The mean value of percent of compound in AD for SAR and QSAR models was 99.9% and 98.6%, respectively. The highest present of compounds in applicability domain displays advantage and better predictive power for SAR models in comparison with QSAR models. **Figure 4B** shows the comparison of RMSE and R^2 values for QSAR models created on K_i and IC_{50} data. Clear features of distribution of these characteristics cannot be seen, but in general, the mean value of R^2 for QSAR models based on K_i data was higher than one for IC_{50} data (0.64 and 0.57, respectively). The mean RMSE value for QSAR models based on IC_{50} data was less than one for K_i data (0.73 and 0.77, respectively). However, if we delete the RMSE value for the QSAR model created based on K_i data for the beta-2 adrenergic receptor, the mean RMSE value also became 0.73 for the other QSAR models created based on K_i data. It means that both K_i and IC_{50} values can be reliably used to predict interactions with antitargets. We may compare (Q)SAR models based on K_i and IC_{50} values only in general view because of they were created on different number of compounds and different structures. Nevertheless, we may reveal some features of the created models. The plots with comparison of Specificity and Sensitivity of (Q)SAR models created based on K_i and IC_{50} data are shown on **Supplementary Figure S1**. These plots display that SAR models based on IC_{50} values have Specificity better than SAR models based on K_i data for approximately half of antitargets. The biggest difference is shown for Mu-type opioid receptor (0.34 for K_i data and 0.97 for IC_{50} data). SAR models based on K_i data for others antitargets have better values of Specificity. The same picture we can see for Sensitivity of SAR models. Analysis of QSAR models revealed that majority of QSAR models based on K_i data had better Specificity value, whereas majority of QSAR models based on IC_{50} data had better Sensitivity value. High value of Sensitivity is more important for revealing possible adverse drug reaction than high value of Sensitivity. Analysis of Accuracy and Balanced Accuracy of (Q)SAR based on IC_{50} and K_i data (**Supplementary Figure S2**) show that the most (Q)SAR models based on K_i values have better values, whereas the values of Balanced Accuracy are higher at the most of QSAR models based on IC_{50} values.

CONCLUSION

The creation of SAR and QSAR models based on the same data of compounds tested as inhibitors of 30 antitargets revealed some features related to the use of qualitative and quantitative data. They are valid to (Q)SAR models related to both K_i and IC_{50} values. SAR models tended to have more balanced prediction results when specificity and sensitivity have the closest values in comparison with QSAR models (**Figure 2**). High values of specificity and low values of sensitivity in QSAR models may be explained by the fact that at the given R^2 values (0.64 and 0.59), prediction results tended to lie closer to the average values of K_i or IC_{50} in the training set. If a threshold of 1 μM divided the training set into different proportions of active and inactive compounds, then a difference between specificity and sensitivity may occur. At the same time, despite the difference of specificity and sensitivity between SAR and QSAR models, the values of accuracy and balanced accuracy for SAR correlated with those of QSAR models (**Figure 3**). This indicated that the prediction results of SAR and QSAR models would complement each other and that the use of both approaches would improve the quality of assessment of interaction between ligands and antitargets.

Another conclusion is that SAR models had advantages in the applicability domain. It may be related to the fact that the use of qualitative data gives SAR models less sensitivity to experimental errors in K_i and IC_{50} values.

In this study, we also displayed that the modern experimental data and methods of (Q)SAR modeling allow for the creation of rather reasonable (Q)SAR models for prediction of interaction between compounds and dozens of antitargets. The used approaches may be applied to the creation of *in silico* panels for estimation of "ligand-antitarget" interactions during the drug design process.

AUTHOR CONTRIBUTIONS

AL designed the study, performed the data analysis, and wrote the manuscript with inputs of all authors. MR, AZ, NK, and BS created and validated (Q)SAR models. PP and SI created datasets and data analysis. DF and VP designed the study, analyzed the results, and wrote the manuscript.

FUNDING

This work was supported by Russian Science Foundation Grant No. 14-15-00449.

REFERENCES

Berman, H. M., Westbrook, J., Feng, Z., Gilliland, G., Bhat, T. N., Weissig, H., et al. (2000). The protein data bank. *Nucleic Acids Res.* 28, 235–242. doi: 10.1093/nar/28.1.235

Böhm, R., and Cascorbi, I. (2016). Pharmacogenetics and predictive testing of drug hypersensitivity reactions. *Front. Pharmacol.* 7:396. doi: 10.3389/fphar.2016.00396

Bowes, J., Brown, A. J., Hamon, J., Jarolimek, W., Sridhar, A., Waldron, G., et al. (2012). Reducing safety-related drug attrition: the use of in vitro pharmacological profiling. *Nat. Rev. Drug Discov.* 11, 909–922. doi: 10.1038/nrd3845

Braga, R. C., Alves, V. M., Silva, M. F., Muratov, E., Fourches, D., Lião, L. M., et al. (2015). Pred-hERG: a novel web-accessible computational tool for predicting cardiac toxicity. *Mol. Inform.* 34, 698–701. doi: 10.1002/minf.201500040

Cortes-Ciriano, I., and Bender, A. (2015). Improved chemical structure-activity modeling through data augmentation. *J. Chem. Inf. Model.* 55, 2682–2692. doi: 10.1021/acs.jcim.5b00570

Filimonov, D., Poroikov, V., Borodina, Y., and Gloriozova, T. (1999). Chemical similarity assessment through multilevel neighborhoods of atoms: definition and comparison with the other descriptors. *J. Chem. Inf. Comput. Sci.* 39, 666–670. doi: 10.1021/ci980335o

Filimonov, D. A., Lagunin, A. A., Gloriozova, T. A., Rudik, A. V., Druzhilovskii, D. S., Pogodin, P. V., et al. (2014). Prediction of the biological activity spectra of organic compounds using the PASS Online web resource. *Chem. Heterocycl. Compd.* 50, 444–457. doi: 10.1007/s10593-014-1496-1

Filimonov, D. A., Zakharov, A. V., Lagunin, A. A., and Poroikov, V. V. (2009). QNA-based 'Star Track' QSAR approach. *SAR QSAR Environ. Res.* 20, 679–709. doi: 10.1080/10629360903438370

Filz, O., Lagunin, A., Filimonov, D., and Poroikov, V. (2008). Computer-aided prediction of QT-prolongation. *SAR QSAR Environ. Res.* 19, 81–90. doi: 10.1080/10629360701844183

Fourches, D., Muratov, E., and Tropsha, A. (2016). Trust, but verify ii: a practical guide to chemogenomics data curation. *J. Chem. Inf. Model.* 56, 1243–1252. doi: 10.1021/acs.jcim.6b00129

García-Sosa, A. T., and Maran, U. (2014). Improving the use of ranking in virtual screening against HIV-1 integrase with triangular numbers and including ligand profiling with antitargets. *J. Chem. Inf. Model.* 54, 3172–3185. doi: 10.1021/ci500300u

Gaulton, A., Hersey, A., Nowotka, M., Bento, A. P., Chambers, J., Mendez, D., et al. (2017). The ChEMBL database in 2017. *Nucleic Acids Res.* 45, 945–954. doi: 10.1093/nar/gkw1074

Hornberg, J. J., Laursen, M., Brenden, N., Persson, M., Thougaard, A. V., Toft, D. B., et al. (2014). Exploratory toxicology as an integrated part of drug discovery. Part I: why and how. *Drug Discov. Today* 19, 1131–1136. doi: 10.1016/j.drudis.2013.12.008

Ivanov, S. M., Lagunin, A. A., and Poroikov, V. V. (2016). In silico assessment of adverse drug reactions and associated mechanisms. *Drug Discov. Today* 21, 58–71. doi: 10.1016/j.drudis.2015.07.018

Ji, Z. L., Han, L. Y., Yap, C. W., Sun, L. Z., Chen, X., and Chen, Y. Z. (2003). Drug adverse reaction target database (DART): proteins related to adverse drug reactions. *Drug Saf.* 26, 685–690. doi: 10.2165/00002018-200326100-00002

Khayrullina, V. R., Gerchikov, A. Y., Lagunin, A. A., and Zarudii, F. S. (2015). Quantitative analysis of structure-activity relationships of tetrahydro-2H-isoindole cyclooxygenase-2 inhibitors. *Biochemistry* 80, 74–86. doi: 10.1134/S0006297915010095

Kochanek, K. D., Murphy, S. L., Xu, J., and Tejada-Vera, B. (2016). Deaths: final data for 2014. *Natl. Vital Stat. Rep.* 65, 100–122.

Lagunin, A., Zakharov, A., Filimonov, D., and Poroikov, V. (2011). QSAR modelling of rat acute toxicity on the basis of PASS prediction. *Mol. Inform.* 30, 241–250. doi: 10.1002/minf.201000151

Lagunin, A. A., Zakharov, A. V., Filimonov, D. A., and Poroikov, V. V. (2007). A new approach to QSAR modelling of acute toxicity. *SAR QSAR Environ. Res.* 18, 285–298. doi: 10.1080/10629360701304253

Politi, R., Rusyn, I., and Tropsha, A. (2014). Prediction of binding affinity and efficacy of thyroid hormone receptor ligands using QSAR and structure-based modeling methods. *Toxicol. Appl. Pharmacol.* 280, 177–189. doi: 10.1016/j.taap.2014.07.009

Poroikov, V., Filimonov, D., Lagunin, A., Gloriozova, T., and Zakharov, A. (2007). PASS: identification of probable targets and mechanisms of toxicity. *SAR QSAR Environ. Res.* 18, 101–110. doi: 10.1080/10629360601054032

Simões, R. S., Maltarollo, V. G., Oliveira, P. R., and Honorio, K. M. (2018). Transfer and multi-task learning in QSAR modeling: advances and challenges. *Front. Pharmacol.* 9:74. doi: 10.3389/fphar.2018.00074

Siramshetty, V. B., Nickel, J., Omieczynski, C., Gohlke, B. O., Drwal, M. N., and Preissner, R. (2016). WITHDRAWN–a resource for withdrawn and discontinued drugs. *Nucleic Acids Res.* 44, D1080–D1086. doi: 10.1093/nar/gkv1192

Starfield, B. (2000). Is US health really the best in the world? *JAMA* 284, 483–485. doi: 10.1001/jama.284.4.483

Wang, Y., Bryant, S. H., Cheng, T., Wang, J., Gindulyte, A., Shoemaker, B. A., et al. (2017). Pubchem bioassay: 2017 update. *Nucleic Acids Res.* 45, 955–963. doi: 10.1093/nar/gkw1118

Whitebread, S., Hamon, J., Bojanic, D., and Urban, L. (2005). Keynote review: in vitro safety pharmacology profiling: an essential tool for successful drug development. *Drug Discov. Today* 10, 1421–1433. doi: 10.1016/S1359-6446(05)03632-9

Wold, S., and Eriksson, L. (1995). "Statistical validation of QSAR results," in *Chemometrics Methods in Molecular Design*, ed. H. van de Waterbeemd (Weinheim: VCH), 309–318.

Zakharov, A. V., Lagunin, A. A., Filimonov, D. A., and Poroikov, V. V. (2012). Quantitative prediction of antitarget interaction profiles for chemical compounds. *Chem. Res. Toxicol.* 25, 2378–2385. doi: 10.1021/tx300247r

Zakharov, A. V., Varlamova, E. V., Lagunin, A. A., Dmitriev, A. V., Muratov, E. N., Fourches, D., et al. (2016). QSAR modeling and prediction of drug-drug interactions. *Mol. Pharm.* 13, 545–556. doi: 10.1021/acs.molpharmaceut.5b00762

Zhang, J. X., Huang, W. J., Zeng, J. H., Huang, W. H., Wang, Y., Zhao, R., et al. (2007). DITOP: drug-induced toxicity related protein database. *Bioinformatics* 23, 1710–1712. doi: 10.1093/bioinformatics/btm139

5

Transfer and Multi-task Learning in QSAR Modeling: Advances and Challenges

*Rodolfo S. Simões[1], Vinicius G. Maltarollo[2], Patricia R. Oliveira[1] and Kathia M. Honorio[1,3]**

[1] School of Arts, Sciences and Humanities, University of São Paulo, São Paulo, Brazil, [2] Department of Pharmaceutical Products, Faculty of Pharmacy, Federal University of Minas Gerais, Belo Horizonte, Brazil, [3] Center for Natural and Human Sciences, Federal University of ABC, Santo André, Brazil

***Correspondence:**
Kathia M. Honorio
kmhonorio@usp.br

Medicinal chemistry projects involve some steps aiming to develop a new drug, such as the analysis of biological targets related to a given disease, the discovery and the development of drug candidates for these targets, performing parallel biological tests to validate the drug effectiveness and side effects. Approaches as quantitative study of activity-structure relationships (QSAR) involve the construction of predictive models that relate a set of descriptors of a chemical compound series and its biological activities with respect to one or more targets in the human body. Datasets used to perform QSAR analyses are generally characterized by a small number of samples and this makes them more complex to build accurate predictive models. In this context, transfer and multi-task learning techniques are very suitable since they take information from other QSAR models to the same biological target, reducing efforts and costs for generating new chemical compounds. Therefore, this review will present the main features of transfer and multi-task learning studies, as well as some applications and its potentiality in drug design projects.

Keywords: drug design, medicinal chemistry, QSAR, machine learning, transfer learning, multi-task learning

INTRODUCTION

The drug design process, since the discovery/identification of bioactive compounds until the approval of its clinical use by a regulatory agency, is very complex and demands time and financial support (Tufts Center for the Study of Drug Development [CSDD], 2014). There are several well-known bottlenecks in this process, such as finding out a suitable and validated molecular target, designing and/or discovering of a lead compound, pharmacokinetic and toxicity optimization, besides commercial reasons, efficacy and clinical safety (Khanna, 2012; Medina-Franco et al., 2013). In this scenario, the use of computational techniques in drug discovery is rapidly increasing.

Computer-aided drug design (CADD) techniques are broadly employed in order to reduce costs and time involved in drug design. Among the important CADD techniques, molecular docking, similarity search and QSAR studies could be highlighted. Molecular docking and virtual screening are considered structure-based drug design (SBDD) strategies since it requires 3D structure of a molecular target and consists of predicting a binding mode of molecules and its binding energy (Walters et al., 1998; Shoichet, 2004; Andricopulo et al., 2008). As the docking simulations consider both structures (ligands and targets), its calculations are more computationally expensive. Considering these aspects, similarity searches and pharmacophore modeling are alternatives to faster calculations (Brogi et al., 2009; Tresadern et al., 2009) and are defined as ligand-based drug design (LBDD) strategies since they do not require the biological target structure

(Turki et al., 2017). **Figure 1** illustrates the main steps in a drug design process, including the use of computational tools.

Another LBDD strategy is known as quantitative structure-activity relationships (QSAR) and it has been widely employed in drug design, mainly aiming to predict the biological activity of a compound set against a specific target to optimize the binding affinity (Du et al., 2008; Gertrudes et al., 2012). QSAR models provide accurate predictions of measured endpoints instead of an independent ranking of biological activity. These quantitative approaches have also been used in other tasks, such as optimization of pharmacokinetics and toxicity profile (Maltarollo et al., 2015; Egeghy et al., 2016; Chemi et al., 2017) and virtual screening (Brogi et al., 2013; Melo-Filho et al., 2016; Neves et al., 2016; Zaccagnini et al., 2017).

Several important QSAR studies can be found in literature, which include the description of successful computational methods and algorithms (Sliwoski et al., 2014; Raies and Bajic, 2016), validation techniques (Gramatica and Sangion, 2016), applications (Cherkasov et al., 2014; Fang and Xiao, 2016) as well-challenges and how those have been addressed (Cronin and Schultz, 2003; Arthur, 2008; Dearden et al., 2009; Scior et al., 2009; Wang et al., 2015; Ponzoni et al., 2017).

In many recent studies, machine learning (ML) methods have been largely applied to QSAR analyses. This growth has been mainly motivated by the increasing availability of data in public repositories, the use of numerous and diverse chemical descriptors and the proposal of accurate predictive algorithms, such as support vector machines (SVMs) and artificial neural networks (Gertrudes et al., 2012; Maltarollo et al., 2013; Mitchell, 2014; Lima et al., 2016). A common application of ML techniques in CADD refers to forecast new compound class labels (e.g., "active" *versus* "inactive") using models previously derived from available training sets (Lavecchia, 2015). In such specific situation, ML techniques are said to perform a classification learning task. In addition, other sort of learning tasks can also be considered in CADD, such as clustering and ranking (Agarwal et al., 2010).

Despite of the widespread use of ML methods in QSAR modeling, the success of such approaches critically depends on the availability of a great amount of data, which remains challenging in drug discovery. This problem is strongly related to issues involving the quality of public data sources, including imprecise representation of chemical structures and inaccurate activity information (Zhao et al., 2017). Furthermore, the nature of different experimental protocols can usually lead to data belonging to different probability distributions, which makes the use of traditional ML techniques impracticable.

The data sets available in public repositories are usually obtained from single structure-activity relationship (SAR) campaigns. This explains the several particular and linear sets of compounds that are commonly used to generate only specialized QSAR models. In most of cases, biological activities of two datasets are measured under different experimental conditions, making the link among chemical spaces difficult to be analyzed (Richter and Ecker, 2015). Furthermore, a large chemical space has activity cliffs naturally: regions in a structure/activity surface where there is a discontinuous SAR (Cruz-Monteagudo et al., 2014).

In 2014, a review on QSAR (Cherkasov et al., 2014) stated that the transferability of QSAR models is one of the challenges in QSAR modeling, since the traditional approaches have been typically designed for each target property individually. Aiming to take advantage of diverse but related available experimental data, transfer and multi-task learning techniques have been recently developed. The novelty behind these approaches is related to their ability to exploit knowledge from other related tasks to improve the learning performance, especially when a small data set is available for training.

TRANSFER AND MULTI-TASK LEARNING

For QSAR purposes, the data space under analysis is characterized by biological and chemical properties. In such scenario, changes in the distribution of data force the model to be rebuilt, implying to collect new training data. However, in many real-world applications, it is expensive or impossible to recollect data required to reconstruct these models. In such situations, transfer learning (or knowledge transfer) among related domains would be desirable (Pan and Yang, 2010).

Transfer learning can be defined as the ability of a system to recognize and apply the knowledge learned in previous (source) tasks for the solution of new (target) problems. The development of such approach was motivated by the fact that one can apply the knowledge acquired previously to solve new problems more quickly and with better solutions. The goal here relies on extracting the knowledge obtained by a model from one or more source tasks and to apply it to a target task. However, one of the premises for using transfer learning technique is that the source and the destination domains must be related. In this sense, Tan et al. (2015) suggest that such relationship can be expressed by instances (Bickel et al., 2009) or characteristics (Satpal and Sarawagi, 2007). If no direct relationship is found, the forced transfer will not work, resulting in no improvement or even degenerating the performance in the target domain (Fitzgerald and Thomaz, 2015). Multi-task learning is closely related to knowledge transfer, but they have also a clear distinction. In multi-task approaches, a number of tasks are learned simultaneously, without involving designated source and target tasks. **Figure 2** illustrates the overall schemes for transfer and multi-task learning.

The methods used for transfer learning can be summarized into four categories, depending on which aspect of knowledge will be transferred, i.e., "what to transfer" (Pan and Yang, 2010). The first category refers to instance-based transfer learning, which assumes that some data from the source set can be selected for training in the target set by re-weighting. Importance sampling and instance reweighting are the two most commonly techniques used (Dai et al., 2007). The second category refers to transfer learning methods by feature representation, which focuses on encoding the structural information carried by molecules into a numerical representation that can be effectively exploited by learning processes in other related problems. In this case, the intuitive idea consists in learning a suitable representation of characteristics for use in the target set, i.e., the transfer learning is coded in the representation of the new characteristics (Raina et al., 2007). The third category refers to the transfer learning techniques by parameters (Lawrence and Platt, 2004), in which it is assumed that the source and the target tasks share some parameters or prior distributions of the hyper-parameters of the respective QSAR models. In this case, knowledge can be transferred between the tasks by discovering these shared parameters or priors. The last category consists of methods that deal with the problem of relational knowledge transfer, which refers to transfer learning in related domains (Mihalkova et al., 2007). In this condition, the knowledge can be transferred by mapping the data from the source set to the destination one. The statistical methods of relational learning are the most applied in this case (Mihalkova et al., 2007; Davis and Domingos, 2009). A scheme illustrating how the transfer learning approaches can be applied to obtain predictive models is presented in **Figure 3**.

To apply transfer learning techniques, it is assumed that two sets of related data are available and the knowledge will be transferred from the dataset with the largest volume to the set with the least amount of available data. However, this assumption in the chemical datasets is not always sufficient, requiring the opinion of an expert to define the source datasets. To overcome this limitation, Girschick et al. (2012) proposed an approach to select a source dataset in a repository containing target-related sets by following a data-driven methodology. The main idea behind such proposal is based on calculating a measure for the activity overlap between the target set and each related set available in PubChem database. As result, a ranking of all related sets according to their similarity to the target set is obtained. In order to find the similarity values, Tanimoto coefficient is calculated using the categorization of the chemical compounds (active/inactive) in each dataset. Therefore, the objective is to select the set that has the distribution of instances (compounds) closest to the distribution (number of instances categorized as active and inactive) of the target set.

One can find out many situations where transfer learning adds benefits, for example, molecules could be classified as active or inactive according to a biological data for a defined endpoint (e.g., IC_{50} values). For this classification task, it is initially necessary to collect several experimentally tested samples and, next, to train a classifier for the collected data with their respective labels. Since the probability distribution of the comments on other endpoints can be very different, a new classifier has to be trained to each dataset in order to maintain a satisfactory performance. To reduce this effort, it would be desirable to use the knowledge from a classification model that is already trained on some related endpoints to improve the classification performance of other tasks with small samples or datasets (Turki et al., 2017). **Table 1** illustrates examples of transfer learning in drug design.

In general, transfer learning approaches have shown to be promising for combining the knowledge previously obtained in related tasks into a single predictive model, whether for classification, regression, or grouping (Pan and Yang, 2010). In particular, researches in medicinal chemistry with focus in drug discovery have been benefited with the use of transfer learning, as can be seen in previous studies (Girschick et al., 2012; Rosenbaum et al., 2013; Saha et al., 2016). Next, applications of transfer and multi-task learning in medicinal chemistry studies will be presented.

SOME APPLICATIONS OF TRANSFER AND MULTI-TASK LEARNING

Many machine learning methods are based on the assumption that similar drugs may share the same side effects, but measuring the similarity of these drugs is still a challenge. However, the use of data from various sources (similar drugs) provides important information for the analysis of side effects and should be integrated for obtaining a highly accurate prediction. Zhang et al. (2016) discussed the problem of predicting side effects

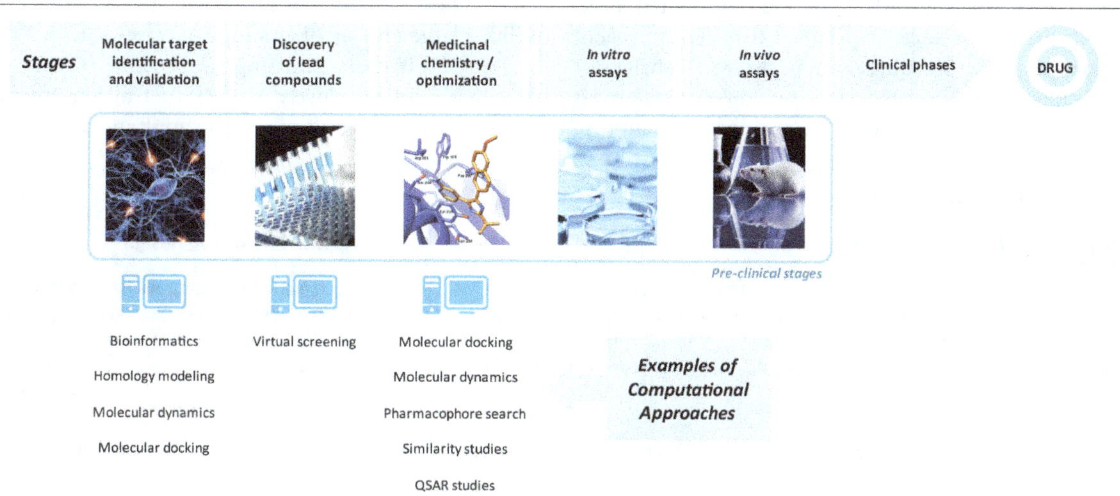

FIGURE 1 | Main steps involved in drug design, highlighting the use of computational approaches.

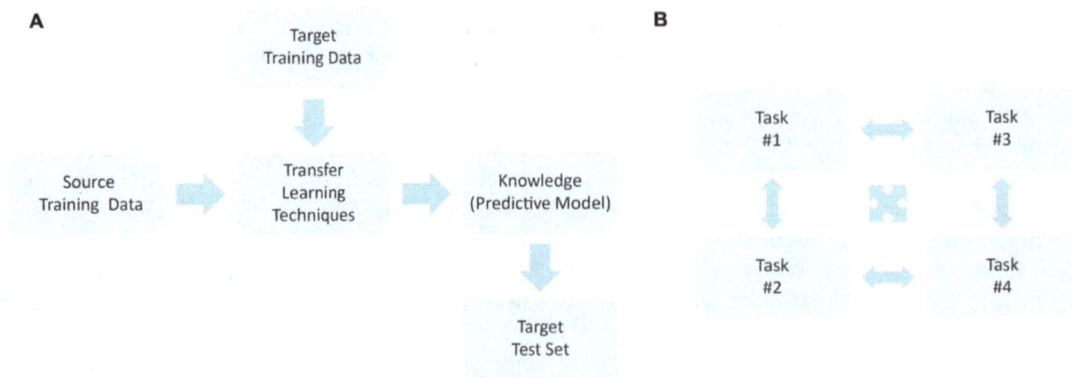

FIGURE 2 | General framework used to plan a study using **(A)** transfer learning techniques and **(B)** multi-task learning.

caused by drugs through linear neighbor approaches and the integration of data from various sources. The authors argued that auxiliary data can bring additional and diverse information (such as drug substructures, drug targets, drug transporters, drug enzymes, drug pathways) that should be integrated to the side-effect prediction, aiming at improving its performance. Analyses on multi-label classification showed that the proposed transfer learning approaches achieved better performance than state-of-art-methods (Pauwels et al., 2011; Liu et al., 2012; Cheng et al., 2013) applied to benchmark datasets.

The task of relating chemical structure to biological activity in QSAR studies is usually based on the notion of chemical similarity to predict the molecular behavior of close compounds. So, techniques that provide similarity measures among chemical compounds are increasingly important (Floris et al., 2014). Lately, relevant solutions have been proposed, which comprise distance learning (Biehl et al., 2014) and inductive transfer (Garcke and Vanck, 2014) methods. Distance learning aims at learning an appropriate distance measure to reflect the underlying relationship between instances in the training set, while inductive transfer refers to the process of transferring knowledge learned from one task into another related task. Girschick et al. (2012) presented an adapted transfer approach, which combines distance learning and inductive transfer by learning the distances on a related task and then transferring them to the target learning task. Additionally, the authors developed a method for selecting a related task that can be used as source task for transfer learning. This technique consists in applying an activity overlap similarity measure to two datasets to find out a suitable source task. This approach was evaluated on five distinct datasets found in PubChem BioAssay (Wang et al., 2009) repository. The results showed that both proposals worked well for large and small amounts of training data.

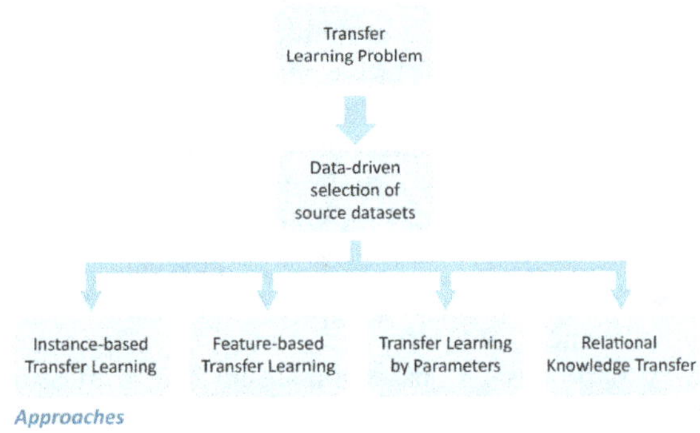

FIGURE 3 | Schemes used for applying transfer learning approaches.

The multi-task learning approach (Caruana, 1998) is considered to be closely related to transfer learning, since it attempts to learn multiple tasks simultaneously even when they

TABLE 1 | Examples of potential applications of transfer learning methods in drug design.

Transfer learning approach	Concept	Application in drug design
Instance-based	Uses the same ML technique for modeling but apply some changes to the parameters of the target model.	Source and target datasets have the same endpoint (e.g., same molecular target) but the training data can be colleted at different experimental conditions.
Feature representation	Based on some mathematical transformations of data.	Source and target datasets have different but related endpoints, e.g., same classes of molecular target (kinases, nuclear receptors, proteases, etc.).
Parameters	It is assumed that both datasets share some properties.	Source and target datasets have the same or related endpoints.
Relational knowledge transfer	Based on technique for mapping the data in the target domain.	The endpoints of the source and target datasets are different but the domains (the independent variable in QSAR models) are related; e.g., cellular permeability and log P.

are different. Rosenbaum et al. (2013) introduced two multi-task methods and evaluated the performance of such approaches by inferring multi-target QSAR models on a subset of human kinome. The authors assumed that the taxonomical relationship of the kinase targets should correspond to the relatedness of the QSAR problems on these targets. The multi-task techniques were compared to SVMs models independently trained for each target and an SVM model that assumed all targets to be identical. The results demonstrated that the multi-target learning can over perform baseline (pure SVM) methods if knowledge can be transferred from a target with a lot of data to a similar target with little domain knowledge.

Varnek et al. (2009) applied different inductive transfer and multi-task learning approaches to model tissue-air partition coefficients. The authors found that these techniques improved the prediction accuracy of the obtained models when compared to single task learning. Finally, this study indicated that inductive transfer learning is very suitable when single modeling is unable to generate reliable QSAR models using diverse data sets and with small amount of samples.

Brown et al. (2014) presented some challenges involved with chemogenomic data, since high-throughput assays give us a large number of information from multi-ligand and multi-target data (Pereira and Williams, 2007). So, the authors assert that computational techniques, in particular inductive transfer and explicit learning, can help to construct more robust models when compared to target-specific (classical) QSAR ones.

The study of Zhang et al. (2013) discussed the use of single- and multi-task learning to construct QSAR models for predicting the binding affinity of a compound database by estrogen receptors (ERs), which are involved with endocrine disruption by chemicals and the construction of predictive models can contribute to design safer substances. The authors concluded that multi-task learning provided better results for a small dataset (ERβ ligands) than single learning, indicating that this approach can be considered as a good tool to understand the action mechanism of endocrine disruption and to predict the ER activity of unknown compounds as endocrine disrupting chemicals.

Another interesting application of multi-task techniques was performed by Liu et al. (2011), which used multi-task learning to construct multi-target QSAR models employing three human immunodeficiency virus (HIV) inhibitor datasets together with other six subsets containing two hepatitis C virus (HCV) inhibitors. The main conclusions of this study included the fact that the integration of all databases (HIV and HCV) improved the rate of the discovery of lead HIV-HCV inhibitors, helping the design of new co-inhibitors for these important infections. Other achievement is related to the successful use (considering efficiency in convergence speed and learning accuracy) of a multi-task learning technique to construct multi-target QSAR models.

DISCUSSION

The main issue of transfer and multi-task learning approaches is to employ the knowledge generated (e.g., features, subset of variables, weights of equations) from available ML models and other datasets in the construction of models for related endpoints. In this sense, it is possible to use different datasets with the same biological activities but measured at different experimental conditions. Other important consequence of applying transfer and multi-task learning is the decrease on computational costs related to the faster convergence obtained by using the knowledge derived from a model previously built from a related endpoint.

From a literature review taking into to account the transfer learning applications on medicinal chemistry, one can note that there is still a great potentiality to be explored in this sense. Other emerging approaches as deep learning methods (Zhang et al., 2017), which basically use complex neural networks architectures, also have promising applications in the era of big data.

Among the main challenges on applying transfer and multi-task learning methods is that they require an artificial intelligence expert to code them since there are no chemical and/or pharmaceutical packages with a graphical user interface. Depend on the source data and on the learning method, transfer and multi-task learning could be also considered as "black-boxes," making the interpretability of QSAR models difficult. And, finally, the transfer of knowledge could be inappropriately employed if the assumption of "equivalent" endpoints is not valid.

CONCLUSION

Nowadays one can observe increasing number of applications of transfer and multi-task learning in medicinal studies. There are also current challenges in the QSAR field that comprise the integration of different datasets (even from different experiments) aiming the same or similar endpoints (Maltarollo et al., 2017) and the development of universal QSAR models using very large datasets (Alves et al., 2017). Therefore, good examples of dataset that could be benefited from transfer and multi-task learning are: (i) compounds with same endpoint measured under different experimental conditions; (ii) antimicrobial activities against genetically similar microorganisms; (iii) compounds with the same mechanism of action in homologous targets and high degree of similarity in the binding pocket; (iv) non-specific endpoints as toxicity against a cell line or permeability rates determined by different models. In this complex scenario, transfer and multi-task learning techniques can be considered powerful tools for drug design.

AUTHOR CONTRIBUTIONS

RS, KH, VM, and PO designed this article. All authors wrote and revised the manuscript. Also, all authors read and approved the final version of the manuscript.

ACKNOWLEDGMENTS

The authors would like to thank FAPESP, CNPq, CAPES, and IBM for funding.

REFERENCES

Agarwal, S., Dugar, D., and Sengupta, S. (2010). Ranking chemical structures for drug discovery: a new machine learning approach. *J. Chem. Inf. Model.* 50, 716–731. doi: 10.1021/ci9003865

Alves, V. M., Muratov, E. N., Zakharov, A., Muratov, N. N., Andrade, C. H., and Tropsha, A. (2017). Chemical toxicity prediction for major classes of industrial chemicals: Is it possible to develop universal models covering cosmetics, drugs, and pesticides? *Food Chem. Toxicol.* doi: 10.1016/j.fct.2017.04.008 [Epub ahead of print].

Andricopulo, A. D., Guido, R. V. C., and Oliva, G. (2008). Virtual screening and its integration with modern drug design technologies. *Curr. Med. Chem.* 15, 37–46. doi: 10.2174/092986708783330683

Arthur, M. D. (2008). QSAR: dead or alive? *J. Comput. Aided Mol. Des.* 22, 81–89. doi: 10.1007/s10822-007-9162-7

Bickel, S., Sawade, C., and Scheffer, T. (2009). Transfer learning by distribution matching for targeted advertising. *Adv. Neural Inf. Proces. Syst.* 21, 145–152.

Biehl, M., Hammer, B., and Villmann, T. (2014). "Distance measures for prototype based classification," in *Brain-Inspired Computing. BrainComp 2013. Lecture Notes in Computer Science*, eds L. Grandinetti, T. Lippert, and N. Petkov (Cham: Springer), doi: 10.1007/978-3-319-12084-3_9

Brogi, S., Kladi, M., Vagias, C., Papazafiri, P., Roussis, V., and Tafi, A. (2009). Pharmacophore modeling for qualitative prediction of antiestrogenic activity. *J. Chem. Inf. Model.* 49, 2489–2497. doi: 10.1021/ci900254b

Brogi, S., Papazafiri, P., Roussis, V., and Tafi, A. (2013). 3D-QSAR using pharmacophore-based alignment and virtual screening for discovery of novel MCF-7 cell line inhibitors. *Eur. J. Med. Chem.* 67, 344–351. doi: 10.1016/j.ejmech.2013.06.048

Brown, J. B., Okuno, Y., Marcou, G., Varnek, A., and Horvath, D. (2014). Computational chemogenomics: Is it more than inductive transfer? *J. Comput. Aided Mol. Des.* 28, 597–618. doi: 10.1007/s10822-014-9743-1

Caruana, R. (1998). "Multitask learning," in *Learning to Learn*, eds S. Thrun and L. Pratt (Boston, MA: Springer), 95–133. doi: 10.1007/978-1-4615-5529-2_5

Chemi, G., Gemma, S., Campiani, G., Brogi, S., Butini, S., and Brindisi, M. (2017). Computational tool for fast *in silico* evaluation of *hERG* K^+ channel affinity. *Front. Chem.* 5:7. doi: 10.3389/fchem.2017.00007

Cheng, F., Li, W., Wang, X., Zhou, Y., Wu, Z., Shen, J., et al. (2013). Adverse drug events: database construction and in silico prediction. *J. Chem. Inf. Model.* 53, 744–752. doi: 10.1021/ci4000079

Cherkasov, A., Muratov, E. N., Fourches, D., Varnek, A., Baskin, I. I., Cronin, M., et al. (2014). QSAR modeling: where have you been? Where are you going to? *J. Med. Chem.* 57, 4977–5010. doi: 10.1021/jm4004285

Cronin, M. T. D., and Schultz, T. W. (2003). Pitfalls in QSAR. *J. Mol. Struct. Theochem* 622, 39–51. doi: 10.1016/S0166-1280(02)00616-4

Cruz-Monteagudo, M., Medina-Franco, J. L., Perez-Castillo, Y., Nicolotti, O., Cordeiro, M. N. D., and Borges, F. (2014). Activity cliffs in drug discovery: Dr Jekyll or Mr Hyde? *Drug Discov. Today* 19, 1069–1080. doi: 10.1016/j.drudis.2014.02.003

Dai, W., Yang, Q., and Yu, Y. (2007). "Boosting for transfer learning," in *Proceedings of the 24th international conference on Machine learning*, (New York, NY: ACM), 193–200. doi: 10.1145/1273496.1273521

Davis, J., and Domingos, P. (2009). "Deep transfer via second-order markov logic," in *Proceedings of the 26th Annual International Conference on Machine Learning*, (New York, NY: ACM), 217–224. doi: 10.1145/1553374.1553402

Dearden, J. C., Cronin, M. T. D., and Kaiser, K. L. E. (2009). How not to develop a quantitative structure-activity or structure-property relationship (QSAR/QSPR). *SAR QSAR Environ. Res.* 20, 241–266. doi: 10.1080/10629360902949567

Du, Q.-S., Huang, R.-B., and Chou, K.-C. (2008). Recent advances in QSAR and their applications in predicting the activities of chemical molecules, peptides and proteins for drug design. *Curr. Protein Pept. Sci.* 9, 248–259. doi: 10.2174/138920308784534005

Egeghy, P. P., Sheldon, L. S., Isaacs, K. K., Özkaynak, H., Goldsmith, M. R., Wambaugh, J. F., et al. (2016). Computational exposure science: an emerging discipline to support 21st-century risk assessment. *Environ. Health Perspect.* 124, 697–702. doi: 10.1289/ehp.1509748

Fang, C., and Xiao, Z. (2016). Receptor-based 3D-QSAR in drug design: methods and applications in kinase studies. *Curr. Top. Med. Chem.* 16, 1463–1477. doi: 10.2174/1568026615666150915120943

Fitzgerald, T., and Thomaz, A. L. (2015). "Skill demonstration transfer for learning from demonstration," in *Proceedings of the Tenth Annual ACM/IEEE International Conference on Human-Robot Interaction Extended Abstracts*, (New York, NY: ACM), 187–188. doi: 10.1145/2701973.2702728

Floris, M., Manganaro, A., Nicolotti, O., Medda, R., Mangiatordi, G. F., and Benfenati, E. (2014). A generalizable definition of chemical similarity for read-across. *J. Cheminform.* 6:39. doi: 10.1186/s13321-014-0039-1

Garcke, J., and Vanck, T. (2014). Importance weighted inductive transfer learning for regression. *Lect. Notes Comput. Sci.* 8274, 466–481. doi: 10.1007/978-3-662-44848-9_30

Gertrudes, J. C., Maltarollo, V. G., Silva, R. A., Oliveira, P. R., Honorio, K. M., and Da Silva, A. B. F. (2012). Machine learning techniques and drug design. *Curr. Med. Chem.* 19, 4289–4297. doi: 10.2174/092986712802884259

Girschick, T., Ruckert, U., and Kramer, S. (2012). Adapted transfer of distance measures for quantitative structure-activity relationships and data-driven selection of source datasets. *Comput. J.* 56, 274–288. doi: 10.1093/comjnl/bxs092

Gramatica, P., and Sangion, A. (2016). A historical excursus on the statistical validation parameters for QSAR models: a clarification concerning metrics and terminology. *J. Chem. Inf. Model.* 56, 1127–1131. doi: 10.1021/acs.jcim.6b00088

Khanna, I. (2012). Drug discovery in pharmaceutical industry: productivity challenges and trends. *Drug Discov. Today* 17, 1088–1102. doi: 10.1016/j.drudis.2012.05.007

Lavecchia, A. (2015). Machine-learning approaches in drug discovery: methods and applications. *Drug Discov. Today* 20, 318–331. doi: 10.1016/j.drudis.2014.10.012

Lawrence, N. D., and Platt, J. C. (2004). "Learning to learn with the informative vector machine," in *Proceedings of the Twenty-rst International Conference on Machine Learning*, (New York, NY: ACM), 65. doi: 10.1145/1015330.1015382

Lima, A. N., Philot, E. A., Trossini, G. H. G., Scott, L. P. B., Maltarollo, V. G., and Honorio, K. M. (2016). Use of machine learning approaches for novel drug discovery. *Exp. Opin. Drug Discov.* 11, 225–239. doi: 10.1517/17460441.2016.1146250

Liu, M., Wu, Y., Chen, Y., Sun, J., Zhao, Z., Chen, X. W., et al. (2012). Large-scale prediction of adverse drug reactions using chemical, biological, and phenotypic properties of drugs. *J. Am. Med. Inform. Assoc.* 19, e28–e35. doi: 10.1136/amiajnl-2011-000699

Liu, Q., Zhou, H., Liu, L., Chen, X., Zhu, R., and Cao, Z. (2011). Multi-target QSAR modelling in the analysis and design of HIV-HCV co-inhibitors: an in-silico study. *BMC Bioinformatics* 12:294. doi: 10.1186/1471-2105-12-294

Maltarollo, V. G., Gertrudes, J. C., Oliveira, P. R., and Honorio, K. M. (2015). Applying machine learning techniques for ADME-Tox prediction: a review. *Expert Opin. Drug Metab. Toxicol.* 11, 259–271. doi: 10.1517/17425255.2015.980814

Maltarollo, V. G., Honorio, K. M., and da Silva, A. B. F. (2013). "Applications of artificial neural networks in chemical problems," in *Artificial Neural Networks-Architectures and Applications*, ed. K. Suzuki (Rijeka: InTech), 203–223. doi: 10.5772/51275

Maltarollo, V. G., Kronenberger, T., Wrenger, C., and Honorio, K. M. (2017). Current trends in quantitative structure–activity relationship validation and applications on drug discovery. *Future Sci. OA* 3, FSO214–FSO216. doi: 10.4155/fsoa-2017-0052

Medina-Franco, J. L., Giulianotti, M. A., Welmaker, G. S., and Houghten, R. A. (2013). Shifting from the single to the multitarget paradigm in drug discovery. *Drug Discov. Today* 18, 495–501. doi: 10.1016/j.drudis.2013.01.008

Melo-Filho, C. C., Dantas, R. F., Braga, R. C., Neves, B. J., Senger, M. R., Valente, W. C., et al. (2016). QSAR-driven discovery of novel chemical scaffolds active against *Schistosoma mansoni*. *J. Chem. Inf. Model.* 56, 1357–1372. doi: 10.1021/acs.jcim.6b00055

Mihalkova, L., Huynh, T., and Mooney, R. J. (2007). "Mapping and revising markov logic networks for transfer learning," in *Proceedings of the.* 22nd Association for the advancement of Artificial Intelligence (AAAI) Conference. Artificial Intelligence, (Vancouver, BC: AAAI), 608–614.

Mitchell, J. B. O. (2014). Machine learning methods in chemoinformatics. *WIREs Comput. Mol. Sci.* 4, 468–481. doi: 10.1002/wcms.1183

Neves, B. J., Dantas, R. F., Senger, M. R., Melo-Filho, C. C., Valente, W. C., De Almeida, A. C., et al. (2016). Discovery of new anti-schistosomal hits by integration of QSAR-Based virtual screening and high content screening. *J. Med. Chem.* 59, 7075–7088. doi: 10.1021/acs.jmedchem.5b02038

Pan, S. J., and Yang, Q. (2010). A survey on transfer learning. *IEEE Trans. Knowl. Data Eng.* 22, 1345–1359. doi: 10.1109/TKDE.2009.191

Pauwels, E., Stoven, V., and Yamanishi, Y. (2011). Predicting drug side-effect profiles: a chemical fragment-based approach. *BMC Bioinformatics* 12:169. doi: 10.1186/1471-2105-12-169

Pereira, D. A., and Williams, J. A. (2007). Origin and evolution of high throughput screening. *Br. J. Pharmacol.* 152, 53–61. doi: 10.1038/sj.bjp.0707373

Ponzoni, I., Sebastián-Pérez, V., Requena-Triguero, C., Roca, C., Martínez, M. J., Cravero, F., et al. (2017). Hybridizing feature selection and feature learning approaches in QSAR modeling for drug discovery. *Sci. Rep.* 7:2403. doi: 10.1038/s41598-017-02114-3

Raies, A. B., and Bajic, V. B. (2016). *In silico* toxicology: computational methods for the prediction of chemical toxicity. *Wiley Interdiscip. Rev. Comput. Mol. Sci.* 6, 147–172. doi: 10.1002/wcms.1240

Raina, R., Battle, A., Lee, H., Packer, B., and Ng, A. Y. (2007). "Self-taught learning: transfer learning from unlabeled data," in *Proceedings of the 24th International Conference on Machine learning, ICML 2007,* (Corvalis, OR: ACM), 759–766. doi: 10.1145/1273496.1273592

Richter, L., and Ecker, G. F. (2015). Medicinal chemistry in the era of big data. *Drug Discov. Today* 14, 37–41. doi: 10.1016/j.ddtec.2015.06.001

Rosenbaum, L., Dörr, A., Bauer, M. R., Boeckler, F. M., and Zell, A. (2013). Inferring multi-target qsar models with taxonomy-based multi-task learning. *J. Cheminform.* 5:33. doi: 10.1186/1758-2946-5-33

Saha, B., Gupta, S., Phung, D., and Venkatesh, S. (2016). "Transfer learning for rare cancer problems via discriminative sparse gaussian graphical model," in *Proceedings of the 23rd International Conference on Pattern Recognition (ICPR),* (Cancun: IEEE - Institute of Electrical and Electronics Engineers, Inc), 537–542. doi: 10.1109/ICPR.2016.7899689

Satpal, S., and Sarawagi, S. (2007). "Domain adaptation of conditional probability models via feature subsetting," in *Knowledge Discovery in Databases: PKDD* 2007, eds J. N. Kok, J. Koronacki, R. Lopez de Mantaras, S. Matwin, D. Mladenic, and A. Skowron (Berlin: Springer), 224–235. doi: 10.1007/978-3-540-749 76-9_23

Scior, T., Medina-Franco, J. L., Do, Q. T., Martínez-Mayorga, K., Yunes Rojas, J. A., and Bernard, P. (2009). How to recognize and workaround pitfalls in QSAR studies: a critical review. *Curr. Med. Chem.* 16, 4297–4313. doi: 10.2174/092986709789578213

Shoichet, B. K. (2004). Virtual screening of chemical libraries. *Nature* 432, 862–865. doi: 10.1038/nature03197

Sliwoski, G., Kothiwale, S. K., Meiler, J., Lowe, E. W., and Barker, E. L. (2014). Computational methods in drug discovery. *Pharmacol. Rev.* 66, 334–395. doi: 10.1124/pr.112.007336

Tan, B., Song, Y., Zhong, E., and Yang, Q. (2015). "Transitive transfer learning," in *Proceedings of the 21th ACM SIGKDD International Conference on Knowledge Discovery and Data Mining,* (New York, NY: ACM), 1155–1164. doi: 10.1145/2783258.2783295

Tresadern, G., Bemporad, D., and Howe, T. (2009). A comparison of ligand based virtual screening methods and application to corticotropin releasing factor 1 receptor. *J. Mol. Graph. Model.* 27, 860–870. doi: 10.1016/j.jmgm.2009.01.003

Tufts Center for the Study of Drug Development [CSDD] (2014). *Cost to Develop and Win Marketing Approval for a New Drug Is $2.6 Billion.* Available at: http://csdd.tufts.edu/news/complete_story/pr_tufts_csdd_2014_cost_study

Turki, T., Wei, Z., and Wang, J. T. (2017). Transfer learning approaches to improve drug sensitivity prediction in multiple Myeloma patients. *IEEE Access* 5, 7381–7393. doi: 10.1109/ACCESS.2017.2696523

Varnek, A., Gaudin, C., Marcou, G., Baskin, I., Pandey, A. K., and Tetko, I. V. (2009). Inductive transfer of knowledge: application of multi-task learning and feature net approaches to model tissue-air partition coefficients. *J. Chem. Inf. Model.* 49, 133–144. doi: 10.1021/ci8002914

Walters, W. P., Stahl, M. T., and Murcko, M. A. (1998). Virtual screening—an overview. *Drug Discov. Today* 3, 160–178. doi: 10.1016/S1359-6446(97)01163-X

Wang, T., Wu, M. B., Lin, J. P., and Yang, L. R. (2015). Quantitative structure-activity relationship: promising advances in drug discovery platforms. *Expert Opin. Drug Discov.* 11, 1–18. doi: 10.1517/17460441.2015.1083006

Wang, Y., Bolton, E., Dracheva, S., Karapetyan, K., Shoemaker, B. A., Suzek, T. O., et al. (2009). An overview of the PubChem BioAssay resource. *Nucleic Acids Res.* 38, D255–D266. doi: 10.1093/nar/gkp965

Zaccagnini, L., Brogi, S., Brindisi, M., Gemma, S., Chemi, G., Legname, G., et al. (2017). Identification of novel fluorescent probes preventing PrP Sc replication in prion diseases. *Eur. J. Med. Chem.* 127, 859–873. doi: 10.1016/j.ejmech.2016.10.064

Zhang, L., Sedykh, A., Tripathi, A., Zhu, H., Afantitis, A., Mouchlis, V. D., et al. (2013). Identification of putative estrogen receptor-mediated endocrine disrupting chemicals using QSAR- and structure-based virtual screening approaches. *Toxicol. Appl. Pharmacol.* 272, 67–76. doi: 10.1016/j.taap.2013.04.032

Zhang, L., Tan, J., Han, D., and Zhu, H. (2017). From machine learning to deep learning: progress in machine intelligence for rational drug discovery. *Drug Discov. Today* 22, 1680–1685. doi: 10.1016/j.drudis.2017.08.010

Zhang, W., Chen, Y., Tu, S., Liu, F., and Qu, Q. (2016). "Drug side effect prediction through linear neighborhoods and multiple data source integration," in *Proceedings of the IEEE International Conference on Bioinformatics and Biomedicine* (Shenzhen: IEEE), 427–434. doi: 10.1109/BIBM.2016.7822555

Zhao, L., Wang, W., Sedykh, A., and Zhu, H. (2017). Experimental errors in QSAR modeling sets: what we can do and what we cannot do. *ACS Omega* 2, 2805–2812. doi: 10.1021/acsomega.7b00274

6

vNN Web Server for ADMET Predictions

Patric Schyman*, Ruifeng Liu, Valmik Desai and Anders Wallqvist*

DoD Biotechnology High Performance Computing Software Applications Institute, Telemedicine and Advanced Technology Research Center, U.S. Army Medical Research and Materiel Command, Fort Detrick, MD, United States

***Correspondence:**
Patric Schyman
pschyman@bhsai.org
Anders Wallqvist
sven.a.wallqvist.civ@mail.mil

In drug development, early assessments of pharmacokinetic and toxic properties are important stepping stones to avoid costly and unnecessary failures. Considerable progress has recently been made in the development of computer-based (*in silico*) models to estimate such properties. Nonetheless, such models can be further improved in terms of their ability to make predictions more rapidly, easily, and with greater reliability. To address this issue, we have used our vNN method to develop 15 absorption, distribution, metabolism, excretion, and toxicity (ADMET) prediction models. These models quickly assess some of the most important properties of potential drug candidates, including their cytotoxicity, mutagenicity, cardiotoxicity, drug-drug interactions, microsomal stability, and likelihood of causing drug-induced liver injury. Here we summarize the ability of each of these models to predict such properties and discuss their overall performance. All of these ADMET models are publically available on our website (https://vnnadmet.bhsai.org/), which also offers the capability of using the vNN method to customize and build new models.

Keywords: ADME, toxicology, QSAR, machine learning, applicability domain, online web platform, open access

INTRODUCTION

Drug discovery is a risky, lengthy, and resource-intensive process with high attrition rates. In recent years, the development of assays and computer-based (*in silico*) models to assess absorption, distribution, metabolism, and excretion (ADME) properties has greatly reduced the attrition rate (Waring et al., 2015). The ability to predict these properties quickly and reliably facilitates the exclusion of compounds with potential ADME issues, and thereby helps investigators prioritize which compounds to synthesize and evaluate. However, toxicity remains a hurdle, with an attrition rate of 40% among new compounds identified in the drug discovery phase (Waring et al., 2015). This necessitates careful selection of compounds during drug development to avoid late-stage attrition. As such, there is an urgent need for *in silico* methods that make fast, easy, and reliable predictions of ADME and toxicity (ADMET) properties, which has resulted in several online tools and web-platforms for ADMET predictions (Walker et al., 2010; Sushko et al., 2011; Cheng et al., 2012; Maunz et al., 2013; Manganaro et al., 2016; Daina et al., 2017).

Here we provide an overview of our versatile variable nearest neighbor (vNN) method (Liu et al., 2012) and the 15 models we constructed using this method to predict the ADMET properties of potential target compounds. The vNN method has several advantages over existing *in silico* methods. First, it calculates the similarity distance between molecules in terms of their structure, and uses a distance threshold to define a domain of applicability (i.e., all nearest neighbors that meet a minimum similarity threshold constraint).

This applicability domain, while limiting vNN-based models to making predictions only for molecules that are similar to the reference molecules, ensures that the predictions they generate are reliable. Second, vNN-based models can be built within minutes and require no re-training when new assay information becomes available—an important feature when keeping quantitative structure—activity relationship (QSAR) models up-to-date to maintain their performance levels. Finally, as we show throughout this work, the performance characteristics of our vNN-based models are comparable, and often superior, to those of other more elaborate model constructs.

We have developed a publically available vNN website (https://vnnadmet.bhsai.org/). This website provides users with ADMET prediction models that we have developed, as well as a platform for using their own experimental data to update these models or build new ones from scratch. Although we use the vNN method here for predicting ADMET properties, the vNN website can be used to build a variety of classification or regression models.

MATERIALS AND METHODS

The vNN Method

The k-nearest neighbor (k-NN) method is widely used to develop QSAR models (Zheng and Tropsha, 2000). This method rests on the premise that compounds with similar structures have similar activities. The simplest form of the k-NN method takes the average property values of the k nearest neighbors as the predicted value. However, because structurally similar compounds tend to show similar biological activity, it is reasonable to weight the contributions of neighbors so that closer neighbors contribute more to the predicted value. One notable feature of the k-NN method is that it always gives a prediction for a compound, based on a constant number, k, of nearest neighbors no matter how structurally dissimilar they are from the compound. An alternative approach is to use a predetermined similarity criterion. We developed the aforementioned vNN method, which uses all nearest neighbors that meet a structural similarity criterion to define the model's applicability domain (Liu et al., 2012, 2015; Liu and Wallqvist, 2014). When no nearest neighbor meets the criterion, the vNN method makes no prediction.

One of the most widely used measures of the similarity distance between two small molecules is the Tanimoto distance, d, which is defined as:

$$d = 1 - \frac{n(P \cap Q)}{n(P) + n(Q) - n(P \cap Q)}, \quad (1)$$

where $n(P \cap Q)$ is the number of features common to molecules p and q, and $n(P)$ and $n(Q)$ are the total numbers of features for molecules p and q, respectively. The features used to calculate molecular similarity are often based on atom type (connectivity and chemical properties), such as element, charge, donor, acceptor, and aromatic, but they can also be based on holistic molecular properties, such as molecular weight and partition coefficient (LogP). The predicted biological activity y is then given by a weighted average across structurally similar neighbors:

$$y = \frac{\sum_{i=1}^{v} y_i e^{-\left(\frac{d_i}{h}\right)^2}}{\sum_{i=1}^{v} e^{-\left(\frac{d_i}{h}\right)^2}}, \quad d_i \leq d_0 \quad (2)$$

where d_i denotes the Tanimoto distance between a query molecule for which a prediction is made and a molecule i of the training set; y_i is the experimentally measured activity of molecule i; h is a smoothing factor, which dampens the distance penalty; d_0 is a Tanimoto-distance threshold, beyond which two molecules are no longer considered to be sufficiently similar to be included in the average; and v denotes the total number of molecules in the training set that satisfy the condition $d_i \leq d_0$. The values of h and d_0 are determined from cross-validation studies.

To identify structurally similar compounds, we used Accelrys extended-connectivity fingerprints with a diameter of four chemical bonds (ECFP4) (Rogers and Hahn, 2010). For the vNN website, we chose ECFP4 fingerprints, which have previously been reported to show satisfactory overall performance in retrieving the active compounds of diverse datasets (Hert et al., 2004; Duan et al., 2010; Schyman et al., 2016). We emphasize that h and d_0 are unique, and need to be optimized for each set of fingerprints and training set.

Model Validation

We used the 10-fold cross-validation (CV) procedure to validate the model and determine the values of h and d_0. We randomly divided the data into 10 sets, 9 of which we used to develop the model and the 10th to validate the model. We repeated this process 10 times, leaving each set of molecules out once. In the next section, we report averages of the 10-fold CV as the performance measures.

Performance Measures

We used the following metrics to assess the quality of the classification models:

$$\text{sensitivity} = \frac{\text{TP}}{\text{TP} + \text{FN}} \quad (3)$$

$$\text{specificity} = \frac{\text{TN}}{\text{FP} + \text{TN}} \quad (4)$$

$$\text{accuracy} = \frac{\text{TP} + \text{TN}}{\text{TP} + \text{TN} + \text{FP} + \text{FN}} \quad (5)$$

$$\text{kappa} = \frac{\text{accuracy} - \Pr(\text{e})}{1 - \Pr(\text{e})} \quad (6)$$

where TP, TN, FP, and FN denote the numbers of true positives, true negatives, false positives, and false negatives, respectively. The metric kappa assesses the quality of binary classifiers (Dunn and Everitt, 1995). Pr(e) is an estimate

Abbreviations: Pgp, permeability glycoprotein; MDR, multidrug resistance.

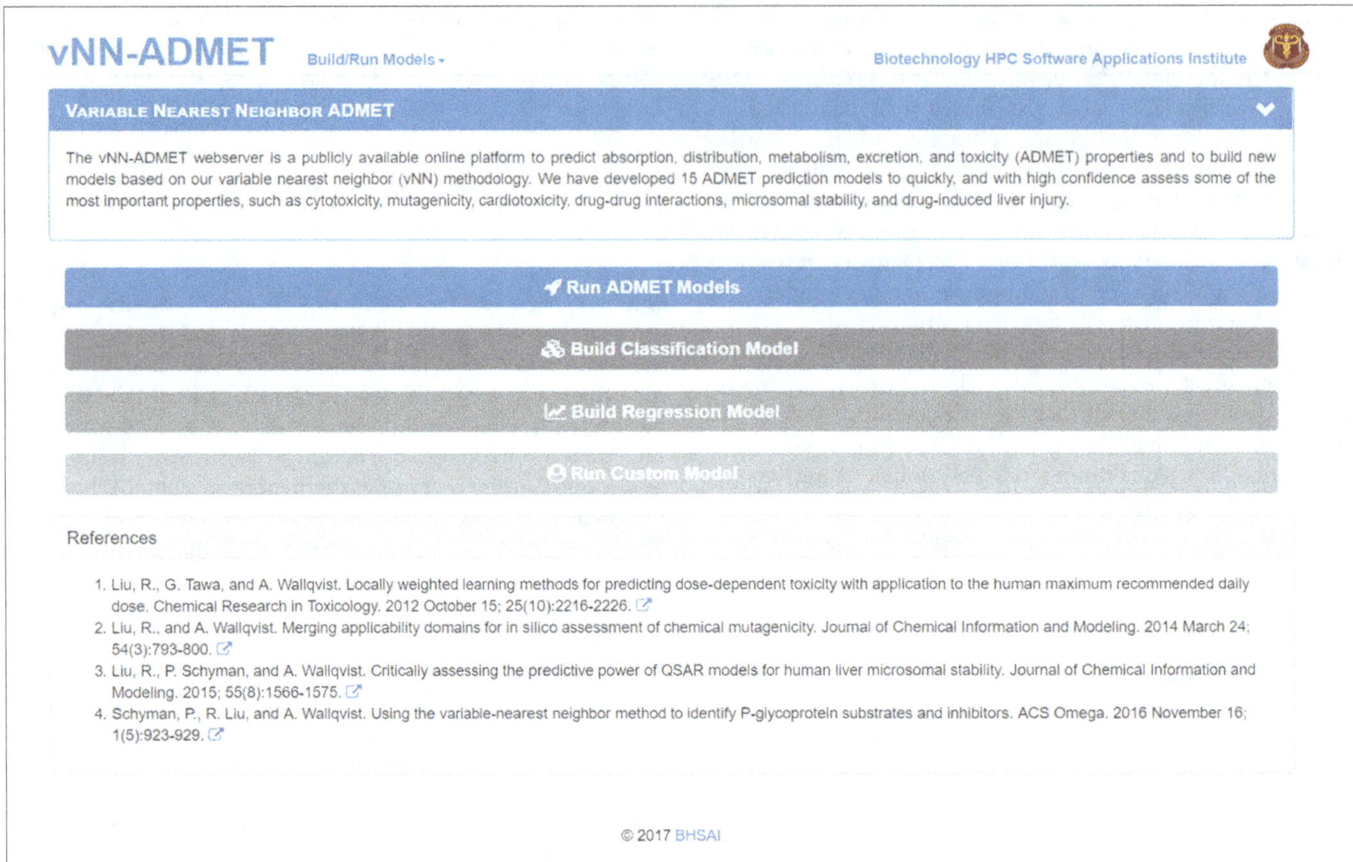

FIGURE 1 | The vNN-ADMET main page. From this page, users can run ADMET models or build their own models.

of the probability of a correct prediction by chance. It is calculated as:

$$\Pr(e) = \frac{(TP + FN)(TP + FP) + (FP + TN)(TN + FN)}{(TP + FN + FP + TN)^2} \tag{7}$$

The sensitivity measures a model's ability to correctly detect true positives, whereas the specificity measures its ability to detect true negatives. Kappa compares the probability of correct predictions to the probability of correct predictions by chance. Its value ranges from +1 (perfect agreement between model prediction and experiment) to −1 (complete disagreement), with 0 indicating no agreement beyond that expected by chance.

The performance measure for regression models is given by the Pearson's correlation coefficient (Adler and Parmryd, 2010):

$$R = \frac{\sum_{i=1}^{n}(x_i - \bar{x})(y_i - \bar{y})}{\sqrt{\sum_{i=1}^{n}(x_i - \bar{x})^2}\sqrt{\sum_{i=1}^{n}(y_i - \bar{y})^2}} \tag{8}$$

where n is the sample size, x_i and y_i are samples, and $\bar{x}$ and $\bar{y}$ are sample means. The correlation coefficient provides a measure of the interrelatedness of numeric properties. Its value ranges from −1 (highly anticorrelated) to +1 (highly correlated), and is 0 when uncorrelated.

We also calculated the coverage, which we define as the proportion of test molecules with at least one nearest neighbor that meets the similarity criterion. For all other molecules that do not meet the criterion, we do not make any predictions. In this case, the coverage is a measure of the size of the applicability domain of a prediction model.

RESULTS

The vNN Platform

The main purpose of the vNN-based platform is to provide users with a tool to make ADMET predictions and a user-friendly environment to build new models. Hence, the platform offers users two main capabilities that are accessible from the main webpage (https://vnnadmet.bhsai.org/) (**Figure 1**): (1) to run prebuilt ADMET models and (2) to build and run customized models.

To use prebuilt ADMET models, users need only provide one or more query molecules as the input (**Figure 2**). They can do this either by drawing the molecule, entering the molecular SMILES string (Weininger, 1988) directly on the website, or uploading a text file (csv or txt format) with query molecules in SMILES format. The text file should contain column headers labeled as NAME and SMILES. Once users upload the query molecules, they can submit the job. The application will then automatically

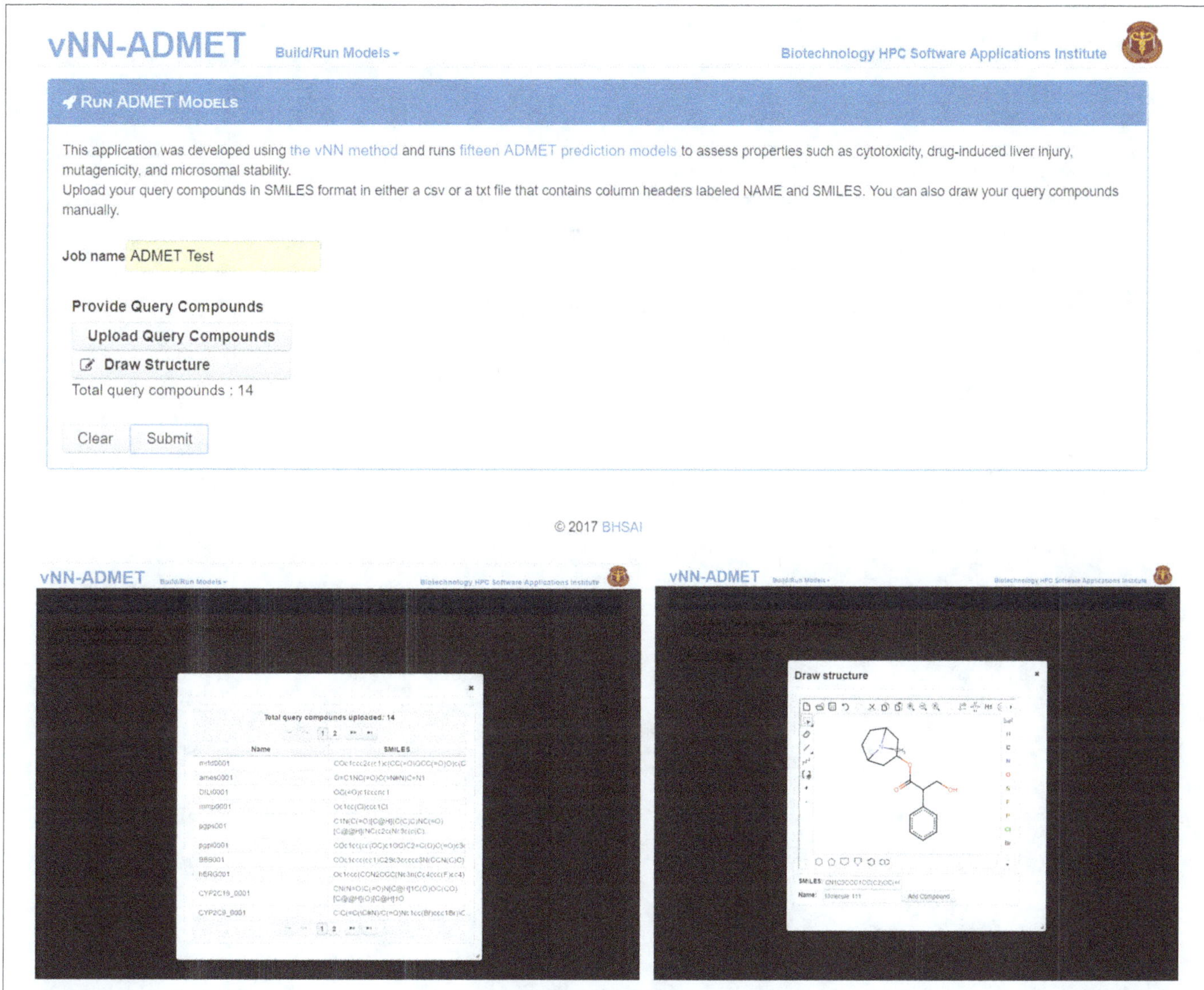

FIGURE 2 | Submit ADMET predictions. On the *Run ADMET Models* page **(top)** users can upload a list of query compounds in SMILES format **(lower left)** or manually enter compounds by using the draw structure feature **(lower right)**.

run all ADMET prediction models. The output will be displayed once all predictions are completed and a temporary link to the result page will be sent to the user's e-mail address. The results can be downloaded as a table to the user's computer (**Figure 3**). By default, the user will see the ADMET results for our models, which use a restricted applicability domain. However, there is an option to include the results for the remaining compounds, using our unrestricted applicability domain models. The time required to run 100 query compounds is ~5 min on the server. However, this may vary depending on the size of the molecules and whether or not the job has been queued.

Users can build their own models by either selecting *Build Classification Model* or *Build Regression Model* on the main webpage (**Figure 1**). On the *Build Classification Model* page (**Figure 4**), users are asked to upload a list of molecules in SMILES format and the property of interest, with column headers labeled as NAME, SMILES, and PROPERTY. The value of the property should be set to 1 or 0 for classification models and real numbers for regression models. The vNN platform will then automatically run 10-fold CV by varying the Tanimoto distance (d) from 0.1 to 1.0 in increments of 0.1, and the smoothing factor (h) from 0.1 to 1.0 at each value of d. Once the calculations are completed, a temporary link to the result page will be sent to the user's e-mail address. The results will be displayed on an interactive webpage where users can select the values for d and h (Equation 2), depending on the optimal performance measures and coverage (**Figure 4**). The time required to build a model with a dataset of 1,000 compounds is ~10 min.

Users can then select the *Run Custom Model* option to predict the activity of new test molecules (**Figure 5**), using the previously selected values for the *Tanimoto Distance* and *Smoothing Factor*, and add the same molecules as those used to train the model in the *Upload Compounds with Property* data field. They then need to add the new query molecule(s) in SMILES format in the

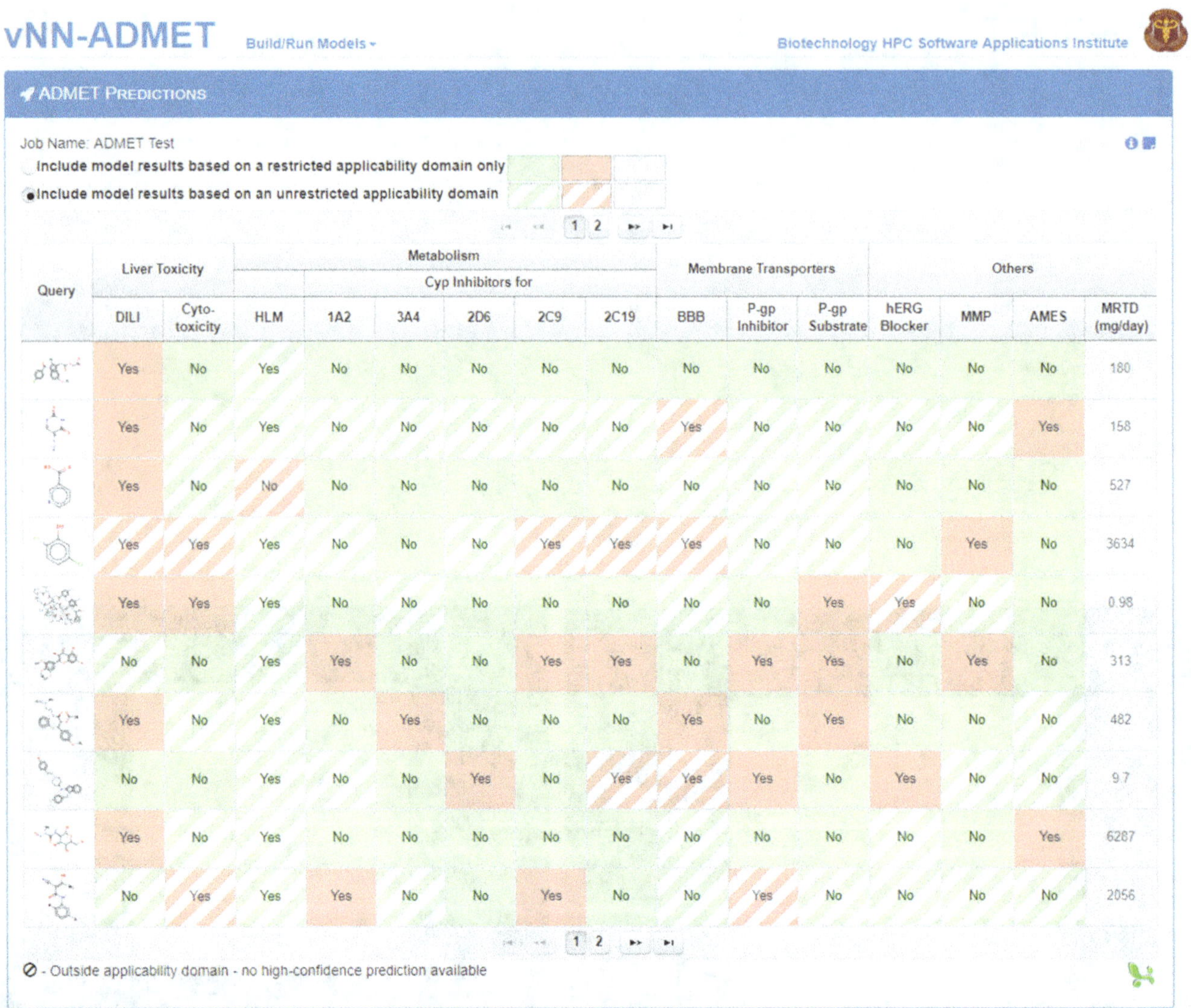
vNN-ADMET
Build/Run Models
Biotechnology HPC Software Applications Institute
ADMET Predictions
Job Name: ADMET Test
Include model results based on a restricted applicability domain only
Include model results based on an unrestricted applicability domain
⊘ - Outside applicability domain - no high-confidence prediction available

Query	Liver Toxicity		Metabolism						Membrane Transporters			Others			
				Cyp Inhibitors for											
	DILI	Cyto-toxicity	HLM	1A2	3A4	2D6	2C9	2C19	BBB	P-gp Inhibitor	P-gp Substrate	hERG Blocker	MMP	AMES	MRTD (mg/day)
	Yes	No	Yes	No	No	No	No	No	No	No	No	No	No	No	180
	Yes	No	Yes	No	No	No	No	No	Yes	No	No	No	No	Yes	158
	Yes	No	No	No	No	No	No	No	No	No	No	No	No	No	527
	Yes	Yes	Yes	No	No	No	Yes	Yes	Yes	No	No	No	Yes	No	3634
	Yes	Yes	Yes	No	No	No	No	No	No	No	Yes	Yes	No	No	0.98
	No	No	Yes	Yes	No	No	Yes	Yes	No	Yes	Yes	No	Yes	No	313
	Yes	No	Yes	No	Yes	No	No	No	Yes	No	Yes	No	No	No	482
	No	No	Yes	No	No	Yes	No	Yes	Yes	Yes	No	Yes	No	No	9.7
	Yes	No	Yes	No	No	No	No	No	No	No	No	No	No	Yes	6287
	No	Yes	Yes	Yes	No	No	Yes	No	No	Yes	No	No	No	No	2056

FIGURE 3 | The ADMET predictions result page. The 15 ADMET predictions for each query molecule are presented on a separate row. Predictions based on models using a restricted applicability domain are shown in solid colors and those based on models using an unrestricted applicability domain are shown in striped colors. Users can download the results from the website into a single file.

Upload Query Compounds field. The result will be displayed on a new webpage, and a temporary link to that page will also be sent to the user's e-mail address (**Figure 5**).

Available ADMET Predictions

The available ADMET prediction models, including their performance measures for the restricted applicability domain model, are summarized in **Table 1**. The performance measures for the models using an unrestricted applicability domain are presented in Table S1 in the Supplementary Material and on our website (https://vnnadmet.bhsai.org/). The 15 models cover a diverse set of ADMET endpoints. We will briefly describe these models and their performance measures, as well as the sources from which we retrieved the data. All datasets are available in SMILES format on the vNN web server or in Structure Data Format (SDF) in the Supplementary Material (Datasheet 1). Some of the models have already been published (Liu et al., 2012, 2015; Liu and Wallqvist, 2014; Schyman et al., 2016). We also present several new models here for the first time.

Blood-Brain Barrier

The blood-brain barrier (BBB) is a highly selective barrier that separates the circulating blood from the central nervous system (CNS) (Abbott et al., 2006). It allows the passage of water molecules and water-soluble lipid molecules, as well as the selective transport of glucose and amino acids. The benefit of predicting BBB-permeable compounds is two-fold: (1) to identify toxicants that could harm the brain, and (2) to design drug molecules that can pass the BBB and reach their target in the CNS.

We developed a vNN-based BBB model, using 353 compounds whose BBB permeability values (log *BB*) were obtained from the literature (Muehlbacher et al., 2011; Naef,

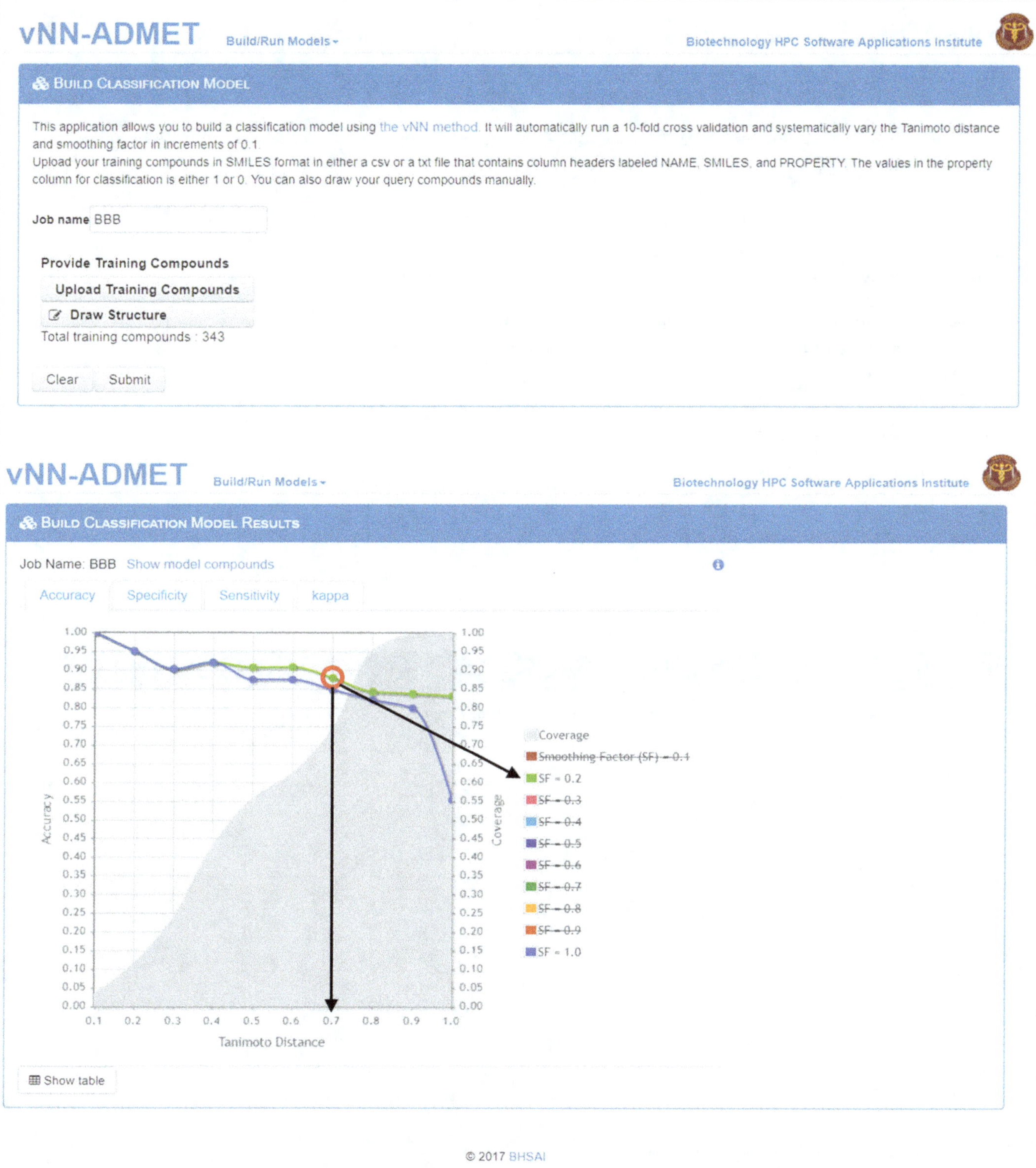

FIGURE 4 | Build a classification model. On the *Build Classification Model* page **(top)**, users can upload their training data and/or draw structures. On the *Build Classification Model Results* page **(bottom)**, users can interactively select/deselect different smoothing factors for comparison. The graph shows accuracy of performance on the 10-fold cross validation test at different Tanimoto distances, where smoothing factors 0.2 and 1.0 are highlighted in green and blue, respectively (strikethrough smoothing factors indicate deselected values). The coverage is shown in gray. The red circle indicates the "best" model performance based on accuracy and coverage, where the black arrows show the corresponding Tanimoto-distance threshold ($d_0 = 0.7$) and smoothing factor ($h = 0.2$). Although the accuracy is reduced to 88 from 90% at $d_0 = 0.6$, the number of compounds predicted increases from 60 to 75%, which may be worth the loss in accuracy.

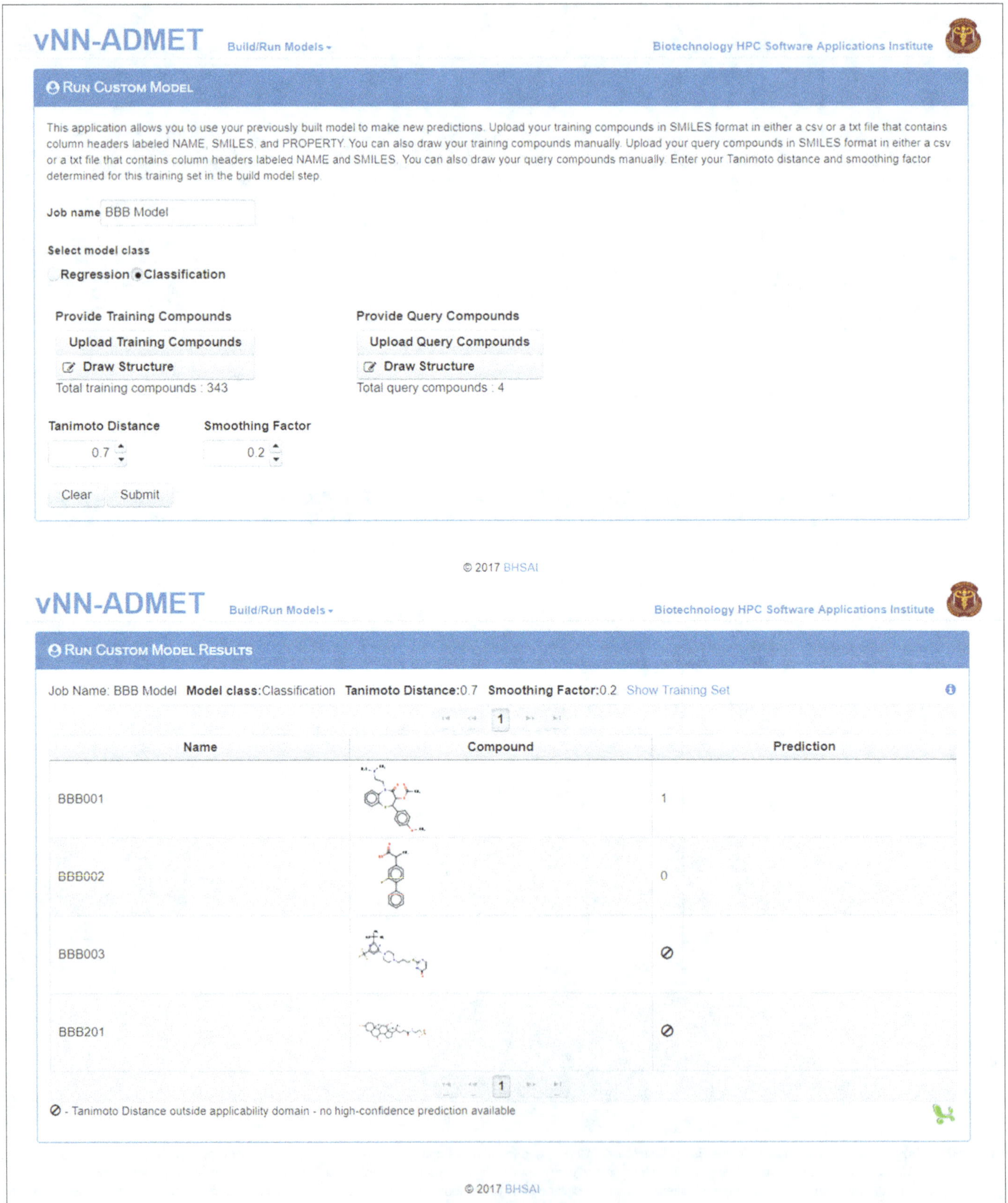
vNN-ADMET
Build/Run Models
Biotechnology HPC Software Applications Institute
Run Custom Model
This application allows you to use your previously built model to make new predictions. Upload your training compounds in SMILES format in either a csv or a txt file that contains column headers labeled NAME, SMILES, and PROPERTY. You can also draw your training compounds manually. Upload your query compounds in SMILES format in either a csv or a txt file that contains column headers labeled NAME and SMILES. You can also draw your query compounds manually. Enter your Tanimoto distance and smoothing factor determined for this training set in the build model step.
Job name BBB Model
Select model class
Regression Classification
Provide Training Compounds
Upload Training Compounds
Draw Structure
Total training compounds : 343
Provide Query Compounds
Upload Query Compounds
Draw Structure
Total query compounds : 4
Tanimoto Distance
0.7
Smoothing Factor
0.2
Clear
Submit
© 2017 BHSAI
vNN-ADMET
Build/Run Models
Biotechnology HPC Software Applications Institute
Run Custom Model Results
Job Name: BBB Model Model class:Classification Tanimoto Distance:0.7 Smoothing Factor:0.2 Show Training Set
Name
Compound
Prediction
BBB001
1
BBB002
0
BBB003
BBB201
- Tanimoto Distance outside applicability domain - no high-confidence prediction available
© 2017 BHSAI

FIGURE 5 | Run a customized model. The first step to run a customized model is to upload the training dataset, as well as the selected Tanimoto distance and smoothing factor from **Figure 4**. The second step is to upload query compounds. The results can be downloaded from the *Run Custom Model Results* page (bottom).

TABLE 1 | Performance measures of vNN models in 10-fold cross validation, using a restricted applicability domain.

Model	Data[a]	d_0[b]	h[c]	Accuracy	Sensitivity	Specificity	Kappa	R[d]	Coverage
DILI	1,427	0.60	0.50	0.71	0.70	0.73	0.42		0.66
Cytotox (hep2g)	6,097	0.40	0.20	0.84	0.88	0.76	0.64		0.89
HLM	3,219	0.40	0.20	0.81	0.72	0.87	0.59		0.91
CYP 1A2	7,558	0.50	0.20	0.90	0.70	0.95	0.66		0.75
CYP 2C9	8,072	0.50	0.20	0.91	0.55	0.96	0.54		0.76
CYP 2C19	8,155	0.50	0.20	0.87	0.64	0.93	0.58		0.76
CYP 3A4	10,373	0.50	0.20	0.88	0.76	0.92	0.68		0.78
CYP 2D6	7,805	0.50	0.20	0.89	0.61	0.94	0.57		0.75
BBB	353	0.60	0.20	0.90	0.94	0.86	0.80		0.61
Pgp Substrate	822	0.60	0.20	0.79	0.80	0.79	0.58		0.66
Pgp Inhibitor	2,304	0.50	0.20	0.85	0.91	0.73	0.66		0.76
hERG	685	0.70	0.70	0.84	0.84	0.83	0.68		0.80
MMP	6,261	0.50	0.40	0.89	0.64	0.94	0.61		0.69
AMES	6,512	0.50	0.40	0.82	0.86	0.75	0.62		0.79
MRTD[e]	1,184	0.60	0.20					0.79	0.69

[a]Number of compounds in the dataset; [b]Tanimoto-distance threshold value; [c]Smoothing factor; [d]Pearson's correlation coefficient; [e]Regression model.

2015). We classified compounds with log *BB* values of <−0.3 and >+0.3 as BBB non-permeable and permeable, respectively. To calculate performance measures, we classified BBB permeable and BBB non-permeable compounds as positives and negatives, respectively.

The model predicted whether or not a given compound would pass the BBB, but only for compounds within the applicability domain defined by the training set. The performance measures in **Table 1** were calculated from 10-fold CV. The model showed a high overall accuracy of 90% and a kappa value of 0.80, with a coverage of 61%. The size of the dataset limited the applicability domain of the model. However, if new data become available, they can easily be added to the model to increase the applicability domain.

The model performed on par with the best of the BBB models published thus far. Most of the latter models, which used small datasets, are global models applied to any molecule. However, all models have a finite applicability domain (Cherkasov et al., 2014). Indeed, modeling BBB permeability is complicated because there are different possible routes across the barrier, via passive diffusion or protein transport, and no model singlehandedly accounts for all factors associated with this property. Our vNN model only makes predictions for compounds that are structurally similar enough to the test set molecules to ensure that they have the same type of transport mechanism. Thus, our vNN method accounts for multiple transport routes.

MMP Disruption (Mitochondrial Toxicity)

Given the fundamental role of mitochondria in cellular energetics and oxidative stress, mitochondrial dysfunction has been implicated in cancer, diabetes, neurodegenerative disorders, and cardiovascular diseases (Pieczenik and Neustadt, 2007). Many pharmaceuticals and environmental toxicants cause mitochondrial dysfunction (Meyer et al., 2013). Therefore, the ability to predict the impact of chemicals on mitochondrial function would be useful. However, predicting mitochondrial toxicants is complicated because mitochondrial dysfunction can result from impairing any of the following: (1) the electron transport chain (ETC), (2) the mitochondrial transport pathway, (3) fatty acid oxidation, (4) the citric acid cycle, (5) mtDNA replication, (6) and mitochondrial protein synthesis.

There are several common experimental techniques to measure mitochondrial function. We used the largest dataset of chemical-induced changes in mitochondrial membrane potential (MMP), based on the assumption that a compound that causes mitochondrial dysfunction is also likely to reduce the MMP. We developed a vNN-based MMP prediction model, using 6,261 compounds collected from a previous study that screened a library of 10,000 compounds (~8,300 unique chemicals) at 15 concentrations, each in triplicate, to measure changes in the MMP in HepG2 cells (Attene-Ramos et al., 2015). The study found that 913 compounds decreased the MMP, whereas 5,395 compounds had no effect. We classified compounds that decreased the MMP as positives and those that did not affect the MMP as negatives.

Our MMP model predicted whether a given compound had the potential to affect the MMP and thereby cause mitochondrial dysfunction. It made predictions for compounds that were well represented in the applicability domain, but not for any other compound. The model showed a high overall accuracy of 89% and a kappa value of 0.61, with a coverage of 69% (**Table 1**).

Cytotoxicity (HepG2)

Cytotoxicity is the degree to which a chemical causes damage to cells. Cytotoxicity assays are widely used to screen compounds for unwanted cell damage, and to identify compounds that could be used, for example, to kill cancer cells. As such, the ability to identify cytotoxic compounds is highly desirable.

We developed a cytotoxicity prediction model, using a training dataset of *in vitro* toxicity against HepG2 cells for

TABLE 2 | Performance measures of vNN DILI models compared with deep learning.

	NCTR[a] 10-fold CV	NCTR[a] Test	Green[a] Test	Xu[a] Test	Combined[a] 10-fold CV
Accuracy (%)	87 (81)	75 (70)	61 (65)	60 (62)	85 (85)[b]
Sensitivity (%)	65 (70)	64 (80)	51 (75)	52 (62)	83 (84)[b]
Specificity (%)	95 (88)	86 (60)	75 (46)	70 (62)	88 (85)[b]
Coverage (%)	40	50	46	41	67
No of Compounds	190	185	320	236	475

[a]*Values in parentheses are the deep learning results from Xu et al. (2015).*
[b]*Values averaged over 60 runs of 10-fold CV.*

6,097 structurally diverse compounds, which we collected from Chemical European Biology Laboratory (ChEMBL) (Bento et al., 2014). In developing our model, we considered compounds with an IC_{50} of $10\,\mu M$ or less in the *in vitro* assay as cytotoxic. We classified cytotoxic compounds as positives and non-toxic compounds as negatives.

The cytotoxicity model performed well, with an overall accuracy of 84% and a kappa value of 0.64 (**Table 1**). Because compounds in the dataset achieved only sparse coverage of the chemical space, the model only predicted compounds that were well represented in the dataset. It did not give predictions for other compounds, and thereby avoided misleading results. When using 10-fold CV, the model reliably predicted 89% of the compounds in our dataset.

Drug-Induced Liver Injury

Over the last 50 years, drug-induced liver injury (DILI) has been the most commonly cited reason for drug withdrawals from the market (Assis and Navarro, 2009). As a result, current drug development efforts are devoted to identifying and eliminating potential DILI compounds. Therefore, a model that predicts at an early stage whether a compound causes liver injury would be highly desirable. However, the mechanisms of DILI are complicated and diverse, making toxicology studies difficult. For example, compounds that cause DILI in humans do not necessarily induce clear liver injury in animal studies.

We collected DILI data from four sources used by Xu et al. (2015): (1) the U.S. FDA's National Center for Toxicological Research (NCTR dataset) (Chen M. et al., 2011), as well as the datasets of (2) Greene (Greene et al., 2010), (3) Xu (Xu et al., 2008), and (4) Liew (Liew et al., 2011). In the first three datasets, which included pharmaceuticals, we classified a compound as causing DILI if it was associated with a high risk of DILI and not if there was no such risk. We excluded low-risk DILI compounds. In the Liew dataset, which contained both pharmaceuticals and non-pharmaceuticals, we classified a compound as causing DILI if it was associated with any adverse liver effect. DILI-associated compounds were classified as positives and non-DILI compounds as negatives.

The performance measures of the vNN model, using 10-fold CV of the entire dataset excluding duplicated compounds, showed an overall accuracy of 71% and a coverage of 66% (**Table 1**). We also used the same datasets and compared our models with some previously published deep learning models (Xu et al., 2015; **Table 2**). Considering the complexity and computational time investment involved in training these deep learning models, our vNN models performed relatively well; they performed on-par with the deep learning models, albeit with a coverage ranging from 40 to 65%.

Cytochrome P450 Inhibition (Drug-Drug Interaction)

Cytochrome P450 enzymes (CYPs) constitute a superfamily of proteins that play an important role in the metabolism and detoxification of xenobiotics (Brown et al., 2008). A drug should not be rapidly metabolized by CYPs if it is to maintain an effective concentration. In addition, it should not inhibit drug-metabolizing CYPs, because such an effect could elevate the concentration of a co-administered drug and potentially lead to drug overdose—an effect known as a drug-drug interaction (Murray, 2006). In drug development, *in vitro* assays are routinely used to assess interactions between drug candidates and CYPs. However, there is a need for *in silico* models that assess potential interactions with CYPs in the early stages of drug development.

We collected data for five main drug-metabolizing CYPs: 1A2, 2D6, 2C9, 2C19, and 3A4. We retrieved CYP inhibitors from ChEMBL (Bento et al., 2014) and classified them as inhibitors if the IC_{50} was below $10\,\mu M$. We removed from the dataset any duplicates or compounds tested multiple times with contradicting results, in which the reported IC_{50} values were below and above the $10\,\mu M$ threshold value. For all CYPs, we classified inhibitors and non-inhibitors as positives and negatives, respectively.

The performance measures for the five CYP models are presented in **Table 1**. All models achieved high accuracy (87–91%) and kappa values (0.54–0.68) while maintaining high coverage (75–78%).

hERG Blockers

The human ether-à-go-go-related gene (hERG) codes for a potassium ion channel involved in the normal cardiac repolarization activity of the heart (Sanguinetti and Tristani-Firouzi, 2006). Drug-induced blockade of hERG function can cause long QT syndrome, which may result in arrhythmia and death (De Ponti et al., 2001). For this reason, hERG liability is one of the toxicology screens that drug candidates must pass during early pre-clinical studies. Therefore, *in silico* models that identify hERG blockers in the early stages of drug design are of considerable interest.

We retrieved 282 known hERG blockers from the literature and classified compounds with an IC_{50} cutoff value of $10\,\mu M$ or less as blockers (Wang et al., 2012). We also collected a set of 404 compounds with IC_{50} values $>10\,\mu M$ from ChEMBL (Bento et al., 2014) and classified them as non-blockers (Czodrowski, 2013). We classified hERG blockers and non-blockers as positives and negatives, respectively.

The hERG model performed with an overall accuracy of 84%, well-balanced sensitivity and specificity values (84 and 83%, respectively), and a kappa value of 0.68 (**Table 1**). The model reliably predicted 80% of the compounds in our dataset when using 10-fold CV. However, the coverage of chemical space by the non-hERG blockers in the dataset was sparse, and only compounds well represented in the dataset were predicted with confidence. Because the model did not give predictions for other compounds, it avoided misleading results. Therefore, users should use this model to flag potential hERG blockers rather than to identify non-hERG blockers.

Pgp Substrates and Inhibitors

P-glycoprotein (Pgp) is an essential cell membrane protein that extracts many foreign substances from the cell (Ambudkar et al., 2003). As such, it is a critical determinant of the pharmacokinetic properties of drugs. Cancer cells often overexpress Pgp, which increases the efflux of chemotherapeutic agents from the cell and prevents treatment by reducing the effective intracellular concentrations of such agents—a phenomenon known as multidrug resistance (Borst and Elferink, 2002). For this reason, identifying compounds that can either be transported out of the cell by Pgp (substrates) or impair Pgp function (inhibitors) is of great interest. Therefore, using the vNN method, we developed models to predict both Pgp substrates and Pgp inhibitors.

The Pgp substrate dataset was collected by Hou and co-workers (Li et al., 2014). This dataset included measurements for 422 substrates and 400 non-substrates. To generate a large Pgp inhibitor dataset, we combined two datasets (Broccatelli et al., 2011; Chen L. et al., 2011), and removed duplicates to form a combined dataset consisting of a training set of 1,319 inhibitors and 937 non-inhibitors. We classified the Pgp inhibitors (substrates) and non-inhibitors (non-substrates) as positives and negatives, respectively.

The vNN models for identifying Pgp substrates and inhibitors gave accurate and reliable results, showing overall accuracies of 79 and 85%, respectively, when using 10-fold CV, with corresponding kappa values of 0.58 and 0.66. These models reliably predicted 65 and 76% of the compounds in their datasets to be Pgp substrates and inhibitors, respectively. The performance characteristics of these models were comparable, or at times superior, to those of other model constructs (Schyman et al., 2016).

Chemical Mutagenicity (AMES Test)

Mutagens are chemicals that cause abnormal genetic mutations leading to cancer. A common way to assess a chemical's mutagenicity is the Ames test (Ames et al., 1973). This test has become the standard for assessing the safety of chemicals and drugs, and has been used to test thousands of molecules. We examined whether the vNN method could effectively use existing data to predict mutagenicity.

We retrieved an Ames mutagenicity dataset consisting of 6,512 compounds, of which 3,503 were Ames-positive (Hansen et al., 2009), and developed a vNN Ames mutagenicity prediction model. The model performed well, with an overall accuracy of 82%; sensitivity and specificity values of 86 and 75%, respectively; and a high kappa value of 0.62 (**Table 1**). The model also reliably predicted 79% of the compounds in the Ames dataset when using 10-fold CV. Further details of the model and its prediction performance can be found elsewhere (Liu and Wallqvist, 2014).

Maximum Recommended Therapeutic Dose

A basic principle of toxicology is that "the dose makes the poison." For most drugs, the therapeutic dose is limited by toxicity, and the maximum recommended therapeutic dose (MRTD) is an estimated upper daily dose that is safe (Contrera et al., 2004). Investigators carry out toxicological experiments on animals to determine the toxic effects of a drug and the initial dose for human clinical trials. Unfortunately, there is a lack of correlation between animal and human toxicity data. Therefore, we investigated whether the vNN method could predict the MRTD values of new compounds based on known human MRTD data. If so, the values could be used to estimate the starting dose in phase I clinical trials, while significantly reducing the number of animals used in preliminary toxicology studies.

We obtained a dataset of MRTD values publically disclosed by the FDA, mostly of single-day oral doses for an average adult with a body weight of 60 kg, for 1,220 compounds (most of which are small organic drugs). For modeling purposes we converted the MRTD unit from mg/kg-body weight/day to mol/kg-body weight/day via the molecular weight of the compound. However, the predicted values on the website are reported in mg/day based upon an average adult weighing 60 kg. We excluded organometallics, high-molecular weight polymers (>5,000 Da), nonorganic chemicals, mixtures of chemicals, and very small molecules (<100 Da). We used an external test set of 160 compounds, which was collected by the FDA for validation. The total dataset for our model contained 1,184 compounds (Liu et al., 2012).

The MRTD model reliably predicted 69% of the FDA MRTD dataset, with a Pearson's correlation coefficient (R) of 0.79 between the predicted and measured *log*(MRTD) values, and a mean deviation (mDev) of 0.56 *log* units, using 40-fold CV (Liu et al., 2012). For comparison, we used two popular QSAR regression methods—the partial least square (PLS) and support vector machine (SVM) methods—to develop two global models to fit the training dataset. We evaluated the model performance, using 40-fold CV of the training set. The best PLS model achieved an R-value of 0.50 and an mDev of 0.79. The results for the SVM model were at best comparable to those of the best PLS model, with an R-value of 0.53 and an mDev of 0.63. For further details of the model, we refer the reader to our previous paper (Liu et al., 2012).

Human Liver Microsomal Stability

The human liver is the most important organ for drug metabolism. For a drug to achieve effective therapeutic concentrations in the body, it cannot be metabolized too rapidly by the liver. Otherwise, it would need to be administered at high doses, which are associated with high toxicity. To identify and exclude rapidly metabolized compounds (Di et al., 2003), pharmaceutical companies commonly use the human liver microsomal (HLM) stability assay. This has led to the accumulation of a substantial body of HLM stability data in publicly accessible databases.

However, our knowledge of how enzymes in the HLM assay metabolize drugs remains fragmentary. Therefore, we examined whether the vNN method could effectively predict drugs that are

TABLE 3 | Tox21 assays with PubChem assay identification number.

Assay ID	Assay	PubChem AID
AhR	Aryl hydrocarbon receptor	743122
Aromatase	Aromatase	743139
AR	Androgen receptor	743040
AR-LBD	Androgen receptor LBD	743053
ER	Estrogen receptor alpha	743079
ER-LBD	Estrogen receptor alpha LBD	743077
PPAR-g	Peroxisome proliferator-activated receptor gamma	743140
ARE	Nuclear factor antioxidant responsive element	743219
ATAD5	ATAD5	720516
HSE	Heat shock factor response element	743228
MMP	Mitochondrial membrane potential	720637
p53	p53	720552

rapidly metabolized by the liver. We retrieved HLM data from the ChEMBL database (Bento et al., 2014), manually curated the data, and classified compounds as stable or unstable based on the reported half-life [T1/2 > 30 min was considered stable, and T1/2 < 30 min unstable (Liu et al., 2015)]. The final dataset contained 3,219 compounds. Of these, we classified 2,047 as stable and 1,166 as unstable.

The HLM model performed with an overall accuracy of 81%; sensitivity and specificity values of 71 and 87%, respectively; and a high kappa value of 0.60 (**Table 1**). The HLM model reliably predicted 91% of the compounds in the HLM dataset when using 10-fold CV. We refer the reader to our original paper for further details of the model and its prediction performance (Liu et al., 2015).

Implementation Aspects

The vNN-ADMET web-application is hosted on an Apache Tomcat Web server that is accessible via a secure service over Hypertext Transfer Protocol Secure (https). We developed the application on the basis of a three-tiered architecture, composed of a backend database, controller, and presentation tiers. The first tier consists of a PostgreSQL 9.5.7 database that stores user account information, uploaded files, constructed models, and model predictions. The second (controller) tier provides access to the prediction engine and implements the functionality required to create and manage multiple predictions. We implemented this tier, using Pipeline Pilot protocols hosted on a local Pipeline Pilot server. The third (presentation) tier provides for visualization of the results, with plotting capabilities for multiple predictions. The controller and presentation tiers were developed using Java Platform, Enterprise Edition 7, Spring Framework 4.2.2, JavaServer Faces 2.2, PrimeFaces 6.0, and BootsFaces 1.0.2. The graphical user interface in the presentation tier uses Web standards supported by modern Web browsers, including Microsoft Edge 38, Chrome version 58, and Firefox version 53, without any need for plugins.

To use the system, the user must register for an account at https://vnnadmet.bhsai.org/. Once logged in, the user can build custom models, and run pre-built ADMET and custom models. The data corresponding to a user (login credentials, compounds, models, results, etc.) are not shared with any other user within or outside the system. The uploaded compounds, constructed models, and model predictions are purged from the system every 2 weeks.

DISCUSSION

We have presented a web-based vNN prediction platform, with which a user can build and test models as well as predict the ADMET properties of a compound by using our existing tools.

All vNN models performed well with accuracies of >71% (see **Table 1** for further details). On average, the models predicted 75% of the compounds in their datasets, using 10-fold CV.

Achieving fair comparisons between a new model and a competing model is always difficult because such comparisons require the same training data, validation data, and performance measures. An important advantage of our platform is that it offers an opportunity for developers to compare their methods with our vNN method, using their training and validation data.

For demonstrative purposes, we quantitatively compared our vNN method with the winning method of the Tox21 challenge (Huang et al., 2016). This challenge was issued in 2014 by the U.S. Toxicology in the twenty-first Century (Tox21) program, which aims to improve toxicity prediction methods. The Tox 21 consortium solicited models that could best predict the toxicity of 10,000 compounds it had tested in 12 different assays (**Table 3**). It used a final evaluation dataset that was concealed to determine the winners.

Table 4 shows the area under the curve for the receiver operating characteristic (AUC-ROC) of the 18 leading research teams with their best-performing model for each of the 12 assays. To compare our models with those in **Table 4**, we set d to 1.0 so that we could predict all compounds. The vNN method performed reasonably well in predicting most of the Tox21 assays. We note that the grand challenge winner used data from PubChem (Wang et al., 2009) and ChEMBL (Bento et al., 2014), in addition to the Tox21 data, which makes it impossible for us to directly compare our results with their results.

The MMP data we used for our mitochondrial dysfunction model were the same as those used in the Tox21 challenge (Attene-Ramos et al., 2015; Huang et al., 2016). Our MMP model was the seventh best performing model, with an AUC-ROC value of 0.882 (with $h = 0.3$ and $d = 1.0$). This was comparable to the values of more elaborate and computationally time-consuming methods, such as deep learning (**Table 4**).

Some QSAR methods do not use an applicability domain to determine whether their predictions are reliable. This could lead to the misperception that a model can predict the activity of any molecule. The applicability domain is vital to the vNN method. The user of our platform can adjust it by varying the Tanimoto distance threshold value. Although this could be set to 1 so that the model predicts the activity of any molecule, no model is likely to have an unlimited applicability domain (Liu et al., 2015).

A more reasonable approach to improve a vNN-based model is to increase the applicability domain by adding more reference

TABLE 4 | AUC-ROCs of vNN models and the best 18 models on the final evaluation test of the Tox21 Challenge.

Team	AhR	AR	AR-LBD	ARE	Aromatase	ATAD5	ER	ER-LBD	HSE	MMP	p53	PPARg
GrandWinner	0.928	0.807	0.879	0.840	0.834	0.793	0.810	0.814	0.865	0.942	0.862	0.861
AMAZIZ	0.913	0.770	0.846	0.805	0.819	0.828	0.806	0.806	0.842	0.95	0.843	0.830
dmlab	0.781	0.828	0.819	0.768	0.838	0.800	0.766	0.772	0.855	0.946	0.880	0.831
T	0.913	0.676	0.848	0.801	0.825	0.814	0.784	0.805	0.811	0.937	0.847	0.822
Microsomes	0.901	–	–	0.804	–	0.812	0.785	0.827	–	–	0.826	0.717
FilipsPL	0.893	0.736	0.743	0.758	0.776	–	0.771	–	0.766	0.928	0.815	–
Charite	0.896	0.688	0.789	0.739	0.781	0.751	0.707	0.798	0.852	0.880	0.834	0.7
RCC	0.872	0.763	0.747	0.761	0.792	0.673	0.781	0.762	0.755	0.920	0.795	0.637
Frozenarm	0.865	0.744	0.722	0.700	0.740	0.726	0.745	0.790	0.752	0.859	0.803	0.803
ToxFit	0.862	0.744	0.757	0.697	0.738	0.729	0.729	0.752	0.689	0.862	0.803	0.791
CGL	0.866	0.742	0.566	0.747	0.749	0.737	0.759	0.727	0.775	0.880	0.817	0.738
SuperToX	0.854	–	0.560	0.711	0.742	–	–	–	–	0.862	0.732	–
Kibutz	0.865	0.750	0.694	0.708	0.729	0.737	0.757	0.779	0.587	0.838	0.787	0.666
MML	0.871	0.693	0.660	0.701	0.709	0.749	0.750	0.710	0.647	0.854	0.815	0.645
NCI	0.812	0.628	0.592	0.783	0.698	0.714	0.483	0.703	0.858	0.851	0.747	0.736
VIF	0.827	0.797	0.610	0.636	0.671	0.656	0.732	0.735	0.723	0.796	0.648	0.666
Toxic Avg	0.715	0.721	0.611	0.633	0.671	0.593	0.646	0.640	0.465	0.732	0.614	0.682
Swamidass	0.353	0.571	0.748	0.372	0.274	0.391	0.680	0.738	0.711	0.828	0.661	0.585
vNN	0.883	0.716	0.626	0.727	0.786	0.699	0.738	0.770	0.793	0.882	0.808	0.690
vNN rank	7	12	13	11	6	13	12	9	7	7	10	11

The vNN parameters were set to $h = 0.3$ and $d_0 = 1.0$. Gray cells indicate models showing performance inferior to the vNN models.

compounds. A good test of the power of a model to generate prospective predictions is time-split validation, which divides the data into "old" and "new" data and uses the former to train the model and the latter "new" data for validation (Sheridan, 2013; Liu et al., 2015). We have previously shown in a time-split validation that, whereas the accuracy of a vNN model is roughly maintained, the number of "new" compounds that it can predict is significantly reduced. However, by simply adding a few "new" compounds, the coverage increases significantly (Liu et al., 2015).

The lack of training data poses an important limitation to the vNN approach. When a dataset is too small, there is a high probability that a target molecule will have no qualified near neighbors in the dataset, and hence a high-quality prediction cannot be made. However, the lack of training data is a limitation for all machine learning methods. The difference is that most such methods build a model no matter how small the training dataset, and will always make a prediction for any input molecule without considering the reliability of the predicted result. In our view, it is better not to give a prediction at all if it is unreliable. This also alerts users to use alternative methods, including experimental measurements, to derive a reliable answer. As more experimental data become available over time, the performance of the vNN method will improve without retraining. This is in contrast to most other machine learning methods, which cannot take advantage of new data without retraining a model.

This finding is especially significant for drug discovery labs because the chemical space is restricted by the target candidates they are investigating. For example, when exploring a new drug target, it is crucial to continuously update the model with new data to ensure that the applicability domain is relevant for the new target. In a vNN-based model, this can be done easily by adding the SMILES strings of the new compounds to the reference dataset. For this reason, we believe that our web-based vNN platform has the potential to greatly accelerate the development of drugs.

AUTHOR CONTRIBUTIONS

PS, RL, and AW developed the method, analyzed the data, and wrote the manuscript. VD designed and implemented the web server.

FUNDING

The authors were supported by the U.S. Army Medical Research and Materiel Command (Fort Detrick, MD), and the Defense Threat Reduction Agency grant CBCall14-CBS-05-2-0007.

ACKNOWLEDGMENTS

The opinions and assertions contained herein are the private views of the authors and are not to be construed as official or as reflecting the views of the U.S. Army or of the U.S. Department of Defense. This paper has been approved for public release with unlimited distribution.

REFERENCES

Abbott, N. J., Rönnbäck, L., and Hansson, E. (2006). Astrocyte-endothelial interactions at the blood-brain barrier. *Nat. Rev. Neurosci.* 7, 41–53. doi: 10.1038/nrn1824

Adler, J., and Parmryd, I. (2010). Quantifying colocalization by correlation: the Pearson correlation coefficient is superior to the Mander's overlap coefficient. *Cytometry A* 77, 733–742. doi: 10.1002/cyto.a.20896

Ambudkar, S. V., Kimchi-Sarfaty, C., Sauna, Z. E., and Gottesman, M. M. (2003). P-glycoprotein: from genomics to mechanism. *Oncogene* 22, 7468–7485. doi: 10.1038/sj.onc.1206948

Ames, B. N., Durston, W. E., Yamasaki, E., and Lee, F. D. (1973). Carcinogens are mutagens: a simple test system combining liver homogenates for activation and bacteria for detection. *Proc. Natl. Acad. Sci. U.S.A.* 70, 2281–2285. doi: 10.1073/pnas.70.8.2281

Assis, D. N., and Navarro, V. J. (2009). Human drug hepatotoxicity: a contemporary clinical perspective. *Expert Opin. Drug Metab. Toxicol.* 5, 463–473. doi: 10.1517/17425250902927386

Attene-Ramos, M. S., Huang, R., Michael, S., Witt, K. L., Richard, A., Tice, R. R., et al. (2015). Profiling of the Tox21 chemical collection for mitochondrial function to identify compounds that acutely decrease mitochondrial membrane potential. *Environ. Health Perspect.* 123, 49–56. doi: 10.1289/ehp.1408642

Bento, A. P., Gaulton, A., Hersey, A., Bellis, L. J., Chambers, J., Davies, M., et al. (2014). The ChEMBL bioactivity database: an update. *Nucleic Acids Res.* 42, D1083–D1090. doi: 10.1093/nar/gkt1031

Borst, P., and Elferink, R. O. (2002). Mammalian ABC transporters in health and disease. *Annu. Rev. Biochem.* 71, 537–592. doi: 10.1146/annurev.biochem.71.102301.093055

Broccatelli, F., Carosati, E., Neri, A., Frosini, M., Goracci, L., Oprea, T. I., et al. (2011). A novel approach for predicting P-glycoprotein (ABCB1) inhibition using molecular interaction fields. *J. Med. Chem.* 54, 1740–1751. doi: 10.1021/jm101421d

Brown, C. M., Reisfeld, B., and Mayeno, A. N. (2008). Cytochromes P450: a structure-based summary of biotransformations using representative substrates. *Drug Metab. Rev.* 40, 1–100. doi: 10.1080/03602530701836662

Chen, L., Li, Y., Zhao, Q., Peng, H., and Hou, T. (2011). ADME evaluation in drug discovery. 10. Predictions of P-glycoprotein inhibitors using recursive partitioning and naive Bayesian classification techniques. *Mol. Pharm.* 8, 889–900. doi: 10.1021/mp100465q

Chen, M., Vijay, V., Shi, Q., Liu, Z., Fang, H., and Tong, W. (2011). FDA-approved drug labeling for the study of drug-induced liver injury. *Drug Discov. Today* 16, 697–703. doi: 10.1016/j.drudis.2011.05.007

Cheng, F., Li, W., Zhou, Y., Shen, J., Wu, Z., Liu, G., et al. (2012). admetSAR: a comprehensive source and free tool for assessment of chemical ADMET properties. *J. Chem. Inf. Model.* 52, 3099–3105. doi: 10.1021/ci300367a

Cherkasov, A., Muratov, E. N., Fourches, D., Varnek, A., Baskin, I. I., Cronin, M., et al. (2014). QSAR modeling: where have you been? Where are you going to? *J. Med. Chem.* 57, 4977–5010. doi: 10.1021/jm4004285

Contrera, J. F., Matthews, E. J., Kruhlak, N. L., and Benz, R. D. (2004). Estimating the safe starting dose in phase I clinical trials and no observed effect level based on QSAR modeling of the human maximum recommended daily dose. *Regul. Toxicol. Pharmacol.* 40, 185–206. doi: 10.1016/j.yrtph.2004.08.004

Czodrowski, P. (2013). hERG me out. *J. Chem. Inf. Model.* 53, 2240–2251. doi: 10.1021/ci400308z

Daina, A., Michielin, O., and Zoete, V. (2017). SwissADME: a free web tool to evaluate pharmacokinetics, drug-likeness and medicinal chemistry friendliness of small molecules. *Sci. Rep.* 7:42717. doi: 10.1038/srep42717

De Ponti, F., Poluzzi, E., and Montanaro, N. (2001). Organising evidence on QT prolongation and occurrence of Torsades de Pointes with non-antiarrhythmic drugs: a call for consensus. *Eur. J. Clin. Pharmacol.* 57, 185–209. doi: 10.1007/s002280100290

Di, L., Kerns, E. H., Hong, Y., Kleintop, T. A., McConnell, O. J., and Huryn, D. M. (2003). Optimization of a higher throughput microsomal stability screening assay for profiling drug discovery candidates. *J. Biomol. Screen.* 8, 453–462. doi: 10.1177/1087057103255988

Duan, J., Dixon, S. L., Lowrie, J. F., and Sherman, W. (2010). Analysis and comparison of 2D fingerprints: insights into database screening performance using eight fingerprint methods. *J. Mol. Graph. Model.* 29, 157–170. doi: 10.1016/j.jmgm.2010.05.008

Dunn, G., and Everitt, B. (1995). *Clinical Biostatistics: An Introduction to Evidence-based Medicine*. London: E. Arnold.

Greene, N., Fisk, L., Naven, R. T., Note, R. R., Patel, M. L., and Pelletier, D. J. (2010). Developing structure–activity relationships for the prediction of hepatotoxicity. *Chem. Res. Toxicol.* 23, 1215–1222. doi: 10.1021/tx1000865

Hansen, K., Mika, S., Schroeter, T., Sutter, A., ter Laak, A., Steger-Hartmann, T., et al. (2009). Benchmark data set for *in silico* prediction of Ames mutagenicity. *J. Chem. Inf. Model.* 49, 2077–2081. doi: 10.1021/ci900161g

Hert, J., Willett, P., Wilton, D. J., Acklin, P., Azzaoui, K., Jacoby, E., et al. (2004). Comparison of topological descriptors for similarity-based virtual screening using multiple bioactive reference structures. *Org. Biomol. Chem.* 2, 3256–3266. doi: 10.1039/b409865j

Huang, R., Xia, M., Nguyen, D.-T., Zhao, T., Sakamuru, S., Zhao, J., et al. (2016). Tox21Challenge to build predictive models of nuclear receptor and stress response pathways as mediated by exposure to environmental chemicals and drugs. *Front. Environ. Sci.* 3:85. doi: 10.3389/fenvs.2015.00085

Li, D., Chen, L., Li, Y., Tian, S., Sun, H., and Hou, T. (2014). ADMET evaluation in drug discovery. 13. Development of *in silico* prediction models for P-glycoprotein substrates. *Mol. Pharm.* 11, 716–726. doi: 10.1021/mp400450m

Liew, C. Y., Lim, Y. C., and Yap, C. W. (2011). Mixed learning algorithms and features ensemble in hepatotoxicity prediction. *J. Comput. Aided Mol. Des.* 25, 855. doi: 10.1007/s10822-011-9468-3

Liu, R., Schyman, P., and Wallqvist, A. (2015). Critically assessing the predictive power of QSAR models for human liver microsomal stability. *J. Chem. Inf. Model.* 55, 1566–1575. doi: 10.1021/acs.jcim.5b00255

Liu, R., Tawa, G., and Wallqvist, A. (2012). Locally weighted learning methods for predicting dose-dependent toxicity with application to the human maximum recommended daily dose. *Chem. Res. Toxicol.* 25, 2216–2226. doi: 10.1021/tx300279f

Liu, R., and Wallqvist, A. (2014). Merging applicability domains for *in silico* assessment of chemical mutagenicity. *J. Chem. Inf. Model.* 54, 793–800. doi: 10.1021/ci500016v

Manganaro, A., Pizzo, F., Lombardo, A., Pogliaghi, A., and Benfenati, E. (2016). Predicting persistence in the sediment compartment with a new automatic software based on the k-Nearest Neighbor (k-NN) algorithm. *Chemosphere* 144, 1624–1630. doi: 10.1016/j.chemosphere.2015.10.054

Maunz, A., Gütlein, M., Rautenberg, M., Vorgrimmler, D., Gebele, D., and Helma, C. (2013). lazar: a modular predictive toxicology framework. *Front. Pharmacol.* 4:38. doi: 10.3389/fphar.2013.00038

Meyer, J. N., Leung, M. C., Rooney, J. P., Sendoel, A., Hengartner, M. O., Kisby, G. E., et al. (2013). Mitochondria as a target of environmental toxicants. *Toxicol. Sci.* 134, 1–17. doi: 10.1093/toxsci/kft102

Muehlbacher, M., Spitzer, G. M., Liedl, K. R., and Kornhuber, J. (2011). Qualitative prediction of blood–brain barrier permeability on a large and refined dataset. *J. Comput. Aided Mol. Des.* 25, 1095–1106. doi: 10.1007/s10822-011-9478-1

Murray, M. (2006). Role of CYP pharmacogenetics and drug-drug interactions in the efficacy and safety of atypical and other antipsychotic agents. *J. Pharm. Pharmacol.* 58, 871–885. doi: 10.1211/jpp.58.7.0001

Naef, R. (2015). A generally applicable computer algorithm based on the group additivity method for the calculation of seven molecular descriptors: heat of combustion, logPO/W, logS, refractivity, polarizability, toxicity and logBB of crganic compounds; scope and limits of applicability. *Molecules* 20:18279. doi: 10.3390/molecules201018279

Pieczenik, S. R., and Neustadt, J. (2007). Mitochondrial dysfunction and molecular pathways of disease. *Exp. Mol. Pathol.* 83, 84–92. doi: 10.1016/j.yexmp.2006.09.008

Rogers, D., and Hahn, M. (2010). Extended-connectivity fingerprints. *J. Chem. Inf. Model.* 50, 742–754. doi: 10.1021/ci100050t

Sanguinetti, M. C., and Tristani-Firouzi, M. (2006). hERG potassium channels and cardiac arrhythmia. *Nature* 440, 463–469. doi: 10.1038/nature04710

Schyman, P., Liu, R., and Wallqvist, A. (2016). Using the variable-nearest neighbor method to identify P-glycoprotein substrates and inhibitors. *ACS Omega* 1, 923–929. doi: 10.1021/acsomega.6b00247

Sheridan, R. P. (2013). Time-split cross-validation as a method for estimating the goodness of prospective prediction. *J. Chem. Inf. Model.* 53, 783–790. doi: 10.1021/ci400084k

Sushko, I., Novotarskyi, S., Körner, R., Pandey, A. K., Rupp, M., Teetz, W., et al. (2011). Online chemical modeling environment (OCHEM): web platform for data storage, model development and publishing of chemical information. *J. Comput. Aided Mol. Des.* 25, 533–554. doi: 10.1007/s10822-011-9440-2

Walker, T., Grulke, C. M., Pozefsky, D., and Tropsha, A. (2010). Chembench: a cheminformatics workbench. *Bioinformatics* 26, 3000–3001. doi: 10.1093/bioinformatics/btq556

Wang, S., Li, Y., Wang, J., Chen, L., Zhang, L., Yu, H., et al. (2012). ADMET evaluation in drug discovery. 12. Development of binary classification models for prediction of hERG potassium channel blockage. *Mol. Pharm.* 9, 996–1010. doi: 10.1021/mp300023x

Wang, Y., Xiao, J., Suzek, T. O., Zhang, J., Wang, J., and Bryant, S. H. (2009). PubChem: a public information system for analyzing bioactivities of small molecules. *Nucleic Acids Res.* 37, W623–W633. doi: 10.1093/nar/gkp456

Waring, M. J., Arrowsmith, J., Leach, A. R., Leeson, P. D., Mandrell, S., Owen, R. M., et al. (2015). An analysis of the attrition of drug candidates from four major pharmaceutical companies. *Nat. Rev. Drug Discov.* 14, 475–486. doi: 10.1038/nrd4609

Weininger, D. (1988). SMILES, a chemical language and information system. 1. Introduction to methodology and encoding rules. *J. Chem. Inf. Comput. Sci.* 28, 31–36. doi: 10.1021/ci00057a005

Xu, J. J., Henstock, P. V., Dunn, M. C., Smith, A. R., Chabot, J. R., and de Graaf, D. (2008). Cellular Imaging predictions of clinical drug-induced liver injury. *Toxicol. Sci.* 105, 97–105. doi: 10.1093/toxsci/kfn109

Xu, Y., Dai, Z., Chen, F., Gao, S., Pei, J., and Lai, L. (2015). Deep learning for drug-induced liver injury. *J. Chem. Inf. Model.* 55, 2085–2093. doi: 10.1021/acs.jcim.5b00238

Zheng, W., and Tropsha, A. (2000). Novel variable selection quantitative structure–property relationship approach based on the k-nearest-neighbor principle. *J. Chem. Inf. Comput. Sci.* 40, 185–194. doi: 10.1021/ci980033m

7

Extending *in Silico* Protein Target Prediction Models to Include Functional Effects

Lewis H. Mervin[1], Avid M. Afzal[1], Lars Brive[2], Ola Engkvist[3] and Andreas Bender[1]*

[1] Centre for Molecular Informatics, Department of Chemistry, University of Cambridge, Cambridge, United Kingdom, [2] Cygnal Bioscience, Pixbo, Sweden, [3] Hit Discovery, Discovery Sciences, IMED Biotech Unit, AstraZeneca, Gothenburg, Sweden

***Correspondence:**
Andreas Bender
ab454@cam.ac.uk

In silico protein target deconvolution is frequently used for mechanism-of-action investigations; however existing protocols usually do not predict compound functional effects, such as activation or inhibition, upon binding to their protein counterparts. This study is hence concerned with including functional effects in target prediction. To this end, we assimilated a bioactivity training set for 332 targets, comprising 817,239 active data points with unknown functional effect (binding data) and 20,761,260 inactive compounds, along with 226,045 activating and 1,032,439 inhibiting data points from functional screens. Chemical space analysis of the data first showed some separation between compound sets (binding and inhibiting compounds were more similar to each other than both binding and activating or activating and inhibiting compounds), providing a rationale for implementing functional prediction models. We employed three different architectures to predict functional response, ranging from simplistic random forest models ('Arch1') to cascaded models which use separate binding and functional effect classification steps ('Arch2' and 'Arch3'), differing in the way training sets were generated. Fivefold stratified cross-validation outlined cascading predictions provides superior precision and recall based on an internal test set. We next prospectively validated the architectures using a temporal set of 153,467 of in-house data points (after a 4-month interim from initial data extraction). Results outlined Arch3 performed with the highest target class averaged precision and recall scores of 71% and 53%, which we attribute to the use of inactive background sets. Distance-based applicability domain (AD) analysis outlined that Arch3 provides superior extrapolation into novel areas of chemical space, and thus based on the results presented here, propose as the most suitable architecture for the functional effect prediction of small molecules. We finally conclude including functional effects could provide vital insight in future studies, to annotate cases of unanticipated functional changeover, as outlined by our CHRM1 case study.

Keywords: target prediction, activation, inhibition, cheminformatics, functional effects, mechanism-of-action, chemical space, AD-AUC

INTRODUCTION

Target deconvolution is an important step in the subsequent analysis of data gleaned from phenotypic screenings, to identify the modulated targets of active compounds and enable the continued dissection of the biological processes involved in a system of interest (Terstappen et al., 2007; Raida, 2011; Kotz, 2012; Lee and Bogyo, 2013). One important additional parameter of consideration is the functional modulation of targets, since its activation or inhibition (in the simplest case of allowing only for two types of functional effects) may positively or negatively modulate a pathway, which in turn may relate in different ways to an observed phenotype (Parker et al., 1993; Bauer-Mehren et al., 2009; Dosa and Amin, 2016).

One example of this is Bone morphogenetic protein 1 (BMP1), which was identified as a key target linked to cytostaticity from a screening cascade discerning the cytotoxic and cytostatic tendencies of compounds (Mervin et al., 2016). In the absence of functional information for the respective target, and since activation of BMP signaling in prostate carcinoma cells is known to be cytostatic (hence its inactivation would not explain the observed phenotype) (Wahdan-Alaswad et al., 2012), the authors were forced to hypothesize that cytostatic agents *may* activate BMP1. Another study rationalized the polypharmacology of sleep-inducing compounds in rat, (which, without functional annotation) were forced to stipulate that bioactive compounds with multi-target activity *may* elicit their synergistic sleep parameter activity through inhibition of Histamine Receptor H1 (HRH1) and activation of Cholinergic Receptor Muscarinic 4 (CHRM4) (since the biological evidence at hand for both targets advocates this rationalization) (Drakakis et al., 2017). Sertindole, a withdrawn approved drug, was also experimentally determined within the study to changeover functional activity. Despite profiles linked to prolonged sleep bouts, the compound was linked to hyperactivity, not inhibition, at key targets implicated with increased bouts of sleep, which further demonstrates how the functional behavior of compounds needs to be considered to understand phenotypic response in biological systems.

One approach to target deconvolution is *in silico* target deconvolution, which is a well-established computational technique capable of inferring compound MOA by utilizing known bioactivity information (Koutsoukas et al., 2011; Wang et al., 2013; Lavecchia and Cerchia, 2016). This technique is well established in the areas for the deconvolution of phenotypic screens (Poroikov et al., 2001; Geronikaki et al., 2004; Liggi et al., 2014) and the identification of compound-side effects via bioactivity profiling of off-targets (Lounkine et al., 2012; Barton and Riley, 2016). The characterization of the functional effects of compounds is often a principle shortcoming for current *in silico* methods, since many protocols only provide probability for compound affinity at a target (Drakakis et al., 2013; Koutsoukas et al., 2013; Mervin et al., 2015).

Existing protocols, such as the Similarity Ensemble Approach (SEA) (Keiser et al., 2007) and Prediction of Activity Spectra for Substances (PASS) (Lagunin et al., 2000), provide functional annotation by training on a compound set extracted from the MDL Drug Data Report [MDDR] (2006). These implementations however only utilize active bioactivity data (experimentally validated negative bioactivity data are disregarded), which has been shown to hinder performance. Additional problems with MDDR are inconsistent annotation, since many activity classes are not on the target level (for example the activity class 'anti-helminthic activity') and relatively small numbers of compound-target pairs are available for modeling, compared to other current databases (Lagunin et al., 2000). Other cheminformatics approaches discriminate between agonist from antagonist classifications of ligands at nuclear receptors across targets simultaneously (within a single-model architecture) (Lagarde et al., 2017). This architecture could negatively affect performance due to the imbalance between the functional data and the requirement to assign probability scores across all target proteins.

We have in this work explored various cascaded approaches to predict the functional effects of orphan compounds and contrasted these with a single-model architecture (similar to previous approaches). To this end, we have assimilated a dataset of 22,836,983 compound-target annotations available in the Chemistry Connect (Muresan et al., 2011) repository across a range of G-protein-coupled receptors (GPCRs), Nuclear Hormone Receptors (NHRs), ion channels and transporters. The dataset comprises 817,239 binders (unknown if activating or inhibiting) and 20,761,260 non-binding compounds from binding assays, as well as 226,045 activating and 1,032,439 inhibiting compounds from functional assays, spanning a total of 332 protein targets.

This work explores three different *in silico* architectures for functional target prediction which are summarized in **Figure 1**. **Figure 1A** outlines Architecture 1 (Arch1), a Random Forest (RF) algorithm trained with all functional labels across all targets within a single model [hence, an approach using only active (functional) data], which serves as a baseline to compare the cascaded, and hence more complex, architectures. Architecture 2 (Arch2), outlined in **Figure 1B**, is the first of two cascaded approaches, combining stage 1 target prediction with subsequent stage 2 functional prediction, which we rationalize could improve performance due to the cascaded nature of models. Stage 2 of Arch2 includes a single RF model trained on both activating and inhibiting compounds during stage 2. In comparison, **Figure 1C** depicts Architecture 3 (Arch3), which is based on an ensemble of two independent RFs trained on either activating or inhibiting compounds separately versus an inactive background set.

To establish the optimal model architecture, we conducted fivefold stratified cross validation for the three different modeling approaches. Models were also prospectively validated using an external testing set of 153,467 compounds, spanning 306 targets extracted from all functional in-house AstraZeneca data after a 4-month interim from initial training set extraction. The cross validation and time-split performance of the approaches has provided guidance into the choice of architecture to be deployed in-house for future triage processes.

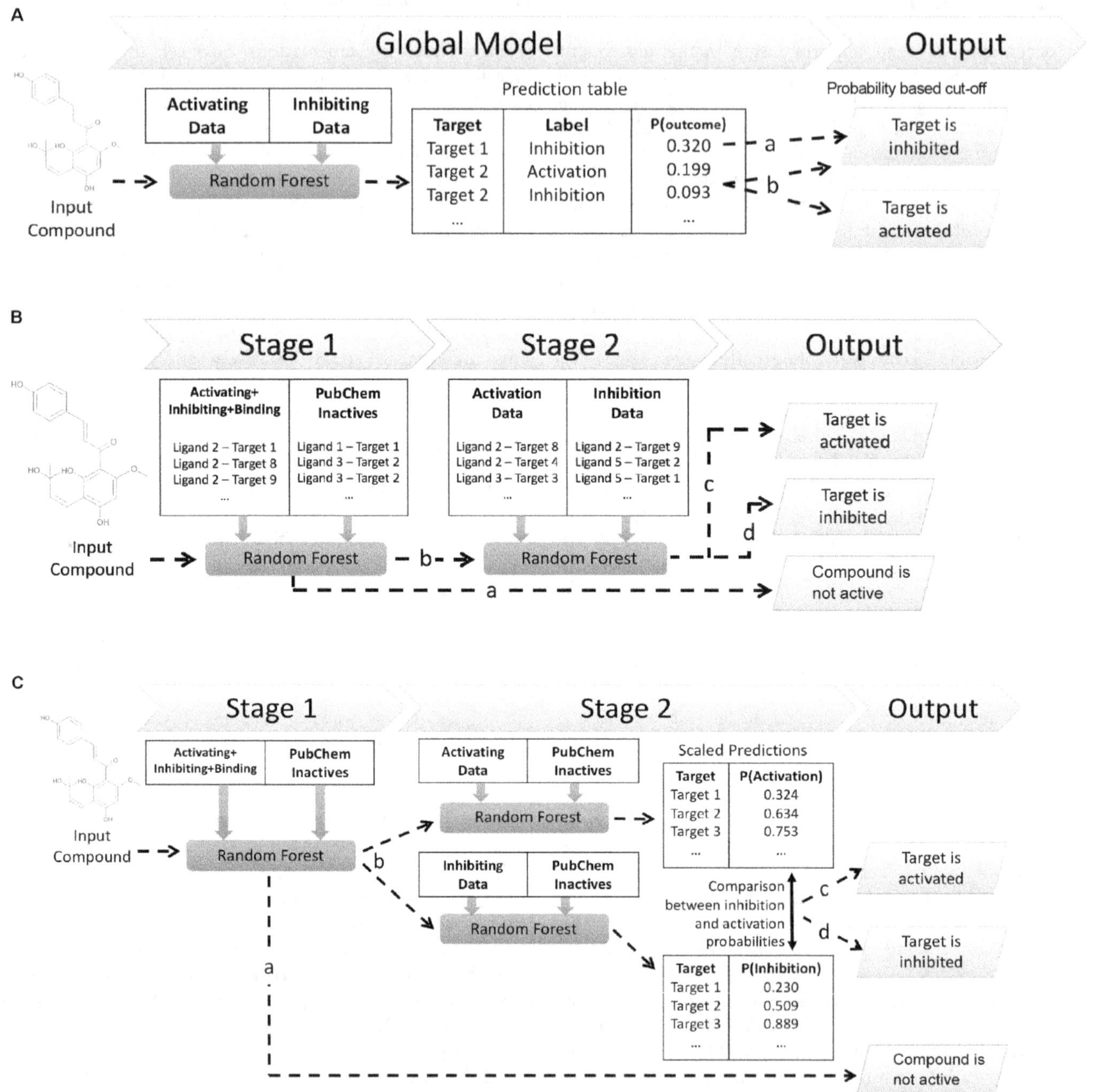

FIGURE 1 | Different architectures employed for functional target prediction in this work. **(A)** Architecture 1 (Arch1). A single random forest (RF) algorithm is trained with the activating and inhibiting compounds across all targets. Model output is a list of functional predictions across all targets, ranked by probability for a target and corresponding functional label, '*p(target_outcome)*'. A probability threshold is employed to generate activating and inhibiting predictions. The functional label with the highest probability is selected if a compound is predicted as both activating and inhibiting, i.e., 'Target 2' (line *b*) is assigned the activating label if using a probability cut-off of 0.092. **(B)** Architecture 2 (Arch2). Stage 1 target prediction utilizes RF target prediction models trained using active (activating, inhibiting or binding only) and inactive compounds on a per target basis. Compounds predicted inactive during Stage 1 (line *a*) are removed from further cascading and annotated as inactive. Compounds predicted to be active during Stage 1 are subsequently profiled using Stage 2 functional prediction (line *b*), comprising RF models trained on the activating and inhibiting compounds on a per-target basis. Compounds are annotated as '*activating'* (line *c*) if the probability of activation is greater than inhibition (line *c*), or '*inhibiting'* if the probability of inhibition is greater than activation (line *d*). **(C)** Architecture 3 (Arch3). Stage 1 target prediction is employed in the same manner as Arch2. Compounds predicted to be active (line *b*) are subsequently profiled at Stage 2 using two independent RF models, trained using either activating or inhibiting compounds and an inactive compound set, and which are Platt scaled to ensure they are directly comparable. The probabilities of activation or inhibition generated by the two models and compared to deduce a functional prediction. A compound is annotated as '*activating'* if the likelihood of activation is greater than inhibition (line *c*), or as '*inhibiting'* if the probability of inhibition is greater than activation (line *d*). Although Arch2 and Arch3 enforce functional prediction in cases of both low activating and inhibiting probabilities, this is preferred for this study rather than the addition of an extra label (e.g., predicted binding only).

MATERIALS AND METHODS

Sources of Compound Training Data

AstraZeneca bioactivity data from Chemistry Connect (Muresan et al., 2011) was mined for functional data with bioactivities (IC_{50} and EC_{50}) better than or equal to 10 μM and annotated with functional terms based on BioAssay Ontology (BAO) assay classifications (Vempati et al., 2012; Abeyruwan et al., 2014). The resulting dataset was filtered for the GPCR, NHR, ion channel and transporter targets, since they are considered to have the highest functional annotation accuracy (in-house) and encompass large numbers of activators which are not given in the case of enzymes.

The full complement of functional annotations includes various mechanisms, such as 'activation,' 'antagonism,' 'inverse agonism,' 'opening,' 'closing' and 'modulation' (full list shown in **Table 1**), which were chosen by BAO as the appropriate units to describe what each assay measures from assay endpoints. As a simple example, the unit EC_{50} was linked to 'activation,' whilst IC_{50} was annotated with 'inhibition.' More complex endpoints were assigned such that the measured activity of NHRs, GPCRs and ligand-gated ion channel mechanism-of-action (MOAs) were annotated as 'agonist,' 'antagonist,' or 'partial antagonist,' whilst voltage-gated ion channel MOAs were assigned 'opening' or 'closing' annotations.

In this study, we classified all compounds into the more simplified binary labels of 'activating' or 'inhibiting' endpoints using an internal mapping scheme (**Table 1**). Although imposing only two (activation and inhibition) functional labels may be an over-simplification, this is preferred to the complex situation resulting from the original complex BAO labeling, since it reduces training data into a binary problem per protein target, ensures larger numbers of compounds are retrained within each MOA, and that generated predictions are easily compared between the complete spectra of functional predictions between targets. It is also less algorithmically difficult to build classification models compared to regression, thereby usually improving performance.

Compounds with conflicting activating and inhibiting annotations were removed from the training data. The resulting functional data set provided 226,045 activating and 1,032,439 inhibiting compounds spanning 320 different targets, the distribution of which is shown in **Figure 2A**, with a median of 186 ± 1,526 activating-target compound pairs and 1,190 ± 5,123 inhibiting-target compound pairs per target. The distribution of ratios between the functional labels (overall median ratio of 5.0 ± 27.4 inhibiting:activating compounds) and distribution of functional set sizes (overall median of 163 ± 1,462 and 948 ± 4,955 for the activating and inhibiting classes, respectively) are shown in **Figures 2B,C**.

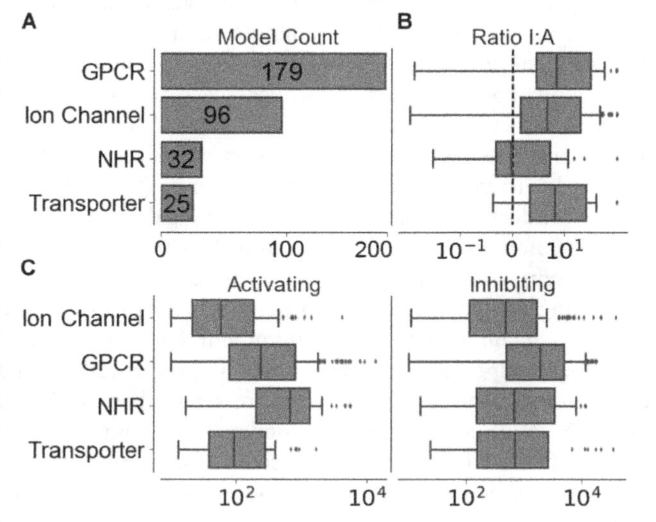

FIGURE 2 | Distribution of training data across individual models in the four target protein classes modeled. **(A)** Number of targets modeled. **(B)** Ratio between inhibiting and activating compound-target data points. **(C)** Distribution of activating and inhibiting compounds available for training.

TABLE 1 | Functional mapping schema employed in this study.

Original BAO label	Simplified label
Activation	Activator
Agonism	Activator
Antagonism	Inhibitor
Blocking	Inhibitor
Closing	Inhibitor
Inhibition	Inhibitor
Inverse agonism	Inhibitor
Opening	Activator

The functional labels of biological screens were reduced into the binary classifications of 'activating' or 'inhibiting' to reduce the complexity of the modeling in this study.

Bioactivity data was also extracted from the same database, for compounds with binding activity (K_i or K_d) better than or equal to 10 μM, as a supplementary source of training data for cascaded Stage 1 target prediction (Arch1 does not cascade predictions and so does not utilize binding information). The resulting data provided 817,239 binding compound-target pairs spanning 300 different targets, comprising a median and standard deviation of 752 ± 4,954 active compounds per target.

Non-binding (inactive) compounds were extracted from PubChem in a same manner as described in Mervin et al. (2015) which involved mapping to NCBI Gene IDs (GIDs) and Protein IDs (PIDs) to the Bioactivity Assay IDs (AIDs) held in the PubChem BioAssay repository for compounds annotated as 'inactive' in deposited bioactivity screens, using the PubChem REST (Kim et al., 2016) and PubChem PUG resources (NCBI, 2007). AstraZeneca high-throughput screens deposited in the HTS DataMart (an internal database of HTS information) were also mined for non-binding compounds from bioactivity screens with bioactivities (K_i, K_d, IC_{50}, and EC_{50}) greater than 10 μM. Compounds with conflicting non-binding annotations were removed from the training data.

To compile additional non-binding compounds for proteins not covered in the internal database or PubChem (hence, for cases where insufficient numbers of confirmed negatives were available), additional putative inactive compounds were sampled from PubChem using a sphere exclusion algorithm. In this protocol, compounds with a Tanimoto similarity coefficient (Tc) value of less than or equal to 0.4 are sampled as a background of putative inactive chemical space. Although sphere exclusion selection leads to artificially inflated performance, this is a necessary step to ensure the existence of a putative negative bioactivity class with sufficient coverage of inactive space to conduct target prediction. The resulting dataset includes 20,761,260 non-binders with a median of 32,320 ± 84,491 non-binding compound-target pairs per protein target.

Training compounds were subjected to pre-processing and filtered to retain targets with a minimum 10 activating and inhibiting compounds, to ensure only targets encompassing sufficient functional chemical space are retained for training. Although not essential for Stage 2 model training, binding data was also filtered for five or more compounds, to ensure the minimum number of binding data is equal to the number of folds used for cross validation. Supplementary Figure 1 shows a Venn diagram of the bioactivity data available for training, comprising 332 models. Overall, the training set includes 20,761,260 non-binding compounds, 817,239 binders, 226,045 activating and 1,032,439 inhibiting data points.

Compound Pre-processing and Fingerprint Generation

RDKit (Landrum, 2006) (Version 2016.09.1) was employed to remove structures not containing carbon from the dataset, and to retain only compounds with atomic numbers between 21–32, 36–52, and greater than 53, as well as with a molecular weight between 100 and 1000 Da, to retain a more 'drug-like' (in the widest sense) chemical space. Compounds were standardized using an in-house (OEChem Toolkits, 2017) script, and RDKit was used to generate 2,048-bit (circular) Morgan fingerprints (Morgan, 1965), with the radius set to 2.

In Silico Modeling

Single Model Functional Prediction (Arch1)

The first model architecture, Arch1 (shown in **Figure 1A**), utilizes a single RF trained using the activating and inhibiting data across all available targets, which is intended to serve as a baseline comparison against similar online web-based approaches such as SEA and PASS, which do not necessarily consider (non-)binding information or consider multiple functional labels within one model.

A RF classifier of 100 trees, with the number of features set to '*auto*' and max depth set to '*20*,' was implemented in Scikit-learn (Pedregosa et al., 2011), and trained using the binary matrix of activating and inhibiting compound fingerprints across all targets. The single-model provides a RF (class) probability (computed as the mean predicted class probabilities of the trees in the forest) of activating or inhibiting a target on an individual compound basis, when considering all other functional predictions for available targets. Generated probabilities are subsequently converted into binary predictions based on a probability cut-off [for example above 0.2 (line a) and 0.09 (line b) in **Figure 1A**], which is described in-depth throughout the next paragraph. The functional label with the highest probability is selected in situations when a target is considered both activating and inhibiting labels. For example, Target 2 would be considered activated when using a cut-off of 0.092 (as indicated by line 'b' in **Figure 1A**).

In order to compare Arch1 to the cascaded methods, a probability cut-off was applied to generate a final set of functional predictions from the probabilities generated. This threshold was defined as the probability providing the optimal F_1-score performance (i.e., target or class performance averaged across the inactive, activating and inhibiting labels) from one percentile increments across the distribution of all scores obtained during cross validation and prospective validation, in a similar procedure to Perezgonzalez (2015). This is an important step since a robust method to fairly compare the different approaches is required, a topic which will be discussed in more detail in the section entitled "*Precision and recall versus. BEDROC and PR-AUC.*"

Stage 1 Target Prediction (Arch2 and Arch3)

Both Arch2 and Arch3 use Stage 1 target prediction. Here, input compounds are subjected to Stage 1 prediction and predicted as binding (or otherwise non-binding) based on the condition that the output probability of binding is greater than non-binding. Compounds predicted non-binding at this point are removed from the further cascaded profiling, whilst compounds predicted to bind are retained for Stage 2 functional prediction.

Stage 1 target prediction employs a similar target prediction protocol to the one described previously by Mervin et al. (2016) utilizing large scale inactive chemical space and active compounds from binding and functional assays. A RF classifier of 100 trees, with the number of features and max depth set to '*auto*' and the '*class_weight*' set to '*balanced*' was implemented in Scikit-learn. The RF was trained using the binary matrix of inactive and active compound fingerprints on a per target bases, whilst supplying the '*sample_weight*' parameter within the '*fit*' method with the ratio of active and inactive training compounds. The implementation of stage 1 target prediction does not differ between Arch2 and Arch3.

Stage 2 prediction (Arch2)

Stage 2 prediction is employed in two different way between the different model architectures of Arch2 and Arch3. Both techniques aim to assign an activating or inhibiting functional prediction to input compounds predicted as active for a particular target during stage 1 prediction.

As visualized in **Figure 1B**, Arch2 employed two cascaded RF models overall (one RF for Stage 1 and one RF for Stage 2). The RF for Stage 2 used the same hyper-parameters as Stage 1, and was trained using the activating and inhibiting compound fingerprints on a per-target basis. This RF was calibrated using Platt Scaling using the Scikit-learn '*calibrate_classification_cv*' method, with the number of calibration and validation folds set to '*3*'. Thus, the predictions generated by the Stage 2 RF can be directly interpreted as a likelihood that an input compound is an activator or inhibitor.

A functional prediction is made for the functional label with the largest probability output from the second cascaded model, i.e., if the probability of activation is higher than that for inhibition, then the compound is classified as an activator (and *vice-versa)*. Thus, this procedure does not distinguish for instances when no confident prediction can be made for the second cascaded prediction. This behavior is preferred for the purpose of this study, since enforcing a prediction for the highest label regardless of confidence ensures the output between Arch1, Arch2, and Arch3 can be compared within this study.

Stage 2 prediction (Arch3)

Figure 1C illustrates Arch3, which employed three RF models overall (one for Stage 1 and *two* independent RF models for Stage 2). Both Stage 2 RFs utilize the same parameters as in Stage 1, and are trained separately for activating and inhibiting compounds, respectively, versus a set of inactive compounds. Probabilities generated by both algorithms were calibrated using Platt Scaling via the Scikit-learn '*calibrate_classification_cv*' method, with the number of calibration and validation folds set to '3'. Scaling the independent probabilities in this manner enables the comparison between the activating and inhibiting probabilities from both algorithms, even though the two are distinct models. Functional predictions are made for input compounds by selecting the activating or inhibiting label with the largest probability.

Performance Measures: Precision and Recall versus BEDROC and PR-AUC

Although the Boltzmann-Enhanced Discrimination of the Receiver Operating Characteristic (BEDROC) (Truchon and Bayly, 2007) and Precision-Recall Area Under the Curve (PR-AUC) scores are frequently used to describe virtual screening performance, this is not an appropriate metric to compare the outputs between all the models benchmarked in this study. Such metrics are based on the distribution of probabilities for the classes for each method; however these are not comparable between the three architectures explored, since they are on different scales, represent different likelihoods, and are processed to generate an overall functional prediction in different ways.

For example, Arch1 is a *single model* with multiple labels hence the generated scores are low, since they are distributed over all 664 target-function effects which overall must sum to '1.0'. In comparison, Arch2 uses a binary classifier on a *per-target* basis for Stage 2, with hence only two probabilities are produced for activating or inhibiting, whose output sum to '1.0'. Thus, these values comprise comparatively higher values since they are shared between two output labels. Furthermore, Arch3 uses *two* different binary classifiers to deduce a final prediction in Stage 2, using the activating and inhibiting labels normalized with a background of inactive compounds. Thus, the probabilities of these activating and inhibiting labels do not sum to '1.0', since they are distinct models. Therefore, we considered that precision, recall and F_1-score (i.e., the actual output expected from the deployed models) are the most suitable and robust metrics to compare the performance of methods in the current situation.

Cross Validation Methodology

Fivefold stratified cross validation was employed in Scikit-learn using the '*StratifiedKFold*' method, ensuring training data is randomly shuffled and seeded. In this procedure, the non-binding and binding (only available for Arch2 and Arch3), and activating and inhibiting training data is split into five folds, whilst maintaining the ratio between compounds with different labels in each split. Each fold is used as a test and train set for cascaded Stage 1 and Stage 2 training and prediction. Binding data is only utilized within training sets for Stage 1 in the cascaded approaches, since it is only used to supplement Stage 1 training data and not employed during Stage 2.

The ranked list of functional compound predictions is used to calculate the optimal threshold for Arch1 (as discussed above) and used to generate precision, recall, and F_1-score for Arch1, whilst the predicted outcome for the activating and inhibiting compounds from each test set is used to calculate the corresponding performance of the cascaded models. **Figure 2** gives details into the size of targets in terms of the data points available for modeling and ratio of inhibiting to activating compounds, which is known to influence the predictivity of target prediction models (Koutsoukas et al., 2013).

Prospective Validation Data Set

AstraZeneca bioactivity data was mined in the same manner as described above after a 4-month interim (exactly the 4 months after extracting training data) to obtain an external dataset of compounds to prospectively validate the models. Compounds with affinities better or equal to 10 μM were extracted and employed for cascaded Stage 1 and Stage 2 prediction. The dataset includes a total of 63,640 activating and 89,827 inhibiting compounds for 306 targets (with the number of compounds per target classification shown in Supplementary Table 1), spanning both similar and dissimilar chemical space compared to the training set (prospective validation chemical space analysis shown in Supplementary Figure 2), with overall median Tc values of 0.51 ± 0.21 and 0.62 ± 0.19, respectively. Class-averaged precision, recall and F_1-score were calculated for each architecture during temporal validation, since some targets comprise only very few test set compounds, which would hence produce unreliable performance metrics.

RESULTS

Functional Data Available in AstraZeneca

We first analyzed the nearest-neighbor similarity distribution per-target for each classification, to explore the chemical space of the functional dataset and to rationalize to what extent the different sets of compounds can be distinguished in chemical similarity space and thus a rationale for implementing and evaluating functional target prediction models.

Figure 3 shows the results of the nearest-neighbor similarity distribution per-target for each classification. The overall distributions highlight that binding (active) and inhibiting compounds ("B-I") are more similar to each other (median of 0.958) than both binding and activating ("B-A") and activating and inhibiting ("A-I") compounds (median similarities of 0.841 and 0.835, respectively). Overall, this analysis indicated there is some separation between the activating and inhibiting classes

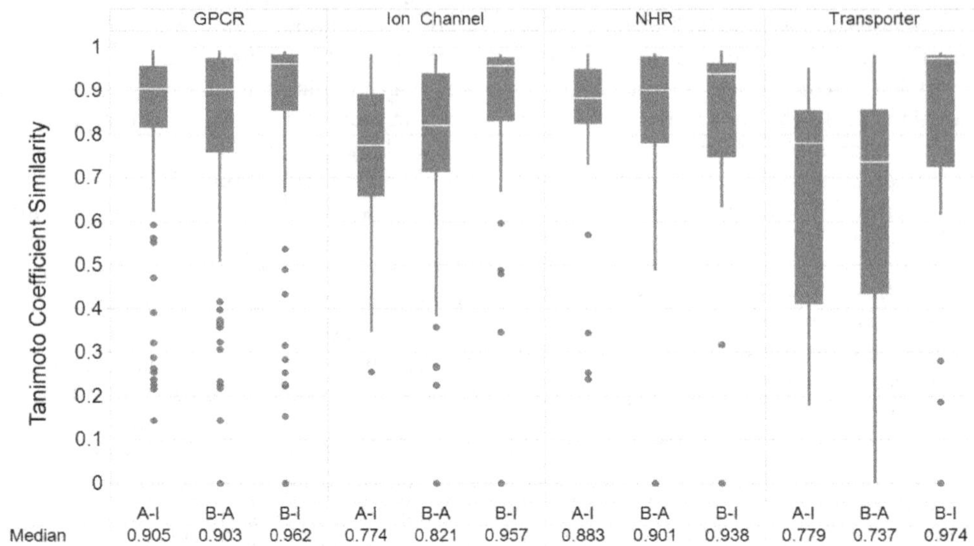

FIGURE 3 | Nearest-neighbor Tanimoto similarity of active, activating and inhibiting compounds. ECFP_4 fingerprint similarity of the compounds to compare the three different bioactivity types, including comparison between activating versus inhibiting compounds (*A-I*), ligand binding-only (active) versus activating (*B-A*) and binding-only (active) versus inhibiting (*B-I*). The most similar compound was retained per-compound, per-target to indicate the nearest neighbor similarity. The overall distribution indicates that inhibiting compounds are more similar to their binding counterparts (*B-I*), in comparison to the other *A-B* and *B-A* comparisons.

of compounds in chemical space, giving us a rationale for implementing and evaluating functional target prediction models (statistical analysis of chemical similarity between the target classes shown in Supplementary Table 2).

The GPCR class comprises the highest median NN similarity between the activating and inhibiting compounds of 0.905 (and an overall median of 0.923 between the three sets), a finding that is corroborated in literature since small structural modifications to GPCR-targeted ligands are known to convey major changes in their functional activity, converting agonists into antagonists and *vice-versa* (Dosa and Amin, 2016). Changes in certain moieties are shown to affect binding outcome more than others; for example, one study highlighted that steric modifications near a basic nitrogen, methylation of indoles, and aniline nitrogen substitutions appeared to play important roles in determining functional activity while keeping overall structure (as captured in the fingerprints employed in the current work) rather similar (Dosa and Amin, 2016). The close proximity between functional labels may be reflected in the performance of the models, since the overlap of features present in both sets confounds the separation between labels (Koutsoukas et al., 2013).

Nuclear hormone receptors are ranked as the second most similar target class based on the NN similarity between activating and inhibiting compounds, with a median Tc of 0.883. A range of ligand modifications can inter-convert functional activity due to changes in the directions in which these ligand R-groups are positioned within the ligand-binding domains (LBDs) of NHR cores (Huang et al., 2010). For example, one study explicitly outlined which ring system extensions alter the functional effects of activating compounds at the NHR estrogen receptor (ER), due to the protrusion of additional groups displacing the agonist conformation of α-helices in the LBD (Parker et al., 1993). In comparison, ion channels and transporters comprise comparatively dissimilar chemistry between compound sets, with median Tanimoto similarities of 0.774 and 0.779, respectively, between the activating and inhibiting compounds, giving rise to the expectation of better classification performance for those datasets.

Cross Validation Results

We next performed stratified fivefold cross-validation (as described in the section "Materials and Methods") and calculated precision, recall and F_1-score metrics for 332 targets averaged over the fivefolds. Overall performance for each of the architectures was next calculated using the class-average precision and recall for the three functional labels (namely non-binding, inhibiting and activating) obtained over the 332 targets, the results of which are shown in **Table 2**.

It can be seen that the Archl architecture optimized for F_1-score performed with overall class-averaged precision and recall performance of 84.5 ± 12.1 and 68.7 ± 17.5, respectively, which provides a baseline performance for what we expected to be superior (or certainly more complex) model architectures. This was indeed found to be the case, since Arch2 and Arch3 performed with target averaged precision and recall scores of 89.4 ± 9.8 and 79.2 ± 11.4, and 92.0 ± 9.1 and 82.9 ± 11.6, respectively (using a cut-off for the label with the largest probabilities as described in the section "Materials and Methods").

In order to understand the performance distribution across different protein class labels, we next averaged precision, recall and F_1-scores across the three functional labels for each of the GPCR, NHR, Ion Channel and NHR target classifications, as illustrated in the second row of **Table 2**. Overall, results from

TABLE 2 | Target-averaged and class-averaged performance across the inactive, activating and inhibiting labels.

		Arch1 (optimal F_1-score cut-off)		Arch2		Arch3	
		Precision	**Recall**	**Precision**	**Recall**	**Precision**	**Recall**
Cross validation	Target averaged	84.5 ± 12.1	68.7 ± 17.5	89.4 ± 9.8	79.2 ± 11.4	92.0 ± 9.1	82.9 ± 11.6
	Class averaged	76.1 ± 0.2	68.6 ± 0.9	89.3 ± 1.9	79.5 ± 2.7	91.9 ± 1.7	82.9 ± 3.4
Prospective validation	Class averaged	59.5 ± 3.2	48.1 ± 1.3	70.9 ± 4.0	52.9 ± 3.6	70.8 ± 3.5	53.1 ± 3.6
	Class averaged (Correct at Stage 1)	–	–	72.4 ± 3.3	71.0 ± 2.0	72.3 ± 2.8	71.3 ± 2.5

Performance metrics are calculated by averaging the scores obtained over all targets or classes, for each of the three labels (inactive, activating, inhibiting), which are then averaged.

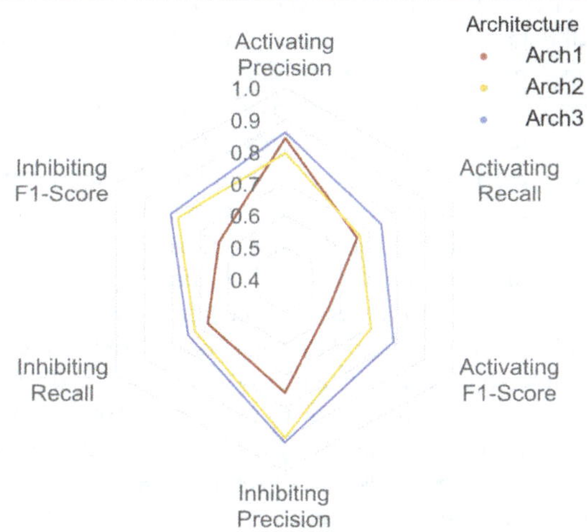

FIGURE 4 | Inhibiting and activating class averaged performance of the three architectures during cross validation. The inactive, activating and inhibiting label performance for Arch1 (red), Arch2 (yellow) and Arch3 (blue) are shown. The performance profile of the three models illustrate that the two cascaded models outperform the single-model architecture. Arch3 is also shown to outperform Arch2, which is particularly evident for the activating recall and precision labels. Arch1 performance was calculated using the threshold comprising the highest overall F_1-score.

this analysis outlined that the baseline model performed with the lowest class averaged precision and recall scores of 76.1 ± 0.2 and 68.6 ± 0.9, whilst Arch2 performed with target class averaged precision and recall of 89.3 ± 1.9 and 79.5 ± 2.7, and Arch3 performed with the best scores of 91.9 ± 1.7 and 82.9 ± 3.4, respectively.

A detailed breakdown of the protein target class averaged performance for the activating and inhibiting labels is shown in **Figure 4**. Overall, the inhibiting (more often majority) label performed with an overall class-averaged precision and recall of 75.5 and 67.3 for Arch1, 89.5 and 72.0 for Arch2 and 91.0 and 74.5 for Arch3. In comparison, the activating (more often minority) label performed with precision and recall scores of 84.2 and 65.8 for Arch1, 79.6 and 66.7 for Arch2, and 86.1 and 74.4 for Arch3, respectively. Hence, we conclude that Arch3 provides the optimal performance across the architectures assessed here.

Our results indicate models frequently perform with higher precision than recall (i.e., they are more certain about positive predictions they *do* make, than being able to identify compounds with the respective label across all of chemical space). Although Arch2 and Arch3 provide overall superior performance profiles, Arch1 exhibits superior activating precision (84.2) over Arch2 (79.6). We attribute this to the fact that Arch1 relies solely on activating or inhibiting compounds, and hence a more simplistic input space compared to Arch 2 and Arch3, which results in a larger number of incorrectly predicted activating compounds with fewer positive predictions with a greater propensity to be correct.

Arch2 and Arch3 also exhibit lower recall compared to precision, which is a consequence of the two-stage functional prediction, when false-negative binding predictions from Stage 1 are not used as input for Stage 2 prediction. Our findings also indicate that Arch3 can best handle the imbalance between inhibiting and activating labels compared to Arch2, to obtain higher activating recall and precision performance, a trend which will be discussed in more detail in the following.

In order to test if the activating and inhibiting performance of Arch3 models lie above that of the Arch2 approach (and hence there is statistical value in normalizing the models using a background of inactive compounds when cascading predictions), we next conducted a two-sample Kolmogorov–Smirnov (KS) test for the precision, recall and F_1-score values obtained for Arch2 and Arch3 (overall results are summarized in the following, more detailed results are shown in Supplementary Table 3). The KS test produces p-values less than 0.05 (5% confidence threshold) for the activating precision, recall and F_1-score (3.96^{E-04}, 7.90^{E-05}, and 1.95^{E-05}, respectively) and inhibiting F_1-score (4.93^{E-03}), indicating that Arch3 performance is statistically improved for these performance parameters, compared to the Arch2 model architecture.

Overall, ~50% (166) of the Arch2 and ~64% (214) of the Arch3 models performed with precision and recall values greater than or equal to 0.8, as shown in **Figure 5**. Thus, functional effects of compounds can be predicted with respectable performance for over half the target modeled. Conversely, only ~40% (133) of the Arch1 models performed with equivalent precision and recall values above 0.8, as shown by the lower distribution of scores.

In total, eight targets failed to predict activating or inhibiting molecules using Arch2 and hence received precision and recall values of '0' (shown as outliers in **Figure 5**). Seven of the eight targets were assigned such scores since no predictions were generated for the activating label, with five of these targets

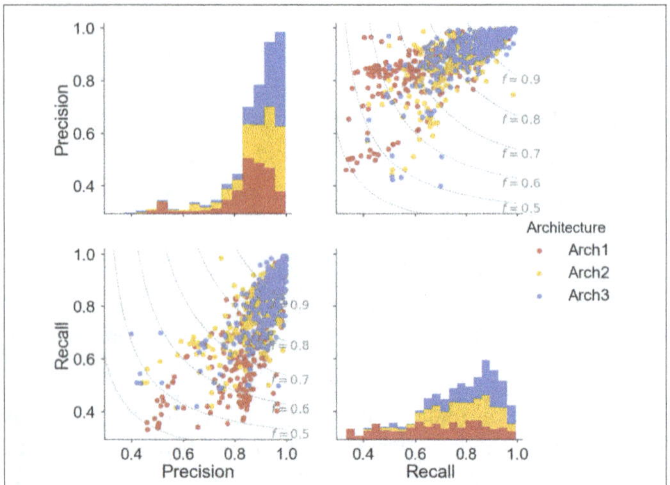

FIGURE 5 | Pairwise distribution of the relationship between precision and recall scores for each architecture. Subplot grids in the upper right and lower left cells visualize a scatter plot of the relationship between recall and precision along with F_1-score boundaries (*f*). Diagonal plots in upper left and lower right show stacked histograms of the precision or recall scores achieved by the Arch1 (red), Arch2 (yellow), and Arch3 (blue) architecture. Our results show that Arch3 provides the highest performance, for models with both high precision and recall, with a higher distribution of scores above the F_1-score 0.9 boundary line.

comprising fewer than 25 activating training instances and an average of 92.7 inhibiting compounds for every activating compound (92.7:1 ratio). In comparison, there was an equivalent ratio of 15.6:1 for the models that *worked*, with F_1-score above 0.8. Hence, we conclude here that the poor performance in these situations was due to the domination of the inhibition class and lack of sufficient data points for the minority (activating) class, and conclude that datasets comprising 25 compounds constitute the minimum to generate bioactivity models with the architectures employed here.

We next analyzed how the Arch3 architecture handles class imbalance with superior class averaged precision, recall and F_1-score performance, which is shown in Supplementary Figure 3. It can be seen that this architecture performs with superior performance than Arch2 and Arch1, with all models comprising one or more inhibiting predictions, and only one model with relatively few activators (18) failing to predict any activating molecules. Since this observation is likely a result of the independent comparison of activating or inhibiting compounds with an inactive background set and the subsequent comparison of Platt scaled probabilities, our most likely explanation is that this, combined with the Platt scaling, enables the minority (more often activating) class to assign higher confidence to predictions to surpass the majority (more often inhibiting) functional label predictions.

We next sought to identify the performance of the activating and inhibiting labels for the Arch2 and Arch3 architectures separated by the individual target classifications, as shown in Supplementary Figure 4. Our results demonstrate that the distribution of performance differs between classes, where the high performance of the GPCRs and NHRs (averaged median F_1-scores of 86.8 and 84.3, respectively) can be contrasted with transporters, and comparatively poorly performing ion channels (with averaged median F_1-scores of 77.5). Although the poor performance for ion channels and transporters may be unexpected due to the overall rather high separation in chemical space between activating and inhibiting training compounds (**Figure 3**), the large imbalance between the labels (as previously outlined by the median activating versus inhibiting ratios of 6.95 and 6.58, highlighted in **Figure 2B**) is likely one reason for the poor performance of these classes, particularly when considering activating label performance.

In order to identify further factors influencing performance of the predictivity of models, we next explored the impact of training set size of data points with functional annotations, the similarity of the five nearest intra-target neighbors and overall cross-validation F_1-score performance as depicted in Supplementary Figure 5. The figure demonstrates both increasing nearest-neighbor similarity within activating and inhibiting compounds and overall model size are shown to improve model performance, with a large proportion of data points clustered toward the top right hand corner of the 3D plot. The intra-target similarity of the models is shown to increase in accordance with training set size, with increased likelihood to cover similar compounds in the train and test set (which hence leads to increased performance). In comparison, small models (with fewer than 100 compounds) perform with more diverse performance (standard deviation of 18), due to the decreased chance of retaining similar compounds throughout the cross validation.

The models also exhibit higher variance in nearest neighbor similarity due to the reduced coverage of chemical space (as previously shown in Supplementary Figures). Smaller target models below 100 compounds with similar nearest neighbors (Tanimoto similarity above 0.6) are shown to perform better, supporting the view that targets with few activating or inhibiting compounds can be reliably utilized in functional target prediction models, providing similar chemistry to the compounds which predictions are made for is represented within the training set. These findings are at least partly due to the nature of cross-validation, and the fact that data is comprised from a single source and that in larger classes there is greater chance to have analogs (which are then easier to predict).

This analysis (Supplementary Figure 5) also highlights the influence of the modeling approach on the cross validated performance of the models, with blue and red markers denoting the Arch2 and Arch3 approaches, respectively. 97 (~30%) of the cascaded models have an F_1-score greater than 0.95, with 63 (~65%) of these originating from the Arch3 approach, illustrating the superior performance of this method compared to the Arch2 method. The figure illustrates both Arch2 and Arch3 approaches perform erratically in situations with low intra-target similarity and small size.

Prospective Validation

The performance of the functional prediction protocols was next analyzed using an external data set extracted from functional screens available at AstraZeneca after a 4-month intermission from the initial date of training data mining. The overall class averaged precision and recall results for the non-binding, binding and inhibiting labels achieved during prospective validation are shown in **Table 2**. Arch1 performed with a class-averaged precision and recall of 59.5 ± 3.2 and 48.1 ± 1.3. In agreement with cross-validation results, the cascaded models performed with superior precision and recall, where Arch2 achieved a precision and recall of 70.9 ± 4.0 and 52.9 ± 3.6, whilst Arch3 performed with values of 70.8 ± 3.5 and 53.1 ± 3.6, respectively. Therefore, a cascaded model architecture produces more predictive models both during cross validation, as well as when applied to a prospective data set comprising novel areas of chemical space (Supplementary Figure 2).

The class-averaged precision, recall and F_1-score performance split between functional labels for prospective validation is shown in **Figure 6**. Our findings show that although the Arch1 architecture outperforms Arch2 and Arch3 based on activating precision (by a margin of ~0.90 and ~0.12 respectively), the cascaded models far outperform the inhibiting precision score obtained by Arch1, by a margin of ~0.35 for both architectures. The inhibiting and activating recall are also higher for the Arch2 and Arch3 models, and hence produce higher F_1-scores for both cascaded architectures compared to Arch1, with scores of ~0.19 and ~0.26 for the activating label and ~0.47 and ~0.46 for the inhibiting compounds, respectively. These findings are likely due to the single model architecture of Arch1, since the single-model architecture creates many false inhibiting predictions due many large classes with inhibiting data, which hence dominate the model with higher probabilities.

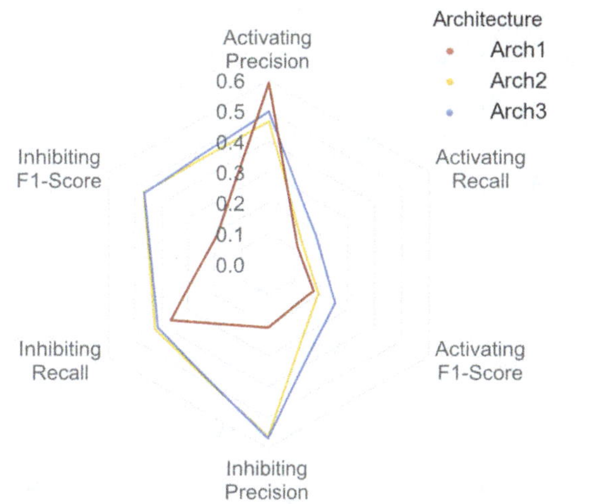

FIGURE 6 | Inhibiting and activating class averaged performance during prospective validation. Arch1 (red) generates a distinct performance profile separate from the cascaded architectures, where Arch2 (yellow) and Arch3 (blue) exhibit significantly reduced class averaged inhibiting precision (and hence markedly lower F_1-score these labels). This is likely due the inability of the single model architecture to counter for the imbalance between the majority (inhibiting) and minority (activating) labels, since Arch1 is forced to consider all functional labels across all targets at once. This factor ranks inhibiting labels higher within the ranked list of predictions, producing higher numbers of false positive inhibiting predictions, and thus reduces the precision of the inhibiting label for this architecture.

In comparison to cross validation, the difference in Arch2 and Arch3 precision, recall and F_1-score performance is narrowed for prospective validation. For example, cross validation results showed a margin of ~0.40 and ~0.51 between activating and inhibiting target class averaged precision and recall values, which are reduced to ~0.19 and ~0.20 during external validation testing.

The cascaded models have fewer compounds for Stage 1, with hence less chemical space, and hence more false negatives. This is shown *via* the striking distribution of poor Arch2 and Arch3 recall, particularly for the activating compounds, where 87 targets (~59% of these belong to the GPCR class) failed to predict true-positive active compounds (i.e., 'predicted to bind') during Stage 1 target prediction. The removal of testing instances are consequently assigned recall scores of '0'. This problem is further exacerbated by the imbalance of the external testing set between functional compounds, as indicated by the ratio between prospective validation compounds, which is applied to already imbalanced models.

Given this observation, we next assessed only *the fraction of active compounds predicted to be positives at Stage 1* for Arch2 and Arch3 (according to the protocol outlined in **Figure 1**), to give a better indication for the benchmarked performance between the two different cascaded methods of Stage 2 prediction (i.e., only compounds predicted active at line *b* in **Figures 1B,C** were considered for this part of the analysis). As shown in **Table 2**, this analysis produces class averaged recall scores for Arch2 and Arch3 of 72.4 ± 3.3 and 71.0 ± 2.0 versus 72.3 ± 2.8 and 71.3 ± 2.5, respectively, indicating the recall and F_1-score performance of is higher for Arch3 than Arch2 when benchmarking cascaded Stage 2 performance by considering only true positives from Stage 1 predictions.

To further explore in more detail the performance of different target classifications between Arch2 and Arch3, we analyzed the distribution of F_1-score prospective validation performance when only active compounds predicted to be positives at Stage 1 are considered. Supplementary Figure 7 also shows, in a similar trend to cross validation, that the ion channels and transporter class have a distribution of activating scores lower than the GPCR and NHR classes due to the imbalance between the activating and inhibiting compounds also represented in the external testing set, whilst there is higher performance for the inhibiting classification of compounds due to the domination of this label.

We finally assessed the applicability domain (AD) of all model architectures using 'distance to the training set' as a method (Gadaleta et al., 2016; Hanser et al., 2016), the results of which are shown in **Figure 7**. The averaged five nearest neighbors ($k = 5$) in the training set and the true positive rate (TPR) (defined by the frequency of correct predictions within activating and inhibiting testing compounds) are shown for Arch1, Arch2 and Arch3. We see that the TPR decreases in accordance with increasing dissimilarity from the nearest compound in the respective label of training data across all architectures, as expected, with Arch3 performing with the highest area under the applicability domain curve (AD-AUC) of 0.30. This analysis enables us to assign confidence to novel predictions as follows; for example, an input

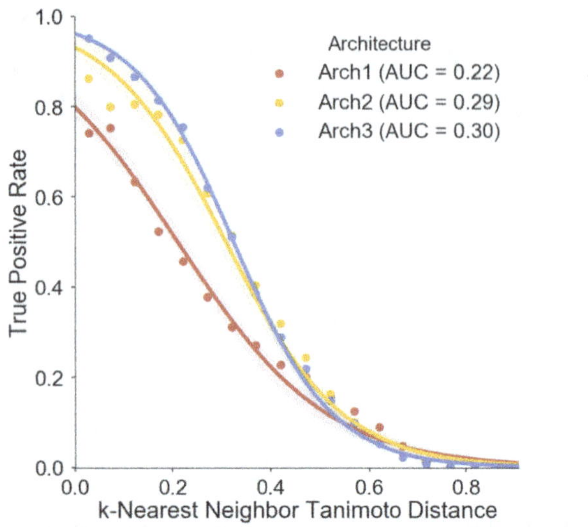

FIGURE 7 | Prospective validation distance-based applicability domain (AD) analysis. AD curves are shown for Arch1 (red), along with Arch2 (yellow) and Arch3 (red). Each line performs with AUC scores of 0.22, 0.29, 0.30, respectively, indicating that Arch3 performs with overall superior AUC when considering the true positive rate achieved and increasing distance between training and prospective validation compounds. The Arch1 architecture produces similar true positive rates to the cascaded architectures for distances beyond 0.6, indicating that all three model architectures have difficulty in extrapolating into novel areas of the chemical space. True positive rate is defined as the recall of the activating and inhibiting data points for each distance bin.

compound with a near neighbor similarity between 0.8 and 0.85 would have an anticipated true-positive rate of ~35% for Arch1, ~78% for Arch2 and ~81% for Arch3. We can also see that although Arch1 performs with a comparatively low AD-AUC of 0.22, all architectures obtain comparatively similar TPR rates throughout increasing dissimilarity scores from 0.6 onward, and hence models are unable to extrapolate into these dissimilar areas of chemical space.

In a final case study, we analyzed the aforementioned study of Drakakis et al. (2017), to illustrate a scenario where functional prediction would have added value to a computational study. In this work, target prediction profiles were related to prolonged sleep bouts, where changing functional effects on receptors was related to the change on the sleep effect of compounds. Contrary to the reasoning gained from the *in silico* mechanism-of-action analysis, Sertindole, which was expected to increase sleep bouts, actually increased wakefulness by 44.9 min. In the absence of functional prediction, the authors hypothesized that the compound switched functional activity at one of the key receptors (CHRM1), compared to the other sleep inducing compounds (Alcaftadine, Ecopipam, Cyproheptadine, and Clopenthixol), leading to hyperactivity and promoted wakefulness. We hence suggest that our method could improve similar analyses by providing vital insight into cases of unanticipated functional changeover.

To illustrate this, we profiled the functional activity of Sertindole at the CHRM1 receptor using Arch1, Arch2, and Arch3. Arch2 and Arch3 predictions both indicate target specific *activation* of CHRM1, compared to the four sleep inducing compounds above. Arch1 however, did not predict CHRM1 activation or inhibition, and thus would not have predicted any functional activity against the CHRM1 receptor.

We conclude that this case study highlights how cascaded functional models provide vital insight into this previous work, and that the unanticipated functional activity could have helped to direct resources toward the experimental functional testing of CHRM1, which was not conducted in the original study.

DISCUSSION

In this study, we present an in-depth analysis of functional bioactivity data available in-house. We first analyzed the chemical space of functional data, to rationalize whether the functional sets of compounds can be distinguished using chemical similarity. Binding and inhibiting compounds were more similar to each other [median Tanimoto Similarity (Tc) of 0.958] than both binding and activating or activating and inhibiting compounds (median Tc of 0.841 and 0.835, respectively). There was separation between functional sets giving us a rationale for implementing and evaluating functional prediction models. We first generated Architecture 1 (Arch1), which uses a simplistic RF similar to existing approaches, and contrasted this with two forms of cascaded models, namely Arch2; comprising a Stage 2 model trained directly on the activating and inhibiting compounds, and Arch3; comprising two independent Stage 2 models trained on either activating or inhibiting compounds, and a set of inactive compounds, respectively. Fivefold cross validation and temporal validation was performed using data available at AstraZeneca after a 4-month interim. Cross validation highlighted Arch3 achieved the highest precision, recall and F_1-scores, which we attributed to the independent comparison of activating or inhibiting compounds with the inactive background sets, and the subsequent comparison of Platt scaled probabilities. In comparison, Arch1 had the lowest precision and recall performance which we attributed to the single-model architecture. Prospective validation indicated that Arch2 and Arch3 outperform the Arch1 overall and hence outlined there is benefit in cascading predictions using a more complex model architecture. Distance-based applicability domain (AD) analysis outlined Arch3 achieved superior AD-AUC (area under the AD curve) and hence superior extrapolation into novel areas of chemical space. Models will be deployed in-house to aid with future phenotypic screening analyses. We conclude that predicting functional effects could provide vital insight for future studies, to annotate cases of unanticipated functional changeover, as outlined by our CHRM1 case study.

AUTHOR CONTRIBUTIONS

LM assimilated the functional data sets, implemented and evaluated the algorithms presented in this work, and wrote this manuscript. AMA helped to implement design model architectures and benchmarking. LB curated the BAO functional dataset. AB and OE conceived the main theme on which the work was performed and made sure that scientific aspect of the study was rationally valid. All authors contributed to revising the final draft of the manuscript.

FUNDING

LM thanks the Biotechnology and Biological Sciences Research Council (BBSRC) (BB/K011804/1); and AstraZeneca, grant number RG75821.

ACKNOWLEDGMENTS

The authors thank Luise Scheidt for proof reading the manuscript.

REFERENCES

Abeyruwan, S., Vempati, U. D., Küçük-McGinty, H., Visser, U., Koleti, A., Mir, A., et al. (2014). Evolving BioAssay Ontology (BAO): modularization, integration and applications. *J. Biomed. Semantics* 5(Suppl. 1 Proceedings of the Bio-Ontologies Spec Interest G):S5. doi: 10.1186/2041-1480-5-S1-S5

Barton, P., and Riley, R. J. (2016). A new paradigm for navigating compound property related drug attrition. *Drug Discov. Today* 21, 72–81. doi: 10.1016/j.drudis.2015.09.010

Bauer-Mehren, A., Furlong, L. I., and Sanz, F. (2009). Pathway databases and tools for their exploitation: benefits, current limitations and challenges. *Mol. Syst. Biol.* 5:290. doi: 10.1038/msb.2009.47

Dosa, P. I., and Amin, E. A. (2016). Tactical approaches to interconverting GPCR agonists and antagonists. *J. Med. Chem.* 59, 810–840. doi: 10.1021/acs.jmedchem.5b00982

Drakakis, G., Koutsoukas, A., Brewerton, S. C., Evans, D. D., and Bender, A. (2013). Using machine learning techniques for rationalising phenotypic readouts from a rat sleeping model. *J. Cheminform.* 5(Suppl. 1):P34.

Drakakis, G., Wafford, K. A., Brewerton, S. C., Bodkin, M. J., Evans, D. A., and Bender, A. (2017). Polypharmacological *in silico* bioactivity profiling and experimental validation uncovers sedative-hypnotic effects of approved and experimental drugs in rat. *ACS Chem. Biol.* 12, 1593–1602. doi: 10.1021/acschembio.7b00209

Gadaleta, D., Mangiatordi, G. F., Catto, M., Carotti, A., and Nicolotti, O. (2016). Applicability domain for QSAR models: where theory meets reality. *Int. J. Quant. Struct.* 1, 45–63. doi: 10.4018/IJQSPR.2016010102

Geronikaki, A. A., Dearden, J. C., Filimonov, D., Galaeva, I., Garibova, T. L., Gloriozova, T., et al. (2004). Design of new cognition enhancers: from computer prediction to synthesis and biological evaluation. *J. Med. Chem.* 47, 2870–2876. doi: 10.1021/jm031086k

Hanser, T., Barber, C., Marchaland, J. F., and Werner, S. (2016). Applicability domain: towards a more formal definition. *SAR QSAR Environ. Res.* 27, 893–909. doi: 10.1080/1062936X.2016.1250229

Huang, P., Chandra, V., and Rastinejad, F. (2010). Structural overview of the nuclear receptor superfamily: insights into physiology and therapeutics. *Annu. Rev. Physiol.* 72, 247–272. doi: 10.1146/annurev-physiol-021909-135917

Keiser, M. J., Roth, B. L., Armbruster, B. N., Ernsberger, P., Irwin, J. J., and Shoichet, B. K. (2007). Relating protein pharmacology by ligand chemistry. *Nat. Biotechnol.* 25, 197–206. doi: 10.1038/nbt1284

Kim, S., Thiessen, P. A., Bolton, E. E., Chen, J., Fu, G., Gindulyte, A., et al. (2016). PubChem Substance and Compound databases. *Nucleic Acids Res.* 44, D1202–D1213. doi: 10.1093/nar/gkv951

Kotz, J. (2012). Phenotypic screening, take two. *SciBX* 5, 1–3. doi: 10.1038/scibx.2012.380

Koutsoukas, A., Lowe, R., Kalantarmotamedi, Y., Mussa, H. Y., Klaffke, W., Mitchell, J. B., et al. (2013). In silico target predictions: defining a benchmarking data set and comparison of performance of the multiclass Naïve Bayes and Parzen-Rosenblatt window. *J. Chem. Inf. Model.* 53, 1957–1966. doi: 10.1021/ci300435j

Koutsoukas, A., Simms, B., Kirchmair, J., Bond, P. J., Whitmore, A. V., Zimmer, S., et al. (2011). From *in silico* target prediction to multi-target drug design: current databases, methods and applications. *J. Proteomics* 74, 2554–2574. doi: 10.1016/j.jprot.2011.05.011

Lagarde, N., Delahaye, S., Jérémie, A., Ben Nasr, N., Guillemain, H., Empereur-Mot, C., et al. (2017). Discriminating agonist from antagonist ligands of the nuclear receptors using different chemoinformatics approaches. *Mol. Inform.* 36:1700020. doi: 10.1002/minf.201700020

Lagunin, A., Stepanchikova, A., Filimonov, D., and Poroikov, V. (2000). PASS: prediction of activity spectra for biologically active substances. *Bioinformatics* 16, 747–748. doi: 10.1093/bioinformatics/16.8.747

Landrum, G. (2006). *RDKit: Open-Source Cheminformatics [Online].* Available: http://www.rdkit.org/

Lavecchia, A., and Cerchia, C. (2016). *In silico* methods to address polypharmacology: current status, applications and future perspectives. *Drug Discov. Today* 21, 288–298. doi: 10.1016/j.drudis.2015.12.007

Lee, J., and Bogyo, M. (2013). Target deconvolution techniques in modern phenotypic profiling. *Curr. Opin. Chem. Biol.* 17, 118–126. doi: 10.1016/j.cbpa.2012.12.022

Liggi, S., Drakakis, G., Koutsoukas, A., Cortes-Ciriano, I., Martínez-Alonso, P., Malliavin, T. E., et al. (2014). Extending *in silico* mechanism-of-action analysis by annotating targets with pathways: application to cellular cytotoxicity readouts. *Future Med. Chem.* 6, 2029–2056. doi: 10.4155/fmc.14.137

Lounkine, E., Keiser, M. J., Whitebread, S., Mikhailov, D., Hamon, J., Jenkins, J. L., et al. (2012). Large-scale prediction and testing of drug activity on side-effect targets. *Nature* 486, 361–367. doi: 10.1038/nature11159

MDL Drug Data Report [MDDR] (2006). *MDL Drug Data Report [MDDR].* San Leandro, CA: MDL Information Systems Inc.

Mervin, L. H., Afzal, A. M., Drakakis, G., Lewis, R., Engkvist, O., and Bender, A. (2015). Target prediction utilising negative bioactivity data covering large chemical space. *J. Cheminform.* 7:51. doi: 10.1186/s13321-015-0098-y

Mervin, L. H., Cao, Q., Barrett, I. P., Firth, M. A., Murray, D., McWilliams, L., et al. (2016). Understanding cytotoxicity and cytostaticity in a high-throughput screening collection. *ACS Chem. Biol.* 11, 3007–3023. doi: 10.1021/acschembio.6b00538

Morgan, H. L. (1965). The generation of a unique machine description for chemical structures – a technique developed at Chemical Abstracts Service. *J. Chem. Doc.* 5, 107–113. doi: 10.1021/c160017a018

Muresan, S., Petrov, P., Southan, C., Kjellberg, M. J., Kogej, T., Tyrchan, C., et al. (2011). Making every SAR point count: the development of Chemistry Connect for the large-scale integration of structure and bioactivity data. *Drug Discov. Today* 16, 1019–1030. doi: 10.1016/j.drudis.2011.10.005

NCBI (2007). *PubChem PUG Help [Online].* Available at: http://pubchem.ncbi.nlm.nih.gov/pug/pughelp.html

OEChem Toolkits (2017). *OEChem Toolkits, Version 2.0.* Santa Fe, NM: OpenEye Scientific Software.

Parker, L. L., Walter, S. A., Young, P. G., and Piwnica-Worms, H. (1993). Phosphorylation and inactivation of the mitotic inhibitor Weel by the nim1/cdr1 kinase. *Nature* 363, 736–738. doi: 10.1038/363736a0

Pedregosa, F., Varoquaux, G., Gramfort, A., Michel, V., Thirion, B., Grisel, O., et al. (2011). Scikit-learn: machine learning in Python. *J. Mach. Learn. Res.* 12, 2825–2830.

Perezgonzalez, J. D. (2015). P-values as percentiles. Commentary on: "Null hypothesis significance tests. A mix-up of two different theories: the basis for widespread confusion and numerous misinterpretations." *Front. Psychol.* 6:341. doi: 10.3389/fpsyg.2015.00341

Poroikov, V., Akimov, D., Shabelnikova, E., and Filimonov, D. (2001). Top 200 medicines: can new actions be discovered through computer-aided prediction? *SAR QSAR Environ. Res.* 12, 327–344. doi: 10.1080/10629360108033242

Raida, M. (2011). Drug target deconvolution by chemical proteomics. *Curr. Opin. Chem. Biol.* 15, 570–575. doi: 10.1016/j.cbpa.2011.06.016

Terstappen, G. C., Schlüpen, C., Raggiaschi, R., and Gaviraghi, G. (2007). Target deconvolution strategies in drug discovery. *Nat. Rev. Drug Discov.* 6, 891–903. doi: 10.1038/nrd2410

Truchon, J. F., and Bayly, C. I. (2007). Evaluating virtual screening methods: good and bad metrics for the "early recognition" problem. *J. Chem. Inf. Model.* 47, 488–508. doi: 10.1021/ci600426e

Vempati, U. D., Przydzial, M. J., Chung, C., Abeyruwan, S., Mir, A., Sakurai, K., et al. (2012). Formalization, annotation and analysis of diverse drug and probe screening assay datasets using the BioAssay Ontology (BAO). *PLoS One* 7:e49198. doi: 10.1371/journal.pone.0049198

Wahdan-Alaswad, R. S., Bane, K. L., Song, K., Shola, D. T., Garcia, J. A., and Danielpour, D. (2012). Inhibition of mTORC1 kinase activates Smads 1 and 5 but not Smad8 in human prostate cancer cells, mediating cytostatic response to rapamycin. *Mol. Cancer Res.* 10, 821–833. doi: 10.1158/1541-7786.MCR-11-0615

Wang, L., Ma, C., Wipf, P., Liu, H., Su, W., and Xie, X. Q. (2013). TargetHunter: an *in silico* target identification tool for predicting therapeutic potential of small organic molecules based on chemogenomic database. *AAPS J.* 15, 395–406. doi: 10.1208/s12248-012-9449-z

Decoys Selection in Benchmarking Datasets: Overview and Perspectives

*Manon Réau†, Florent Langenfeld†, Jean-François Zagury, Nathalie Lagarde and Matthieu Montes**

Laboratoire GBA, EA4627, Conservatoire National des Arts et Métiers, Paris, France

***Correspondence:**
Matthieu Montes
matthieu.montes@cnam.fr

†These authors have contributed equally to this work.

Virtual Screening (VS) is designed to prospectively help identifying potential hits, i.e., compounds capable of interacting with a given target and potentially modulate its activity, out of large compound collections. Among the variety of methodologies, it is crucial to select the protocol that is the most adapted to the query/target system under study and that yields the most reliable output. To this aim, the performance of VS methods is commonly evaluated and compared by computing their ability to retrieve active compounds in benchmarking datasets. The benchmarking datasets contain a subset of known active compounds together with a subset of decoys, i.e., assumed non-active molecules. The composition of both the active and the decoy compounds subsets is critical to limit the biases in the evaluation of the VS methods. In this review, we focus on the selection of decoy compounds that has considerably changed over the years, from randomly selected compounds to highly customized or experimentally validated negative compounds. We first outline the evolution of decoys selection in benchmarking databases as well as current benchmarking databases that tend to minimize the introduction of biases, and secondly, we propose recommendations for the selection and the design of benchmarking datasets.

Keywords: virtual screening, benchmarking databases, benchmarking, decoy, structure-based drug design, ligand-based drug design

INTRODUCTION

Computer-aided drug design (CADD) is now a commonly integrated tool in drug discovery processes (Sliwoski et al., 2014). It represents a way to predict ligands bioactivity *in silico*, and help focusing the drug discovery efforts on a limited number of promising compounds, saving both time and money in this very competitive field. Among these computational methods, Virtual Screening (VS) is designed to prospectively help identifying potential hits, i.e., compounds able to interact with the target and to modulate its activity, out of large compound collections (Tanrikulu et al., 2013). VS approaches can be Ligand-Based (LBVS) when they rely only on the structure/properties of known active compounds to retrieve promising molecules from compound collections (using similarity search, QSAR or 2D/3D pharmacophore, etc.), or Structure-Based (SBVS) if the structural information of the target is used (like in molecular docking studies).

The evaluation of VS methods is crucial prior to large library prospective screening to select the appropriate methodology, and subsequently generate reliable outcome on real-life project. Thus, software and workflows must be thoroughly evaluated retrospectively using benchmarking datasets. Such datasets are composed of known active data together with inactive compounds referred to as "decoys" (Irwin, 2008). Ideally, both active and inactive compounds should be selected on the basis of experimental data. However, the documentation on inactive data is scarce, and putative inactive compounds are generally used instead. Among the common metrics used to estimate the performance of VS methods we find receiver operating characteristics (ROC) curves, the area under the ROC curve (ROC AUC) (Triballeau et al., 2005), Enrichment Curves (EC), Enrichment Factors (EF) and predictiveness curves (Empereur-mot et al., 2015). While conceptually different, they all share the same objective: assess the ability of a given method to identify active compounds as such, and discriminate them from the decoy compounds.

However, since the publication of the first benchmarking database in the early 2000s, the composition in both active and decoy compounds have been pointed out to crucially impact VS methods evaluation; several biases have been shown to incline VS assessment outcomes positively or negatively. The difference between the two chemical spaces defined by the active compounds on the one hand and the decoy compounds on the other hand may lead to artificial overestimation of the enrichment (Bissantz et al., 2000). On the contrary, the possible presence of active compounds in the decoy compounds set may introduce an artificial underestimation of the enrichment (Verdonk et al., 2004; Good and Oprea, 2008) since decoys are usually assumed to be inactive rather than proved to be true inactive compounds (i.e., confirmed inactive through experimental bioassays). New databases were designed to minimize those biases (Rohrer and Baumann, 2009; Vogel et al., 2011; Mysinger et al., 2012; Ibrahim et al., 2015a). Finally, many studies pointed out that the VS performance depends on the target and its structural properties (structural flexibility, binding site physicochemical properties, etc.; Cummings et al., 2005). Taking this into consideration, and despite the growing number of protein families represented in databases, decoy datasets generation tools were made publicly available in order to allow any scientist to fine-tune target-dependant and reliable benchmarking datasets (Mysinger et al., 2012; Ibrahim et al., 2015a).

In this review, we first present how the notion of decoy compounds evolved from randomly selected putative inactive compounds to rationally selected putative inactive compounds and finally true negative compounds. We develop the successive benchmarking datasets that were published in the literature and their basic to highly refined decoys selection workflows together with the resulting positive or negative biases due to their design. We then detail 5 benchmarking databases or decoy sets generator tools along with their detailed decoy compounds selection that represent the current state-of-the-art as of 2017: their respective composition tend to minimize such biases. Finally, we propose recommendations to select minimally biased benchmarking datasets containing putative inactive compounds as decoy compounds and introduce guidelines to design true inactive compounds containing databases.

THE HISTORY OF DECOYS SELECTION

Randomly Selected Decoys

The first use of a benchmarking database to evaluate virtual screening tools dates back to 2000, with the pioneering work of Bissantz et al. (2000). The objective of their study was to evaluate the ligands enrichment, i.e., the ability of docking programs to associate active compounds with the best scores within a compound collection. Three docking programs [Dock (Kuntz et al., 1982), FlexX (Rarey et al., 1996), Gold (Jones et al., 1997)] combined with 7 scoring functions [ChemScore (Eldridge et al., 1997), Dock, FlexX, Fresno (Rognan et al., 1999), Gld, Pmf (Muegge and Martin, 1999), Score (Wang et al., 1998)] were evaluated on two different target proteins: Thymidine Kinase (TK) and the ligand binding domain of the Estrogen Receptor α subtype (ER α).

For each target, a dataset containing 10 known ligands and 990 molecules assumed to be inactive (decoy compounds) was created. The decoy compounds were selected following a two-step scheme: (1) the Advanced Chemical Directory (ACD v.2000-1, Molecular Design Limited, San Leandro) was filtered to eliminate undesired compounds (chemical reagents, inorganic compounds and molecules with unsuitable molecular weights), (2) 990 molecules were randomly selected out of the filtered dataset. The datasets were used to evaluate and compare several docking and scoring schemes. The authors eventually recommended a calibration of docking/consensus scoring schemes on reduced data sets prior to large dataset screens. Later on, Bissantz et al. (2003) applied the same protocol to three human GPCRs to investigate whether their homology models were suitable for virtual screening experiments.

A growing interest for virtual screening benchmarking databases soon emerged from the community (Kellenberger et al., 2004; Brozell et al., 2012; Neves et al., 2012; Repasky et al., 2012; Spitzer and Jain, 2012). New databases were designed with an increasing complexity in the decoys selection methodologies (see section Benchmarking Databases). Nowadays, benchmarking databases are widely used to evaluate various VS tools (Kellenberger et al., 2004; Warren et al., 2006; McGaughey et al., 2007; von Korff et al., 2009; Braga and Andrade, 2013; Ibrahim et al., 2015a; Pei et al., 2015) and to support the identification of hit/lead compounds using LBVS and SBVS (Allen et al., 2015; Ruggeri et al., 2015).

Integration of Physicochemical Filters to the Decoy Compounds Selection

In the early 2000s, Diller's group incorporated filters in the decoys selection to ensure that the discrimination they observed was not solely based on the size of the decoy compounds (Diller and Li, 2003). In addition to the 1,000 kinases inhibitors they retrieved from the literature for 6 kinases (EGFr, VEGFr1, PDGFrβ, FGFr1, SRC, and p38), 32,000 compounds were randomly selected from a filtered version of the MDL Drug Data Report (MDDR). The filters were designed to select decoy compounds displaying similar polarity and molecular weight. Similarly, in 2003, a benchmarking database derived from the MDDR was constructed by McGovern et al. (McGovern and Shoichet, 2003). Compounds with unwanted functional groups were removed, leading to 95,000 compounds. The targets of the MDDR for which at least 20 known ligands were available constituted a target dataset (CA II, MMP-3, NEP, PDF, and XO). The remaining compounds were used as decoy compounds. The addition of rational filters was a considerable step forward in the improvement of decoys selection, but due to the commercial licensing of the MDDR, its use was limited (http://www.akosgmbh.de/accelrys/databases/mddr.htm[1]).

The first benchmarking databases were composed as follows: (1) true active compounds consisted in known ligands extracted from the literature while (2) decoy compounds consisted in putative inactive compounds randomly selected from large databases possibly filtered to be compliant to specific criteria (drug likeness, molecular weight, topological polar surface area…). Since the decoy compounds were pseudo-randomly selected, they were assumed to be inactive on the defined targets.

Despite the use of the MDDR and the filtering of the decoy compounds, these benchmarking databases displayed a major drawback: the significant differences occurring between the physicochemical properties of the active compounds and decoy compounds led to obvious discrimination and then artificially good enrichments (Verdonk et al., 2004; Huang et al., 2006).

In 2006, Irwin et al. proposed that the decoy compounds should be similar to the known ligands regarding their physicochemical properties to reduce the introduction of bias while being structurally dissimilar to the known ligands to reduce their probability to be active on the defined target. Following these recommendations, they created the DUD database (Huang et al., 2006) that was immediately considered as the gold standard for the evaluation of VS methods.

The DUD database is composed of 2,950 ligands and 95,326 decoys for a total of 40 proteins from 6 classes (nuclear hormone receptors, kinases, serine proteases, metalloenzymes, folate enzymes and others). The decoy compounds were extracted from the drug-like subset of the ZINC database (Irwin and Shoichet, 2005). The 2D-similarity between known ligands and decoy compounds was computed by calculating the Tanimoto distance based on the CACTVS type 2 substructure keys and 5 physicochemical properties. For each active compound, the 36 molecules sharing the most similar properties while being topologically dissimilar (Tanimoto < 0.9) were conserved. The evaluation of the performance of DOCK (Meng et al., 1992; Wei et al., 2002; Lorber and Shoichet, 2005; Huang et al., 2006) confirmed that uncorrected databases such as the MDDR led to over-optimistic enrichments compared to corrected databases such as the DUD.

Benchmarking Database Biases

Despite the precautions taken to build the DUD database, several remaining biases have been reported in the literature.

The "analogous bias" (Good and Oprea, 2008) lies in the limited chemical space of active compounds that is restricted to the chemical series that have been explored and referenced in databases. The discrimination of the active compounds from decoy compounds can be simplified since the decoy sets would display a larger structural variability that could induce an overestimation of the performance of VS methods. The lack of diversity in the structures of known active compounds limits the training and evaluation of LBVS methods to perform scaffold-hopping, i.e., the identification of active hit compounds that structurally differ from reference molecules while retaining similar activity.

The "complexity bias" (Stumpfe and Bajorath, 2011) or "artificial enrichment bias": active compounds and decoy compounds often display differences in their respective structural complexity since active compounds are often optimized compounds extracted from large series in the scientific and patent literature, which is not necessarily the case for the structures of pseudo-randomly selected decoy compounds.

The "false negative bias" (Vogel et al., 2011; Bauer et al., 2013) lies in the presence of active compounds in the decoy set. Unlike the analogous and complexity biases, it induces an underestimation of the performance of the VS methods that could be particularly dramatic for the evaluation of LBVS methods (Irwin, 2008).

The need for less biased benchmarking databases to objectively evaluate VS methods favored the emergence of new strategies to eradicate or at least minimize those biases. Two decoys selection strategies arose from benchmarking databases improvement attempts: (1) the use of highly refined decoys selection strategies and (2) the integration of true negative compounds in the decoy set.

Highly Refined Putative Inactive Compounds Selection

The reported biases pointed out that the composition of both active compounds and decoy compounds sets has a huge impact on the evaluation of the performance of VS methods (Verdonk et al., 2004; Good and Oprea, 2008). Therefore, particular efforts were performed in the selection strategies for active compounds and decoy compounds.

To address analogous bias, a strategy consists in modifying the receiver operating characteristics (ROC) curves (i.e., the fraction of actives among the top fraction x of the data set) (Triballeau et al., 2005) by weighting the rank of each active compound with the size of its corresponding lead series (Clark and Webster-Clark, 2008). This allows an equal contribution of each active chemotype to the ROC curve (rather than each active compound). Another widely used method is to fine-tune the active compounds dataset prior to screen to ensure an intrinsic structural diversity. To this aim, the MUV datasets (Rohrer and Baumann, 2009) were designed using the Kennard Jones algorithm to obtain an optimal spread of the active compounds in the decoy compounds chemical space while ensuring a balance between the active compounds self-similarity and separation from the decoy compounds. Despite these observations, the most used strategy in the literature still consists in clustering ligands based on 2D descriptors and retain only cluster representatives in the final dataset (Good and Oprea, 2008; Mysinger et al., 2012; Bauer et al., 2013).

To reduce artificial enrichment, efforts were made to match as much as possible the physicochemical properties of the decoys to the physicochemical properties of the active compounds. To this aim, the Maximum Unbiased Validation database (MUV) (Rohrer and Baumann, 2009) was designed to ensure embedding of active compounds in the decoy compounds

[1]MDDR licensed by Molecular Design, Ltd., San Leandro, CA.

chemical space based on an embedding confidence distance cut-off calibrated on multiple drug-like compounds banks' chemical space. Active compounds that were poorly embedded in the decoy set were discarded. A way to ensure the availability of potential decoy compounds for any ligand is to generate decoys that ignore synthetic feasibility (Wallach and Lilien, 2011). Other databases select decoys that match active compounds in a multiple physicochemical properties space. The DEKOIS 2.0 (Ibrahim et al., 2015a) proposed a workflow that used 8 physicochemical properties while the DUD-E added net charge to the 5 physicochemical properties already considered in the original DUD.

To address the risk of including false negatives in the decoy set, a common strategy is to select decoy compounds topologically different to any active compound. For this purpose, Bauer et al. introduced the LADS score to guide decoys selection (Vogel et al., 2011). In the DUD-E, potential false decoys are avoided by applying a stringent FCFP_6 fingerprints Tanimoto-based filter. It is important to note that since the evaluation of LBVS methods requires that decoy compounds should not be discriminated using basic 2D-based similarity tools, the use of 2D-based dissimilarity filters to avoid false negatives in the decoy set makes the concerned databases inappropriate for the evaluation of the performance of LBVS methods. Therefore, Xia et al. developed a method to select adequate decoys for both SBVS and LBVS (Xia et al., 2014) by favoring physicochemical similarity as well as topological similarity between active compounds and decoy compounds that passed a primary topological dissimilarity filter.

With these improvements, the notion of decoys remained the same—putative inactive compounds—but their selection critically evolved. Ever since, the main progress achieved in the literature lies in the diversification of the protein targets represented in benchmarking databases. The growing need for datasets dedicated to a given target led to (1) an increasing diversity of targets in benchmarking databases [the DUD-E (Mysinger et al., 2012) contains datasets against 102 targets while the previous DUD (Huang et al., 2006) contained datasets only for 40 targets] and (2) highly specialized benchmarking databases focused on a particular class of targets. Such specialized datasets exist for GPCRs [GPCR ligand library (GLL)/Decoy Database (GDD) (Gatica and Cavasotto, 2012)], histone deacetylases [maximal unbiased benchmarking data sets for HDACs—MUBD-HDACs (Xia et al., 2015)], or nuclear receptors [NRLiSt BDB (Lagarde et al., 2014a)]. As a notice, DUD-E or DecoyFinder (Cereto-Massagué et al., 2012) offer automated decoy set generation tools based on the properties of active compounds, enabling the community to easily design and tune their own dataset for a particular target.

Toward True Negative Compounds

A common issue about decoys is the lack of data regarding their potential bioactivity against the target. Most methods assume that the absence of data means an absence of activity, which may lead to include unknown active ligands into a decoy set. To eliminate such false negatives from decoy sets, one solution is to use referenced true negative compounds that can be either true inactive or compounds displaying an undesirable activity.

True inactive compounds, i.e., compounds that displayed no experimental binding affinity against the target of interest, can be used to identify binders. Inactive data is made available in several public activity and/or affinity annotated compound repositories and high throughput screening (HTS) initiatives such as: ChEMBL (Bento et al., 2014), Drugbank (Wishart et al., 2008) that provides annotations for approved drugs; PDBBind (Wang et al., 2004, 2005), Binding MOAD (Benson et al., 2008) and AffinDB (Block et al., 2006) that contain binding affinity data for protein–ligand complexes available in the Protein Data Bank (PDB) (Berman et al., 2000); PDSP Ki database (Roth et al., 2000) that stores screening data from the National Institute of Mental Health's Psychoactive Drug Screening Program; BRENDA (Placzek et al., 2017) that provides binding constants for enzymes; IUPHAR (Southan et al., 2016) that contains binding information for receptors and ion channels; GLIDA (Okuno et al., 2006) and GPCRDB (Munk et al., 2016) that contains binding data for G-protein-coupled receptors; D3R datasets (Drug Design Data Resource[2]) that have been provided by pharmaceutical companies and academia and contain affinity data for 7 proteins together with inactive compounds; ToxCast™/Tox21 (Kavlock et al., 2012) and PCBioAssay (Wang et al., 2017) that provide HTS data for various targets.

As an example, the DUD-Enhanced (Mysinger et al., 2012) (DUD-E) integrates some experimentally validated inactive compounds extracted from ChEMBL in the decoy set in addition to putative inactive compounds: an arbitrary 1 μM cutoff is used to classify ligands in the active set while molecules with no measurable activity at 30 μM or higher concentration were classified into the decoy set. Similarly, the Maximum Unbiased Validation (MUV) (Rohrer and Baumann, 2009) datasets are composed of both active and inactive compounds collected from the PubChem BioAssay annotated database.

Unwanted compounds, i.e., compounds that display unwanted activity or binding, can also be used as negatives. For instance, a recent study used ligands of the NRLiSt BDB (Lagarde et al., 2014a) either as active compounds or decoy compounds, depending on their activity for each nuclear receptor; antagonist (or agonist) ligands of a given nuclear receptor were used as decoys to evaluate agonistic (or antagonistic) pharmacophores (Lagarde et al., 2016, 2017). This strategy has shown successful results in the past: Guasch et al. (2012) focused on PPAR γ partial agonists to avoid side effects accompanying full receptor activation and built an anti-pharmacophore model with known full agonist compounds to remove all potential full agonist compounds from their initial set of 89,165 natural products and natural product derivatives. The authors screened the remaining compounds on a partial agonist pharmacophore model and identified 135 compounds as potential PPARγ partial agonists with good ADME properties among which 8 compounds with new chemical scaffolds for PPARγ partial agonistic activity. After

[2] Available at: drugdesigndata.org

BENCHMARKING DATABASES

DB name	Year	Download address	Origin of the ligands	Origin of the decoys	No. of targets / No. of classes	Decoy compounds selection	Remarks
Rognan's decoy set (Bissantz et al., 2000)	2000	http://bioinfo-pharma.u-strasbg.fr/labwebsite/download.html	Literature	ACD	2/2	Random selection	Design of decoy sets to evaluate the performance of 3 docking programs and 7 scoring functions
Shoichet's decoy set (McGovern and Shoichet, 2003)	2003	–	MDDR	MDDR	9/4	Remove compounds with unwanted functional groups	Compare VS performance depending on the binding site definition (apo, holo or homology modeled structures)
Li's decoy set (Diller and Li, 2003)	2003	–	Literature	MDDR	6/1	Fit polarity and MW to known kinases inhibitors	Compare decoys and ligands physicochemical properties to select decoys
Jain's decoy set (Jain and Nicholls, 2008)	2006	http://www.jainlab.org/downloads.html	PDBbind	ZINC "drug-like" and Rognan's decoy set	34/7	1,000 random molecules from the ZINC that comply to MW $\leq$ 500, logP $\leq$ 5, HBA $\leq$ 10, HBD $\leq$ 5 and RB $\leq$ 12 and Rognan's decoys with RB $\leq$ 15	Use of 5 physicochemical properties to match decoy sets to ligands sets
Directory of Useful Decoys (DUD) (Huang et al., 2006)	2006	http://dud.docking.org	Literature and PDBbind	ZINC "drug-like"	40/6	Decoys must be Lipinski-compliant. The selection is based on both the topologically dissimilarity to ligands and the fit of physicochemical properties	Largest decoy data set so far (40 proteins) and first attempt to select decoys topologically dissimilar decoys
DUD Clusters (Meyer, 2007)	2008	http://dud.docking.org/clusters/	DUD	–	40/6	–	DUD clusters more relevant for scaffold hopping
WOMBAT Datasets (Meyer, 2007)	2007	http://dud.docking.org/wombat/	WOMBAT	–	13/4	–	Design to decrease the analog bias on 13 of the 40 DUD targets, enrich DUD active data sets with compounds from WOMBAT database
Maximum Unbiased Validation (MUV) (Rohrer and Baumann, 2009)	2009	–	PubChem	PubChem	18/7	Two functions measure the active-active and decoy-active distances using 2D chemical descriptors. Actives with the maximum spread within the active set were chosen and decoys with similar spatial distribution were selected	Ligands and decoys are from biologically actives and inactive compounds, i.e., are true actives and inactives, respectively
DUD LIB	2009	http://dud.docking.org/jahn/	DUD-cluster	DUD	13/4	Subset of the DUD database, with more stringent criteria on MW ($\leq$450) and AlogP ($\leq$4,5), and a minimal number of chemotypes	Initially designed for "scaffold-hopping" studies

(Continued)

DB name	Year	Download address	Origin of the ligands	Origin of the decoys	No. of targets / No. of classes	Decoy compounds selection	Remarks
Charge Matched DUD	2010	http://dud.docking.org/charge-matched/	DUD	ZINC	40/6	Apply a net charge property match on DUD datasets	
REPROVIS-DB	2011	–	Literature	Literature	–	Extracted from previous successful studies	Designed for LBVS only
Virtual Decoy sets (VDS) (Wallach and Lilien, 2011)	2011	http://compbio.cs.toronto.edu/VDS	DUD	ZINC	40/6	Same as DUD, but does not consider synthetic feasibility	Purely virtual decoys, availability is not considered
DEKOIS (Vogel et al., 2011)	2011	http://dekois.com/dekois_orig.html	BindingDB	ZINC	40/6	Class decoys and ligands into "cells" based on 6 physicochemical properties and select the closest decoys based on (1) a weighted physicochemical similarity and (2) a LADS score based on functional fingerprints similarity elaborated from the active set	Original treatment of the physicochemical similarity, and introduce the concept of *Latent Active in Decoy set*, i.e., false false positives
GPCR Ligand (GLL)/Decoys Database (GDD) (Xia et al., 2014)	2012	http://cavasotto-lab.net/Databases/GDD/	GLIDA and PDB structures and Vilar et al., 2010	ZINC	147/1	Physico-chemical properties fit and topological dissimilarity filter. Final selection based on MW	First extensive database targeting a specific protein family
Decoy Finder (Cereto-Massagué et al., 2012)	2012	http://urvnutrigenomica-ctns.github.io/DecoyFinder/	User	User	–	Same as DUD	Graphical tool to generate decoy data sets with adaptable thresholds for physicochemical properties
DUD Enhanced (DUD-E) (Mysinger et al., 2012)	2012	http://dud.docking.org/r2/	CHEMBL	ZINC	102/8	Physico-chemical properties fit along with a topological dissimilarity filter. Random selection of decoys is then applied	Largest database so far (1,420,433 decoys and 66,695 actives)
DEKOIS 2.0 (Ibrahim et al., 2015a)	2013	http://www.dekois.com	BindingDB	ZINC	81/11	Same as DEKOIS with 3 additional physicochemical properties (nFC, nPC, Ar), a PAINS filter and an improved, weighted LADS score	
NRLiSt BDB (Lagarde et al., 2014a)	2014	http://nrlist.drugdesign.fr	CHEMBL	ZINC and DUD-E decoys generator	27/1	Use the DUD-E decoy generation tool	Ligands can be either agonists or antagonists (other actives are removed), depending on the purpose of the study
MUBD-HDACs (Xia et al., 2015)	2015	–	CHEMBL and literature	ZINC	14/1	Select decoys based a weighted physicochemical similarity (6 physicochemical properties are considered), and ensure a random spatial distribution of the decoys (i.e., decoys should be as distant to the other actives as a reference ligand)	Applicable both to SBVS and LBVS strategies, uses ligands with proved bioactivity

biological tests, 5 compounds were confirmed to be PPAR γ partial agonists.

SELECTED DATABASES

Maximum Unbiased Validation (MUV)

The MUV was designed to propose unbiased datasets in regard to both artificial enrichment and analogous bias by proposing a new approach gleaned from spatial statistics (Rohrer and Baumann, 2009). The authors ensured homogeneity in actives-actives similarity and actives-decoys dispersion in order to reach a random-like distribution of active compounds and decoy compounds in a physicochemical descriptors chemical space. This implies that the molecular properties contained no information about the bioactivities of active and decoy compounds. Datasets were designed for 18 targets with a total of 30 actives and 15,000 decoys for each target.

Initial Compounds Database

Potential active and decoy compounds were extracted from HTS experiments available in PCBioAssay (June 2008) (PubChem BioAssay[3]). In these assays, a primary screen was performed in a large number of compounds (>50,000) and was followed by a low throughput confirmatory screen. Compounds with an experimental EC50 in the confirmatory screen were selected as potential active compounds while inactive compounds from the primary screen were selected as potential decoys.

Actives Selection

A two-step process was applied to rationally select final active compounds for the MUV data sets. (1) Potential active compounds were filtered to eliminate artifacts caused by organic chemicals aggregation in aqueous buffers ("Hill slope filter"), as well as off-targets, cytotoxic effects or interference with optical detection methods ["frequency of hits filter" and "autofluorescence (Simeonov et al., 2008) and luciferase inhibition (Auld et al., 2008) filters"]. (2) A "chemical space embedding filter" was applied to ensure that actives located in regions of the chemical space devoid of decoys were eliminated from the dataset (**Figure 1**). Subsets of 30 actives with the maximum spread per target were generated using a Kennard-Jones algorithm. Selected active compounds were exchanged with remaining potential active compounds until all datasets were adjusted to a common level of spread.

Decoys Selection

To carefully match active and decoys physicochemical properties, Rohrer et al. proposed that the level of self-similarity within the active compounds set [measured using the "nearest neighbor function" $G(t)$] should be equal to the degree of separation between the active compounds set and the decoy compounds set [evaluated with the "empty space function" $F(t)$] (**Figure 1**). Following guideline, the data clumping should be null, ensuring a random-like distribution of decoy and active compounds in the overall chemical space. The distances were computed based on 1D molecular properties (counts of all atoms, heavy atoms, boron, bromine, carbon, chlorine, fluorine, iodine, nitrogen, oxygen, phosphorus, and sulfur atoms in each molecule as well as the number of H-bond acceptors, H-bond donors, the logP, the number of chiral centers, and the number of ring systems). The level of separation between the decoy compounds and the active compounds was adjusted to the same level of spread so that the data clumping is null. In total, 500 decoys were selected per selected active, resulting in 15,000 decoys per dataset.

The minimization of analog bias and artificial enrichment makes the MUV datasets fitted for LBVS. The availability of structures in the PDB (2008) for seven of the MUV targets makes it suitable for SBVS as well (Löwer et al., 2011). Thus, the MUV constituted the first dataset that enabled comparative evaluations of SB and LBVS methods and protocols.

Demanding Evaluation Kits for Objective *in Silico* Screening (DEKOIS)

In 2011, Vogel et al. proposed a new generator of decoy compounds sets called *Demanding Evaluation Kits for Objective In Silico Screening* (DEKOIS) (Vogel et al., 2011). The authors designed their tool to avoid the introduction of well-known and described biases into the decoy sets, i.e., analog bias and artificial enrichment. A first step in their workflow is subsequently to closely match physicochemical properties of both ligand and decoys to limit the analog bias. Then, to deal with the risk of including false negative compounds in the decoy compounds set, a new concept is applied to the decoys selection process: the *latent actives in the decoy set* (LADS). Finally, the structural diversity of the active and decoy compounds structures into the sets is evaluated and maximized, and the embedding of the actives into the decoys chemical is assessed. The whole workflow was further improved in 2013 to produce the current version of this tool, DEKOIS 2.0 (Bauer et al., 2013), and 81 ready-to-use (active and decoys) benchmarking datasets for 11 target classes are currently available through the DEKOIS website (www.dekois.com/, accessed 10/23/2017).

Initial Compounds Database

Decoy compounds from the DEKOIS 2.0 benchmarking datasets are selected from a subset of the ZINC database of 15 million molecules. Eight physicochemical properties are evaluated: molecular weight, octanol–water partition coefficient, hydrogen bonds acceptor and/or donor, number of rotatable bonds, positive and negative charges, and the number of aromatic rings. For each physicochemical property, bins are defined, and all possible combinations of bins are used to split the database compounds into cells. The initial bins are defined so that each bin is equally populated, and each final cell is characterized by a set of 8 physicochemical properties. Each user-provided active compound is associated with the closest cell (in terms of physicochemical properties), and 1,500 decoys are randomly preselected from this parent cell, or from the direct neighbor cells if the parent cell is not populated enough to provide 1,500 decoy compounds (**Figure 1**).

Decoys Selection

The two criteria for the refinement steps are the structural diversity and the low rate of *latent active in decoy set* (LADS). A physicochemical similarity score (PSS) and a LADS score are

[3]Available online at: http://pubchem.ncbi.nlm.nih.gov/sources#assay

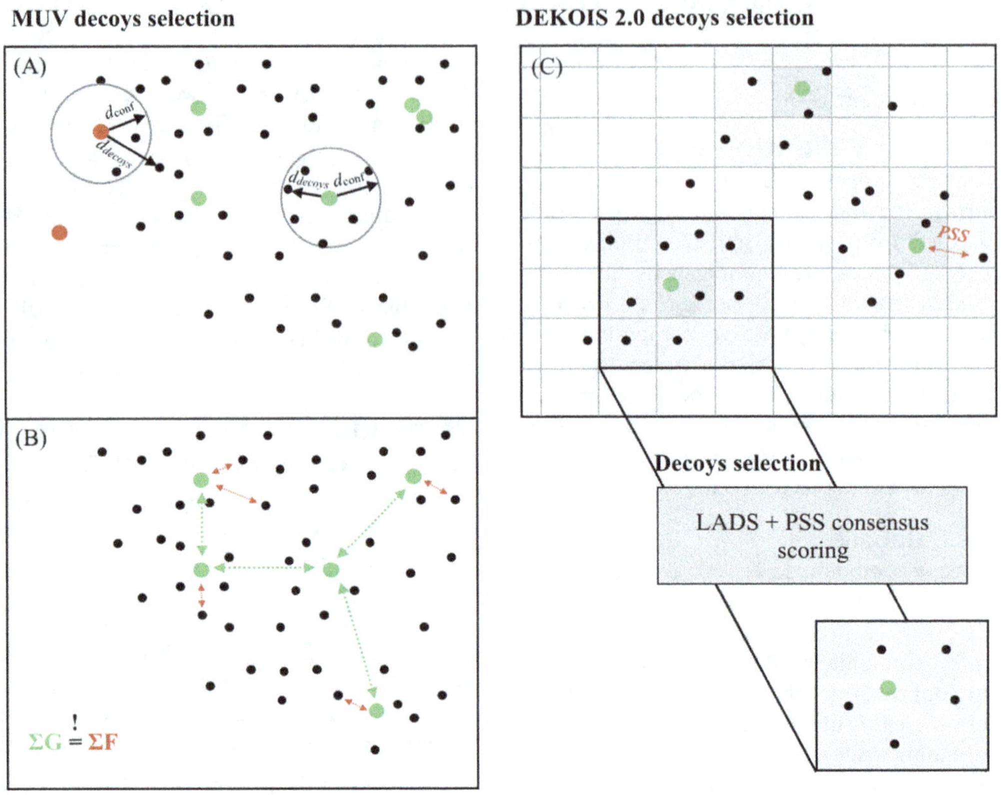

FIGURE 1 | Decoys selection in MUV and DEKOIS 2.0. **(A)** For each active of the MUV, a distance to the 500th nearest neighbor from 100 random samples from multiple drug-like compounds collections was computed. The 90th percentile was recorded as the confidence distance for a good embedding (d_{conf}). Active compounds were accepted only if the 500th nearest neighbor from the decoy compounds (d_{decoys}) set was within the d_{conf}. **(B)** Selected active compounds datasets from the MUV were adjusted to the same level of spread ($\Sigma G \approx$ constant), and decoy compounds sets were, in turn, adjusted to this level of spread ($\Sigma F \approx \Sigma G$). **(C)** The chemical space of both active and decoy compounds was divided into cells characterized by a set of 8 physicochemical properties. Each user-provided compound is associated with its property matching cell, and 1,500 decoys are selected from the same cell, or direct neighboring cells if the parent cell is not populated enough.

computed, normalized and combined to select the final 30 decoys associated with each active ligand:

(1) The PSS score is the arithmetic mean of the normalized distance between a decoy and the reference ligand, for each physicochemical property.
(2) The avoidance of LADS relies on the fingerprints bit strings shared by the active compounds: the fingerprint bit strings of each preselected decoy compound is matched to the fingerprint bit strings of all active compounds using the following:

$$LADS\ score = \frac{\sum_{i=1}^{n}\left(N_{i(HeavyAtoms)} \cdot f_{i(FCFP_6 fragment)}\right)}{N_{FCPC_6 fragments}},$$

with n the number of fingerprint bit strings shared by the decoy and the active set, f_i the frequency of fragment i in the active set, N_i the number of heavy atoms into fragment i, and N the total number of FCPC_6 fragments into the decoy.

The weighting of the LADS score by the frequency of the bit string and the size of the corresponding fragment was added in the second version of DEKOIS (Bauer et al., 2013) to ensure that large bioactive substructures and substructures frequently found exert a greater influence on LADS score compared to smaller and rare functional groups.

(3) The LADS and PSS scores are normalized and combined into a consensus score to sort decoy compounds. The subsequently best 100 decoys are selected. Finally, the fingerprints are used to select the 30 most dissimilar decoys for each active.

Using this enhanced protocol, Bauer et al. showed an improvement of the "deviation from optimal embedding score" (DOE score) (Vogel et al., 2011; Bauer et al., 2013) for DEKOIS 2.0 compared to DEKOIS, and found a good (<0.2) DOE score for 89% out of the 81 targets considered.

Dud-Enhanced (DUD-E)

Despite the extensive use of the DUD, several studies pointed out that some scaffolds were over-represented in the active sets, that the charge was not considered in property-matching for ligand selection, and that true ligands could be found in the decoy sets (Good and Oprea, 2008; Hawkins et al.,

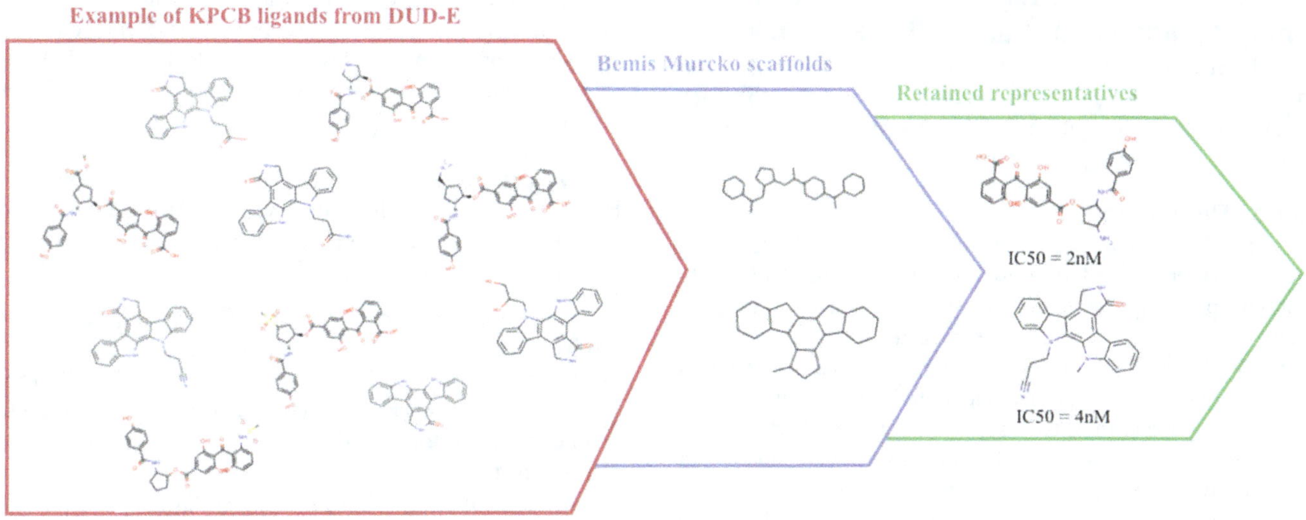

FIGURE 2 | Example of Bemis-Murcko atomic frameworks clustering of Protein kinase C beta type (KPCB) ligands from the DUD-E.

2008; Irwin, 2008; Mysinger and Shoichet, 2010). Shoichet et al. proposed the DUD-E (DUD-Enhanced) to address these weaknesses in both the active and the decoy sets design in the DUD, and extended the number of represented protein families in the database. The DUD-E contains 102 proteins that span diverse target classes. To address analogous bias, ligands were clustered by their Bemis-Murcko atomic frameworks (Bemis and Murcko, 1996) (**Figure 2**), and a topological dissimilarity filter was applied to avoid active compounds in the decoy sets.

Initial Compounds Database

Active compounds assigned to each target of the DUD-E were collected from the ChEMBL09 database if their activity/affinity (Ki, Kd, IC50, EC50, or associated logP) was $\leq 1 \mu M$ (Gaulton et al., 2012). Additionally, 9,219 experimental decoys displaying no measurable affinity up to $30 \mu M$ were included in the decoy sets.

Active Set Preparation

Active compounds were clustered based on their Bemis-Murcko atomic frameworks. When more than 100 frameworks were represented, the highest energy ligand from each cluster is considered, while when less than 100 frameworks are represented, the numbered of considered ligands was raised to obtain more than 100 molecules. Even if this selection protocol could have been optimized for sets with low frameworks diversity, it ensures sufficient diversity and quantity of compounds for the other sets.

Decoys Selection

The decoy compounds were extracted from the ZINC database (Irwin and Shoichet, 2005) and selected by narrowing or widening windows around 6 physicochemical properties: molecular weight, octanol-water partition coefficient, rotatable bonds, hydrogen bonds acceptors, hydrogen bonds donors, and the net charge. To avoid active compounds in the decoy sets, a topological dissimilarity filter was applied. Molecules were sorted according to their Tanimoto distance to any ligands using CACTVS fingerprints, and the 25% most dissimilar decoy molecules were retained. Finally, up to 50 decoys were randomly selected for each ligand and pooled with the 9,219 experimental decoys.

An automated tool was made available online to generate decoys from user-supplied ligands using the same protocol (http://decoys.docking.org). The possibility to generate decoy sets for any target has been revealed successful and is now widely used by the scientific community (Lacroix et al., 2016; Nunes et al., 2016; Allen et al., 2017; Meirson et al., 2017).

Despite the success of the DUD-E, some weaknesses should be corrected in the DUD-E benchmarking database. The 102 targets are defined as a UniProt gene prefix (such as DRD3) and not a full gene_species (such as DRD3_HUMAN or P35462), which can bias the actives selection when the binding site composition differs between species. Additionally, only one single structure was considered for each protein while many docking studies pointed out that the structure selection is crucial for screening and docking, particularly for proteins that accommodate ligands with different binding modes (May and Zacharias, 2005; Ben Nasr et al., 2013; Lionta et al., 2014). A recent study has shown that the ligand pharmacological profile should be considered for both the active set design and the structure selection (Lagarde et al., 2017). For instance, nuclear receptors (NR) can be inhibited by antagonists or activated by agonists that differ in their structure and properties: agonists should be considered in the active set if the screening is performed on an agonist-bound structure while antagonists should be used in the active set if the screening is performed on an antagonist-bound structure.

Nuclear Receptors Ligands and Structures Benchmarking Database (NRLiSt BDB)

The NRLiSt BDB (Nuclear Receptors Ligands and Structures Benchmarking DataBase) was created to address the lack of annotation information and pharmacological profile consideration in existing NR databases.

Ligands Preparation

The NRLiSt BDB is composed of 9,905 active molecules targeting 27 nuclear receptors (NRs). Active compounds are divided into 2 datasets per target according to their agonist or antagonist profile. All active compounds were extracted from the ChEMBL database and included in the NRLiSt after a manual inspection of the corresponding ligands bioactivity data in the original papers. All inverse-agonists, modulators, agonists/antagonists, weak to partial agonists, weak to partial antagonists and ligands with unknown pharmacological profile were discarded.

In addition 339 human holo structures extracted from the PDB are provided, among which 266 are agonists-bound, 17 are antagonists-bound and 56 are others-bound. Valid active compounds extracted from literature were clustered using chemical fingerprints, and a Tanimoto cut-off of 0.5.

Decoys Selection

In total 458,981 decoys generated with the DUD-E online tool were provided, with a mean ratio of 1/51 for each dataset.

In further studies, Lagarde et al. integrated the anti-pharmacological profile ligands in the decoy set to orient the screening toward the desired pharmacological profile (Lagarde et al., 2014b). For instance, antagonists were considered as the decoy compounds set for agonists screening research, while agonists were considered as the decoy compounds set for antagonists screening research. In agreement, the corresponding agonist- and antagonist-bound structures were used for SBVS, when available. Results showed that the enrichment is better when the pharmacological profile is considered prior to screening and should therefore be systematically considered to avoid artificially bad ligands enrichment.

Maximal Unbiased Benchmarking Data Sets for HDACs (MUBD-HDACs)

So far, most of the decoy datasets [such as DUD-E (Mysinger et al., 2012) and DEKOIS (Vogel et al., 2011; Bauer et al., 2013)] or decoys generator [such as DecoyFinder (Cereto-Massagué et al., 2012) or the DUD-E generator server] are designed for SBVS purpose. Few databases [i.e., MUV (Rohrer and Baumann, 2009), NRLiSt BDB] are intended to propose benchmarking datasets for LBVS. Xia et al. thus proposed a workflow to fulfill this need, and built up decoy datasets for LBVS targeting the histone deacetylases protein family (HDACs).

Ligands Preparation

Active compounds were retrieved from the ChEMBL18 database (Gaulton et al., 2012), among molecules annotated with quantitative data (i.e., IC50), manually checked, and filtered (exclusion of salts, molecules with more than 20 rotatable bonds or with a MW of 600 or more). Finally, ligands displaying a Tanimoto coefficient greater than 0.75 based on MACCS fingerprints were removed to exclude analog molecules, and 6 physicochemical properties (MW, logP, HBAs, HBDs, RBs and net Formal Charge–nFC) were computed for all HDACs inhibitors (HDACIs).

Decoys Selection

The "All-Purchasable Molecules" subset of the ZINC database was used as the initial set of molecules before a two-step filtering:

(1) Compounds outside of the bounds of the HDACIs physicochemical properties were removed, as well as molecules with a Tanimoto coefficient ("similarity in structure" or *sims*) greater than 0.75 to any active compounds to circumvent the introduction of potential active structures (false negatives) into the decoy set.
(2) To retain only 39 decoys per HDACI, compounds were further filtered to ensure similar physicochemical properties and a random spatial distribution of the decoys around the ligands. A specific metric was assigned to each step, specifically the *simp* ("similarity in properties") and the *simsdiff* ("*sims* difference"). The *simp* is the Euclidian distance of the physicochemical properties between a target compound and a reference compound. The *simsdiff* between a potential decoy and a query ligand is the average difference between (a) the topological similarity *sims* between the potential decoy and the remaining ligands and (b) the topological similarity *sims* between the query ligands and the remaining ligands. First, a cut-off is applied on the *simp* to ensure properties similarity between ligands and decoy compounds and second, the 39 lowest *simsdiff* decoys for each ligand are selected.

Last, for each ligand, the PDB (Berman et al., 2000) structures of the targeted HDAC isoform were prepared and provided for SBVS data sets. Unlike DUD-E (Mysinger et al., 2012), only Homo sapiens 3D-data were considered.

The MUBD-HDAC datasets for HDAC2 and HDAC8 isoforms were compared to DUD-E (Mysinger et al., 2012) and DEKOIS 2.0 (Ibrahim et al., 2015a) datasets, in terms of structural diversity [Bemis-Murcko atomic frameworks (Bemis and Murcko, 1996)], property matching and ligand enrichment in SB- and LB-VS approaches. The MUBD-HDAC displayed similar to better results in terms of structural diversity and property matching and was more challenging as measured by ligand enrichment using GOLD (Jones et al., 1997) or fingerprints similarity search, in agreement with a higher structural similarity. Finally, the MUBD-HDACs sets displayed small to great improvement in terms of nearer ligands bias (i.e., ligands that are more similar structurally to a ligand than to any decoy), compared to DUD-E and DEKOIS 2.0, respectively. This bias is known to produce artificially positive LBVS evaluation outcomes (Cleves and Jain, 2008) and thus, should be minimized.

Of note, a similar work was done (Xia et al., 2014) on GPCRs using the GLL/GDD database (Gatica and Cavasotto, 2012) as ligands set, and also resulted in reduced artificial enrichment and analog bias compared to the original GLL/GDD sets.

DISCUSSION AND RECOMMENDATIONS

Ideal Benchmarking Database

The ideal VS benchmarking datasets composition should mimic real-life cases, where a small number of diverse active ligands is embedded into a much larger fraction of inactive compounds. Moreover, both sets of molecules are usually indistinguishable using simple descriptors like their physicochemical properties and share common fragments or functional chemical groups; such features should therefore be transposed to benchmarking datasets design, so that the putative inactive compounds constitute good "decoy" compounds in line with the active compounds and ensure a robust evaluation of the VS methods(Good and Oprea, 2008; Lagarde et al., 2015; Xia et al., 2015).

Comparison of Decoys Selection Methods for SBVS

Among the recent tools to help create benchmarking sets (MUV, DEKOIS, DUD-E, and MUBD), the main difference resides in the strategy used to achieve their respective objectives: the DUD-E and DEKOIS data sets are designed for evaluating SBVS methods while MUV and MUBD are conceived for benchmarking LBVS approaches. Following this basic distinction, the respective algorithms to generate decoy datasets differ significantly. In the former case, the topological dissimilarity between ligand compounds and decoy compounds is maximized to avoid inclusion of active compounds into decoy datasets. In the latter case, the proper embedding of decoy compounds into the ligands chemical space is of primary importance.

For the DUD-E, the final decoys were randomly selected from the 25% most topologically dissimilar molecules compared to the ligands to ensure unbiased selection of decoy compounds. However, several studies pointed out that bias are still present into DUD-E data sets. For instance, Chaput et al. recently evidenced that the performance of four VS programs (Glide, Gold, FlexX and Surflex) is biased (over-estimated) using the DUD-E. Good performance (as measure by BEDROC curves) could be achieved for all programs when original DUD-E datasets were used, while only Glide was considered successful when chemical library biases (i.e., datasets whose decoys and active compounds differ for nine physicochemical properties) were removed. While the DUD-E was successfully used for numerous studies, this observation clearly showed that there is still place for improvements.

Boeckler's group proposed a similar workflow in DEKOIS and DEKOIS 2.0. A physicochemical similarity over eight properties (and represented by the physicochemical similarity score PSS) is used and the topological dissimilarity between the active compounds and the future decoy compounds is computed as in the DUD-E. However, two main differences have to be noted: (1) the topological dissimilarity was computed using the more elaborated weighted LADS score rather than a 2D fingerprint based Tanimoto coefficient filter and (2) the LADS score was combined with the PSS prior to final selection of the decoys. Therefore, the final decoys selection was balanced by both parameters (physicochemical similarity and topological dissimilarity) rather than using successive arbitrary (even if widely used) thresholds, and was successfully used by Hamza et al. (2014) for drug repurposing. This balance may come at a cost, as evidenced by Xia et al.: DEKOIS datasets for HDAC2 and HDAC8 were shown to be less efficient in terms of property matching between the active compounds and the decoy compounds (Xia et al., 2015). However, the DUD-E and DEKOIS sets perform similarly in enrichment using Gold and DEKOIS perform significantly worse than DUD-E using 2D based similarity search approaches.

Comparison of Decoys Selection Methods for LBVS

Both DUD-E and DEKOIS databases share the same overall decoy selection procedure by combining topological dissimilarity and physicochemical properties similarity. While adapted to SBVS, this approach may hinder the objective evaluation of LBVS that is very sensitive to topological difference between active and decoy compounds. The MUV datasets (Rohrer and Baumann, 2009) was designed to overcome this specific weakness of the benchmarking datasets. The authors introduced the notion that decoy compounds and active compounds should be homogeneously spread in the chemical space rather than decoy compounds should be topologically dissimilar to the active compounds (as in the DUD-E for instance). The authors tested 18 datasets and claimed that MUV benchmarking datasets displayed neither analogous bias nor artificial enrichment. Furthermore, they noticed that their data sets were SBVS compliant and compared advantageously to the biased DUD sets, leading to a potential broader use of their sets. MUV sets were applied to the evaluation of VS tools (Tiikkainen et al., 2009; Abdo et al., 2010), the training of new QSAR models (Marchese Robinson et al., 2017) or molecular graph convolutions (Kearnes et al., 2016).

As highlighted by Xia et al. "MUV is restricted by the sufficient experimental decoys (chemical space of decoys)" (Xia et al., 2015). Indeed, MUV relies on the availability of experimental data and is restricted to well-studied targets. The authors subsequently proposed the Maximum Unbiased Benchmarking Data sets (MUBD, see section Benchmarking Databases) that was applied to GPCRs (Xia et al., 2014), HDACs (Xia et al., 2015; Hu et al., 2017) and Toll-like receptor 8 (Pei et al., 2015). The MUBD-DecoyMaker algorithm relies on both a minimal and required topological dissimilarity (*sims*) between decoy and active compounds, but makes use of an additional criterion that minimizes the *simsdiff* parameter, i.e., ensures that decoy and active compounds are as similar as possible.

One should note that this additional step (the decoy-actives similarity check) yield datasets also suitable for SBVS; they seemed even more challenging in SBVS (for HDAC2 and HDAC8) as they provided datasets with higher structural similarity (Xia et al., 2015). Thus, these approaches are particularly appealing as they provide benchmarking datasets that (1) are adapted to LB and SB-VS approaches, (2) subsequently allow comparative evaluations of the performance of LB and SB-VS approaches, and (3) may be more challenging for SBVS.

Fine-Tuned Benchmarking Datasets

The quality of an evaluation lies in the consistency between the retrospectively screened benchmarking datasets and the prospectively screened compound collections as well as the target binding site properties (Ben Nasr et al., 2013). The recent trend to publish protein family-specific datasets or user-provided active compounds dependent decoys generation tools paves the way for a valuable and systematic use of benchmarking datasets prior to prospective VS of large compound collections.

In SBVS, tuned datasets should be used to identify the protocol, conformational sampling, and/or scoring methods that induces the best enrichment in active compounds (Allen et al., 2015, 2017; Lacroix et al., 2016; Li et al., 2016; Nunes et al., 2016; Meirson et al., 2017). For instance, Allen et al. (2015, 2017) evaluated different scoring schemes using DUD-E generated decoys and successfully identified dual EFGR/BRD4 inhibitors. In LBVS, the choice of the dataset is crucial to build a reliable model that can be used to distinguish active compounds from decoy compounds. For example, Ruggeri et al. (2015) used DUD-E generated decoys to define and optimize pharmacophore models that led to the identification of 2 dual competitive inhibitors of *P. Falciparum* M1 (*Pf*A-M1) and M17 (*Pf*A-M17) aminopeptidases.

Of note, when using automatic decoy datasets generation tools, the provided active compounds should be carefully selected to avoid the previously detailed biases.

Integration of True Inactive Compounds

Despite the open-data initiatives that should ease the access to data in the near future, the low documentation about negative data (inactive and/or non-binding) is still an open issue. The inclusion of experimental data in a dataset requires great attention since (1) publicly available databases may present annotation errors that should be manually corrected (Lagarde et al., 2014a), and (2) diversity in the type of value and experimental conditions make some data barely comparable. The selection and the use of negative compounds (inactive and/or non-binding) in the evaluation/development of methods is a delicate step that strongly influences the quality of the resulting model. In agreement with Lagarde et al. (2014a) and Kaserer et al. (2015), we recommend that:

(1) Interaction data should be extracted from receptor binding or enzymatic activity assays on isolated or recombinant protein; cell-based assays should be avoided because of the many factors that can influence the outcome of the assay (non-specific binding...).
(2) Low binders or high IC50/EC50 should not be included in the active set and could be either classified as "inactive," as negative data or discarded.
(3) Experimental bias should be minimized by (a) considering the measured affinity/activity confidence based on the number of documented repeated assays and/or convergent values in different studies and (b) filtering compounds which measured activity/affinity may be an artifact caused by organic chemicals aggregation in aqueous buffers, off-targets effects, cytotoxic effects or interference with optical detection methods (auto-fluorescence and luciferase inhibition).
(4) The origin of the protein used in the assay should be considered, favoring 100% identity with the reference.
(5) Attention should be paid to the ligand binding-site, particularly for proteins that possess more than one binding site, and for multiple conformation binding sites.

One should note that the integration of inactive/non-binding compounds comes with new basics for datasets design. This case is particularly challenging since the inactive/non-binding compounds are usually extracted from the same chemical series as the active compounds. In this case, small fragments modification can induce important bioactivity loss or gain, thus, clustering active compounds to guarantee diversity and minimize analogous bias would have no meaning. Since the final objective of using such data is to harshly evaluate ability of VS methods to discriminate active from inactive compounds based on small signals, the proximity between active and inactive compounds within a chemotype should be conserved, as well as the similarity within the active compounds of a chemotype. However the over representation of a given chemotype could hinder the evaluation of VS method by masking the enrichment of low populated chemotypes. We suggest that a work should be made to equally represent chemotypes and/or to weight the resulting ROC curve (Ibrahim et al., 2015b).

CONCLUSION

Benchmarking databases are widely used to evaluate virtual screening methods. They are particularly important to compare performance of virtual screening methods and therefore to select appropriate protocol prior to large compounds collections screening, and to estimate the reliability of the results of a screening. The characterization of the weaknesses of the first published databases helped designing improved benchmarking datasets with minimized bias. The rational selection of decoy compounds is particularly important to avoid artificial enrichment in the evaluation of the different methods. The diversification of public datasets gathering both active and decoy compounds for a given protein family, and the publication of online decoys generation tools contributed to the democratization of the use of benchmarking studies to help identifying protocols adapted for the query/target system under study. Nowadays, experimental data are being integrated in the decoy compounds set to look for a specific activity or to identify methods fitted for highly similar binders/non binders discrimination. Experimentally validated decoys selection requires careful attention to minimize experimental biases that may arise.

AUTHOR CONTRIBUTIONS

All authors listed have made substantial, direct and intellectual contribution to the work, and approved it for publication.

REFERENCES

Abdo, A., Chen, B., Mueller, C., Salim, N., and Willett, P. (2010). Ligand-based virtual screening using Bayesian networks. *J. Chem. Inf. Model.* 50, 1012–1020. doi: 10.1021/ci100090p

Allen, B. K., Mehta, S., Ember, S. W., Schonbrunn, E., Ayad, N., and Schürer, S. C. (2015). Large-scale computational screening identifies first in class multitarget inhibitor of EGFR kinase and BRD4. *Sci. Rep.* 5:srep16924. doi: 10.1038/srep16924

Allen, B. K., Mehta, S., Ember, S. W. J., Zhu, J.-Y., Schönbrunn, E., Ayad, N. G., et al. (2017). Identification of a novel class of BRD4 inhibitors by computational screening and binding simulations. *ACS Omega* 2, 4760–4771. doi: 10.1021/acsomega.7b00553

Auld, D. S., Southall, N. T., Jadhav, A., Johnson, R. L., Diller, D. J., Simeonov, A., et al. (2008). Characterization of chemical libraries for luciferase inhibitory activity. *J. Med. Chem.* 51, 2372–2386. doi: 10.1021/jm701302v

Bauer, M. R., Ibrahim, T. M., Vogel, S. M., and Boeckler, F. M. (2013). Evaluation and optimization of virtual screening workflows with DEKOIS 2.0 – a public library of challenging docking benchmark sets. *J. Chem. Inf. Model.* 53, 1447–1462. doi: 10.1021/ci400115b

Bemis, G. W., and Murcko, M. A. (1996). The properties of known drugs. 1. Molecular frameworks. *J. Med. Chem.* 39, 2887–2893. doi: 10.1021/jm9602928

Ben Nasr, N., Guillemain, H., Lagarde, N., Zagury, J.-F., and Montes, M. (2013). Multiple structures for virtual ligand screening: defining binding site properties-based criteria to optimize the selection of the query. *J. Chem. Inf. Model.* 53, 293–311. doi: 10.1021/ci3004557

Benson, M. L., Smith, R. D., Khazanov, N. A., Dimcheff, B., Beaver, J., Dresslar, P., et al. (2008). Binding MOAD, a high-quality protein-ligand database. *Nucleic Acids Res.* 36, D674–D678. doi: 10.1093/nar/gkm911

Bento, A. P., Gaulton, A., Hersey, A., Bellis, L. J., Chambers, J., Davies, M., et al. (2014). The ChEMBL bioactivity database: an update. *Nucleic Acids Res.* 42, D1083–D1090. doi: 10.1093/nar/gkt1031

Berman, H. M., Westbrook, J., Feng, Z., Gilliland, G., Bhat, T. N., Weissig, H., et al. (2000). The protein data bank. *Nucleic Acids Res.* 28, 235–242. doi: 10.1093/nar/28.1.235

Bissantz, C., Bernard, P., Hibert, M., and Rognan, D. (2003). Protein-based virtual screening of chemical databases. II. Are homology models of G-Protein Coupled Receptors suitable targets? *Proteins* 50, 5–25. doi: 10.1002/prot.10237

Bissantz, C., Folkers, G., and Rognan, D. (2000). Protein-based virtual screening of chemical databases. 1. Evaluation of different docking/scoring combinations. *J. Med. Chem.* 43, 4759–4767. doi: 10.1021/jm001044l

Block, P., Sotriffer, C. A., Dramburg, I., and Klebe, G. (2006). AffinDB: a freely accessible database of affinities for protein-ligand complexes from the PDB. *Nucleic Acids Res.* 34, D522–D526. doi: 10.1093/nar/gkj039

Braga, R. C., and Andrade, C. H. (2013). Assessing the performance of 3D pharmacophore models in virtual screening: how good are they? *Curr. Top. Med. Chem.* 13, 1127–1138. doi: 10.2174/1568026611313090010

Brozell, S. R., Mukherjee, S., Balius, T. E., Roe, D. R., Case, D. A., and Rizzo, R. C. (2012). Evaluation of DOCK 6 as a pose generation and database enrichment tool. *J. Comput. Aided Mol. Des.* 26, 749–773. doi: 10.1007/s10822-012-9565-y

Cereto-Massagué, A., Guasch, L., Valls, C., Mulero, M., Pujadas, G., and Garcia-Vallvé, S. (2012). DecoyFinder: an easy-to-use python GUI application for building target-specific decoy sets. *Bioinformatics* 28, 1661–1662. doi: 10.1093/bioinformatics/bts249

Clark, R. D., and Webster-Clark, D. J. (2008). Managing bias in ROC curves. *J. Comput. Aided Mol. Des.* 22, 141–146. doi: 10.1007/s10822-008-9181-z

Cleves, A. E., and Jain, A. N. (2008). Effects of inductive bias on computational evaluations of ligand-based modeling and on drug discovery. *J. Comput. Aided Mol. Des.* 22, 147–159. doi: 10.1007/s10822-007-9150-y

Cummings, M. D., DesJarlais, R. L., Gibbs, A. C., Mohan, V., and Jaeger, E. P. (2005). Comparison of automated docking programs as virtual screening tools. *J. Med. Chem.* 48, 962–976. doi: 10.1021/jm049798d

Diller, D. J., and Li, R. (2003). Kinases, homology models, and high throughput docking. *J. Med. Chem.* 46, 4638–4647. doi: 10.1021/jm020503a

Eldridge, M. D., Murray, C. W., Auton, T. R., Paolini, G. V., and Mee, R. P. (1997). Empirical scoring functions: I. The development of a fast empirical scoring function to estimate the binding affinity of ligands in receptor complexes. *J. Comput. Aided Mol. Des.* 11, 425–445. doi: 10.1023/A:1007996124545

Empereur-mot, C., Guillemain, H., Latouche, A., Zagury, J.-F., Viallon, V., and Montes, M. (2015). Predictiveness curves in virtual screening. *J. Cheminformatics* 7:52. doi: 10.1186/s13321-015-0100-8

Gatica, E. A., and Cavasotto, C. N. (2012). Ligand and decoy sets for docking to G protein-coupled receptors. *J. Chem. Inf. Model.* 52, 1–6. doi: 10.1021/ci200412p

Gaulton, A., Bellis, L. J., Bento, A. P., Chambers, J., Davies, M., Hersey, A., et al. (2012). ChEMBL: a large-scale bioactivity database for drug discovery. *Nucleic Acids Res.* 40, D1100–D1107. doi: 10.1093/nar/gkr777

Good, A. C., and Oprea, T. I. (2008). Optimization of CAMD techniques 3. Virtual screening enrichment studies: a help or hindrance in tool selection? *J. Comput. Aided Mol. Des.* 22, 169–178. doi: 10.1007/s10822-007-9167-2

Guasch, L., Sala, E., Castell-Auví, A., Cedó, L., Liedl, K. R., Wolber, G., et al. (2012). Identification of PPARgamma partial agonists of natural origin (I): development of a virtual screening procedure and *in vitro* validation. *PLoS ONE* 7:e50816. doi: 10.1371/journal.pone.0050816

Hamza, A., Wagner, J. M., Wei, N.-N., Kwiatkowski, S., Zhan, C.-G., Watt, D. S., et al. (2014). Application of the 4D fingerprint method with a robust scoring function for scaffold-hopping and drug repurposing strategies. *J. Chem. Inf. Model.* 54, 2834–2845. doi: 10.1021/ci5003872

Hawkins, P. C., Warren, G. L., Skillman, A. G., and Nicholls, A. (2008). How to do an evaluation: pitfalls and traps. *J. Comput. Aided Mol. Des.* 22, 179–190. doi: 10.1007/s10822-007-9166-3

Hu, H., Xia, J., Wang, D., Wang, X. S., and Wu, S. (2017). A thoroughly validated virtual screening strategy for discovery of novel HDAC3 inhibitors. *Int. J. Mol. Sci.* 18, 137. doi: 10.3390/ijms18010137

Huang, N., Shoichet, B. K., and Irwin, J. J. (2006). Benchmarking sets for molecular docking. *J. Med. Chem.* 49, 6789–6801. doi: 10.1021/jm0608356

Ibrahim, T. M., Bauer, M. R., and Boeckler, F. M. (2015a). Applying DEKOIS 2.0 in structure-based virtual screening to probe the impact of preparation procedures and score normalization. *J. Cheminformatics* 7:21. doi: 10.1186/s13321-015-0074-6

Ibrahim, T. M., Bauer, M. R., Dörr, A., Veyisoglu, E., and Boeckler, F. M. (2015b). pROC-Chemotype plots enhance the interpretability of benchmarking results in structure-based virtual screening. *J. Chem. Inf. Model.* 55, 2297–2307. doi: 10.1021/acs.jcim.5b00475

Irwin, J. J. (2008). Community benchmarks for virtual screening. *J. Comput. Aided Mol. Des.* 22, 193–199. doi: 10.1007/s10822-008-9189-4

Irwin, J. J., and Shoichet, B. K. (2005). ZINC–a free database of commercially available compounds for virtual screening. *J. Chem. Inf. Model.* 45, 177–182. doi: 10.1021/ci049714+

Jain, A. N., and Nicholls, A. (2008). Recommendations for evaluation of computational methods. *J. Comput. Aided Mol. Des.* 22, 133–139. doi: 10.1007/s10822-008-9196-5

Jones, G., Willett, P., Glen, R. C., Leach, A. R., and Taylor, R. (1997). Development and validation of a genetic algorithm for flexible docking. *J. Mol. Biol.* 267, 727–748. doi: 10.1006/jmbi.1996.0897

Kaserer, T., Beck, K. R., Akram, M., Odermatt, A., and Schuster, D. (2015). Pharmacophore models and pharmacophore-based virtual screening: concepts and applications exemplified on hydroxysteroid dehydrogenases. *Mol. Basel Switz.* 20, 22799–22832. doi: 10.3390/molecules201219880

Kavlock, R., Chandler, K., Houck, K., Hunter, S., Judson, R., Kleinstreuer, N., et al. (2012). Update on EPA's ToxCast program: providing high throughput decision support tools for chemical risk management. *Chem. Res. Toxicol.* 25, 1287–1302. doi: 10.1021/tx3000939

Kearnes, S., McCloskey, K., Berndl, M., Pande, V., and Riley, P. (2016). Molecular graph convolutions: moving beyond fingerprints. *J. Comput. Aided Mol. Des.* 30, 595–608. doi: 10.1007/s10822-016-9938-8

Kellenberger, E., Rodrigo, J., Muller, P., and Rognan, D. (2004). Comparative evaluation of eight docking tools for docking and virtual screening accuracy. *Proteins* 57, 225–242. doi: 10.1002/prot.20149

Kuntz, I. D., Blaney, J. M., Oatley, S. J., Langridge, R., and Ferrin, T. E. (1982). A geometric approach to macromolecule-ligand interactions. *J. Mol. Biol.* 161, 269–288. doi: 10.1016/0022-2836(82)90153-X

Lacroix, C., Fish, I., Torosyan, H., Parathaman, P., Irwin, J. J., Shoichet, B. K., et al. (2016). Identification of novel smoothened ligands using structure-based docking. *PLoS ONE* 11:e0160365. doi: 10.1371/journal.pone.0160365

Lagarde, N., Ben Nasr, N., Jérémie, A., Guillemain, H., Laville, V., Labib, T., et al. (2014a). NRLiSt BDB, the manually curated nuclear receptors ligands and structures benchmarking database. *J. Med. Chem.* 57, 3117–3125. doi: 10.1021/jm500132p

Lagarde, N., Delahaye, S., Jérémie, A., Ben Nasr, N., Guillemain, H., Empereur-Mot, C., et al. (2017). Discriminating agonist from antagonist ligands of the nuclear receptors using different chemoinformatics approaches. *Mol. Inform.* 36:1700020. doi: 10.1002/minf.201700020

Lagarde, N., Delahaye, S., Zagury, J.-F., and Montes, M. (2016). Discriminating agonist and antagonist ligands of the nuclear receptors using 3D-pharmacophores. *J. Cheminformatics* 8:43. doi: 10.1186/s13321-016-0154-2

Lagarde, N., Zagury, J.-F., and Montes, M. (2014b). Importance of the pharmacological profile of the bound ligand in enrichment on nuclear receptors: toward the use of experimentally validated decoy ligands. *J. Chem. Inf. Model.* 54, 2915–2944. doi: 10.1021/ci500305c

Lagarde, N., Zagury, J.-F., and Montes, M. (2015). Benchmarking data sets for the evaluation of virtual ligand screening methods: review and perspectives. *J. Chem. Inf. Model.* 55, 1297–1307. doi: 10.1021/acs.jcim.5b00090

Li, J., Wang, H., Li, J., Bao, J., and Wu, C. (2016). Discovery of a potential HER2 inhibitor from natural products for the treatment of HER2-positive breast cancer. *Int. J. Mol. Sci.* 17:1055. doi: 10.3390/ijms17071055

Lionta, E., Spyrou, G., Vassilatis, D. K., and Cournia, Z. (2014). Structure-based virtual screening for drug discovery: principles, applications and recent advances. *Curr. Top. Med. Chem.* 14, 1923–1938. doi: 10.2174/1568026614666140929124445

Lorber, D. M., and Shoichet, B. K. (2005). hierarchical docking of databases of multiple ligand conformations. *Curr. Top. Med. Chem.* 5, 739–749. doi: 10.2174/1568026054637683

Löwer, M., Geppert, T., Schneider, P., Hoy, B., Wessler, S., and Schneider, G. (2011). Inhibitors of helicobacter pylori protease HtrA found by 'virtual ligand' screening combat bacterial invasion of epithelia. *PLoS ONE* 6:e17986. doi: 10.1371/journal.pone.0017986

Marchese Robinson, R. L., Palczewska, A., Palczewski, J., and Kidley, N. (2017). Comparison of the predictive performance and interpretability of random forest and linear models on benchmark data sets. *J. Chem. Inf. Model.* 57, 1773–1792. doi: 10.1021/acs.jcim.6b00753

May, A., and Zacharias, M. (2005). Accounting for global protein deformability during protein-protein and protein-ligand docking. *Biochim. Biophys. Acta* 1754, 225–231. doi: 10.1016/j.bbapap.2005.07.045

McGaughey, G. B., Sheridan, R. P., Bayly, C. I., Culberson, J. C., Kreatsoulas, C., Lindsley, S., et al. (2007). Comparison of topological, shape, and docking methods in virtual screening. *J. Chem. Inf. Model.* 47, 1504–1519. doi: 10.1021/ci700052x

McGovern, S. L., and Shoichet, B. K. (2003). Information decay in molecular docking screens against holo, apo, and modeled conformations of enzymes. *J. Med. Chem.* 46, 2895–2907. doi: 10.1021/jm0300330

Meirson, T., Samson, A. O., and Gil-Henn, H. (2017). An *in silico* high-throughput screen identifies potential selective inhibitors for the non-receptor tyrosine kinase Pyk2. *Drug Des. Devel. Ther.* 11, 1535–1557. doi: 10.2147/DDDT.S136150

Meng, E. C., Shoichet, B. K., and Kuntz, I. D. (1992). Automated docking with grid-based energy evaluation. *J. Comput. Chem.* 13, 505–524. doi: 10.1002/jcc.540130412

Meyer, K. (2007). WOMBAT—A tool for mixed model analyses in quantitative genetics by restricted maximum likelihood (REML). *J. Zhejiang Univ. Sci. B* 8, 815–821. doi: 10.1631/jzus.2007.B0815

Muegge, I., and Martin, Y. C. (1999). A general and fast scoring function for protein-ligand interactions: a simplified potential approach. *J. Med. Chem.* 42, 791–804. doi: 10.1021/jm980536j

Munk, C., Isberg, V., Mordalski, S., Harpsøe, K., Rataj, K., Hauser, A. S., et al. (2016). GPCRdb: the G protein-coupled receptor database – an introduction. *Br. J. Pharmacol.* 173, 2195–2207. doi: 10.1111/bph.13509

Mysinger, M. M., Carchia, M., Irwin, J. J., and Shoichet, B. K. (2012). Directory of useful decoys, enhanced (DUD-E): better ligands and decoys for better benchmarking. *J. Med. Chem.* 55, 6582–6594. doi: 10.1021/jm300687e

Mysinger, M. M., and Shoichet, B. K. (2010). Rapid context-dependent ligand desolvation in molecular docking. *J. Chem. Inf. Model.* 50, 1561–1573. doi: 10.1021/ci100214a

Neves, M. A., Totrov, M., and Abagyan, R. (2012). Docking and scoring with ICM: the benchmarking results and strategies for improvement. *J. Comput. Aided Mol. Des.* 26, 675–686. doi: 10.1007/s10822-012-9547-0

Nunes, R. R., Costa, M. D., Santos, B. D., Fonseca, A. L., Ferreira, L. S., Chagas, R. C., et al. (2016). Successful application of virtual screening and molecular dynamics simulations against antimalarial molecular targets. *Mem. Inst. Oswaldo Cruz* 111, 721–730. doi: 10.1590/0074-02760160207

Okuno, Y., Yang, J., Taneishi, K., Yabuuchi, H., and Tsujimoto, G. (2006). GLIDA: GPCR-ligand database for chemical genomic drug discovery. *Nucleic Acids Res.* 34, D673–D677. doi: 10.1093/nar/gkj028

Pei, F., Jin, H., Zhou, X., Xia, J., Sun, L., Liu, Z., et al. (2015). Enrichment assessment of multiple virtual screening strategies for Toll-like receptor 8 agonists based on a maximal unbiased benchmarking data set. *Chem. Biol. Drug Des.* 86, 1226–1241. doi: 10.1111/cbdd.12590

Placzek, S., Schomburg, I., Chang, A., Jeske, L., Ulbrich, M., Tillack, J., et al. (2017). BRENDA in 2017: new perspectives and new tools in BRENDA. *Nucleic Acids Res.* 45, D380–D388. doi: 10.1093/nar/gkw952

Rarey, M., Kramer, B., Lengauer, T., and Klebe, G. (1996). A fast flexible docking method using an incremental construction algorithm. *J. Mol. Biol.* 261, 470–489. doi: 10.1006/jmbi.1996.0477

Repasky, M. P., Murphy, R. B., Banks, J. L., Greenwood, J. R., Tubert-Brohman, I., Bhat, S., et al. (2012). Docking performance of the glide program as evaluated on the Astex and DUD datasets: a complete set of glide SP results and selected results for a new scoring function integrating WaterMap and glide. *J. Comput. Aided Mol. Des.* 26, 787–799. doi: 10.1007/s10822-012-9575-9

Rognan, D., Lauemoller, S. L., Holm, A., Buus, S., and Tschinke, V. (1999). Predicting binding affinities of protein ligands from three-dimensional models: application to peptide binding to class I major histocompatibility proteins. *J. Med. Chem.* 42, 4650–4658. doi: 10.1021/jm9910775

Rohrer, S. G., and Baumann, K. (2009). Maximum unbiased validation (MUV) data sets for virtual screening based on PubChem bioactivity data. *J. Chem. Inf. Model.* 49, 169–184. doi: 10.1021/ci8002649

Roth, B. L., Lopez, E., Patel, S., and Kroeze, W. K. (2000). The multiplicity of serotonin receptors: Uselessly diverse molecules or an embarrassment of riches? *Neuroscientist* 6, 252–262. doi: 10.1177/107385840000600408

Ruggeri, C., Drinkwater, N., Sivaraman, K. K., Bamert, R. S., McGowan, S., and Paiardini, A. (2015). Identification and validation of a potent dual inhibitor of the *P. falciparum* M1 and M17 aminopeptidases using virtual screening. *PLoS ONE* 10:e0138957. doi: 10.1371/journal.pone.0138957

Simeonov, A., Jadhav, A., Thomas, C. J., Wang, Y., Huang, R., Southall, N. T., et al. (2008). Fluorescence spectroscopic profiling of compound libraries. *J. Med. Chem.* 51, 2363–2371. doi: 10.1021/jm701301m

Sliwoski, G., Kothiwale, S., Meiler, J., and Lowe, E. W. (2014). Computational methods in drug discovery. *Pharmacol. Rev.* 66, 334–395. doi: 10.1124/pr.112.007336

Southan, C., Sharman, J. L., Benson, H. E., Faccenda, E., Pawson, A. J., Alexander, S. P., et al. (2016). The IUPHAR/BPS guide to PHARMACOLOGY in 2016: towards curated quantitative interactions between 1300 protein targets and 6000 ligands. *Nucleic Acids Res.* 44, D1054–D1068. doi: 10.1093/nar/gkv1037

Spitzer, R., and Jain, A. N. (2012). Surflex-dock: docking benchmarks and real-world application. *J. Comput. Aided Mol. Des.* 26, 687–699. doi: 10.1007/s10822-011-9533-y

Stumpfe, D., and Bajorath, J. (2011). "Applied virtual screening: strategies, recommendations, and caveats," in *Virtual Screening: Principles, Challenges, and Practical Guidelines*, ed C. Sotriffer (Weinheim: Wiley-VCH Verlag GmbH and Co. KGaA), 291–318. doi: 10.1002/9783527633326.ch11

Tanrikulu, Y., Krüger, B., and Proschak, E. (2013). The holistic integration of virtual screening in drug discovery. *Drug Discov. Today* 18, 358–364. doi: 10.1016/j.drudis.2013.01.007

Tiikkainen, P., Markt, P., Wolber, G., Kirchmair, J., Distinto, S., Poso, A., et al. (2009). Critical comparison of virtual screening methods against the MUV data set. *J. Chem. Inf. Model.* 49, 2168–2178. doi: 10.1021/ci900249b

Triballeau, N., Acher, F., Brabet, I., Pin, J.-P., and Bertrand, H.-O. (2005). Virtual screening workflow development guided by the "receiver operating characteristic" curve approach. Application to high-throughput docking on metabotropic glutamate receptor subtype 4. *J. Med. Chem.* 48, 2534–2547. doi: 10.1021/jm049092j

Verdonk, M. L., Berdini, V., Hartshorn, M. J., Mooij, W. T., Murray, C. W., Taylor, R. D., et al. (2004). Virtual screening using protein-ligand docking: avoiding artificial enrichment. *J. Chem. Inf. Comput. Sci.* 44, 793–806. doi: 10.1021/ci034289q

Vilar, S., Karpiak, J., and Costanzi, S. (2010). Ligand and structure-based models for the prediction of ligand-receptor affinities and virtual screenings: development and application to the β2-adrenergic receptor. *J. Comput. Chem.* 31, 707–720. doi: 10.1002/jcc.21346

Vogel, S. M., Bauer, M. R., and Boeckler, F. M. (2011). DEKOIS: Demanding evaluation kits for objective *in silico* screening—a versatile tool for benchmarking docking programs and scoring functions. *J. Chem. Inf. Model.* 51, 2650–2665. doi: 10.1021/ci2001549

von Korff, M., Freyss, J., and Sander, T. (2009). Comparison of ligand- and structure-based virtual screening on the DUD data set. *J. Chem. Inf. Model.* 49, 209–231. doi: 10.1021/ci800303k

Wallach, I., and Lilien, R. (2011). Virtual decoy sets for molecular docking benchmarks. *J. Chem. Inf. Model.* 51, 196–202. doi: 10.1021/ci100374f

Wang, R., Fang, X., Lu, Y., and Wang, S. (2004). The PDBbind database: collection of binding affinities for protein-ligand complexes with known three-dimensional structures. *J. Med. Chem.* 47, 2977–2980. doi: 10.1021/jm030580l

Wang, R., Fang, X., Lu, Y., Yang, C.-Y., and Wang, S. (2005). The PDBbind database: methodologies and updates. *J. Med. Chem.* 48, 4111–4119. doi: 10.1021/jm048957q

Wang, R., Liu, L., Lai, L., and Tang, Y. (1998). SCORE: a new empirical method for estimating the binding affinity of a protein-ligand complex. *Mol. Model. Annu.* 4, 379–394. doi: 10.1007/s008940050096

Wang, Y., Bryant, S. H., Cheng, T., Wang, J., Gindulyte, A., Shoemaker, B. A., et al. (2017). PubChem BioAssay: 2017 update. *Nucleic Acids Res.* 45, D955–D963. doi: 10.1093/nar/gkw1118

Warren, G. L., Andrews, C. W., Capelli, A.-M., Clarke, B., LaLonde, J., Lambert, M. H., et al. (2006). A critical assessment of docking programs and scoring functions. *J. Med. Chem.* 49, 5912–5931. doi: 10.1021/jm050362n

Wei, B. Q., Baase, W. A., Weaver, L. H., Matthews, B. W., and Shoichet, B. K. (2002). A model binding site for testing scoring functions in molecular docking. *J. Mol. Biol.* 322, 339–355. doi: 10.1016/S0022-2836(02)00777-5

Wishart, D. S., Knox, C., Guo, A. C., Cheng, D., Shrivastava, S., Tzur, D., et al. (2008). DrugBank: a knowledgebase for drugs, drug actions and drug targets. *Nucleic Acids Res.* 36, D901–D906. doi: 10.1093/nar/gkm958

Xia, J., Jin, H., Liu, Z., Zhang, L., and Wang, X. S. (2014). An unbiased method to build benchmarking sets for ligand-based virtual screening and its application to GPCRs. *J. Chem. Inf. Model.* 54, 1433–1450. doi: 10.1021/ci500062f

Xia, J., Tilahun, E. L., Kebede, E. H., Reid, T.-E., Zhang, L., and Wang, X. S. (2015). Comparative modeling and benchmarking data sets for human histone deacetylases and sirtuin families. *J. Chem. Inf. Model.* 55, 374–388. doi: 10.1021/ci5005515

9

Development of Matrix Metalloproteinase-2 Inhibitors for Cardioprotection

Péter Bencsik[1,2†], Krisztina Kupai[3†], Anikó Görbe[1,2], Éva Kenyeres[1,2], Zoltán V. Varga[4], János Pálóczi[4], Renáta Gáspár[3], László Kovács[5], Lutz Weber[6], Ferenc Takács[5], István Hajdú[7,8], Gabriella Fabó[7], Sándor Cseh[7], László Barna[8,9], Tamás Csont[3], Csaba Csonka[3], György Dormán[7‡] and Péter Ferdinandy[2,4*‡]*

[1] Cardiovascular Research Group, Department of Biochemistry, Faculty of Medicine, University of Szeged, Szeged, Hungary, [2] Pharmahungary Group, Szeged, Hungary, [3] Department of Biochemistry, Faculty of Medicine, University of Szeged, Szeged, Hungary, [4] Department of Pharmacology and Pharmacotherapy, Faculty of Medicine, Semmelweis University, Budapest, Hungary, [5] Infarmatik, Budapest , Hungary, [6] OntoChem GmbH, Halle (Saale), Germany, [7] Targetex Biosciences, Dunakeszi, Hungary, [8] Research Centre for Natural Sciences, Institute of Enzymology, Hungarian Academy of Sciences, Budapest, Hungary, [9] Microscopy Center at IEM HAS, Institute of Experimental Medicine, Hungarian Academy of Sciences, Budapest, Hungary

***Correspondence:**
György Dormán
dorman@targetex.com
Péter Ferdinandy
peter.ferdinandy@pharmahungary.com

† These authors have contributed equally to this work.

‡ Joint last authors.

The objective of our present study is to develop novel inhibitors for MMP-2 for acute cardioprotection. In a series of pilot studies, novel substituted carboxylic acid derivatives were synthesized based on imidazole and thiazole scaffolds and then tested in a screeening cascade for MMP inhibition. We found that the MMP-inhibiting effects of imidazole and thiazole carboxylic acid-based compounds are superior in efficacy in comparison to the conventional hydroxamic acid derivatives of the same molecules. Based on these results, a 568-membered focused library of imidazole and thiazole compounds was generated *in silico* and then the library members were docked to the 3D model of MMP-2 followed by an *in vitro* medium throughput screening (MTS) based on a fluorescent assay employing MMP-2 catalytic domain. Altogether 45 compounds showed a docking score of >70, from which 30 compounds were successfully synthesized. Based on the MMP-2 inhibitory tests using gelatin zymography, 7 compounds were then selected and tested in neonatal rat cardiac myocytes subjected to simulated I/R injury. Six compounds showed significant cardio-cytoprotecion and the most effective compound (MMPI-1154) significantly decreased infarct size when applied at 1 μM in an *ex vivo* model for acute myocardial infarction. This is the first demonstration that imidazole and thiazole carboxylic acid-based compounds are more efficacious MMP-2 inhibitor than their hydroxamic acid derivatives. MMPI-1154 is a promising novel cardio-cytoprotective imidazole-carboxylic acid MMP-2 inhibitor lead candidate for the treatment of acute myocardial infarction.

Keywords: matrix metalloproteinase, MMP-2 inhibitor, heart, ischemia/reperfusion injury, cardioprotection, lead candidate

INTRODUCTION

Coronary heart disease (CHD) is the number one cause of death globally (Alwan et al., 2010). Recent data show that almost 18 million people died from CVDs in 2015, of which an estimated 7.4 million were due to coronary heart disease (Roth et al., 2017; WHO, 2017). The discovery of endogenous cardioprotective mechanisms (Ischemic pre-, post-, and remote pre- and perconditioning) has allowed for the exploration of several molecular processes of cell injury and survival mechanisms during ischemia/reperfusion (I/R) (Ferdinandy et al., 2014). However, in spite of numerous promising preclinical attempts aiming pharmacological triggering these cardioprotective mechanisms, the dilemma of translation of the results into clinical practice has remained unsolved due to the presence of several additional factors including cardiovascular co-morbidities (e.g., hyperlipidemia or diabetes mellitus) (Ferdinandy et al., 2014). Thus, to improve clinical outcomes, novel therapeutic strategies against myocardial I/R injury are needed, which may preserve their protection even in the presence of cardiovascular co-morbidities (Hausenloy et al., 2017).

Matrix metalloproteinases (MMP) are zinc containing peptidases classified into several subtypes. The gelatinase-type MMP-2 occurs in the heart in physiological conditions and is synthesized by cardiomyocytes, fibroblasts, and endothelial cells (DeCoux et al., 2014). During I/R, MMP-2 is activated and released from the injured myocardium (Cheung et al., 2000), which may contribute to the degradation of contractile proteins (Wang et al., 2002; Sawicki et al., 2005; Sung et al., 2007; Ali et al., 2010), thereby leading to myocardial dysfunction, and in the long run, to heart failure. Furthermore, in patients with ST-elevation myocardial infarction (STEMI), a significant positive correlation has been shown between the circulating levels of MMP-2 measured before and 12 h after recanalization therapy, and infarct size as determined by cardiac MR (D'Annunzio et al., 2009). We have demonstrated that MMP-2 can be a promising biomarker for patients with coronary artery disease (Bencsik et al., 2015). We have previously also reported that pharmacological inhibition of MMP-2 in rats evoked cardioprotection that is equivalent to ischemic preconditioning (Giricz et al., 2006; Bencsik et al., 2010). Our work has also shown that although hyperlipidemia abolished the beneficial effect of ischemic preconditioning, cardioprotection in the presence of hyperlipidemia was preserved during pharmacological inhibition of MMP-2 (Giricz et al., 2006). We can thus conclude that MMP-2 inhibition is a promosing drug target since it works in the presence of a significant cardiovascular co-morbidity, namely hyperlipidemia (see for reviews Andreadou et al., 2017).

To date, several MMP inhibitors have been identified, including hydroxamates, thiols, carbamoylphosphonates, hydroxyureas, hydrazines, β-lactam, squaric acids, and nitrogenous ligands (Durrant et al., 2011). Most of these consist of a metal-coordinating function, called a zinc-binding group (ZBG), which binds to the catalytic zinc ion of the MMPs. Despite the promising features of these potent MMP inhibitor compounds, only one compound has been approved for clinical use by the U.S. Food and Drug Administration Authority, which is Periostat® (doxycycline hyclate), for the treatment of periodontitis (Dormán et al., 2010). In spite of much preclinical evidence about the involvement of MMP-2 in acute myocardial infarction (AMI), surprisingly, only one failed clinical trial was conducted by the administration of a non-selective, hydroxamate type MMP inhibitor, PG-116800, in a relatively high dose (400 mg/day) for 90 days for AMI patients (Hudson et al., 2006).

Consequent research has been focused on the design of selective compounds that can distinguish between different members of the MMP family, thereby exploiting zinc-binding groups other than the hydroxamate group (Fisher and Mobashery, 2006). In addition, we have recently shown that there is no need for complete inhibition of MMP-2 to achieve cardioprotection since a moderate (~20–25%) inhibition of MMP-2 activity was sufficient to reduce infarct size in normo- and hyperlipidemic isolated rat hearts (Giricz et al., 2006) and also in an *in vivo* rat model of AMI (Bencsik et al., 2014).

Consequently, our aims were to develop novel MMP-2 inhibitors with potent anti-ischemic efficacy and moderate MMP-2 selectivity among the MMP-subtypes. Preclinical studies with MMPI's revealed a severe adverse side-effect frequently, referred to as musculoskeletal syndrome. This is primarily due to MMP-1 inhibition (which is considered an anti-target within the MMPs). Selectivity against MMP-1 may be important to avoid such side effects of MMP inhibitors (Papp et al., 2007).

The significant differences in the structural features of the sub-pockets of the binding/active sites allow for easy differentiation and selectivity of the MMP inhibitors. S1' and S2' pockets are responsible for the selectivity of the inhibitors and this can be taken into consideration in the design of selective inhibitors to tailor the occupation of the particular sub-pockets (**Figure 1**). In the case of MMP-2, the S1' pocket is mainly hydrophobic and relatively large, while in MMP-1 it is short and shallow. Increasing bulkiness at the S1' pocket could change the activity profile and allows for some selectivity over MMP-1. This trend was clearly observed in the case of substituted thiazepine MMP inhibitors (Almstead et al., 1999; Papp et al., 2007).

Therefore, we have designed a screening cascade to select potent MMP-2 inhibitors with cardioprotective effects.

MATERIALS AND METHODS

Experimental Design-Screening Cascade

Our group applied a complex screening cascade to identify candidates that may reduce acute cardiac I/R injury via inhibition of MMP-2. During our complex screening protocol, virtual screening was combined with docking calculations followed by medium-throughput screening using MMP-2 catalytic domain. In the next stage, the inhibitory effect was confirmed on full length MMP-2 enzyme isolated from cardiac tissue. Finally, the cardioprotective effects of selected molecules were tested in neonatal cardiac myocytes that were subjected to simulated ischemia and reoxygenation as well as on an isolated rat heart model of AMI (**Figure 2**).

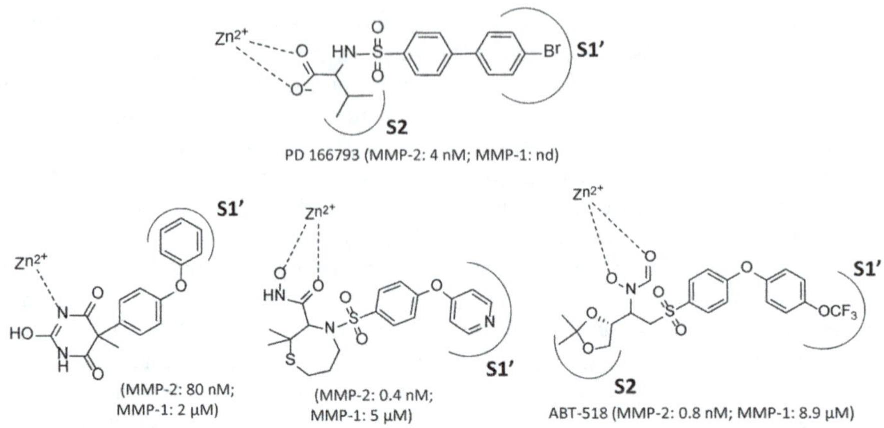

FIGURE 1 | Selected MMP-2 inhibitors and their subpocket occupation leading to selectivity against MMP-1 (Corresponding IC50 values are shown).

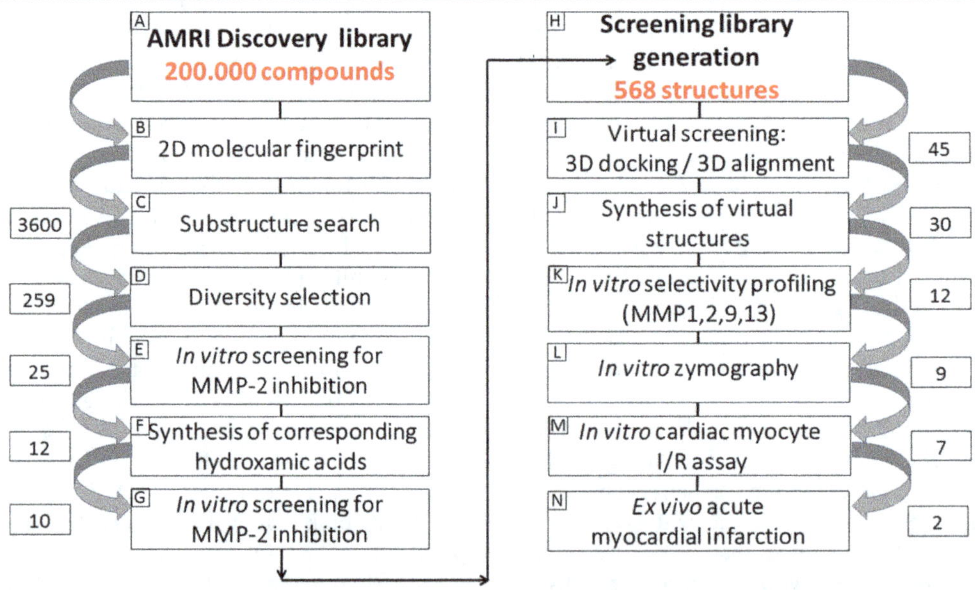

FIGURE 2 | The screening cascade. Complex screening cascade to identify candidates that may reduce acute cardiac I/R injury via inhibition of MMP-2. **(A)** AMRI Chemical Library contains ~200,000 drug-like small molecules (<500 Da) as compound set. We intended to select zinc-binding motif holding molecules, similar to hydroxamic acids. **(B)** For 2D substructure and similarity search. **(C)** Selection of free acids from the AMRI's compound's collection. **(D)** Further focus to compounds holding various motifs around a central core, reflecting the typical MMP inhibitor architecture. **(E)** Selected acids screened in a fluorescent assay using a recombinant human MMP-2 catalytic fragment and a synthetic peptide substrate. **(F)** The synthesis of the thiazole and the isosteric imidazole carboxylic acids. **(G)** The hydroxamic acid pairs of the previously measured acids were tested. **(H)** The novel thiazole carboxylic acid chemotype was the starting point for further structure-based optimization. A 568-membered focused library was *in silico* generated around the AMRI library hits including their bioisosters and some simplified analog. **(I)** Docking studies: Genetic Optimization for Ligand Docking (GOLD) was used to build a 3D model based on the X-ray structure of human MMP-2 and MMP-9. **(J)** Thirty compounds were successfully synthesized for screening combining the *in silico* hits and the additional designed compounds. **(K)** *In vitro* MMP-2 activity was measured using a fluorometric assay. **(L)** Low throughput screening by gelatin zymography technique. **(M)** Cell viability experiments in isolated neonatal cadiac myocytes subjected to simulated ischemia/reperfusion injury. **(N)** Myocardial infarct size was measured after *ex vivo* global ischemia experiments on isolated rat hearts.

Chemistry—MMP-2 Inhibitor Design

Design of Selective MMP-2 Inhibitors

We applied contemporary library design approaches based on the structural features of the known MMP-2 inhibitors (**Figure 2**). Our approach started from a diverse 200k compound library and the multi-step selection procedure consisted of a substructure search for binding motifs of MMP-2 inhibitors and diversity selection.

In Silico Chemisty Approach

Chemical library

The Albany Molecular Research Inc. (AMRI; Albany, NY) Library contains ~200,000 drug-like small molecules (<500

Mwt) synthesized by solution phase parallel synthesis. The compound set contained ~300 medicinal chemistry relevant chemotypes with diverse substitution patterns. The library was succesfully involved in many exclusive drug discovery projects.

2D chemoinformatics methods

According to the Similar Property Principle (Johnson and Maggiora, 1990), molecules that are structurally similar are likely to have similar properties. Applying simple 2D fingerprints is often the method of choice, particularly when numerous reference compounds and multimillion compound databases are available not only "because of its computational efficiency but also because of its demonstrated effectiveness in many comparative studies" (Willett, 2006; Baig et al., 2016). Most frequently the Tanimoto coefficient (Willett and Winterman, 1986) is used for measuring similarity, in spite of its marked size-dependency.

In practice, determining the similarity between known reference structures and each molecule in a database, followed by ranking the database molecules according to the similarities would lead to a potentially active compound set for *in vitro* screening. Similarly, reoccurring (privileged) structural motifs could also be identified and the compounds holding the motifs could represent another screening library.

For 2D substructure and similarity search, we applied standard chemical fingerprints as implemented into InstantJChem software (ChemAxon Ltd. Budapest) in which binary strings encode the presence or absence of substructures.

The physico-chemical parameters [Mwt, clogP, H-bond donors/acceptors,—Lipinski's Rule-5 (Lipinski et al., 2001); rotatable bonds, and topological polar surface area] were calculated by the calculation suit of InstantJChem (ChemAxon Ltd. Budapest).

3D alignment methods

Novel 3D approaches consider not only the molecular topology, but also deal with 3D coordinates of both the active and the potential lead molecules for the similarity comparison and estimate 3D shape similarity (Kalászi et al., 2014).

A rough estimation of the binding behavior of the compounds is to assess their conformational flexibility and the overall statistical representation of such conformational properties would be presented as a 3D structure (ChemAxon Screen3D software) (ChemAxon, 2013).

In flexible alignment, the conformations are created "on-the-fly" during the alignment procedure. Flexible alignment methods, such as used in the present study, have the advantage of not requiring a pre-defined set of initial conformers to sample the conformational space of the molecules. During the alignment procedure we took specific atom-type information such as pharmacophore sites into account. This information would be capable of generating alignments where patterns (With similar binding character) are oriented in a similar fashion as occurs during the real binding to the active site. Therefore, it provides a more realistic picture of the potential bioactive similarity of the molecules.

3D modeling approaches

For docking studies, Genetic Optimization for Ligand Docking (GOLD; version 4.0.1; Jones et al., 1997) was used to build a 3D molecule model based on the X-ray structure of human MMP-2. 1CK7 was the only full length 3D structure found in protein databases but it contained a mutation (E404A). On the other hand, the availability of the 3D structure of the collagenase-like 1-2 catalytic domain is sufficient for virtual screening targeting MMP-2 inhibition, thus 1HOV (NMR), and 1QIB (X-Ray) structures provided feasible alternatives.

Another option was 1EAK (X-Ray), which contains the collagenase-like 1-2 domain together with connecting collagen binding region (propeptides). Comparing the models 1EAK was found to be the particularly reliable for virtual screening even though it also contains the E404A mutation (Supplementary Figure 1). The propeptide regions could be removed without affecting the docking realiability.

The 3D structure of small molecules to be screened were optimized and protonated before docking. The pH was set as 7.2. For docking the standard Gold parameters were used as described in the actual User Guide (Centre, 2017).

The MMP-2 active site was defined containing all the atoms around a sphere with 19 Å radius. We have chosen Zn-ion coordination as octahedral. For all the small molecules 10 independent runs were conducted.

The 1EAK model was validated with three known MMP-2 inhibitors: SC-74020 (Supplementary Figure 2), PD 166793 (**Figure 1**), and ABT-518 (**Figure 1**).

Synthetic Methods

The hydroxamic acids (e.g., AMRI-101H, AMRI-102H, and AMRI-103H) were prepared from the corresponding acids using bromo-tris-pyrrolidino phosphoniumhexafluorophosphate (PyBrOP) and polymer supported hydroxybenzotriazole as activating agent before adding hydroxylamine hydrochloride and a base (see Supplementary Figure 3). The isolated yields were between 10 and 76%, while the purity was higher than 85%.

The synthesis of the thiazole and the isosteric imidazole carboxylic acids were carried out according to standard procedures and as described elsewhere (Ferdinandy et al., 2010).

In order to increase the solubility of the compounds, the benzene ring was replaced with pyridine in various analogs (MMPI-1248, MMPI-1260). Unfortunately, combination of the pyridine ring with the imidazolyl core was synthetically unsuccessful.

In Vitro Pharmacological Testing by MTS Screening

In vitro MMP-2 activity was then measured, using a fluorometric assay in a 384 well format. Human MMP-2 catalytic domain (residues 110-221, 397-455) (Feng et al., 2000) was expressed in *E. coli* in form of inclusion bodies. The protein was refolded and then purified by means of Ni-NTA affinity and anion exchange chromatography. Inhibition assays were carried out in 50 mM Tris, 5 mM $CaCl_2$, 300 mM NaCl, 20 μM $ZnSO_4$, pH = 7.5 buffer. For inhibition studies the catalytic domain of the enzyme was pre-incubated with varying amount of inhibitor for 30 min. Then MMP substrate (Mca-Pro-Leu-Gly-Leu-Dpa-Ala-Arg-NH2) (Papp et al., 2007) was added at 3 μM final concentration. After 1 h incubation at 37°C the fluorescence was detected using a Wallac 1420 Victor2 microplate reader at 320 nm/405 nm Ex/Em wavelength. As an alternative substrate we also used 5-FAM-Pro-Leu-Gly-Leu-Dap(QXL™ 520)-Ala-Arg-NH_2, where the fluorescence was detected at 485 nm/520 nm. For each inhibitor candidate, the percentage of inhibition was determined in duplicate experiments at six inhibitor concentrations, chosen to observe a 5–95% range of inhibition. For validation of the fluorometric assay, Ilomastat [N-[(2R)-2-(Hydroxamidocarbonylmethyl)-4-methylpentanoyl]-L-tryptophan Methylamide, (GM6001)], a non-selective MMP inhibitor, was used as a positive control inhibitor. The measured IC50 values varied between 0.3-1.0 nM which is in line with previous literature data (Galardy et al., 1994; Yamamoto et al., 1998).

Gelatin Zymography Assay to Screen the Efficacy of MMP-Inhibitiors

Gelatin zymography was performed as described previously (Kupai et al., 2010; Bencsik et al., 2017). MMP-2 was isolated from rat heart homogenates as follows: 50 μg protein/lane were loaded and separated by electrophoresis under non-reducing conditions on an 8% SDS-polyacrylamide gels copolymerized with 2 mg/ml gelatin from porcine skin (Sigma-Aldrich; St. Louis, MO). After electrophoresis, gels were washed in 2.5% Triton-X 100 with gentle agitation and then incubated for 20 h at 37°C in zymography development buffer (50 mM Tris-HCl, pH 7.5, containing 5 mM $CaCl_2$, 200 mM NaCl) in the presence or abscence of the MMP inhibitor compounds. Zymographic gels were stained in a 0.05% Coomassie Brilliant Blue R-250 solution followed by destaining, and then zymograms were scanned. MMP activity was detected as a colorless transparent zone on a blue background and the clear bands in the gel were quantified by densitometry using the Quantity One software (Bio-Rad, Hercules, CA). The obtained density values were measured and percentage of inhibition values were then calculated.

Cytoprotective Effect of MMP Inhibitor Compounds in Neonatal Rat Cardiac Myocytes Subjected to Simulated Ischemia/Reperfusion (SI/R)

Simulated Ischemia/Reperfusion Injury Under Hypoxic Cinditions

For our cell viability experiments, 3 day-old cardiomyocytes plated onto 24-well plates were tested under normoxic condition or subjected to simulated ischemia (SI). The normoxic cardiomyocytes were kept under normoxic conditions, i.e., the growth medium was changed to a normoxic solution (in mM: NaCl 125, KCl 5.4, NaH_2PO_4 1.2, $MgCl_2$ 0.5, HEPES 20, glucose 15, taurine 5, $CaCl_2$ 1, creatine 2.5, BSA 0.1%, pH 7.4, 310 mOsm/l) (Li et al., 2004) and the cells were incubated under 95% air and 5% CO_2 at 37°C for 2.5 h. In the second series of experiments, cardiac myocytes were subjected to SI by incubating the cells in hypoxic solution (in mM: NaCl 119, KCl 5.4, $MgSO_4$ 1.3, NaH_2PO_4 1.2, HEPES 5, $MgCl_2$ 0.5, $CaCl_2$ 0.9, Na-lactate 20, BSA 0.1%, 310 mOsm/l, pH = 6.4) (Li et al., 2004) and placing the plates in a humidified 37°C hypoxic chamber exposed to a constant flow of a mixture of 95% N_2 and 5% CO_2 for 4 h. The cells were then subjected to the following treatments during SI or normoxic protocol: vehicle control or MMP inhibitors at different doses calculated according to IC doses *in vitro*. Normoxic and SI treatments were followed by 2 h reoxygenation with growth medium with administration of the same dose of compounds as during normoxia or SI and superfusion with 95% air and 5% CO_2 at 37°C (**Figure 3**).

Cell Viability Assay

Cell viability was assessed by a calcein and propidium iodine assay performed in each group after 2 h reoxygenation. Briefly, the growth medium was removed, the cells were then washed with PBS twice and afterwards were incubated with calcein (1 μM) for 30 min. Then the calcein solution was replaced with fresh PBS and the fluorescence intensity of each well was detected by a fluorescent plate reader (FluoStar Optima, BMG Labtech, Ortenberg, Germany). Fluorescent intensity was then measured in well scanning mode (scan matrix:10 × 10; scan diameter: 10 mm; bottom optic; no of flashes/scan point: 3; temp: 37°C; excitation wavelength: 490 nm; emission wavelength: 520 nm). Then the PBS was removed and the cells were incubated with PI (50 μM) and a digitonin (10^{-4} M) (Sigma-Aldrich; St. Louis, MO) for 7 min. Following that, the PI solution was replaced with fresh PBS and fluorescent intensity was detected using the same settings, excitation wavelength: 544 nm; emission wavelength: 610 nm). Background fluorescent intensity (Cells without staining) was subtracted from the calcein fluorescence intensity (reflecting live cell population) and divided by PI

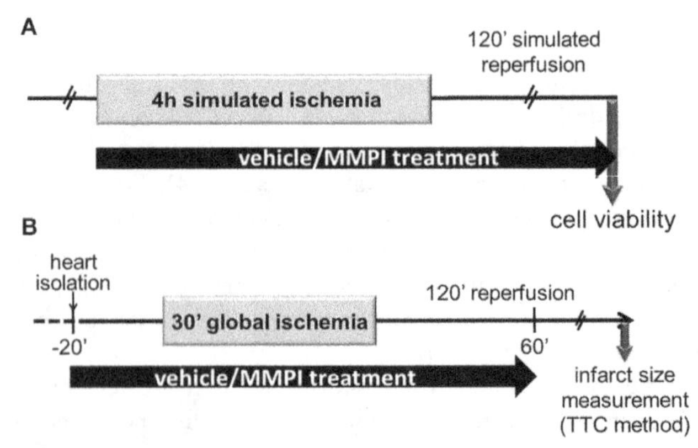

FIGURE 3 | Experimental protocol for cell culture studies and for the *ex vivo* rat heart model of AMI. **(A)** Isolated neonatal rat cardiac myocytes were subjected to 4 h of simulated ischemia followed by 2 h of simulated reperfusion. At the end of the reperfusion, cell viability was determined by using calcein flurescence. **(B)** Isolated adult rat hearts were perfused according to Langendorff and a 30-min global, no-flow ischemia was applied after a 20 min equilibration period. Subsequently, 2 h reperfusion was applied and then infarct size was determined. The hearts were perfused with Krebs-Henseleit solution containing lead candidates or vehicle from 20 min prior to the global ischemia until the 60th min of reperfusion.

fluorescence intensity (reflecting total cell count) and the average intensity of each group was plotted. The cytoprotective effect of different compounds was compared to simulated ischemic control groups.

Myocardial Infarction in Isolated Rat Heart

Ex Vivo Global Ischemia/Reperfusion Injury

Our experiment conforms to the National Institutes of Health Guide for the Care and Use of Laboratory Animals (NIH Pub. No. 85-23, Revised 1996) and also to the EU directive guideline for the care and use of laboratory animals published by the European Union (2010/63/EU) and was approved by the local ethics committee of the University of Szeged. Eight to ten week-old male Wistar rats weighing 300–350 g (Toxicoop Ltd., Budapest, Hungary) were anesthetized intraperitoneally with 60 mg/kg pentobarbital sodium (Euthasol, Produlab Pharma, Raamsdonksveer, The Netherlands). After administration of 500 U/kg heparin through the femoral vein, the heart was isolated and perfused according to Langendorff with oxygenated Krebs-Henseleit buffer at 37°C as previously described (Turan et al., 2006). Briefly, hearts were subjected to 10 min aerobic perfusion for equilibration and stabilization of heart function and then by 30-min global ischemia followed by 120 min reperfusion. Global ischemia was induced by setting a stopcock (B/Braun, Melsungen, Germany) in closed position, and reperfusion was achieved by turning the stopcock in the original (perfusion) position. Heart rate and coronary flow were monitored throughout the perfusion protocol. All the test compounds, their vehicle (DMSO, <0.1% in Krebs-Henseleit solution) as well as the positive control PD166793 (Tocris Bioscience, Cat. No. 2520; Bristol, UK) were applied 20 min before the onset of global ischemia and maintained until the 30th min of reperfusion (**Figure 3**).

Determination of Myocardial Infarct Size

At the end of the 2-h reperfusion, the right ventricle was removed, hearts were frozen, cut into six 1-mm-thick slices, and incubated in 1% triphenyl-tetrazolium chloride (Sigma-Aldrich; St. Louis, MO) at 37°C to delineate infarcted tissue. Slices were then fixed and quantified by planimetry using Infarctsize™ 2.5 software (Pharmahungary, Szeged, Hungary) (Fekete et al., 2013). Infarct size was expressed as a percentage of the left ventricle.

Statistical Analysis

Data were expressed as mean ± SEM. Cell viability were expressed as % of vehicle treated groups. Data were compared to vehicle using ANOVA followed by *post-hoc* tests, e.g., Tukey or Fisher LSD test.

RESULTS

Focused Library Design and MTS Screening

Since hydroxamic acids are reported as the primary zinc-binding motif, we intended to select such a library from the AMRI 200,000 member non-exclusive compound repository as a starting point of our drug discovery efforts. Since only a few compounds were available in the repository as hydroxamic acids and the conversion of acids to hydroxamic acids were not applicable to HT parallel synthesis, we decided first to select free acids from the AMRI's compound collection. This selection supported our initial hypothesis since acids are considered as weaker Zn^{2+} chelators than hydroxamic acids, which might be beneficial for achieving selectivity and in addition could be considered as a good indicator of the MMP-2 inhibitory activity. The substructure search resulted in 3600 acids, which were further focused to a small diverse subset by chemoinformatics methods including 259 compounds, where the compounds hold various motifs around a central core, reflecting the typical MMP inhibitor architecture described above (see **Figure 2**). The selected acids were screened in a fluorescent assay using a recombinant human MMP-2 catalytic fragment and a synthetic peptide substrate. Ilomastat (a non-selective MMP inhibitor) was used for the validation of the assay and in each subsequent experiment as a control compound. The selected compounds (259) were first tested using single point measurements at 10 μM concentration; 6 compounds showed > 70% inhibition, 7 compounds between 60–70%, and 12 compounds between 50–60%. The accumulated hit-rate was 10%. The primary acid hits (12) were attempted to convert to hydroxamic acids. Since two reactions failed 10 hydroxamic acids were prepared successfully for comparative MMP-2 screening. The hydroxamic acid pairs of the previously measured acids were then tested. Comparing the inhibitory activity of the acids and hydroxamic acids, we had an unexpected discovery. Five acids showed higher inhibition than the corresponding hydroxamic acids during catalytic fragment measurement, and among them 3 belonged to the same chemotype: thiazolyl-carboxylic acid (**Table 1**).

Furthermore, we found that the thiazole ring (MMPI-1157) to the isosteric imidazole (MMPI-1154) increased the selectivity to 1.5-fold over MMP-1 (**Table 2**) while the overall inhibitory profile was similar. The 3D similarity score was also high (3D-T = 0.85). The thiazole-imidazole replacement also made the compounds less lipophilic (cLogP was reduced from 3.3 to 2.9). Interestingly, 4- (or para)-fluoro-phenyl substitution in the shorter side chain (MMPI-1157, 1154, 1260, 1248) is favored over the 3- (or meta)-fluoro-phenyl substitution. It showed higher selectivity and MMP-2 inhibitory effect even if the 3D similarity scores were high. The 4- benzyl-phenyl ether or 4-pyridyl-phenyl ether side chain was also favored over the other groups in the longer side chain. On the other hand, if the benzene ring was replaced with pyridine in the shorter side chain, it reduced the MMP-9 inhibition significantly, thus MMP-2/9 selectivity was increased (MMP 9 inhibition: MMPI-1252, 1253 ≥ 500 μM). One compound (MMPI-1140) that lacks the heterocyclic ring but contains the corresponding side chains showed similar activity profile as the parent thiazole carboxylic acid, MMPI-1133, even though the 3D similarity alignment was relatively low (0.56). In summary, the entire screening cascade (**Figure 2**) including library design, selection, virtual screening, and *in vitro* biological screening resulted in a novel thiazole/imidazole carboxylic acid chemotypes, which could be suitable starting points for further structure-based optimization.

As a next step we started to explore the chemical space around this chemotype using 2D/3D structure-based *in silico* methods. First, a 568-membered focused library was *in silico* generated

TABLE 1 | Comparing the inhibitory activity of the acids and hydroxamic acids.

Structure	Type	Code	IC_{50} on MMP-2 (μM)	Structure	Type	Code	IC_{50} on MMP-2 (μM)
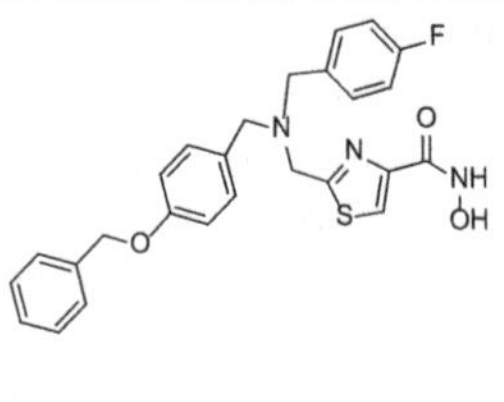	hydroxamic acid	AMRI-101H	12	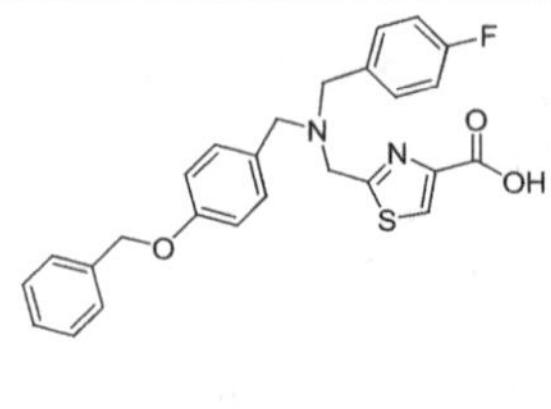	carboxylic acid	AMRI-101A/ MMPI-1157	3.4
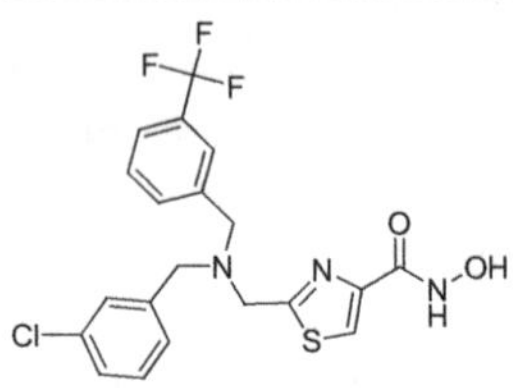	hydroxamic acid	AMRI-102H	11	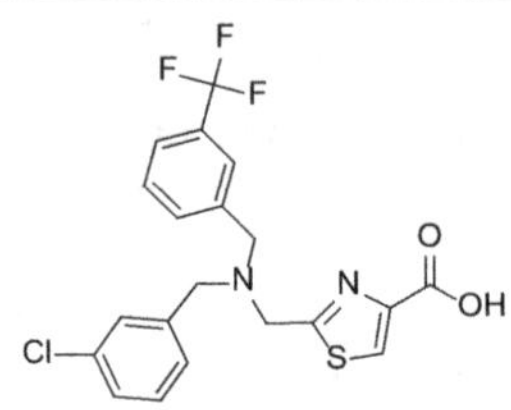	carboxylic acid	AMRI-102A	6.2
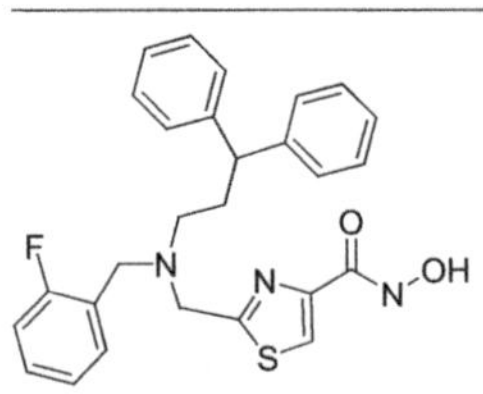	hydroxamic acid	AMRI-103H	17.6	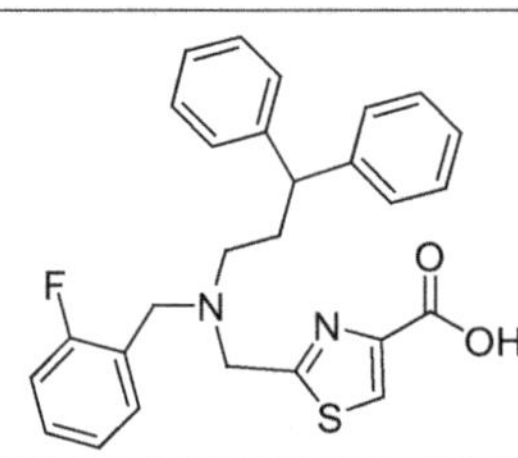	carboxylic acid	AMRI-103A	7.6

around the AMRI library hits including their bioisosters and some simplified analogs and then the library members were docked to the 3D model of MMP-2.

Virtual 3D docking of potential MMP inhibitors was executed using GOLD. The protein structure coordinates were obtained from Protein Data Bank using the highest available resolution (preferably co-crystallized with ligand). We used (MMP-2: 1QIB), (Dhanaraj et al., 1999). The region of interest used for GOLD docking was defined as all the protein residues within the 19 Å radius sphere with the midpoint of the Zinc ion in the catalytic center. GOLD default parameters were used, which were set to 200,000. The complexes were submitted to 20 genetic algorithm runs using the GOLDScore fitness function.

As a result, 45 compounds were considered as virtual hits (docking score > 70) and proposed for chemical synthesis. The synthesizable compound set was completed with several close analogs by rational design. For instance, in order to increase the solubility of the compounds, the benzene ring was successively replaced with pyridine (see MMPI-1252, 1253, 1248, and 1260). Altogether 30 compounds were successfully synthesized for screening combining the *in silico* hits and the additional designed compounds.

The compounds were measured for MMP-1, 2, 9, 13 to determine their inhibitory profile. Efficiency Index amplifies the two major required effects, selectivity against MMP-1 and the inhibitory activity.

Table 2 shows the IC_{50} values of the hit compounds (hit criteria: 100% MMP-2 inhibition at 100 microM). The Gold docking scores are shown for those hits that are coming from virtual screening.

In addition, 3D flexible alignment studies were performed between the novel hit compounds and the initial AMRI library best hit (AMRI-101A/MMPI-1157) compounds. The measure of the alignment was characterized by 3D similarity scores (3D Tanimoto coefficient, ChemAxon Screen3D software). It was postulated that high 3D similarity score could reveal similar conformation and binding mode which could result in similar bioactivities. Finally, cLogP was calculated for each compound. The lower values showing less lipophilicity which is expected to accelerate the passage through the cell membrane leading to higher bioavailability.

MMPI-1154 was investigated more deeply in 3D docking studies. **Figure 4** shows the interaction of the compound to the active site of MMP-2. In MMPI-1154 (Containing an imidazole-carboxylic acid moiety), the acid residue had a chelating interaction to the Zn^{2+} with the contribution of one of the N-hetero atoms of the heterocyclic ring. This relatively weak Zn^{2+} chelation dynamically and statistically gives an allosteric binding feature of this inhibitor.

The Effect of MMP Inhibitors on Cardiac MMP-2 Activity Measured by Zymography

To confirm the MTS screen results, we tested the potential MMP inhibitor molecules on MMP-2 enzyme isolated from rat heart *in vitro*. Therefore, we applied the MMPIs at 1 and 100 μM final concentration in the enzyme's development buffer (**Table 3**).

TABLE 2 | Results of thiazole carboxylic acid (TCA) and imidazole carboxylic acids (ICA) and related analogs.

Structure	Code	IC_{50} on MMP-1 (μM)	IC_{50} on MMP-2 (μM)	IC_{50} on MMP-9 (μM)	IC_{50} on MMP-13 (μM)	3D alignment to 1157	cLogP
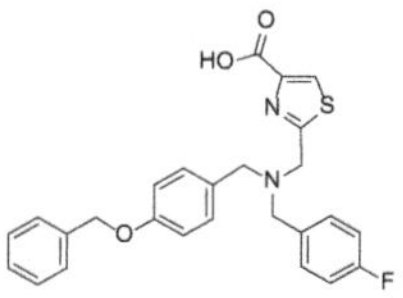	MMPI-1157 (TCA)	3.6	3.4	15	1.6	1.00	3.33
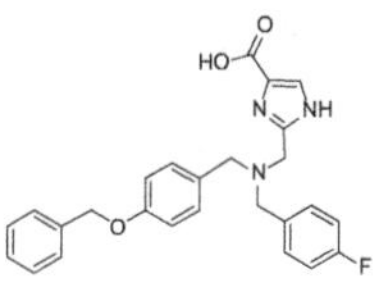	*MMPI-1154 (ICA)*	10	6.6	13	1.8	0.85	2.91
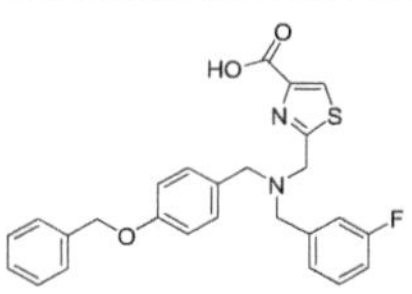	MMPI-1133 (TCA)	6.8	25	9,8	4.7	0.932	3.37
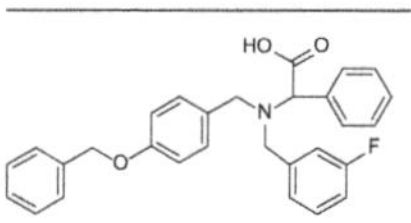	*MMPI-1140*	12	20	39	2.6	0.56	2.91
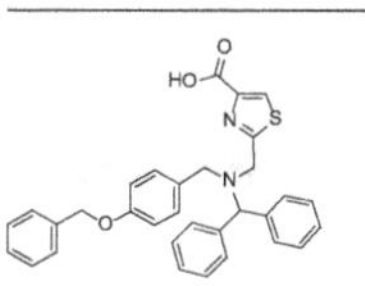	MMPI-1155 (TCA)	26	25	10	1.76	0.663	4.77
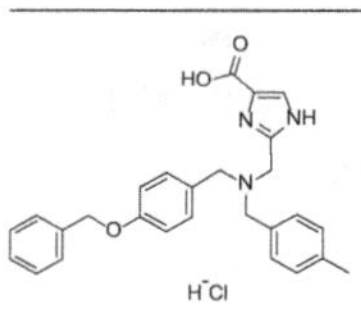	MMPI-1247 (ICA)	33	15	100	3.3	0.843	3.11
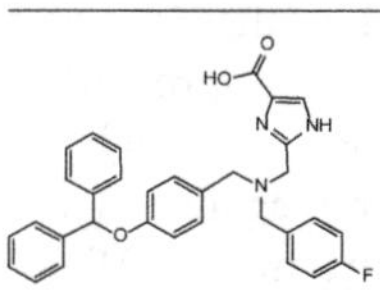	MMPI-1245 (ICA)	16	35	8	0.28	0.673	4.70
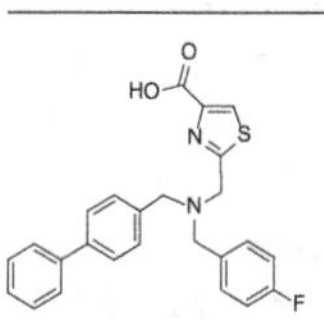	*MMPI-1254 (TCA)*	17	30	20	3	0.739	3.39

(Continued)

TABLE 2 | Continued

Structure	Code	IC_{50} on MMP-1 (μM)	IC_{50} on MMP-2 (μM)	IC_{50} on MMP-9 (μM)	IC_{50} on MMP-13 (μM)	3D alignment to 1157	cLogP
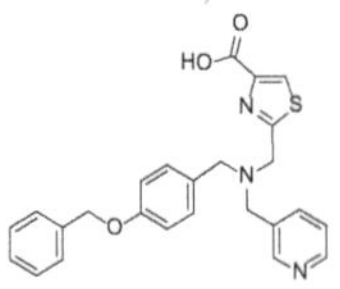	MMPI-1253 (TCA)	240	90	>500	8	0.927	2.22
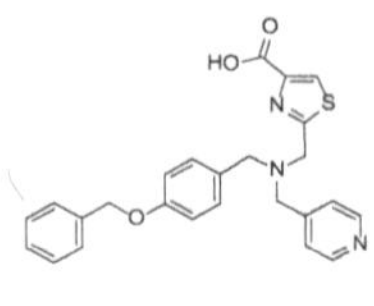	MMPI-1252 (TCA)	115	54	>500	1.5	0.948	2.20
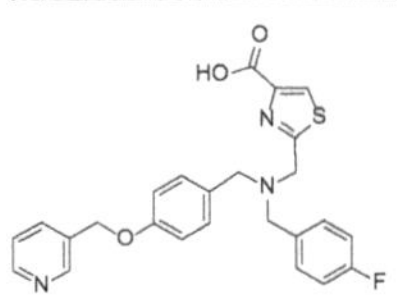	MMPI-1260 (TCA)	51	5.7	37	2.5	0.916	2.16
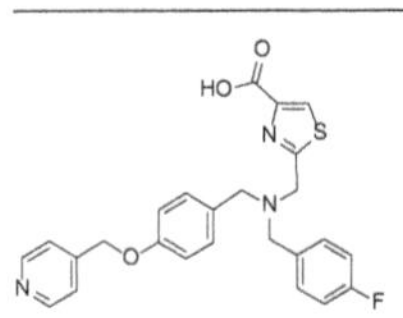	MMPI-1248 (TCA)	47	8	8.8	1.24	0.962	2.24

Cardio-Cytoprotection by MMPIs in Cell Culture Model of I/R Injury

Some doses of MMPIs affected cell viability significantly in normoxic conditions (Supplementary Figure 4). Since the vehicle for MMPIs was DMSO, aerobic cardiac myocytes were treated with 0.1% (v/v%) DMSO and their viability was also assessed. Vehicle treatment did not affect cell viability in comparison to non-treated cardiomyocytes (Supplementary Figure 5).

Hypoxia is one of the numerous influences on cardiac matrix remodeling, via ECM turnover and induction of MMPs. In addition, I/R injury is also a critical modulator of MMP expression through alternative mechanisms (Jun et al., 2011).

The 4-h hypoxic exposure and 2-h reoxygenation caused a marked cell death (Supplementary Figure 5), which was attenuated by MMPI treatment. To investigate whether MMPIs treatment influences cardiac myocite survival after simulated I/R, we selected 6 MMPIs that were available at that time and, which showed significant MMP inhibitory effect during pre-screening. We tested those compounds in cultured neonatal cardiac myocytes subjected to simulated I/R studies. Ilomastat served as positive control (Supplementary Figure 6). The tested compounds showed significant cytoprotection, between 17 and 47% (**Figure 5**). The supplementary figures show all inhibitor testing data (Supplementary Figure 4).

Cardioprotection by MMPI-1154 in Isolated Rat Heart Model of I/R Injury

Finally, based on the results of cell culture experiments, we selected the most potent cardioprotective compound, MMPI-1154 for testing in an isolated rat heart model of AMI. MMPI-1154 reduced myocardial infarct size significanly at 1 μM as compared to the vehicle-treated group (**Figure 6**).

DISCUSSION

In our study, we have successfully demonstrated the development of a novel, selective MMP-2 inhibitor for cardioprotection from an *in silico* compound library selection, through to the testing of the most promising compound against acute myocardial infarction, in an isolated rat heart model. We've found that the MMP-inhibiting effects of imidazole and thiazole carboxylic acid-based compounds are superior to the conventional hydroxamic acid type derivatives of the same molecules. We have thus shown for the first time in the literature that the acute application of MMPI-1154 (An imidazole carboxylic acid-based compound) has a protective effect for the heart against acute myocardial infarction. We achieved *ex vivo* cardioprotection via a moderate MMP-2 inhibition, since MMPI-1154 was applied at around the concentration of its IC_{20} value.

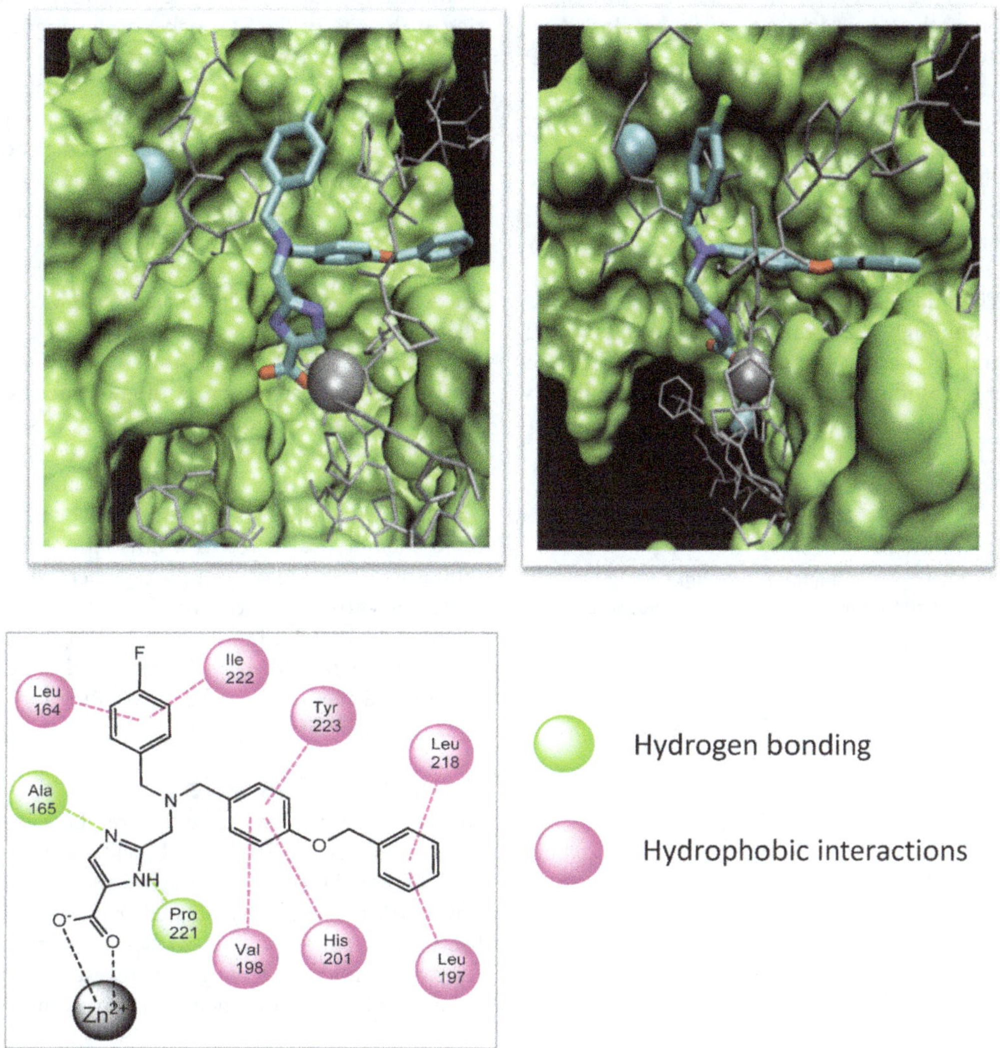

FIGURE 4 | Two different views of the 3D structure of MMP-1154 docked to the active site of MMP-2 together with the major binding interactions.

MMP Inhibitor Development Strategy

Currently, ~500 papers investigating the role of MMP inhibition in myocardial ischemia are available from the last 2 decades in PubMed database. There are several papers that describe the non-zinc binding, allosteric (e.g., π-π stacking) interactions of MMP-2 with selected inhibitors (Di Pizio et al., 2013; Agamennone et al., 2016; Ammazzalorso et al., 2016; Adhikari et al., 2018). Most of these papers employ MMP-2 as a potential biomarker for ischemic heart diseases or as a therapeutic target to evoke cardioprotection. However, early clinical trials targeting MMP-2 for improving cardiovascular outcomes after acute myocardial infarction have failed (e.g., PREMIER study, Hudson et al., 2006). The likely reason for failure was the lesser selectivity of the applied MMP inhibitors as well as the chronic and relatively high-dose administration regimen. Therefore, in our present study, we aimed to develop novel MMP-2 inhibitor lead candidates, which possess high selectivity and lead only to a moderate MMP-2 inhibition in accordance to our previous findings (Giricz et al., 2006; Bencsik et al., 2014).

Novel Structural Findings Regarding MMP-2 Inhibitor Development

Several hydroxamic acid compounds are known as non-selective MMP inhibitors. Therefore, we started our inhibitor development with selecting hydroxamic acid compounds from the AMRI library. We also selected their carboxylic acid derivatives. We identified thiazole and imidazole substituted carboxylic acid molecules, in which MMP-2 inhibitory effect was superior to the corresponding hydroxamic acid derivatives. Furthermore, we found that changing the thiazole ring (MMPI-1157) to the isosteric imidazole (MMPI-1154) increased the selectivity over MMP-1, although the overall inhibitory profile and the structure were similar. This feature was an advantageous factor during molecular designing process since MMP-1 inhibition was responsible for the development of musculoskeletal syndrome, the most severe adverse effect of early MMP inhibitors.

The relatively weak Zn^{2+} chelation derived from the imidazole-carboxylic acid moiety interacting to the Zn^{2+} dynamically and statistically gave an allosteric binding feature for MMPI-1154. It is also assumed that the additional electron donating heteroatom being in close proximity to the acid moiety (thiazole/imidazole ring) would also contribute to the chelation of the Zn^{2+} ion. The bulky side chain is deep inside in the S1' pocket as expected, although some rotational movements would be permitted around the central tertiary N atom. This option would allow different binding modes and activity profiles as well.

TABLE 3 | Screening of molecules on cardiac MMP-2 with gelatin zymography.

Code	Inhibition (%)±SEM at 100 μM final MMP inhibitor concentration
MMPI-1133	11.14 ± 1.58
MMPI-1140	81.08 ± 3.88
MMPI-1154	100
MMPI-1155	46.95 ± 19.06
MMPI-1157	100
MMPI-1245	100
MMPI-1247	100
MMPI-1248	100
MMPI-1252	100
MMPI-1253	100
MMPI-1254	100
MMPI-1260	100

Most importantly, the pyridine moiety instead of the phenyl ring at the end of the S1' pocket occupying longer side chain of the molecules increased the selectivity of the inhibition for MMP-2 against MMP-1 (MMPI-1260, 1248). This is most likely due to the increased polarity of the tail group (such as pyridine), which is exposed to the aqueous environment at the end of the S1' pocket. Similar compounds are described in Duan et al. (2007), where non-zinc chelating MMP-2 inhibitors with a similar bulky side chain were reported. This finding supported our hypothesis that weak or negligible Zn^{2+} chelation with bulky and partially polar side chains lead to selective and active MMP-2 inhibitors. The phenyl-pyridine exchange is also beneficial to the cell penetration since the calculated octanol-water partition (cLogP) decreased in one order of magnitude. Although this change did not cause significant conformational changes, the 3D similarities were high between these compounds and the initial hit (MMPI-1157).

In conclusion, the biological data and the docking studies together with the 3D alignment modeling confirmed that these chemotypes represent a novel promising class of MMP-2 inhibitors. The bulky groups together with a weaker Zn^{2+}-chelating carboxylic acid residue allowed us to achieve low micromolar MMP-2 inhibition, often together with an apparent selectivity against MMP-1. Finally, all the hit compounds meet the drug-likeness criteria (Lipinski Rule of 5.), which predicts high developability prognosis.

Screening Cascade

After the chemical optimization of the novel MMP inhibitor lead candidates, we determined their IC_{50} values by using gelatin zymography. During zymographic analysis, we used full-length, active MMP-2 enzymes isolated from healthy young adult rat hearts. Subsequently, the cardio-cytoprotective effects of the selected candidates having the lowest IC_{50} values to MMP-2 were tested in cultured neonatal cardiac myocytes subjected to

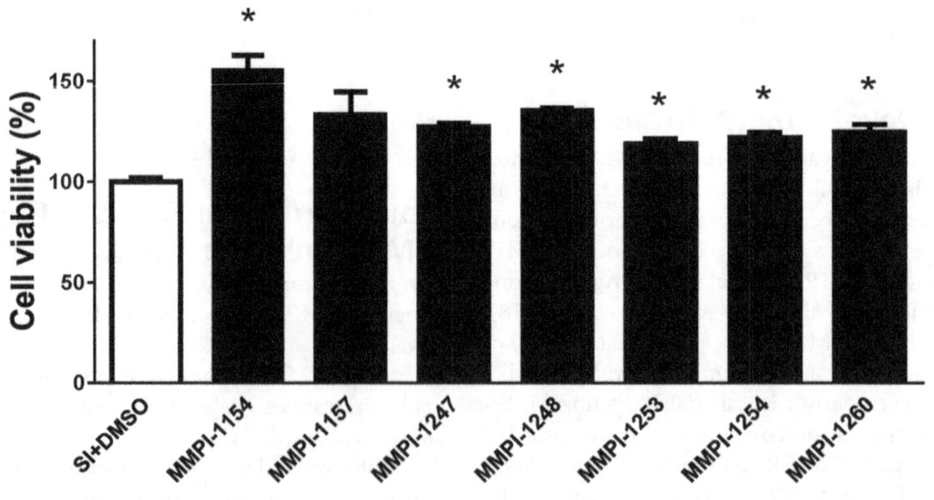

FIGURE 5 | Cardioprotective effects of MMPI lead candidates on neonatal rat cardiac myocytes subjected to simulated I/R. Cell viability was measured after 4 h simulated ischemia followed by 2 h of simulated reperfusion. Data are expressed in the ratio of vehicle (DMSO) control in percentage. Positive data (more than 100%) shows higher viability compared to the control. *$p < 0.05$ vs. Vehicle, $n = 5$–6 (One-way ANOVA followed by Dunnett *post-hoc* test). The most effective doses of the series of experiments are presented in the case of all compounds (for more detailed results see for Supplementary materials, Figure 4).

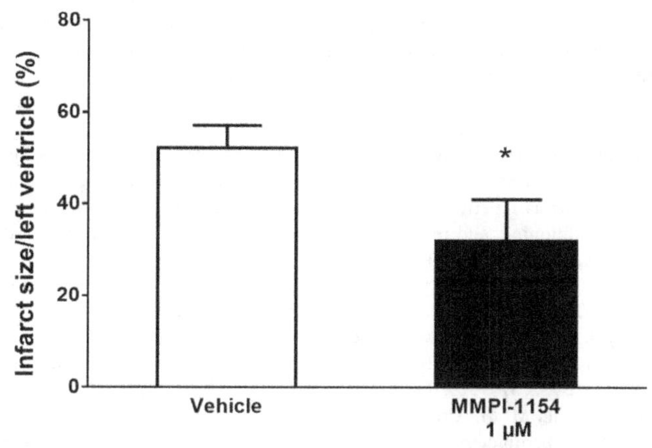

FIGURE 6 | MMPI-1154 is cardioprotective. The effect of MMPI-1154 on myocardial infarct size in isolated rat hearts subjected to 30 min global ischemia followed by 120 min reperfusion. $^{*}p < 0.05$ vs. Vehicle, $n = 6–8$ (One-way ANOVA followed by Fisher LSD *post-hoc* test).

simulated I/R injury. Cardiac myocyte cell culture assay allowed a relatively high throughput biological efficacy testing (Gorbe et al., 2010) of the selected lead candidates in several dose ranges at different levels of inhibition of MMP-2 activity. Our cell culture test system revealed several biologically efficacious doses beyond the IC_{50} values of the selected lead candidates (see data Supplementary Figure 1 for details).

Cardio-Cytoprotection by MMPI-1154

Based on the results of the abovementioned cell culture experiments, we selected MMPI-1154 (The lead candidat) which showed the highest increase in cell viability during simulated I/R experiments. We then used it for cardioprotection in an *ex vivo* rat heart model of acute myocardial infarction. To approximate the moderate 20% inhibition of MMP-2 activity by MMPI-1154 (based on our previous findings, Giricz et al., 2006; Bencsik et al., 2014), in the *ex vivo* model of AMI, we used the 1 μM concentration (IC_{20} value) instead of the most effective 2.5 μM (IC_{50} value) concentration seen during cell culture experiments. Although MMPI-1154 is not highly selective to MMP-2, it seems to be one of the most efficient MMP-2 inhibitors as shown in **Table 2** (efficiency index). In the present study, the *in silico* and subsequent *in vitro* chemical efficiency has been confirmed in the isolated heart experiments since MMPI-1154 in 1 μM showed a significant cardioprotection effect by decreasing myocardial infarct size during acute global ischemia/reperfusion injury. Further research in *in vivo* models of AMI can shed light on its cardioprotective properties as well as on its safety derived from the optimal selectivity toward different MMP isoforms.

CONCLUSIONS

This is the first demonstration that imidazole and thiazole carboxylic acid-based compounds are more efficacious than their hydroxamic acid derivatives in MMP-2 inhibition. MMPI-1154 is a promising novel cardio-cytoprotective imidazole-carboxylic acid MMP-2 inhibitor lead candidate for the treatment of acute myocardial infarction.

AUTHOR CONTRIBUTIONS

PB: Study management and paper writing; KK: Gelatine zymography and *ex vivo* experiments; AG and ZV: Cell culture experiments; ÉK: Paper writing, statistics, data, and figure management; JP and RG: Cell culture and *ex vivo* experiments; LK: *In silico* drug design, synthesis of analogs; LW: MMP inhibitor design, medical chemistry advising; FT: Synthesis of analogs; IH, GF, SC, and LB: Molecular docking and high troughput screening; TC and CC: Supervising zymography and *ex vivo* experiments; GD: Supervising *in silico* and HT screening, granting, paper writing; PF: Supervising whole project, paper writing, and granting.

ACKNOWLEDGMENTS

This work was supported by the National Research, Development and Innovation Office (TÉT_15_IN-1-2016-0068) and by the former National Development Agency (NKFP_06_A1-MMP_2006). PB was supported by the János Bolyai Research Scholarship of the Hungarian Academy of Sciences. We are grateful to ChemAxon Ltd. (Budapest) providing the Screen3D software for the present study and to Miklós Szabó, Adrián Kalászi for their advice.

REFERENCES

Adhikari, N., Sk Abdul, A., Achintya, S., and Tarun, J. (2018). Structural exploration for the refinement of anticancer matrix metalloproteinase-2 inhibitor designing approaches through robust validated multi-QSARs. *J. Mol. Struct.* 1156, 501–515. doi: 10.1016/j.molstruc.2017.12.005

Agamennone, M., Belov, D. S., Laghezza, A., Ivanov, V. N., Novoselov, A. M., Andreev, I. A., et al. (2016). Fragment-based discovery of 5-Arylisatin-based inhibitors of matrix metalloproteinases 2 and 13. *ChemMedChem* 11, 1892–1898. doi: 10.1002/cmdc.201600266

Ali, M. A., Cho, W. J., Hudson, B., Kassiri, Z., Granzier, H., and Schulz, R. (2010). Titin is a target of matrix metalloproteinase-2: implications in myocardial ischemia/reperfusion injury. *Circulation* 122, 2039–2047. doi: 10.1161/CIRCULATIONAHA.109.930222

Almstead, N. G., Bradley, R. S., Pikul, S., De, B., Natchus, M. G., Taiwo, Y. O., et al. (1999). Design, synthesis, and biological evaluation of potent thiazine- and thiazepine-based matrix metalloproteinase inhibitors. *J. Med. Chem.* 42, 4547–4562. doi: 10.1021/jm990330y

Alwan, A., Maclean, D. R., Riley, L. M., d'Espaignet, E. T., Mathers, C. D., Stevens, G. A., et al. (2010). Monitoring and surveillance of chronic non-communicable diseases: progress and capacity in high-burden countries. *Lancet* 376, 1861–1868. doi: 10.1016/S0140-6736(10)61853-3

Ammazzalorso, A., De Filippis, B., Campestre, C., Laghezza, A., Marrone, A., Amoroso, R., et al. (2016). Seeking for non-zinc-binding MMP-2 inhibitors: synthesis, biological evaluation and molecular modelling studies. *Int. J. Mol. Sci.* 17:E1768. doi: 10.3390/ijms17101768

Andreadou, I., Iliodromitis, E. K., Lazou, A., Gorbe, A., Giricz, Z., Schulz, R., et al. (2017). Effect of hypercholesterolaemia on myocardial function, ischaemia-reperfusion injury and cardioprotection by preconditioning, postconditioning and remote conditioning. *Br. J. Pharmacol.* 174, 1555–1569. doi: 10.1111/bph.13704

Baig, M. H., Ahmad, K., Roy, S., Ashraf, J. M., Adil, M., Siddiqui, M. H., et al. (2016). Computer aided drug design: success and limitations. *Curr. Pharm. Des.* 22, 572–581. doi: 10.2174/1381612822666151125000550

Bencsik, P., Bartekova, M., Gorbe, A., Kiss, K., Paloczi, J., Radosinska, J., et al. (2017). MMP activity detection in zymograms. *Methods Mol. Biol.* 1626, 53–70. doi: 10.1007/978-1-4939-7111-4_6

Bencsik, P., Kupai, K., Giricz, Z., Gorbe, A., Pipis, J., Murlasits, Z., et al. (2010). Role of iNOS and peroxynitrite-matrix metalloproteinase-2 signaling in myocardial late preconditioning in rats. *Am. J. Physiol. Heart Circ. Physiol.* 299, H512–H518. doi: 10.1152/ajpheart.00052.2010

Bencsik, P., Paloczi, J., Kocsis, G. F., Pipis, J., Belecz, I., Varga, Z. V., et al. (2014). Moderate inhibition of myocardial matrix metalloproteinase-2 by ilomastat is cardioprotective. *Pharmacol. Res.* 80, 36–42. doi: 10.1016/j.phrs.2013.12.007

Bencsik, P., Sasi, V., Kiss, K., Kupai, K., Kolossvary, M., Maurovich-Horvat, P., et al. (2015). Serum lipids and cardiac function correlate with nitrotyrosine and MMP activity in coronary artery disease patients. *Eur. J. Clin. Invest.* 45, 692–701. doi: 10.1111/eci.12458

Centre, C. C. D. (2017). *Hermes User Guide, A Component of the GOLD Suite 5.6.* Available online at: https://www.ccdc.cam.ac.uk/support-and-resources/ccdcresources/aec7ea64e7974961877c1b09e7506970.pdf.

ChemAxon (2013). Available online at: https://www.chemaxon.com/app/uploads/2013/03/screen3d_2013-02-12.pdf.

Cheung, P. Y., Sawicki, G., Wozniak, M., Wang, W., Radomski, M. W., and Schulz, R. (2000). Matrix metalloproteinase-2 contributes to ischemia-reperfusion injury in the heart. *Circulation* 101, 1833–1839. doi: 10.1161/01.CIR.101.15.1833

D'Annunzio, V., Donato, M., Erni, L., Miksztowicz, V., Buchholz, B., Carrion, C. L., et al. (2009). Rosuvastatin given during reperfusion decreases infarct size and inhibits matrix metalloproteinase-2 activity in normocholesterolemic and hypercholesterolemic rabbits. *J. Cardiovasc. Pharmacol.* 53, 137–144. doi: 10.1097/FJC.0b013e318197c5e9

DeCoux, A., Lindsey, M. L., Villarreal, F., Garcia, R. A., and Schulz, R. (2014). Myocardial matrix metalloproteinase-2: inside out and upside down. *J. Mol. Cell. Cardiol.* 77, 64–72. doi: 10.1016/j.yjmcc.2014.09.016

Dhanaraj, V., Williams, M. G., Ye, Q. Z., Molina, F., Johnson, L. L., Ortwine, D. F., et al. (1999). X-ray structure of gelatinase A catalytic domain complexed with a hydroxamate inhibitor. *Croat. Chem. Acta* 72, 575–591.

Di Pizio, A., Laghezza, A., Tortorella, P., and Agamennone, M. (2013). Probing the S1' site for the identification of non-zinc-binding MMP-2 inhibitors. *ChemMedChem* 8, 1475–1482, 1421. doi: 10.1002/cmdc.201300186

Dormán, G., Cseh, S., Hajdu, I., Barna, L., Konya, D., Kupai, K., et al. (2010). Matrix metalloproteinase inhibitors: a critical appraisal of design principles and proposed therapeutic utility. *Drugs* 70, 949–964. doi: 10.2165/11318390-000000000-00000.

Duan, J. J., Chen, L., Lu, Z., Jiang, B., Asakawa, N., Sheppeck, J. E. II., et al. (2007). Discovery of low nanomolar non-hydroxamate inhibitors of tumor necrosis factor-alpha converting enzyme (TACE). *Bioorg. Med. Chem. Lett.* 17, 266–271. doi: 10.1016/j.bmcl.2006.09.048

Durrant, J. D., de Oliveira, C. A., and McCammon, J. A. (2011). Pyrone-based inhibitors of metalloproteinase types 2 and 3 may work as conformation-selective inhibitors. *Chem. Biol. Drug Des.* 78, 191–198. doi: 10.1111/j.1747-0285.2011.01148.x

Fekete, V., Murlasits, Z., Aypar, E., Bencsik, P., Sarkozy, M., Szenasi, G., et al. (2013). Myocardial postconditioning is lost in vascular nitrate tolerance. *J. Cardiovasc. Pharmacol.* 62, 298–303. doi: 10.1097/FJC.0b013e3182993ae0

Feng, Y., Likos, J., Zhu, L., Woodward, H., McDonald, J., Stevens, A., et al. (2000). 1H, 13C and 15N resonance assignments for a truncated and inhibited catalytic domain of matrix metalloproteinase-2. *J. Biomol. NMR* 17, 85–86.

Ferdinandy, P., Csont, T. B., Csonka, C., Kupai, K. K., Kovács, L., Kis-Tamás, A., et al. (2010). *Novel Inhibitors of Matrix Metalloproteinases.* WO_2012/080762_A1.

Ferdinandy, P., Hausenloy, D. J., Heusch, G., Baxter, G. F., and Schulz, R. (2014). Interaction of risk factors, comorbidities, and comedications with ischemia/reperfusion injury and cardioprotection by preconditioning, postconditioning, and remote conditioning. *Pharmacol. Rev.* 66, 1142–1174. doi: 10.1124/pr.113.008300

Fisher, J. F., and Mobashery, S. (2006). Recent advances in MMP inhibitor design. *Cancer Metastasis Rev.* 25, 115–136. doi: 10.1007/s10555-006-7894-9

Galardy, R. E., Cassabonne, M. E., Giese, C., Gilbert, J. H., Lapierre, F., Lopez, H., et al. (1994). Low molecular weight inhibitors in corneal ulceration. *Ann. N. Y. Acad. Sci.* 732, 315–323. doi: 10.1111/j.1749-6632.1994.tb24746.x

Giricz, Z., Lalu, M. M., Csonka, C., Bencsik, P., Schulz, R., and Ferdinandy, P. (2006). Hyperlipidemia attenuates the infarct size-limiting effect of ischemic preconditioning: role of matrix metalloproteinase-2 inhibition. *J. Pharmacol. Exp. Ther.* 316, 154–161. doi: 10.1124/jpet.105.091140

Gorbe, A., Giricz, Z., Szunyog, A., Csont, T., Burley, D. S., Baxter, G. F., et al. (2010). Role of cGMP-PKG signaling in the protection of neonatal rat cardiac myocytes subjected to simulated ischemia/reoxygenation. *Basic Res. Cardiol.* 105, 643–650. doi: 10.1007/s00395-010-0097-0

Hausenloy, D. J., Garcia-Dorado, D., Erik Botker, H., Davidson, S. M., Downey, J., Engel, F. B., et al. (2017). Novel targets and future strategies for acute cardioprotection: position paper of the European Society of Cardiology Working Group on Cellular Biology of the Heart. *Cardiovasc. Res.* 113, 564–585. doi: 10.1093/cvr/cvx049

Hudson, M. P., Armstrong, P. W., Ruzyllo, W., Brum, J., Cusmano, L., Krzeski, P., et al. (2006). Effects of selective matrix metalloproteinase inhibitor (PG-116800) to prevent ventricular remodeling after myocardial infarction: results of the PREMIER (Prevention of Myocardial Infarction Early Remodeling) trial. *J. Am. Coll. Cardiol.* 48, 15–20. doi: 10.1016/j.jacc.2006.02.055

Johnson, M. A., and Maggiora, G. M. (1990). *Concepts and Applications of Molecular Similarity.* New York, NY: Wiley.

Jones, G., Willett, P., Glen, R. C., Leach, A. R., and Taylor, R. (1997). Development and validation of a genetic algorithm for flexible docking. *J. Mol. Biol.* 267, 727–748. doi: 10.1006/jmbi.1996.0897

Jun, J. H., Cho, J. E., Shim, Y. H., Shim, J. K., and Kwak, Y. L. (2011). Effects of propofol on the expression of matric metalloproteinases in rat cardiac fibroblasts after hypoxia and reoxygenation. *Br. J. Anaesth.* 106, 650–658. doi: 10.1093/bja/aer006

Kalászi, A., Szisz, D., Imre, G., and Polgar, T. (2014). Screen3D: a novel fully flexible high-throughput shape-similarity search method. *J. Chem. Inf. Model.* 54, 1036–1049. doi: 10.1021/ci400620f

Kupai, K., Szucs, G., Cseh, S., Hajdu, I., Csonka, C., Csont, T., et al. (2010). Matrix metalloproteinase activity assays: importance of zymography. *J. Pharmacol. Toxicol. Methods* 61, 205–209. doi: 10.1016/j.vascn.2010.02.011

Li, X., Heinzel, F. R., Boengler, K., Schulz, R., and Heusch, G. (2004). Role of connexin 43 in ischemic preconditioning does not involve intercellular communication through gap junctions. *J. Mol. Cell. Cardiol.* 36, 161–163. doi: 10.1016/j.yjmcc.2003.10.019

Lipinski, C. A., Lombardo, F., Dominy, B. W., and Feeney, P. J. (2001). Experimental and computational approaches to estimate solubility and permeability in drug discovery and development settings. *Adv. Drug Deliv. Rev.* 46, 3–26. doi: 10.1016/S0169-409X(00)00129-0

Papp, A., Szommer, T., Barna, L., Gyimesi, G., Ferdinandy, P., Spadoni, C., et al. (2007). Enhanced hit-to-lead process using bioanalogous lead evolution and chemogenomics: application in designing selective matrix metalloprotease inhibitors. *Expert Opin. Drug Discov.* 2, 707–723. doi: 10.1517/17460441.2.5.707

Roth, G. A., Johnson, C., Abajobir, A., Abd-Allah, F., Abera, S. F., Abyu, G., et al. (2017). Global, regional, and national burden of cardiovascular diseases for 10 causes, 1990 to 2015. *J. Am. Coll. Cardiol.* 70, 1–25. doi: 10.1016/j.jacc.2017.04.052

Sawicki, G., Leon, H., Sawicka, J., Sariahmetoglu, M., Schulze, C. J., Scott, P. G., et al. (2005). Degradation of myosin light chain in isolated rat hearts subjected to ischemia-reperfusion injury: a new intracellular target for matrix metalloproteinase-2. *Circulation* 112, 544–552. doi: 10.1161/CIRCULATIONAHA.104.531616

Sung, M. M., Schulz, C. G., Wang, W., Sawicki, G., Bautista-Lopez, N. L., and Schulz, R. (2007). Matrix metalloproteinase-2 degrades the cytoskeletal protein alpha-actinin in peroxynitrite mediated myocardial injury. *J. Mol. Cell. Cardiol.* 43, 429–436. doi: 10.1016/j.yjmcc.2007.07.055

Turan, N., Csonka, C., Csont, T., Giricz, Z., Fodor, G., Bencsik, P., et al. (2006). The role of peroxynitrite in chemical preconditioning with 3-nitropropionic acid in rat hearts. *Cardiovasc. Res.* 70, 384–390. doi: 10.1016/j.cardiores.2005.12.012

Wang, W., Schulze, C. J., Suarez-Pinzon, W. L., Dyck, J. R., Sawicki, G., and Schulz, R. (2002). Intracellular action of matrix metalloproteinase-2 accounts for acute myocardial ischemia and reperfusion injury. *Circulation* 106, 1543–1549. doi: 10.1161/01.CIR.0000028818.33488.7B

WHO (2017). *Cardiovascular Diseases (CVDs) Fact Sheet*. Available online at: http://www.who.int/mediacentre/factsheets/fs317/en/.

Willett, P. (2006). Similarity-based virtual screening using 2D fingerprints. *Drug Discov. Today* 11, 1046–1053. doi: 10.1016/j.drudis.2006.10.005

Willett, P., and Winterman, V. (1986). A comparison of some measures for the determination of intermolecular structural similarity measures of intermolecular structural similarity. *Quant. Struct. Act. Relat.* 5, 18–25. doi: 10.1002/qsar.19860050105

Yamamoto, M., Tsujishita, H., Hori, N., Ohishi, Y., Inoue, S., Ikeda, S., et al. (1998). Inhibition of membrane-type 1 matrix metalloproteinase by hydroxamate inhibitors: an examination of the subsite pocket. *J. Med. Chem.* 41, 1209–1217. doi: 10.1021/jm970404a

10

Multi-Target Screening and Experimental Validation of Natural Products from *Selaginella* Plants against Alzheimer's Disease

Yin-Hua Deng [1], *Ning-Ning Wang* [1], *Zhen-Xing Zou* [1,2], *Lin Zhang* [3], *Kang-Ping Xu* [1], *Alex F. Chen* [1,4], *Dong-Sheng Cao* [1,4]* *and Gui-Shan Tan* [1,2]*

[1] Xiangya School of Pharmaceutical Sciences, Central South University, Changsha, China, [2] Pharmacy Department, Xiangya Hospital, Central South University, Changsha, China, [3] College of Food Science and Technology, Central South University of Forestry and Technology, Changsha, China, [4] Center for Vascular Disease and Translational Medicine, Third Xiangya Hospital, Central South University, Changsha, China

***Correspondence:**
Dong-Sheng Cao
oriental-cds@163.com
Gui-Shan Tan
tgs395@csu.edu.cn

Alzheimer's disease (AD) is a progressive and irreversible neurodegenerative disorder which is considered to be the most common cause of dementia. It has a greater impact not only on the learning and memory disturbances but also on social and economy. Currently, there are mainly single-target drugs for AD treatment but the complexity and multiple etiologies of AD make them difficult to obtain desirable therapeutic effects. Therefore, the choice of multi-target drugs will be a potential effective strategy inAD treatment. To find multi-target active ingredients for AD treatment from *Selaginella* plants, we firstly explored the behaviors effects on AD mice of total extracts (TE) from *Selaginella doederleinii* on by Morris water maze test and found that TE has a remarkable improvement on learning and memory function for AD mice. And then, multi-target SAR models associated with AD-related proteins were built based on Random Forest (RF) and different descriptors to preliminarily screen potential active ingredients from *Selaginella*. Considering the prediction outputs and the quantity of existing compounds in our laboratory, 13 compounds were chosen to carry out the *in vitro* enzyme inhibitory experiments and 4 compounds with BACE1/MAO-B dual inhibitory activity were determined. Finally, the molecular docking was applied to verify the prediction results and enzyme inhibitory experiments. Based on these study and validation processes, we explored a new strategy to improve the efficiency of active ingredients screening based on trace amount of natural product and numbers of targets and found some multi-target compounds with biological activity for the development of novel drugs for AD treatment.

Keywords: Alzheimer, *Selaginella* plants, multi-target screening, multi-target SAR, BACE1, MAO-B

INTRODUCTION

Alzheimer's disease (AD) is a progressive and irreversible neurodegenerative disorder which is considered to be the most common cause of dementia. With the acceleration of aging process in human society, AD prevalence is expected to reach the epidemic levels (Mount and Downton, 2006). Commonly, a majority of AD patients often have both of behavioral and psychological symptoms of dementia (BPSD). The behavioral characteristic includes the progressive loss of memory, the decline of cognitive function, the decrease of physical function and ultimately problems with communication, time and space disorientation and so on. The psychological symptom includes psychosis, depression, agitation and anxiety (Gauthier et al., 2010; Okura et al., 2011; Borisovskaya et al., 2014). Furthermore, the presence of BPSD usually exacerbates the morbidity and mortality associated with dementia. In more advanced stages, BPSD has a greater impact on social and economic than on the learning and memory disturbances and it has become the major impetus to force patients choosing primary home care and specialized psychogeriatric units. Unfortunately, the existing therapeutic approaches for BPSD are usually efficacy-limited and associated with serious adverse effects, such as the increasing risk of death (Cummings, 2000; U.S. Food and Drug Administration, 2005, 2008).

Although the molecular mechanism of AD pathogenesis has not been clearly understood, several hypotheses have been proposed for AD pathogenesis and their interconnections aggravate this disease a complex disorder (Šimić et al., 2017). The amyloid hypothesis (Goedert and Spillantini, 2006) is hallmarked by the neuropathological accumulation of amyloid beta (Aβ) plaques in the extracellular compartment and the intracellular accumulation of hyper-phosphorylated tau protein in the form of neurofibrillary tangles. The cholinergic hypothesis proposed a decreased level of acetylcholine in certain areas of brain (Craig et al., 2011). Oxidative stress hypothesis proposed the deregulation of endogenous detoxification redox systems and over-production of radical species leading to lipid peroxidation and nucleic acid mutations (Pratico, 2008). In addition, some other hypotheses, such as glutamatergic hypothesis (Bezprozvanny and Mattson, 2008), metal hypothesis (Bonda et al., 2011), and inflammatory hypothesis (Trepanier and Milgram, 2010) have also been proposed. Based on these pathogenesis, there are more than 200 enzymes or proteins related to AD, such as AchE, BACE1, GSK3β, MAO-B, GABA-A receptor, Glutamate receptor, and so on (Saura et al., 1994; Sathya et al., 2012; Fang et al., 2015; Yan et al., 2016). At present, licensed drugs approved for AD treatment are always based on single-target pharmacology. Now, there are two main categories of drugs for AD treatment: one is AchE inhibitor, including donepezil, rivastigmine, and galantamine. They can improve ACh level in the brain by decreasing the hydrolysis of ACh and are mainly used for mild to moderate AD treatment. The other one is N-methyl-D-aspartate antagonist (NMDA). The representative drug, memantine, is mainly used for the treatment of moderate to severe AD, but it is only licensed in several countries because of serious adverse drug reaction (Cummings, 2004; Standridge, 2004). Until now, the limitation of therapeutic treatments and their poor effectiveness make AD treatment become the current biggest medical problem in neurology. In fact, as described before, the complexity and multiple etiologies of AD make the single-target strategy difficult to obtain desirable therapeutic effects. Therefore, the choice of multi-target drugs will be a potential effective strategy in the treatment of AD and consequently the new chemical skeletons or active precursors with multi-target activities for AD therapy are inspired to be found.

As we all know, natural product is a highly valuable resource in searching for chemical precursors with potential bioactivity and few adverse effects because of their structural diversity. For example, biflavonoid glycosides from *Impatiens balsamina* show potential neuroprotective activity (Kim et al., 2017) and apigenin, quercetin show potent anti-Aβaggregation activity which is one of the major culprits in AD (Espargaró et al., 2017). Huperzine A (Hup A) is a highly selective, reversible and potent AChEI extracted from the Chinese medicinal herb *Huperzia serrata*. Compared with tacrine and donepezil, it has a higher bioavailability and potency but is less active toward BChE (Silva et al., 2014; Pisani et al., 2016). Nowadays, the purification of new chemical skeletons and activity screening from natural products still maintain sightless and accidental. Although more and more trace elements have been purified with the development of separation technology, it is still scarcely possible to carry out large-scale activity screening due to the contingency and trace outputs of separation. In recent years, with the rapid development of computer science and the accumulation of chemogenomics data, multi-target SAR model for active-ingredient screening was proposed as a useful method for seeking active compounds and target identification (Cao et al., 2012, 2014; He et al., 2013; Yao et al., 2016). As to the multi-target SAR, the SAR predictive model for each target protein is built based on the relationship between the chemical structure of active and inactive compound. This *in silico* method can give a preliminary screening and target identification for a large number of natural compounds with a prediction probability before the *in vitro* activity test is carried out.

Based on the previous researches, flavonoids show extensive pharmacological activities including anti-AD efficiency. In 2015, Duan SW has identified silibinin, a flavonoid, as a dual inhibitor of AChE and Aβ peptide aggregation for AD treatment (Duan et al., 2015). And then, Song X also proved that Silibinin can attenuate the inflammatory responses, increase glutathione (GSH) levels, decrease malondialdehyde (MDA) levels and upregulate autophagy levels in the $A\beta_{25-35}$-injected rats (Song et al., 2017). What's more, Baicalein, *Scutellaria barbata* flavonoids, *Capparis spinose* flavonoids, and 4-dimethylamine flavonoid derivatives all show some degree of anti-AD activities in animal experiments or *in vitro* tests (Gu et al., 2016; Luo et al., 2016; Mohebali et al., 2016; Wu et al., 2016). Therefore, it's highly valuable and feasible to screen multi-target ingredients from flavonoids extracts for the treatment of AD.

In this study, we aimed to find multi-targets active ingredients for AD treatment from the flavonoids extracts of *Selaginella* plants. Firstly, we explored behavioral effects on AD mice of total extracts (TE) from *Selaginella doederleinii* by Morris water maze test. And then, we screened our home-database consisted of compounds extracted from *Selaginella* plants to hunt ingredients with anti-AD activity through multi-target SAR models *in silico*. Finally, the *in vitro* enzyme activity inhibitory test and the molecular docking experiment were applied to verify the prediction results and to find the potential active ingredients for the AD multi-targets treatment.

MATERIALS AND METHODS

Total Extracts of *Selaginella* Plants

Two hundred and fifty seven compounds were purified from *Selaginella* plants, including *Selaginella tamariscina*, *Selaginella pulvinata* Maxim, *Selaginella braunii* Baker, *Selaginella delicatula* (Desv.) Alston, *Selaginella moellendorfii* hieron, *Selaginella uncinate*, *Selaginella involven Spring*, *Selaginella doederleinii* Hieron. Total extracts (TE) were extracted using 75% ethanol and then freeze-dried into extractum. The suspensions of saline and freeze-dried extractum after ultrasonic vibration was orally administrated for AD mice.

Morris Water Maze Test

The learning and memory ability of AD mice were evaluated by Morris water maze test. Male specific-pathogen-free (SPF) grade male ICR mice (body weighing 18–22 g) were purchased from Hunan Provincial Experimental Animal Centers [Changsha, Hunan, China, Certificate No. SYXK (Xiang) 2012-0004] (Sun et al., 2009).

Mice were randomly divided into five groups (10 mice for each group), namely normal control group (NCG), model control group (MCG), low dose group (LDG, 50 mg/kg), middle dose group (MDG, 100 mg/kg) and high dose group (HDG, 200 mg/kg). To build the AD mice model, mice in MCG, LDG, MDG, and HDG were treated with D-gal (120 mg/kg, intraperitoneally) for 56 days (8 weeks), and the mice in normal group were treated with saline of the same volume for 56 days (8 weeks; dorsonuchal subcutaneous injection). After that, the TE suspensions of saline and freeze-dried extractum after ultrasonic vibration was orally administrated to the mice in LDG, MDG, and HDG for 42 days (6 weeks), and the mice in NCG and MCG were orally treated with saline of the same volume for 42 days (6 weeks). Finally, the spatial learning and memory ability of all the mice were tested by Morris water maze.

The equipment of Morris Water Maze were purchased from Anhui Zheng-hua biological equipment corporation and the test process followed to the relevant laboratory manual. Two indexes, the place navigation and spatial probe, were chosen as the main monitor elements to evaluate the spatial learning and memory ability of all the mice. The experimental method is divided into two parts: acquisition phase and probe trial. In the acquisition phase, we randomly put the head of the mouse into the wall of the pool and fix the starting position. After that, the time of finding the underwater platform was recorded. On the day after acquisition phase, the platform was removed and the probe trial began. The time of finding the position where the platform is located, the swimming distance and the number of crossing through the area where the platform is located were recorded as the spatial memory test indexes.

This study was carried out in accordance with the recommendations of "Laboratory Animals-Guideline of welfare and ethics, Ethics Committee of Hunan Provincial Experimental Animal Centers." The protocol was approved by the "Ethics Committee of Hunan Provincial Experimental Animal Centers."

Multi-Target SAR Model and Prediction of 257 Compounds

According to previous studies published in recent years, we finally found 19 significant proteins related to AD (Cavalli et al., 2008; Fang et al., 2015). For these important AD-related proteins, we collected their ligands that are small, drug-like molecules from Binding database[1]. For each protein, activity data were filtered to keep only activity end-point points that have half-maximum inhibitory concentration (IC_{50}), half-maximum effective concentration (EC_{50}) or Ki values. A compound would be considered as a positive sample when its activity value was below 10 μM. Otherwise, this compound would be considered as a negative sample. Following this step, maybe some AD-related proteins have very little number of negative samples. To balance the number between positive samples and negative samples, we randomly selected certain number of compounds from other AD-related proteins to generate the negative samples for these AD-related proteins. The number of these selected negative samples together with inactive samples should be basically equal to the number of the active samples for these AD-related proteins. These prepared positive sets and negative sets were used for the subsequent model building. The detailed information of AD-related proteins and these datasets used for model building can be seen in Supporting Information (Supplementary Material).

For each protein, a series of high confidence SAR models were built by Random Forest (RF) and different fingerprint representations (FP2, MACCS, Daylight, ECFP2, ECFP4, and ECFP6). RF was introduced by Breiman and Cutler for regression and classification modeling in 2001 firstly (Breiman, 2001). The method is based upon an ensemble of decision trees, from which the prediction of a classification task is provided as the majority vote of the predictions of all trees. Recent studies have suggested that RF offers several striking features which make it very attractive for QSAR/QSPR studies. These include relatively high accuracy of prediction, built-in descriptor selection, and a method for assessing the importance of each descriptor to the model (Cao et al., 2011a,b; Yun et al., 2016). RFs were trained using the RF library in the statistical computing environment, R. All the fingerprints were calculated by some tools developed by our group: ChemDes, BioTriangle webserver and ChemoPy package (Cao et al., 2013; Dong et al., 2015, 2016). To improve the prediction ability of the SAR model, we assembled all fingerprint models to obtain the consensus models with average output. All the assembled models were validated by 5-fold cross validation and test set validation to demonstrate their prediction performance. In this part, some popular statistic parameters were applied to evaluate the performance of these

[1] http://www.bindingdb.org/bind/index.jsp

classification models: true positive (TP); false negative (FN); true negative (TN); false positive (FP); sensitivity (SE); specificity (SP); accuracy (ACC); area under receiver operating characteristic curve (AUC). These classification evaluation parameters are defined as follows:

$$SE = \frac{TP}{TP + FN}$$

$$SP = \frac{TN}{TN + FP}$$

$$ACC = \frac{TP + TN}{TP + FP + TN + FN}$$

After a series of modeling and validation processes, we aimed to obtain reliable SAR models for above-mentioned AD-related proteins. And then, 257 compounds purified from *Selaginella* plants were predicted by these robust and practical models and their inhibitory activities were identified preliminarily for further study.

Target Enzyme Inhibitory Activity *In vitro*

For the compounds that have been regarded as active ingredients by the multi-target SAR models, the *in vitro* target enzyme inhibitory activity test was applied to verify their actual activity for AD treatment. The inhibitory activities were determined by fluorimetric method on Infinite M200 Multi scan Spectrum (Tecan, Swiss). Each concentration was analyzed in triplicate and IC_{50} values were determined by nonlinear regression of inhibition vs. log concentration plots, using GraphPad Prism 7 for Windows, Version 7.00 (GraphPad Software Inc.). BACE1 fluorescence resonance energy transfer assay kits were purchased from the Pan Vera Co and Monoamine Oxidase B (MAO-B) inhibitor screening kits were purchased from Bio Vision Inc.

In the BACE1 inhibition test, the assay was performed in 384-well plates. The assay solution was consisted of 10 μL test compounds (concentrations: 0.017, 0.050, 0.167, 0.500, 1.667, 5.000, 16.667, and 50.000 μM), 10 μL BACE1 substrate and 10 μL BACE1 enzyme. LY2811376 was selected as the reference compound with $IC_{50} = 0.242$ μM and the blank buffer was set as the negative control. The mixture was incubated for 60 min at room temperature. At the end, 10 μL BACE1 stop solution was added to stop the reaction and the fluorescence was detected at the Ex/Em = 545/585 (12 nm bandwidth) settings on Multi scan Spectrum.

In the MAO-B inhibition test, the assay was performed in 96-well plates. The assay solution was consisted of 10 μL test compounds(concentrations: 0.2, 0.4, 0.8, 1.6, 3.2, 6.4, 12.8, and 25.6 μM), 37 μL MAO-B assay buffer, 1 μL MAO-B substrate, 1 μL developer and 1 μL OxiRed Probe. Selegiline was used as the reference control with $IC_{50} = 0.028$ μM and the blank buffer was set as the negative control. The mixture was incubated for 10 min at 37°C. The fluorescence was measured at Ex/Em = 535/587 nm kinetically at 37°C for 10–40 min. Two points (T1 and T2) in the linear range of the plot were chosen and the corresponding fluorescence values (RFU1 and RFU2) were obtained to calculate the slope for all samples. The Calculation of % relative inhibition was following the manual of MAO-B inhibitor screening kit.

Molecular Docking Simulation

To further verify the results of multi-target SAR prediction and enzyme inhibitory experiments, the molecular docking process was applied to simulate the binding position and binding affinity between the active compounds and target proteins. Generally speaking, docking is a computer simulation modeling technique used to predict the interaction between a ligand and a receptor active site, and is an important tool in structure-based drug design. The technique of docking is to position the ligand in different orientations and conformations within the binding site to calculate optimal binding geometries and energies. In this part, the molecular operating environment (MOE, version 2014.) was applied to carry out the molecular docking process. MOE's dock application searches for favorable binding modes between small- to medium-sized ligands and a not-too-flexible macromolecular target. For each ligand, a number of placements called poses are generated and scored. The score can be calculated as either a free energy of binding including among others solvation and entropy terms, or enthalpy based on polar interaction terms including metal ligation, or as qualitative shaped-based numerical value. According to the score values, ligands with different conformations can be ranked and the optimal structural conformation will be affirmed (Wang J. et al., 2015). To make the interactions with the binding site easy to see, the ligand interaction was carried out. It will automatically be loaded with a 2D diagram of the original ligand and a schematic representation of the binding site residues, with the important interactions between ligand and binding site shown. In this study, we selected two proteins as the docking acceptors: BACE1 (PDB ID: 1TQF) (Cobum et al., 2004); MAO-B (PDB ID: 2V5Z) (Binda et al., 2007). As a control, the original ligand included in the crystal structure should also be docked. A series of parameters were set: Dock: rescoring 1 = ASE; retain = 100; rescoring 2 = ASE; retain = 100. Configure force field: final gradient = 0.0001; maximum iterations = 1,000; force constant = 10; radius offset = 0.4. For rest parameters, the default treatment was applied.

RESULTS AND DISCUSSION

Behavioral Evaluation of AD Mice Dealt with Total Extracts

Learning and memory ability of AD mouse was evaluated by Morris water maze test in which the navigation and space exploration are used as indexes. There were five groups of mice under study and the behavioral results can be seen in **Table 1** and **Figure 1**. In the **Table 1**, the residence time and residence distance of each quadrant, the total distance and the number through platform for each group of mice were listed. From the table, we can see that the residence time of MCG was significantly decreased ($P < 0.05$) in 1st and 4th quadrant compared with NCG. The stay intervals in 1st quadrant for MCG group were significantly lower than NCG ($P < 0.05$). However, the residence distance in 3rd quadrant increased prominently ($P < 0.05$). HDG showed longer distance in 1st quadrant ($P < 0.05$) and opposite trends in 3rd quadrant ($P < 0.05$) compared with MCG after 42 days' dosage. With respect to the total distance and

TABLE 1 | The effects of TE on AD mice's behavior ($\bar{x} \pm s$, $n = 10$).

Group	Dose (mg/kg)	1st quadrant		2nd quadrant		3rd quadrant		4th quadrant		Total distance	Speed	Crossing through number
		Time	Distance	Time	Distance	Time	Distance	Time	Distance			
NCG	–	46.5 ± 6.2	906.1 ± 307.2	24.1 ± 6.5	741.5 ± 145.9	24.1 ± 6.5	419.0 ± 109.2	23.0 ± 4.3	544.5 ± 78.8	2778.4 ± 269.8	22.2 ± 0.8	4.0 ± 1.1
MCG	–	30.4 ± 2.3*	707.5 ± 122.0*	28.2 ± 1.8	750.4 ± 97.3	29.2 ± 1.8	580.7 ± 116.7*	18.9 ± 0.4*	421.1 ± 97.3	2459.9 ± 303.4*	20.5 ± 4.2	1.0 ± 0.0*
LDG	50	31.5 ± 5.4	833.1 ± 396.3	25.7 ± 3.4	685.7 ± 142.4	25.7 ± 4.0	706.9 ± 107.3	14.0 ± 0.1	723.6 ± 20.9	2420.7 ± 768.8	23.2 ± 5.6	1.5 ± 0.7
MDG	100	36.3 ± 1.9^{+}	835.6 ± 295.4	30.4 ± 1.2	837.5 ± 49.8	30.4 ± 1.2	535.9 ± 110.2	29.8 ± 5.3^{+}	349.3 ± 49.9	2659.7 ± 100.7	22.8 ± 1.6	2.0 ± 1.4^{+}
HDG	200	39.9 ± 1.5^{+}	854.6 ± 110.5^{+}	35.8 ± 4.9	692.2 ± 262.2	16.8 ± 1.9^{+}	453.5 ± 95.4^{+}	29.3 ± 1.4^{+}	468.8 ± 104.0	2729.4 ± 188.3^{+}	20.2 ± 6.4	3.0 ± 1.4^{+}

*Compared with NCG *P < 0.05, compared with MCG $^{+}$P < 0.05; Crossing through number, the number of crossing through the area where the platform is located; time, s; distance, cm; speed, cm/s.*

numbers through platform, they were significantly reduced for MCG ($P < 0.05$) compared with NCG. They were increased significantly for HDG ($P < 0.05$) compared with MCG after 42 days' dosage. What's more, the crossing through number for MDG were also significantly increased ($P < 0.05$).

Figure 1 shows the navigation and space exploration for different groups of mice. From the figure, we can see that the spatial learning and memory ability of NCG were significantly increased, but there was an opposite trend for MCG and mice in MCG mainly ran along the cell wall. What's more, all the low, medium and high dose of TE can significantly increase the numbers of exploration platform. Considering both results in **Table 1** and **Figure 1**, TE of *Selaginella* has a remarkable improvement on learning and memory function for AD mice. This result inspires us to further explore the effect of the chemical ingredients from *Selaginella* on AD treatment.

Performance Evaluation and the Inhibitory Activity Prediction

Based on the results of the Morris water maze test, the TE of *Selaginella* plants show a potential benefit for AD treatment. To quickly screen the active ingredients from a number of compounds preliminarily, multi-target SAR models associated with AD-related proteins were constructed as described before. In this part, we finally obtained a series of ensemble predictive models for AD-related proteins. Their statistic results of 5-fold cross validation and test set validation were listed in **Table 2**. From this table, we can see that for each predictive model, the accuracy is good enough not only for cross validation (0.808–0.955) but also the test set validation (0.846–0.970). With respect to other statistic parameters, the similar results were obtained and it can be strong evidence for the good predictive ability of this model. Therefore, we have reasons to believe that these ensemble models are robust and practical and can be used to predict the inhibitory activity for a new compound in the early stage of drug discovery.

To evaluate the probability of inhibitory activity for the 19 AD-related targets, 257 compounds were purified from the TE including 143 flavonoids, 9 selaginellins and some other compounds. Before the inhibitory activity prediction by SAR models, the preliminary druggability evaluation was carried out to exclude some compounds that have no beneficial property for further drug development process. In this part, we mainly evaluated the molecular weight and two important ADME (absorption, distribution, metabolism, elimination) properties for druggability by corresponding QSAR models developed by our group: $\log D_{7.4}$ (the distribution coefficients at pH = 7.4) (Wang J. B. et al., 2015; Wang et al., 2017), and logPapp (the Caco-2 membrane permeability) (Wang et al., 2016). Based on previous studies, a good drug candidate should have a $\log D_{7.4}$ value smaller than 5, a logPapp value larger than −5.15 and a molecular weight smaller than 500. After excluding compounds that perform very poorly in at least two of three aforementioned

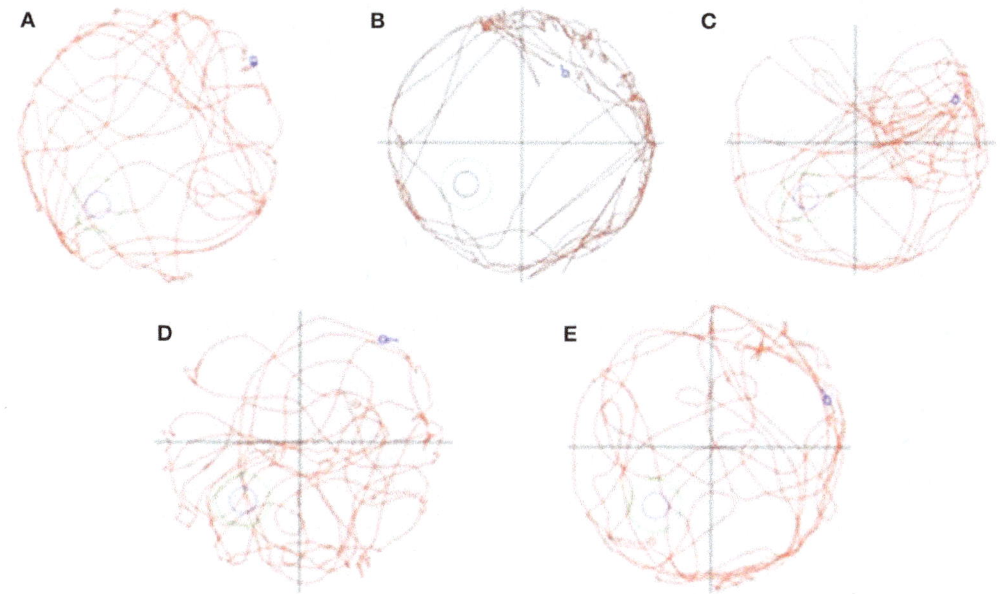

FIGURE 1 | The spatial learning and memory ability of AD mice tested by Morris water maze [**(A)** NCG: normal control group; **(B)** MCG: model control group; **(C)** LDG: low dose group; **(D)** MDG: middle dose group; **(E)** HDG: high dose group]. This figure shows that TE has a remarkable improvement on learning and memory function for AD mice which mainly lies in the increased distance and this functional improvement is dose-dependent.

TABLE 2 | The statistic results of these predictive models (5-fold cross validation and test set validation).

Uniprot_ID	Gene name	5-fold cross validation				Test set validation			
		AUC	ACC	SE	SP	AUC	ACC	SE	SP
P08908	HTR1A	0.950	0.904	0.884	0.924	0.961	0.921	0.911	0.931
Q9Y5N1	HRH3	0.985	0.955	0.944	0.967	0.991	0.970	0.967	0.973
P50406	HTR6	0.969	0.930	0.918	0.942	0.986	0.953	0.932	0.974
P22303	ACHE	0.892	0.845	0.818	0.871	0.944	0.903	0.886	0.922
Q99720	SIGMAR1	0.967	0.918	0.897	0.938	0.979	0.949	0.944	0.955
P11229	CHRM1	0.864	0.808	0.798	0.818	0.938	0.882	0.882	0.883
P49841	GSK3B	0.892	0.821	0.786	0.856	0.963	0.903	0.902	0.905
P06276	BCHE	0.879	0.820	0.797	0.842	0.926	0.855	0.862	0.848
P56817	BACE1	0.961	0.930	0.919	0.942	0.971	0.942	0.951	0.934
P27338	MAOB	0.888	0.826	0.809	0.842	0.941	0.877	0.860	0.895
P36544	CHRNA7	0.875	0.824	0.791	0.857	0.916	0.846	0.792	0.899
Q07343	PDE4B	0.957	0.914	0.884	0.945	0.974	0.942	0.953	0.930
P27815	PDE4A	0.951	0.917	0.911	0.924	0.962	0.922	0.910	0.934
Q13639	HTR4	0.963	0.943	0.921	0.965	0.976	0.950	0.920	0.977
P46098	HTR3A	0.894	0.853	0.810	0.896	0.928	0.892	0.833	0.949
Q96BI3	APH1B	0.942	0.899	0.917	0.882	0.973	0.948	0.963	0.935
P05067	APP	0.973	0.915	0.881	0.950	0.944	0.912	0.867	0.961
Q9NZ42	PSENEN	0.945	0.924	0.946	0.903	0.951	0.914	0.953	0.880
Q8WW43	APH1B	0.937	0.920	0.938	0.902	0.952	0.935	0.924	0.944

properties, there were 238 compounds left for further activity screening.

As described before, the inhibitory activity of these 238 compounds were predicted by the multi-target SAR model. The predictive result for a new compound was outputted as a probability value. For each compound that was classified as active ingredient by SAR models, if its probability value >0.5, it is considered to be active, otherwise, it is inactive. From the predictive result, it can be seen that 54 flavonoids and 4 selaginellins present a good inhibitory correlation with MAO-B, 21 flavonoids may show BACE1 inhibitory activity. However, to improve the reliability of prediction, we apply the prediction probability of 0.8 as a cut-off value to select the active compounds for some related targets. As a result, 18 compounds

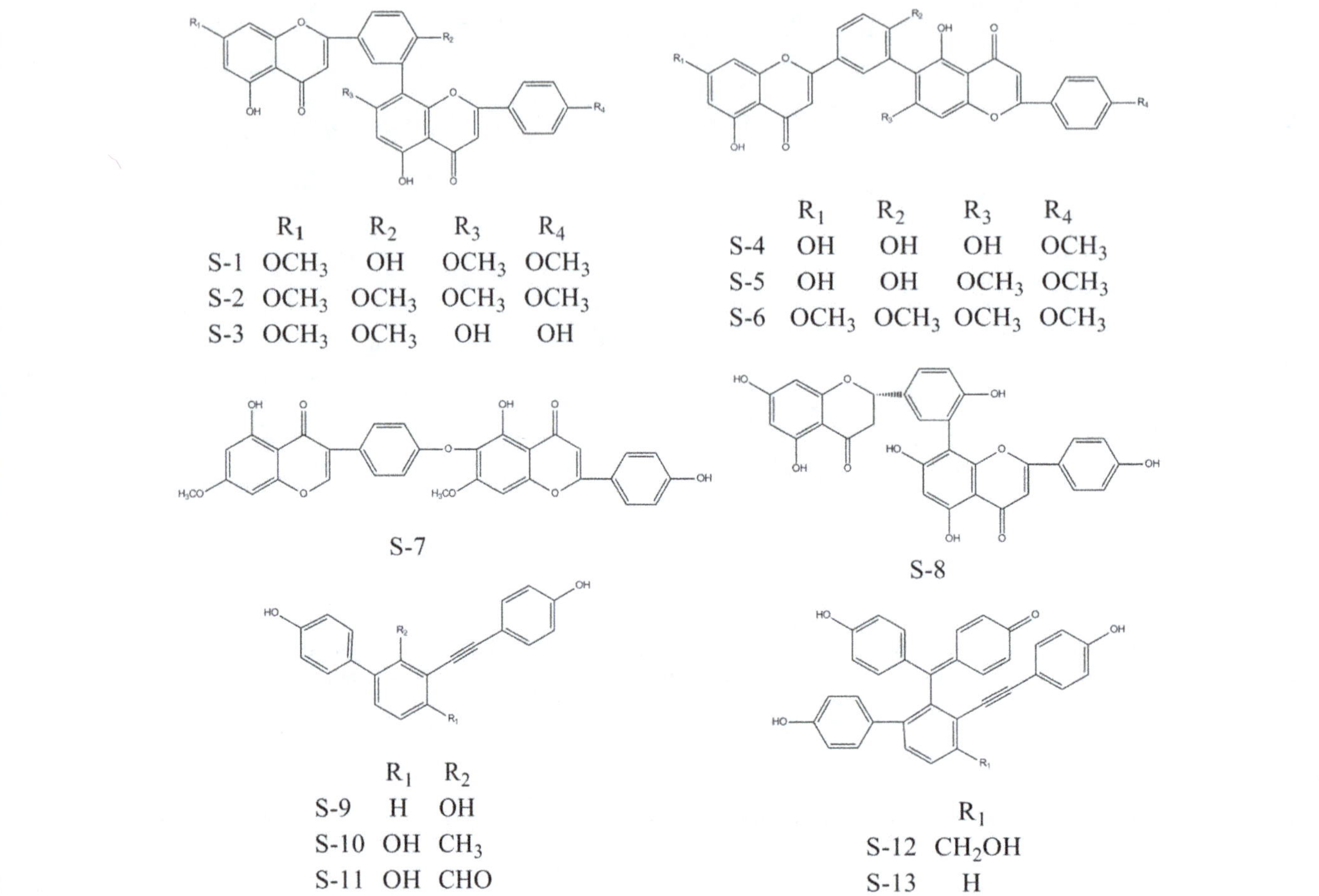

FIGURE 2 | The chemical structures of 13 compounds that with inhibitory activity after multi-target SAR model prediction. Among them, eight are biflavones and the left five are selaginellins.

TABLE 3 | The IC_{50} values of 13 compounds under study.

Compound		S-1	S-2	S-3	S-4	S-5	S-6	S-7	S-8	S-9	S-10	S-11	S-12	S-13	Z-factor
IC_{50} (μM)	BACE1	70.89	17.20	2.75	81.93	7.58	20.70	3.97	0.75	4.32	3.40	2.27	2.82	2.72	0.93
	MAO-B	–[a]	15.74	11.72	13.89	2.91	8.81	23.17	3.62	18.21	10.24	–[a]	3.52	3.42	0.89

[a]*The IC_{50} value cannot be calculated in the predetermined concentration range.*

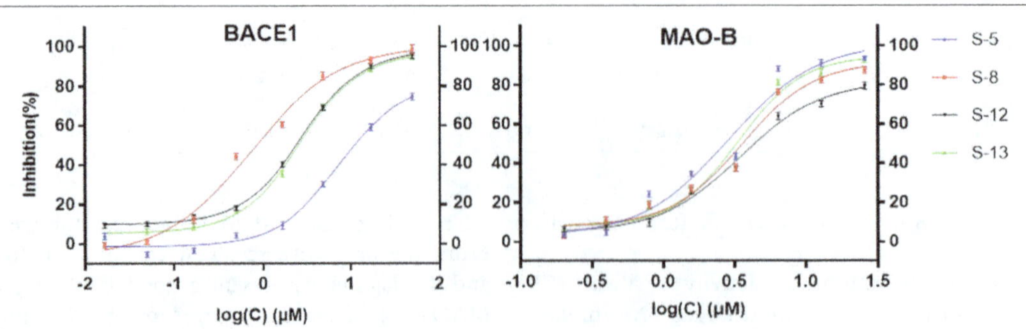

FIGURE 3 | Verification of BACE1 and MAO-B Inhibition. This figure shows that all these four compounds (S-5, S-8, S-12, S-13) have good inhibitory activity in the *in vitro* validation test.

TABLE 4 | Four active compounds and their docking results.

Compound	BACE1			MAO-B		
	Score	Binding residues	Binding force	Score	Binding residues	Binding force
S-5	−29.7	THR (232A); GLN (12A);THR (232A)	H-acceptor; pi-H; pi-H	−44.0	CYS (397A); GLY (13A)	H-donor; pi-H
S-8	−32.7	ASP (32A); THR (231A)	H-donor; pi-H	−38.4	TYR (398A)	H-pi
S-12	−27.8	THR (231A)	pi-H	−35.4	TRP (388A)	H-pi
S-13	−28.4	GLN (73A); ARG (307A)	H-donor; H-acceptor	−34.1	TRP (388A)	H-pi
Ligand	−35.8	–	–	−51.7	–	–

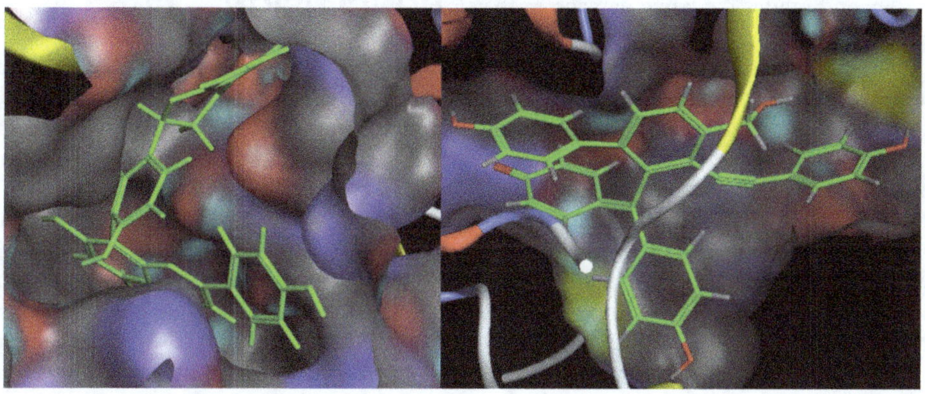

FIGURE 4 | The docking results of S-8 bounding to BACE1 (**left**, PDB ID: 1TQF) and MAO-B (**right**, PDB ID: 2V5Z). The structure of S-8 is rendered green and the docking pocket surface was adjected to a suitable transparency.

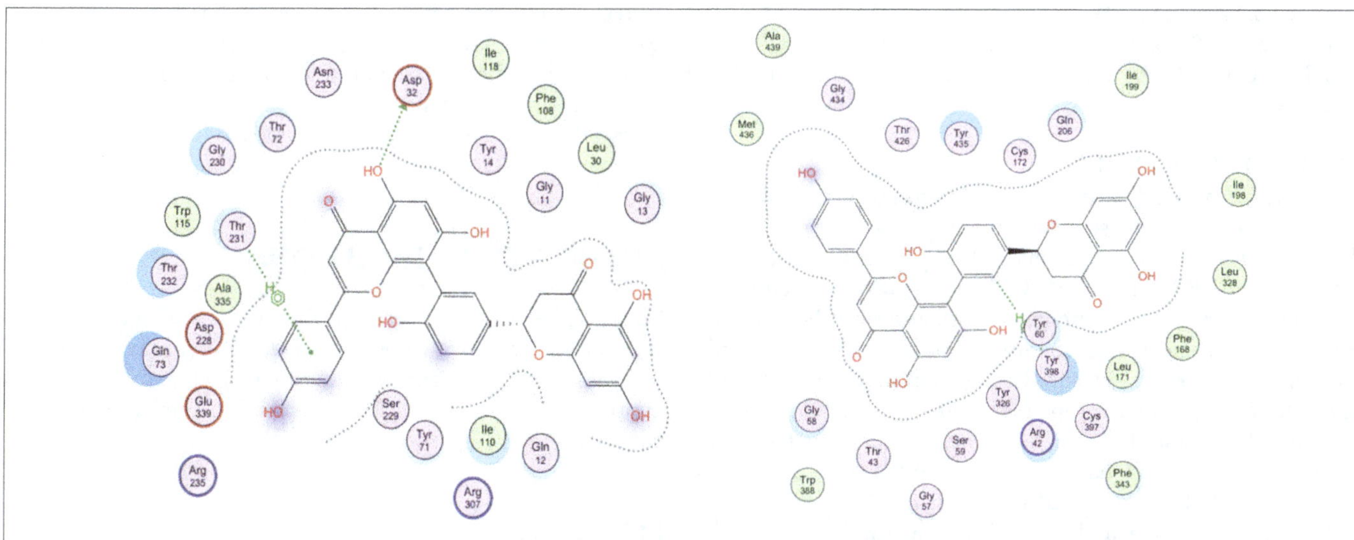

FIGURE 5 | The ligand interaction diagram of S-8 bounding to BACE1 (**left**, PDB ID: 1TQF) and MAO-B (**right**, PDB ID: 2V5Z). It is a 2D diagram of the original ligand and a schematic representation of the binding site residues, with the important interactions between ligand and binding site shown. For BACE1, the main binding force is the hydrogen bond force and pi-bond force with ASP (232A) and THR (231A); for MAO-B, the main binding force is the hydrogen bond force and pi-bond force with CYS (397A) and GLY (13A).

with a probability value larger than 0.8 were extracted. These compounds were prepared for further validation in the inhibitory activity test and their detailed information can be seen in the Supporting Information (Supplementary Material).

In vitro Validation of Inhibitory Activity for Target Enzyme

Based on the prediction outputs, we focused on the screening of BACE1/MAO-B dual inhibitory activity of flavonoids and selaginellins. The enzyme BACE1 is considered as a prime target to design therapeutics for AD mainly because of that the catalysis process by BACE1 is the rate-limiting step in APP proteolysis and the BACE1 knock-out mice lacking Aβ production survives with normal physiology (Roberds et al., 2001). As the majorβ-secretase enzyme that initiates the generation of Aβ, BACE1 is undoubtedly a prime target for anti-Aβtherapy in AD (Ohno, 2016). The increase of MAO-B activity is associated with gliosis, which can result in higher levels of H_2O_2 and oxidative free radicals (Nebbioso et al., 2012). Thus, the MAO-B inhibitors are potential candidates for anti-AD drugs due to their capacity to regulate neurotransmitters and inhibit oxidative damage in the central nervous system.

Considering the quantity of existing compounds in our laboratory, 13 compounds were chosen to carry out the inhibitory activity validation experiments. Their chemical structures were displayed in **Figure 2** and their IC_{50} values can be seen in **Table 3**. To evaluate the inhibitory activity of these compounds, a threshold value of $IC_{50} = 10$ μM was applied. If a compound has a IC_{50} values smaller than 10 μM, it would be considered to be active. Otherwise, it is inactive. We can find that nine of them show good inhibition on BACE1 with IC_{50} values ranged from 0.7454 to 7.578 μM and five of them show good inhibition on MAO-B with IC_{50} values ranged from 2.913 to 8.813 μM. Among them, S-8, S-5, S-13, and S-12 all have significant dual BACE1/MAO-B inhibitory activities with IC_{50} values in the micromole magnitude and S-8 has been proved to be the most potent against BACE1 and MAO-B with IC_{50} values of 0.7454 and 3.619 μM, respectively. Among them, S-5 and S-8 are biflavones, S-12 and S-13 are selaginellins. The inhibitory curves for these four compounds were summarized in **Figure 3**.

Molecular Docking

As described before, for each structural conformation of S-5, S-8, S-12, and S-13, a score value was obtained to evaluate the binding affinity between this active compound and each target protein (BACE1 and MAO-B). Generally, a lower score is better. Therefore, the optimal conformation can be decided from a series of generated conformations for each compound according to their score values. Combining the result of ligand interaction, four active compounds and their docking results were listed in **Table 4**. From the table, we can see that four compounds indeed all have some degree of interaction with BACE1 and MAO-B compared with their original ligands. For BACE1, the most active molecule is S-8 for which the score value is −32.7 and the main binding force is the hydrogen bond force and pi-bond force with ASP (232A) and THR (231A). As to the rest three molecules, the mainly binding force are also the hydrogen bond and pi-bond force with different residues. For MAO-B, the most active molecule is S-5 for which the score value is −44.0 and the main binding force is the hydrogen bond force and pi-bond force with CYS (397A) and GLY (13A). In summary, the molecular docking results were consistent with the results of aforementioned inhibitory experiments that S-8 has the strongest inhibition activity for BACE1 and S-5/S-8 performs better than S-12/S-13 in the inhibition of MAO-B. Therefore, as the conclusion obtained from above *in intro* inhibitory test, S-5, S-8, S-12, S-13 all have significant dual BACE1/MAO-B inhibitory activities and S-8 promises to be the most potent against BACE1 and MAO-B. The docking results and corresponding 2D ligand interaction diagram of S-8 bound to BACE1 and MAO-B can be seen in **Figures 4, 5**. The detailed information of all conformations and docking results for other three compounds can be seen in the Supporting Information (Supplementary Material).

CONCLUSION

In this study, we explored that the TE extracted from *Selaginella* plants has a remarkable improvement on learning and memory function for AD mice by Morris water maze test. And then, we preliminarily screened our home-database consisting of flavonoids compounds by multi-target SAR models *in silico*. After that, the *in vitro* enzyme activity inhibitory test was applied to evaluate 13 compounds that were considered to be active by multi-target SAR models and finally 4 compounds (S-8, S-5, S-13, and S-12) were found to have significant inhibitory activities on both BACE1 and MAO-B. Among them, S-8 has been proved to be the most potent ingredient against BACE1 and MAO-B with IC_{50} values of 0.745 and 3.619 μM, respectively. What's more, the molecular docking experiment was applied to verify the prediction results and to find the binding position and binding strength between the active ingredient and AD-related proteins. All in all, after these study and validation processes, we explored a new strategy to improve the efficiency of screening the active ingredients based on trace amount of natural product and numbers of targets and finally obtained some multi-targets potential compounds for the development of novel drugs for AD treatment.

AUTHOR CONTRIBUTIONS

YD, NW, DC, and GT designed this study. YD and NW wrote and revised the manuscript. ZZ helped in preparing figures and tables. LZ, AC, and KX helped in giving suggestions to improve the manuscript. All authors read and approved the final manuscript.

FUNDING

This work is financially supported by the National Natural Science Foundation of China (Grants No. 81402853, 31370370, 81501619), the National Key Basic Research Program (2015CB910700), the Central South University Innovation Foundation for Postgraduate (2016zzts498), the Project of Innovation-driven Plan in Central South University, and the Postdoctoral Science Foundation of Central South University, the Chinese Postdoctoral Science Foundation (2014T70794, 2014M562142). The studies meet with the approval of the university's review board.

SUPPLEMENTARY MATERIAL

Supporting Information SI1 lists 19 AD-related proteins and their detail information, the information including their gene names, uniport ID, protein name, and the number of samples for modeling process. Supporting Information SI2 lists the structural information of 18 compounds selected by multi-target SAR models. Supporting Information SI3 shows the detailed information of all conformations and docking results for S-5, S-12, and S-13.

REFERENCES

Bezprozvanny, I., and Mattson, M. P. (2008). Neuronal calcium mishandling and the pathogenesis of Alzheimer's disease. *Trends Neurosci.* 31, 454–463. doi: 10.1016/j.tins.2008.06.005

Binda, C., Wang, J., Pisani, L., Caccia, C., Carotti, A., Salvati, P., et al. (2007). Structures of human monoamine oxidase B complexes with selective noncovalent inhibitors: safinamide and coumarin analogs. *J. Med. Chem.* 50, 5848–5852. doi: 10.1021/jm070677y

Bonda, D. J., Lee, H. G., Blair, J. A., Zhu, X., Perry, G., and Smith, M. A. (2011). Role of metal dyshomeostasis in Alzheimer's disease. *Metallomics* 3, 267–270. doi: 10.1039/c0mt00074d

Borisovskaya, A., Pascualy, M., and Borson, S. (2014). Cognitive and neuropsychiatric impairments in Alzheimer's disease: current treatment strategies. *Curr. Psychiatry Rep.* 16, 1–9. doi: 10.1007/s11920-014-0470-z

Breiman, L. (2001). Random forests. *Mach. Learn.* 45, 5–32. doi: 10.1023/A:1010933404324

Cao, D. S., Liang, Y. Z., Xu, Q. S., Zhang, L. X., Hu, Q. N., and Li, H. D. (2011a). Feature importance sampling-based adaptive random forest as a useful tool to screen underlying lead compounds. *J. Chemometrics* 25, 201–207. doi: 10.1002/cem.1375

Cao, D. S., Hu, Q. N., Xu, Q. S., Yang, Y. N., Zhao, J. C., Lu, H. M., et al. (2011b). *In silico* classification of human maximum recommended daily dose based on modified random forest and substructure fingerprint. *Anal. Chim. Acta* 692, 50–56. doi: 10.1016/j.aca.2011.02.010

Cao, D. S., Liu, S., Xu, Q. S., Lu, H. M., Huang, J. H., Hu, Q. N., et al. (2012). Large-scale prediction of drug-target interactions using protein sequences and drug topological structures. *Anal. Chim. Acta* 752, 1–10. doi: 10.1016/j.aca.2012.09.021

Cao, D. S., Xu, Q. S., Hu, Q. N., and Liang, Y. Z. (2013). ChemoPy: freely available python package for computational biology and chemoinformatics. *Bioinformatics* 29, 1092–1094. doi: 10.1093/bioinformatics/btt105

Cao, D. S., Zhang, L. X., Tan, G. S., Xiang, Z., Zeng, W. B., Xu, Q. S., et al. (2014). Computational prediction of drug target interactions using chemical, biological, and network features. *Mol. Inform.* 33, 669–681. doi: 10.1002/minf.201400009

Cavalli, A., Bolognesi, M. L., Minarini, A., Rosini, M., Tumiatti, V., Recanatini, M., et al. (2008). Multi-target-directed ligands to combat neurodegenerative diseases. *J. Med. Chem.* 51, 347–372. doi: 10.1021/jm7009364

Cobum, C. A., Stachel, S. J., Li, Y. M., Rush, D. M., Steele, T. G., Chen-Dodson, E., et al. (2004). Identification of a small molecule nonpeptide active site β-secretase inhibitor that displays a nontraditional binding mode for aspartyl proteases. *J. Med. Chem.* 47, 6117–6119. doi: 10.1021/jm049388p

Craig, L. A., Hong, N. S., and McDonald, R. J. (2011). Revisiting the cholinergic hypothesis in the development of Alzheimer's disease. *Neurosci. Biobehav. Rev.* 35, 1397–1409. doi: 10.1016/j.neubiorev.2011.03.001

Cummings, J. L. (2000). The role of cholinergic agents in the management of behavioural disturbances in Alzheimer's disease. *Int. J. Neuropsychopharmacol.* 4, 21–29. doi: 10.1017/S1461145700001917

Cummings, J. L. (2004). Treatment of Alzheimer's disease: current and future therapeutic approaches. *Rev. Neurol. Dis.* 1, 60–69.

Dong, J., Cao, D. S., Miao, H. Y., Liu, S., Deng, B. C., Yun, Y. H., et al. (2015). ChemDes: an integrated web-based platform for molecular descriptor and fingerprint computation. *J. Cheminform.* 7:60. doi: 10.1186/s13321-015-0109-z

Dong, J., Yao, Z. J., Wen, M., Zhu, M. F., Wang, N. N., Miao, H. Y., et al. (2016). BioTriangle: a web-accessible platform for generating various molecular representations for chemicals, proteins, DNAs/RNAs and their interactions. *J. Cheminform.* 8:34. doi: 10.1186/s13321-016-0146-2

Duan, S., Guan, X., Lin, R., Liu, X., Yan, Y., Lin, R., et al. (2015). Silibinin inhibits acetylcholinesterase activity and amyloid β peptide aggregation: a dual-target drug for the treatment of Alzheimer's disease. *Neurobiol. Aging* 36, 1792–1807. doi: 10.1016/j.neurobiolaging.2015.02.002

Espargaró, A., Ginex, T., Vadell, M. D., Busquets, M. A., Estelrich, J., Mu-oz-Torrero, D., et al. (2017). Combined *in vitro* cell-based/*in silico* screening of naturally occurring flavonoids and phenolic compounds as potential Anti-Alzheimer drugs. *J. Nat. Prod.* 80, 278–289. doi: 10.1021/acs.jnatprod.6b00643

Fang, J. S., Li, Y. J., Liu, R., Pang, X. C., Li, C., Yang, R. Y., et al. (2015). Discovery of multitarget-directed ligands against Alzheimer's disease through systematic prediction of chemical–protein interactions. *J. Chem. Inf. Model* 55, 149–164. doi: 10.1021/ci500574n

Gauthier, S., Cummings, J., Ballard, C., Brodaty, H., Grossberg, G., Robert, P., et al. (2010). Management of behavioral problems in Alzheimer's disease. *Int Psychogeriatr.* 22, 346–372. doi: 10.1017/S1041610209991505

Goedert, M., and Spillantini, M. G. (2006). A century of Alzheimer's disease. *Science* 314, 777–781. doi: 10.1126/science.1132814

Gu, X. H., Xu, L. J., Liu, Z. Q., Wei, B., Yang, Y. J., Xu, G. G., et al. (2016). The flavonoid baicalein rescues synaptic plasticity and memory deficits in a mouse model of Alzheimer's disease. *Behav. Brain Res.* 311, 309–321. doi: 10.1016/j.bbr.2016.05.052

He, M., Cao, D. S., Liang, Y. Z., Li, Y. P., Liu, P. L., Xu, Q. S., et al. (2013). Pressor mechanism evaluation for phytochemical compounds using *in silico* compound–protein interaction prediction. *Regul. Toxicol. Pharmacol.* 67, 115–124. doi: 10.1016/j.yrtph.2013.07.010

Kim, C. S., Bae, M., Oh, J., Subedi, L., Suh, W. S., Choi, S. Z., et al. (2017). Anti-neurodegenerative biflavonoid glycosides from impatiens balsamina. *J. Nat. Prod.* 80, 471–478. doi: 10.1021/acs.jnatprod.6b00981

Luo, W., Wang, T., Hong, C., Yang, Y. C., Chen, Y., Cen, J., et al. (2016). Design, synthesis and evaluation of 4-dimethylamine flavonoid derivatives as potential multifunctional anti-Alzheimer agents. *Eur. J. Med. Chem.* 122, 17–26. doi: 10.1016/j.ejmech.2016.06.022

Mohebali, N., Shahzadeh Fazeli, S. A., Ghafoori, H., Farahmand, Z., MohammadKhani, E., Vakhshiteh, F., et al. (2016). Effect of flavonoids rich extract of Capparisspinosa on inflammatory involved genes in amyloid-beta peptide injected rat model of Alzheimer's disease. *Nutr. Neurosci.* 25, 1–8. doi: 10.1080/1028415X.2016.1238026

Mount, C., and Downton, C. (2006). Alzheimer disease: progress or profit? *Nat. Med.* 12, 780–784. doi: 10.1038/nm0706-780

Nebbioso, M., Pascarella, A., Cavallotti, C., and Pescosolido, N. (2012). Monoamine oxidase enzymes and oxidative stress in the rat optic nerve: age-related changes. *Int. J. Exp. Pathol.* 93, 401–405. doi: 10.1111/j.1365-2613.2012.00832.x

Ohno, M. (2016). Alzheimer's therapy targeting the β-secretase enzyme BACE1: Benefits and potential limitations from the perspective of animalmodel studies. *Brain Res. Bull.* 126(Pt 2), 183–198. doi: 10.1016/j.brainresbull.2016.04.007

Okura, T., Plassman, B. L., Steffens, D. C., Llewellyn, D. J., Potter, G. G., and Langa, K. M. (2011). Neuropsychiatric symptoms and the risk of institutionalization and death: the aging, demographics, and memory study. *J. Am. Geriatr. Soc.* 59, 473–481. doi: 10.1111/j.1532-5415.2011.03314.x

Pisani, L., Farina, R., Soto-Otero, R., Denora, N., Mangiatordi, G. F., Nicolotti, O., et al. (2016). Searching for multi-targeting neurotherapeutics against Alzheimer's: discovery of potent AChE-MAO B inhibitors through the decoration of the 2H-chromen-2-one structural motif. *Molecules* 21, 362–375. doi: 10.3390/molecules21030362

Pratico, D. (2008). Oxidative stress hypothesis in Alzheimer's disease: a reappraisal. *Trends Pharmacol. Sci.* 29, 609–615. doi: 10.1016/j.tips.2008.09.001

Roberds, S. L., Anderson, J., Basi, G., Bienkowski, M. J., Branstetter, D. G., Chen, K. S., et al. (2001). BACE knockout mice are healthy despite lacking the primary β-secretase activity in brain: implications for Alzheimer's disease therapeutics. *Hum. Mol. Genet.* 10, 1317–1324. doi: 10.1093/hmg/10.12.1317

Sathya, M., Premkumar, P., Karthick, C., Moorthi, P., Jayachandran, K. S., and Anusuyadevi, M. (2012). BACE1 in Alzheimer's disease. *Clin. Chim. Acta* 414, 171–178. doi: 10.1016/j.cca.2012.08.013

Saura, J., Luque, J. M., Cesura, A. M., Da Prada, M., Chan-Palay, V., Huber, G., et al. (1994). Increased monoamine oxidase B activity in plaque-associated astrocytes of Alzheimer brains revealed by quantitative enzyme radioautography. *Neuroscience* 62, 15–30. doi: 10.1016/0306-4522(94)90311-5

Silva, T., Reis, J., Teixeira, J., and Borges, F. (2014). Alzheimer's disease, enzyme targets and drug discovery struggles: from natural products to drug prototypes. *Ageing Res. Rev.* 15, 116–145. doi: 10.1016/j.arr.2014.03.008

Šimić, G., Babić Leko, M., Wray, S., Harrington, C. R., Delalle, I., Jovanov-Milošević, N., et al. (2017). Monoaminergic neuropathology in Alzheimer's disease. *Prog. Neurobiol.* 151, 101–138. doi: 10.1016/j.pneurobio.2016.04.001

Song, X., Zhou, B., Cui, L., Lei, D., Zhang, P., Yao, G., et al. (2017). Silibinin ameliorates Aβ25-35-induced memory deficits in rats by modulating autophagy and attenuating neuroinflammation as well as oxidative stress. *Neurochem. Res.* 42, 1073–1083. doi: 10.1007/s11064-016-2141-4

Standridge, J. B. (2004). Pharmacotherapeutic approaches to the prevention of Alzheimer's disease. *Am. J. Geriatr. Pharmacother.* 2, 119–132. doi: 10.1016/S1543-5946(04)90017-7

Sun, Z. Z., Chen, Z. B., Jiang, H., Li, L. L., Li, E. G., and Xu, Y. (2009). Alteration of Aβ metabolismrelated molecules in predementia induced by AlCl3 and D-galactose. *Age (Dordr)* 31, 277–284. doi: 10.1007/s11357-009-9099-y

Trepanier, C. H., and Milgram, N. W. (2010). Neuroinflammation in Alzheimer's disease: are NSAIDs and selective COX-2 inhibitors the next line of therapy? *J. Alzheimers Dis.* 21, 1089–1099. doi: 10.3233/JAD-2010-090667

U.S. Food and Drug Administration (2005). *Public Health Advisory: Deaths with Antipsychoticsin Elderly Patients with Behavioral Disturbances.* Rockville, MD: Center for Drug Evaluation and Research. Available online at: http://www.fda.gov/drugs/drugsafety/postmarketdrugsafetyinformationforpatientsandproviders/ucm053171 (Accessed April 04, 2016).

U.S. Food and Drug Administration (2008). *Information on Conventional Antipsychotics.* Rockville, MD: Center for Drug Evaluation and Research. Available online at: http://www.fda.gov/Drugs/DrugSafety/PostmarketDrugSafetyInformationforPatientsandProviders/ucm107211.htm (Accessed April 04, 2016).

Wang, J., Li, Y., Yang, Y., Du, J., Zhang, S., and Yang, L. (2015). *In silico* research to assist the investigation of carboxamide derivatives as potent TRPV1 antagonists. *Mol. Biosyst.* 11, 2885–2899. doi: 10.1039/C5MB00356C

Wang, J. B., Cao, D. S., Zhu, M. F., Yun, Y. H., Xiao, N., and Liang, Y. Z. (2015). *In silico* evaluation of logD7.4 and comparison with other prediction methods. *J. Chemometr.* 29, 389–398. doi: 10.1002/cem.2718

Wang, N. N., Dong, J., Deng, Y. H., Zhu, M. F., Wen, M., Yao, Z. J., et al. (2016). ADME properties evaluation in drug discovery: prediction of caco-2 cell permeability using a combination of NSGA-II and boosting. *J. Chem. Inf. Model.* 56, 763–773. doi: 10.1021/acs.jcim.5b00642

Wang, N. N., Huang, C., Dong, J., Yao, Z. J., Zhu, M. F., Deng, Z. K., et al. (2017). Predicting human intestinal absorption with modified random forest approach: a comprehensive evaluation of molecular representation, unbalanced data, and applicability domain issues. *RSC Adv.* 7, 19007–19018. doi: 10.1039/C6RA28442F

Wu, X. G., Wang, S. S., Miao, H., Cheng, J. J., Zhang, S. F., and Shang, Y. Z. (2016). Scutellariabarbata flavonoids alleviate memory deficits and neuronal injuries induced by composited Aβ in rats. *Behav. Brain Funct.* 12:33. doi: 10.1186/s12993-016-0118-8

Yan, R. Q., Fan, Q. Y., Zhou, J., and Vassar, R. (2016). Inhibiting BACE1 to reverse synaptic dysfunctions in Alzheimer's disease. *Neurosci. Biobehav. Rev.* 65, 326–340. doi: 10.1016/j.neubiorev.2016.03.025

Yao, Z. J., Dong, J., Che, Y. J., Zhu, M. F., Wen, M., Wang, N. N., et al. (2016). TargetNet: a web service for predicting potential drug–target interaction profiling via multi-target SAR models. *J. Comput. Aided Mol. Des.* 30, 413–424. doi: 10.1007/s10822-016-9915-2

Yun, Y. H., Deng, B. C., Cao, D. S., Wang, W. T., and Liang, Y. Z. (2016). Variable importance analysis based on rank aggregation with applications in metabolomics for biomarker discovery. *Anal. Chim. Acta* 911, 27–34. doi: 10.1016/j.aca.2015.12.043

11

Advanced Activity-Based Protein Profiling Application Strategies for Drug Development

Shan Wang[1], Yu Tian[1], Min Wang[1], Gui-bo Sun[1] and Xiao-bo Sun[1]**

[1] *Beijing Key Laboratory of Innovative Drug Discovery of Traditional Chinese Medicine (Natural Medicine) and Translational Medicine, Institute of Medicinal Plant Development, Chinese Academy of Medical Sciences and Peking Union Medical College, Beijing, China,* [2] *Life and Environmental Science Research Center, Harbin University of Commerce, Harbin, China*

***Correspondence:**
Gui-bo Sun
gbsun@implad.ac.cn
Xiao-bo Sun
sun_xiaobo163@163.com

Drug targets and modes of action remain two of the biggest challenges in drug development. To address these problems, chemical proteomic approaches have been introduced to profile targets in complex proteomes. Activity-based protein profiling (ABPP) is one of a growing number chemical proteomic approaches that uses small-molecule chemical probes to understand the interaction mechanisms between compounds and targets. ABPP can be used to identify the protein targets of small molecules and even the active sites of target proteins. This review focuses on the overall workflow of the ABPP technology and on additional advanced strategies for target identification and/or drug discovery. Herein, we mainly describe the design strategies for small-molecule probes and discuss the ways in which these probes can be used to identify targets and even validate the interactions of small molecules with targets. In addition, we discuss some basic strategies that have been developed to date, such as click chemistry-ABPP, competitive strategies and, recently, more advanced strategies, including isoTOP-ABPP, fluoPol-ABPP, and qNIRF-ABPP. The isoTOP-ABPP strategy has been coupled with quantitative proteomics to identify the active sites of proteins and explore whole proteomes with specific amino acid profiling. FluoPol-ABPP combined with HTS can be used to discover new compounds for some substrate-free enzymes. The qNIRF-ABPP strategy has a number of applications for *in vivo* imaging. In this review, we will further discuss the applications of these advanced strategies.

Keywords: ABPP, isoTOP-ABPP, fluoPol-ABPP, qNIRF-ABPP, drug targets

INTRODUCTION

Two major challenges in the field of drug discovery are drug development and target identification (Schenone et al., 2013). The identification of drug targets, which is important for elucidating the mode of action, is of great significance in the process of drug discovery. Two drug discovery strategies are currently used: phenotype-based drug discovery and target-based drug discovery (Samsdodd, 2005). Phenotype-based drug discovery refers to the screening of small molecules or polypeptides in cells, tissues, or organs based on existing pharmacology. Target-based drug discovery involves first determining the targets and then identifying active molecules. With the rapid development of molecular biology, target-based drug discovery paradigm replaced the traditional phenotype-based approach, because it allowed an increased screening capacity and the definition of rational drug discovery programs. However, analysis of the process of target-based drug discovery showed that this screening platform did not effectively improve the productivity of pharmaceutical industry, but the time and cost increased significantly (Samsdodd, 2005). Due to the complexity of biological systems, phenotype-based strategies can provide more comprehensive evaluation of potential drugs and play an important role in drug development. In recent years, phenotype-based strategies have received increasing attention and have become the main method for drug discovery. These screening strategies are more efficient, effective and economical than other screening platforms.

Numerous technologies for identifying targets have recently been developed. Experimental approaches such as genomic and proteomic techniques are the primary tools for target identification. To complement experimental methods, a series of computational (*in silico*) tools have also been developed for target identification over the past two decades (Krysiak and Breinbauer, 2012; Yue et al., 2012). With the advancement of molecular biology and the advent of the post-genomic era, these technologies provide a solid technical basis for improving the efficiency of drug discovery; however, there remain many barriers for the identification of drug targets, and we need to overcome these barriers.

Activity-based protein profiling is a technology to identify the binding of small molecule probes with proteins and confirm direct interaction. It combines activity-based probe and proteomics technologies together to help us to understand the mechanisms of compounds and the modes of action (Kozarich, 2003; Cravatt et al., 2008). The ABPP-like experiments were firstly reported in the early 1970s to explore the mechanisms of penicillin (Blumberg and Strominger, 1972; Suginaka et al., 1972).

However, the term proteome was firstly proposed at a scientific conference in Italy in 1994 (Wilkins et al., 1996; Huber, 2003). The development of proteomics allows the use of ABPP in many areas, from studying enzyme classes, including proteases, kinases, phosphatases, glycosidases, and oxidoreductases, to studying uncharacterized enzymes. ABPP has contributed to our understanding of enzyme activity in specific physiological and pathological processes on a proteome-wide scale (Heal et al., 2011; Li et al., 2012). This review will discuss all aspects of the ABPP workflow in greater detail. Appropriate strategies are also very important before beginning ABPP-associated experiments. With the development of this field, an increasing number of advanced strategies have been applied in more areas, and we will discuss these strategies in a later section of this review.

ABPP WORKFLOW

Activity-based protein profiling workflow (**Figure 1**) will be discussed in the section and some important issues will be considered. Small-molecule probes are firstly designed and synthesized before ABPP progress begin, the basic chemical structure of a small-molecule probe consists of three parts: 1, a reactive group; 2, a linker site; and 3, a reporter group (Niphakis and Cravatt, 2014). In principle, the active group of small molecule interacts directly with the target protein and the reporter group to facilitate target fishing. Commonly used reporter groups are fluorescent groups, biotin, alkynes or azide, which can be modified by click chemistry methods to visualize protein targets. Depending on the selected reporting groups, different subsequent experiments can be carried out. For example, fluorescent groups can be used for rapid gel screening and the identification of the localization of small molecules in cells or animals, and biotin can be used for protein enrichment and then detected by mass spectrometry to identify target proteins.

After the probe is obtained, it is firstly subjected to rapid determination of working concentration and reaction time by using SDS-PAGE (Wright and Sieber, 2016). Typical workflows are as follows: (i) incubation of the probe with proteins, live cells, tissues, or animals to react with the target, (ii) for cc-probes, performing CuAAC to catalytically label the protein with a fluorescent group or other detectable labels followed by protein enrichment and pull-down assays, (iii) performing gel electrophoresis and fluorescence scanning or Western blotting (for detection of biotin) or quantitative proteomics to identify the target, and (iv) verifying the targets.

During the course of an ABPP project, there are many conditions that must be carefully considered. First, the probe can be incubated in cell lysates or in tissue homogenates *in vitro*. In this case, the conditions of the lysate are very important because the protein function and folding state must be retained to allow the protein to specifically bind to the probe molecule; Tris buffer or PBS are usually suitable (Speers and Cravatt, 2009). *In situ* labeling of cells in culture or *in vivo* labeling of mice via i.p. injection using an ABPP probe can be used to avoid this problem because in these conditions the probe interacts with the protein in a natural state. The caveat of the *in situ* method is that the probe-labeled protein may be metabolized. Some cytotoxic probes may also reduce the amount of protein recovered by killing the cells. However, these problems can be avoided by shortening the time of probing. Second, the selection of reporters should be considered. Biotin labeling can be used for protein enrichment, target identification, and Western blot verification. However, it has been reported that endogenous biotinylated proteins can enhance the noise signal and cause interference. Fluorescence detection is faster and cleaner than blot-based biotin detection and has no additional endogenous biotinylated protein signals (Charron et al., 2009). Other alternative approaches are emerging, such as IAF (immunoaffinity fluorescent) labeling (Yu et al., 2010), or the direct click-on-resin approach, to avoid the use of biotin (Cassiano et al., 2014). Finally, it is very important to comprehensively identify the potential target, including direct identification by pull-down Western blots and recombinant-protein interaction assays with small molecules. The next step is to confirm the mode of action between the proteins and compounds and to uncover the mechanisms by using SPR, ITC, and FP (fluorescence polarization immunoassay). Several assays of biological function are needed to test the associated pharmacological effects of the compounds.

The Design of the Probe

A typical ABPP probe contains three groups: a reactive group, a linking group or binding group, and a reporter tag. For probe design, the first factor to consider is the reactivity of

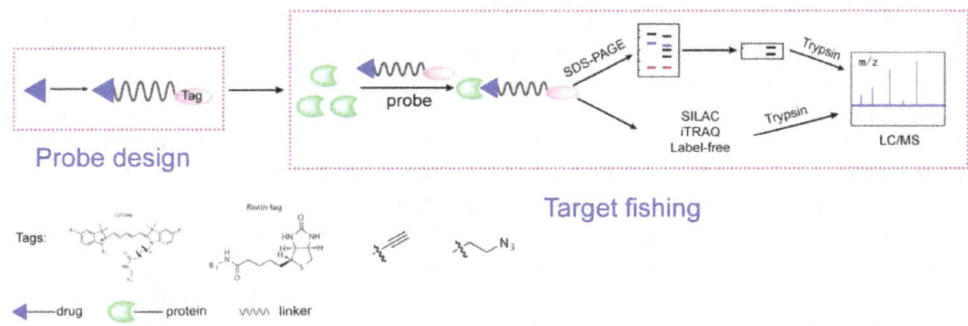

FIGURE 1 | A general representation of the ABPP workflow. The probe is designed based on the structure of the compounds, is added to the proteome and binds to its target protein. Gel-based method or quantitative approaches (label-free, iTRAQ, SILAC) for chemical proteomics experiments.

compound. Most probes are based on bioactive small molecules. So far, many ABPP probes have utilized electrophilic reactive groups, including epoxides, Michael-addition units, disulfides, lactones, β-lactams, and quinone compounds. These groups can react with serine, tyrosine, or glutamine to modulate enzyme activity (Bottcher and Sieber, 2008). However, there are many compounds that react with targets via non-covalent interactions. To overcome this problem, a more intuitive and unbiased strategy for identifying binding partners of unreactive NPs is to use photoaffinity labeling (PAL). PAL makes use of photoreactive moieties that are inert under standard synthetic-chemical and biological conditions but can be activated by UV light, generating highly reactive, transient species. Benzophenone, aliphatic and aromatic diazirines are the most commonly used PAL groups.

In the process of probe design, the choice of linking groups can also be critical. Linking groups can attach the reactive groups with the label groups together and reduce the impact of the label group on the reactive group. The choice of linker group is also significant for reducing non-specificity. In this basic form, a linker can take the form of an extended alkyl or polyethylene glycol (PEG) spacer. Furthermore, of late, the design of cleavable linkers for protein enrichment has received much attention, especially for the isoTOP-ABPP strategy; more details can be found in some other reviews (Leriche et al., 2012; Rudolf et al., 2013).

The other critical challenge in the process of probe design is the reporter group. The widely used reporters are the biotin-streptavidin system for pull-down assays and fluorescent reporters for imaging-based detection. Because of the existence of intrinsically biotinylated proteins, some non-specific background can interfere with the identification of targets; however, fluorescent reporters can be used to avoid this problem. An increasing number of studies are combining these two reporters to identify targets (Liao et al., 2017; Nasheri et al., 2013).

Fishing the Targets

Fishing for targets by using probes is a very critical step, and different platforms have been developed. In this section, we will talk about two commonly used methods: gel-based and gel-free platforms.

Gel-Based Platform for ABPP

To investigate the targets of ABPs, the typical method is to utilize gel electrophoresis to separate proteins by one-dimensional (1D) or two-dimensional (2D) polyacrylamide gel electrophoresis (PAGE) and detect the proteins by Coomassie brilliant blue staining or silver staining to obtain specific bands. The bands are then cut, and LC/MS is used for protein identification. This is the original method for target identification; however, this method can introduce contaminants in the form of other proteins, especially keratin, which makes data analysis more challenging. Non-specific labeling of various proteins, especially of abundant and sticky proteins, in addition to that of the actual target proteins has been a major problem in ABPP. To address this limitation, Seung Park's group have developed a new method called fluorescence difference in two-dimensional gel electrophoresis (FITGE) and employed it in the target identification of the anti-neuroinflammatory agent inflachromene (ICM) (Park et al., 2012; Lee et al., 2014). The platform can simultaneously label two or more different samples, such as control and treatment groups, with different fluorescent labels and then simultaneously perform two-dimensional gel electrophoresis. If one spot was labeled with two fluorescent labels, the labeling can be thought of as being non-specific, and only signals in the treatment group were identified by LC/MS. High-resolution gel electrophoresis can exclude some non-specific targets; however, 2D-PAGE always requires a large amount of protein, which can be difficult to obtain for some precious samples, especially human disease samples.

Gel-Free Approaches

Given the promiscuity of many small molecules and the complexity of the cellular proteome, a high-flux and high-accuracy method is necessary. With the development of mass spectrometers, ABPs coupled with quantitative chemical proteomics has been used to identify drug targets, which can achieve a high-throughput work platform while improving the accuracy of target-protein identification. Quantitative chemical proteomic approaches have been developed, including metabolic labeling (SILAC), chemical labeling (iTRAQ), and the label-free approach (Chen et al., 2017).

SILAC (stable isotope labeling by amino acids in culture) is a stable-isotope-based labeling method, which mainly involves elements of metabolic incorporation. iTRAQ, isobaric tags for relative and absolute quantification, which stands for isobaric tags for relative and absolute quantitation, uses chemical tagging to label different sample populations. These approaches need tags for quantification and identification. These tags result in mass differences that can be detected via MS and enable quantitation and comparison between multiple samples. Some researchers have used ABPP-SILAC and ABPP-iTRAQ to validate some examples. In 2014, Cravatt's group examined the application of ABPP-SILAC to study the protein targets of the kinase inhibitor class of drugs, which includes the Bruton's tyrosine kinase (BTK) inhibitor ibrutinib. A total of 29 probe targets were identified, including epidermal growth factor receptor and BTK (Lanning et al., 2014). Lin's group explored the application of ABPP-iTRAQ to accurately identify the targets and mechanism of action of curcumin, a natural product with anti-inflammatory and anti-cancer properties. In total, 197 proteins were confidently identified from the HCT116 colon cancer cell line as binding targets of curcumin. Ingenuity pathway analysis (IPA) suggested that curcumin may exert its anticancer effects on multiple critical biological pathways, including the EIF2, eIF4/p70S6K, and mTOR signaling and mitochondrial dysfunction pathways (Wang et al., 2016). In iTRAQ-based mass spectrometry the protein is degraded into peptides and labeled at the final step of the entire process; therefore, in the event of an operational error, this process is irreversible. The ability of the ABPP-SILAC approach to identify a wide range of targets in an unbiased manner has been proved, especially for the identification of non-kinase off-target proteins. SILAC is limited by labeling efficiency. SILAC requires cell labeling, and cells often need to grow for at least 3 generations for high labeling efficiency, which is not suitable for some primary cells and tissues.

The label-free approach is another quantitative proteomic approach, which is generally cost-efficient and widely applicable compared to SILAC and iTRAQ. However, it was the need for very high reproducibility to allow run-run comparisons in label-free strategy. Artemisinin is the most potent of the anti-malarial drugs; however, the mechanism of action of artemisinin is not completely understood. Lin's group used an unbiased chemical proteomic analysis to directly explore this mechanism in Plasmodium falciparum. This group designed and synthesized an alkyne-tagged artemisinin probe, combining click chemistry and the label-free method to identify 124 covalently binding protein targets of artemisinin, many of which are involved in essential biological processes of the parasite (Wang et al., 2015).

After the ABPP workflow is finished, the other important issue is to validate the targets. Once potential targets have been identified by ABPP, it is challenging to validate these targets and to verify their modes of action. Many approaches can be taken to assay the interactions between small molecules and targets; some of the commonly used approaches are as follows: (1) if the antibody is available or can be produced, the protein of interest may be enriched and then verified by Western blotting; (2) recombinant proteins can be used to perform the ABPP workflow and verify the interaction; (3) some biophysical methods, such as ITC (isothermal titration calorimetry), FPIA (fluorescence polarization immunoassay), SPR (surface plasmon resonance), and CTSA (cellular thermal shift assay), are should be used (Molina et al., 2013). (4) structural biology can also provide supportive evidence; (5) binding sites can be identified by LC-MS to further validate the direct site of interaction of proteins and small molecules, and if an amino acid modification can be identified, such as Cys or Ser, site-directed mutagenesis can be applied to identify these; and (6) the mode of action of small molecules can be very challenging, and it is necessary to apply many different biological and chemical tools, such as genetic methods and imaging technologies.

ABPP STRATEGIES

In recent years, ABPP technology has developed rapidly. To enhance the specificity and accuracy of this technology, some basic strategies, such as CC-ABPP (click chemistry-ABPP) and competitive-ABPP strategies, have been utilized in most studies. To expand the application of ABPP, some more advanced strategies have been developed, such as isoTOP-ABPP, fluoPol-ABPP and qNIRF-ABPP. These advanced strategies have different characteristics and are used in many areas from active sites identification to new potential compounds discovery and live imaging. The isoTOP-ABPP strategy can be used to directly identify active sites of target proteins; fluoPol-ABPP was used for the discovery of new small molecules based on specific enzymes; and qNIRF-ABPP provides us the opportunity to image the distribution of compounds and promote the development of preclinical diagnosis. We will discuss each strategy in greater detail.

Basic Strategies

CC-ABPP (Click Chemistry-ABPP)

With the development of click chemistry, this method has been introduced into the field of ABPP technology. This method can overcome the limitations of bulky groups and enhance the cell permeability of the probes. By adding smaller alkyne or azide groups to the system, a single probe can be diversified with a variety of reporter groups without the need to develop new synthetic routes. The most widely used click chemistry reaction is the copper (I)-catalyzed azide-alkyne cycloaddition (CuAAC) between an azide and a terminal alkyne to generate a 1,4-disubstituted 1,2,3-triazole (Presolski et al., 2011; Martell and Weerapana, 2014). Concerns about the use of a cytotoxic copper species to catalyze the reaction promoted the development of a copper-free variant of this reaction, which utilizes a strained alkyne to accelerate the reaction (Chang et al., 2010).

To date, the use of CuAAC in living systems has been hindered by the toxicity of copper(I). Considerable cell death occurs when optimized CuAAC conditions that require 1 mM copper(I) are employed. Thus, as presently formulated, CuAAC is of limited use for labeling biomolecules in living systems. Cyclooctyne, the smallest stable cycloalkyne, reacted "like an explosion" when combined with phenylazide and enabled the detection of azides in living systems through strain-promoted [3+2] cycloaddition

(Agard et al., 2004). Moreover, with the aim of improving the kinetics of the process, a series of compounds bearing electron-withdrawing fluorine atoms at the propargylic positions were investigated.

Competitive-ABPP

The non-specific binding is one of the main limitations of ABPP strategies. The photoreactive or electrophilic probes, even probes with higher concentration would in all probability label proteins non-specifically to some extent (i.e., not targets of the parent compound) (Wright and Sieber, 2016). To overcome this problem, the competitive strategy is receiving increasing attention. In competitive ABPP (Leung et al., 2003), a proteome is pre-incubated with parent compounds and subsequently with the activity-based probes, thus decreasing the binding of the probe with the target proteins by competing for the common binding site. The parent compounds are the prototype compounds before transforming to the probes, for example, Liao and his colleagues used SA to compete with the SA-probe to decrease its binding with IMPDH2 which demonstrated that they can interact with the same target (Liao et al., 2017). By this method, non-specific binding can be excluded, and only those sites that interact with the active site of the compound are analyzed. Some review papers have discussed its application and advantages and disadvantages (Willems et al., 2014; Wright and Sieber, 2016). With the development of advanced strategies, it has been applied in these strategies such as isoTOP-ABPP, fluoPol-ABPP and qNIRF-ABPP strategies, so we will discuss its application with these advanced strategies together in the next section.

Advanced Strategies

isoTOP-ABPP

To identify the specific reactive amino acid sites of the target protein by using small molecules, Cravatt and co-workers developed a strategy called isoTOP-ABPP (isotopic tandem orthogonal proteolysis–ABPP) (Weerapana et al., 2010). This method uses isotope-labeled probes to achieve more reliable results compared to other quantitative protein profiling methods. This platform can simultaneously identify probe-labeled proteins and the exact sites of probe modification. Cysteine is the most intrinsically nucleophilic amino acid in proteins, and the activity of the protein is regulated by the modification of cysteine by endogenous and exogenous electrophiles. Iodoacetamide is a reagent classically used to react with cysteine and is often seen in proteomics; so, the Cravatt group used iodoacetamide to design a probe (Backus et al., 2016). The IA probe has an alkyne handle for "click chemistry" conjugation of probe-labeled proteins and isotopically labeled cleavable tags for quantitative mass spectrometry. Using this probe, researchers can quantitatively describe and profile the intrinsic reactivity of cysteine residues in native biological systems. Recently, Weerapana and his colleagues improved this IA probe. These researchers developed a pair of isotopically labeled iodoacetamide-alkyne probes, namely, IA-light and IA-heavy. These probes can be utilized for quantitative analysis of proteome samples and are easy to synthesize, especially compared to the isotopically tagged cleavable linkers (Abo et al., 2017). The iodoacetamide (IA)-based chemical probe has been used to concurrently quantify reactivity changes in hundreds of cysteines within cell lysates. However, the cytotoxicity of the IA group precludes efficient live-cell labeling, which is important for preserving transient cysteine modifications. To overcome this limitation, Weerapana and his colleagues developed a caged bromomethyl ketone (BK) electrophile, which shows minimal cytotoxicity and provides spatial and temporal control of electrophile activation through irradiation. Using this probe, these researchers were the first to describe reactivity changes associated with diverse cysteine modifications in living cells (Abo and Weerapana, 2015).

A competitive isoTOP-ABPP platform expands the application of this strategy for functional cysteines in proteomes. This platform has been used to identify the protein targets of HNE, 15d-PGJ2, and 2-HD and elucidate the cellular functions and mechanisms of action of these compounds (Wang et al., 2014). Fragment-based covalent ligand discovery coupled with competitive isoTOP-ABPP can rapidly lead to the discovery of lead small molecules and the identification of druggable sites. Using this platform, the Nomura group discovered some anti-cancer fragments and revealed the mechanisms of action of these fragments (Anderson et al., 2017; Bateman et al., 2017; Roberts et al., 2017). For example, this group confirmed one compound, DKM 2-93, which impairs pancreatic cancer cell survival and *in vivo* tumor growth, from a fragment-based cysteine-reactive ligand library and identified UBA5 as the target of this compound by covalently modifying the catalytic cysteine, thereby inhibiting the activity of the protein as an activator of the ubiquitin-like protein UFM1 to UFMylate proteins (Roberts et al., 2017).

Recent studies have shown that reactive scaffolds targeting other amino acids such as serine (Bachovchin and Cravatt, 2012), and lysine (Anderson et al., 2017; Hacker et al., 2017), can also be explored by using these platforms to discover unique and novel druggable sites in proteins. Anderson and coworkers developed a screening platform for lysine reactive fragments, which are dichlorotriazine-based covalent ligands, and screened this library to reveal small molecules that impair 231 MFP cancer cell survivals. Using this platform, they identified KEA1-97 and specific targets of KEA1-97 in 231 MFP proteomes and identified that this compound targets lysine 72 of thioredoxin, which disrupts the interaction of thioredoxin with caspase 3, activates caspases, and induces apoptosis.

FluoPol-ABPP

Target-based high-throughput screening (HTS) is essential for the discovery of small-molecule modulators of proteins. Typical screening methods rely on extensively tailored substrate assays for enzyme inhibitors or screens that profile cellular phenotypes. However, for those enzymes whose biochemical activity is not well characterized, such assays are not available. Competitive ABPP studies use SDS-PAGE as readout, limiting the applicability of such studies in HTS. Therefore, Cravatt and colleagues have developed a high-throughput competitive screening platform, namely, the fluopol-ABPP HTS assay, which can be used to select specific enzyme inhibitors, especially for enzymes with poorly characterized substrate or biological functions. The platform also combines high-throughput screening with identification of modes of action (Bachovchin et al., 2009). This strategy, based on a probe tagged with a fluorophore, combines fluorescent probes with competitive inhibition strategies. When the fluorescent probes react with target proteins, the fluorophore signal is strong and consistent; in the presence of a competitor, the probe is released and the signal is decreased. These results can be easily and rapidly measured; therefore, this assay is suitable for HTS. Fluopol-ABPP is a substrate-free approach that is ideally suited for studying enzymes for which no substrates are known.

Using this platform identified specific inhibitors of the substrate-free enzyme RBBP9 and the mechanistically distinct enzyme GSTO1 from a library of small-molecules (Bachovchin et al., 2009). Bachovchin et al. (2009) used the serine hydrolase-directed activity-based probe fluorophosphonate (FP)-rhodamine as the readout probe to select for specific inhibitors to purified RBBP9 from a library of 18,974 small molecules. From this screen, they identified 35 primary hits, and 20 compounds were confirmed via secondary gel-based screens. Finally, they identified emetine as a reversible RBBP9 inhibitor. This fluorophosphonate (FP)-rhodamine probe has also been used to explore other serine hydrolases, such as prolyl endopeptidase-like (PREPL) (Lone et al., 2011), phosphatase methylesterase-1 (PME-1) (Bachovchin et al., 2011a,b), and retinoblastoma-binding protein 9 (RBBP9) (Bachovchin et al., 2010).

Some other probes based on specific enzymes have also been used with the HTS-fluoPol-ABPP strategy. Bryan and his colleagues used a PAD-specific probe, namely, rhodamine-conjugated F-amidine (RFA), to develop an HTS assay. Using these assay conditions, they screened 2,000 compounds (5 μM final concentration) from an NIH validation set at The Scripps Research Institute in La Jolla, CA, United States (Pubchem AID 463073). Finally, they identified streptonigrin as an irreversible PAD4 inactivator (Knuckley et al., 2010). Tsuboi and his colleagues also combined their specific probe, a rhodamine-conjugated phenyl sulfonate ester (SE-Rh), with GSTO1 to identify GSTO1 inhibitors from a 300K+ compound library, and they confirmed an agent, KT53, that inactivates GSTO1 with excellent *in vitro* (IC50 = 21 nM) and *in situ* (IC50 = 35 nM) potency (Tsuboi et al., 2011).

qNIRF-ABPP

qNIRF-ABPP means quenched near-infrared fluorescent ABPP. Imaging agents that enable direct visualization and quantification *in vivo* have great potential value for monitoring chemotherapeutic responses and for early diagnosis and disease monitoring (Edgington et al., 2009; Garland et al., 2016). Fluorescent tags are heavily used in ABPP; however, the main limitation of these tags is the general fluorescence observed both during interaction with enzyme targets and when free in solution. To overcome this limitation, Matthew Bogyo's group engineered probes with a highly efficient quenching group to inhibit the fluorophore group and make the probe intrinsically "dark"; such a probe emits a fluorescent signal only after covalently modifying a specific protease target, resulting in the loss of the quenching group (Blum et al., 2005). Finally, they synthesized the quenched probe GB117, which was attached the large but potentially cell-permeable quenching group QSY7 through a linker to improve the stability and potency of the probe. From fluorescent-imaging studies, they found that GB117 was mainly accumulated in lysosomes. GB117 probes are considered to be tools for cell-based imaging of cysteine cathepsin activity. However, the application of these probes for imaging in animals is limited. Therefore, these researchers combined their method with non-invasive imaging technology and generated a series of near-infrared fluorescent activity-based probes (NIRF-ABPs), which are better suited for *in vivo* imaging and target identification (Blum et al., 2007). These NIRF-ABPs contain Cy5 (646/664 nm excitation/emission), which is better suited for *in vivo* imaging owing to lower background fluorescence, and are insensitive to serum. The researchers synthesized the quenched probe GB137 and unquenched probe GB123 based on GB117 and GBB111 for application in *in vivo* imaging studies. An *in vivo* analysis of the quenched and unquenched probes was conducted to quantify the overall signal-to-background ratios for each probe in multiple animals; the results indicated that GB123 and GB137 generated similar overall signal-to-background ratios. However, some limitations still exist, such as the quenched probe achieved its maximum signal much more rapidly than the unquenched probe. Cathepsin protease activity is highly elevated in macrophages of vulnerable plaques and contributes to plaque instability. The researchers also explored the distribution of cathepsin in an atherosclerosis mouse model by using GB137 and GB123 (Abd-Elrahman et al., 2016). They compared these two probes by *in vivo* imaging and found that both probes showed distinct signals in the macrophage-rich ligated carotids; however, GB123 was also detected in the lymph nodes, aortic arch and heart and exhibited slower signal accumulation than GB137. These cathepsin ABPs represent a rapid diagnostic tool for macrophage detection in atherosclerotic plaque. An improved quenched fluorescent probe containing a phenoxymethyl ketone (PMK) electrophile with greater reactivity and broader selectivity compared to previously reported AOMK-based probes has been synthesized by Matthew Bogyo's group (Verdoes et al., 2013).

DISCUSSION

Drugs that form covalent attachments with their targets have traditionally been considered to be conceptually distinct from conventional non-covalent drugs because the potential off-target reactivity could lead to undesirable side effects. However, covalent drugs have raised various concerns in the field of drug development (Singh et al., 2011; Bauer, 2015; Pichler et al., 2016). ABPP, a very powerful technique in target identification, has generated interest in covalent drugs and allows a more thorough investigation of the modes of action of individual drugs. ABPP is based on the activities of small molecules with a reactive group for binding and covalently modifying the active site of a certain enzyme class. Many ABPP probes have, so far, utilized electrophiles, including fluorophosphonates, sulfonates and epoxides, which exhibit preferences for nucleophilic groups in the active sites of several distinct enzyme classes (Bottcher and Sieber, 2008).

Now, ABPP has been thought as an enormous approach to explore drug targets, with the advanced strategies application, its application expand from drug targets identification to drug discovery. However, it stills exist some limitations, probes labeling non-specific proteins, which is the main issue in this field. Competitive ABPP strategy was commonly used to address this problem by comparison with control. With the quantitative proteomics application, the quantitative data can be used to cut off these background signals, and in general proteins are identified as hits by their enrichment in probe-treated sample over control groups. The other issue is the probe itself, probe-specific hits, which was difficult to deal with. Enrichment in the presence and absence of a competitor (typically the parent NP) is one approach widely used to test whether a protein is a probe-specific hit. Further work in this area may be helpful in providing resources to aid researchers in assessing whether putative targets are genuine or related to the probe moiety itself. To address this issue, follow-up validation of putative targets is very important.

isoTOP-ABPP can enable quantitative analysis of native amino acid reactivity and record changes in enzyme activity directly in native biological systems. It provides information about the post-translational modification of proteins and overcome the deficiency of conventional proteomic or genomic methods, which mainly focus on the expression level. Especially, a fragment-based ligand screening with competitive isoTOP-ABPP platform couples the identification of covalent ligands with the discovery of druggable hotspots. A reactivity-based chemical probe to map reactive, functional, and ligandable hotspots in complex proteomes is firstly needed such as iodoacetamide (IA) probe to label cysteine residues (Weerapana et al., 2010), fluorophosphonate (FP) probe for serine (Liu et al., 1999), sulfotetrafluoropheny (STP) for lysine (Hacker et al., 2017). An isotopically labeled valine for quantitative mass spectrometry (MS) measurements of labeled peptides across multiple proteomes is also important. Probe labeling efficiency is need consideration, for example, FP probes can react with >80% of mammalian metabolic serine hydrolases (Bachovchin and Cravatt, 2012).

FluoPol ABPP is a broadly applicable HTS platform for inhibitor discovery where the ability of compounds to block fluorescent activity-based probe labeling of proteins is monitored by fluorescence polarization and can be readily adapted for use with different classes of enzymes and ABPP probes. However, there are some important issues to be considered. A cognate activity-based probe has been developed before this platform. In addition, fluoPol-ABPP requires a substantial amount of purified protein, which may prove challenging for certain enzymes (e.g., transmembrane enzymes). Regardless, in cases where protein quantity is not limiting, fluoPol-ABPP is quite cheap, since the quantity of probe used per assay is negligible. A library of small molecules is another issue. This platform makes the ABPP technology useful not only for mechanism identification but also for compound discovery and will help us understand more about some poorly characterized enzymes and the inhibitors or activators of these enzymes.

It is important to visualize these diseased cells to enable diagnosis, facilitate surgical resection and monitor therapeutic response. Therefore, there is great opportunity to develop non-invasive imaging technologies for interventional surgical imaging and for diagnostic and therapeutic applications. The qNIRF-ABPP strategy provides a method for *in vivo* imaging. qNIRF-ABPs are potentially valuable novel imaging agents for disease diagnosis and are powerful tools for preclinical and clinical testing of small-molecule therapeutic agents *in vivo*, for the identification of specific therapeutic targets and biomarkers, and for monitoring the efficacy of small-molecule inhibitors (Joyce et al., 2004; Rosenthal et al., 2015; Garland et al., 2016).

CONCLUSION

Activity-based protein profiling can provide an unbiased, global and quantitative analysis of protein binding partners. It has been used with different samples, including cell lysates, live cells, animal lysates, and even live animals. All these applications help us understand the interactions between compounds and organisms. With the applications of advanced strategies, ABPP has expanded its area from drug targets identification to drug discovery. The advanced strategies of ABPP open a new door for us, from target-based high-throughput screening to take images *in vivo*. isoTOP-ABPP strategy can provide us the global analysis of cysteine, serine and lysine reactivity even in living cells, which is important for preserving transient amino acids modifications. Fluopol-ABPP HTS assay overcome the traditional screening methods disadvantages relying on substrate assay and cellular phenotypes. It can be used for some poorly characterized enzymes to explore their inhibitors or activators. qNIRF-ABPP provides a method for *in vivo* imaging and is helpful for diagnosis, surgical resection and therapeutic response. The wide applicability of the above methods will provide more possibility to success for novel drug development, and expand more technical innovation in ABPP field. Finally, with advances in technology and through continuous improvement, chemical proteomic technology will remain at the forefront of drug discovery and target recognition.

AUTHOR CONTRIBUTIONS

SW wrote and edited this paper. YT and MW (third author) gave some convincing advice. MW (fourth author) checked and edited this paper. G-bS and X-bS designed this review.

FUNDING

This work was supported by the National Science and Technology Major Project (Grant No. 2015ZX09501004-001-003), the Special Research Project for TCM (Grant No. 201507004), the CAMS Innovation Fund for Medical Science (CIFMS) (Grant No. 2016-I2M-1-012), and Peking Union Medical College Graduate Student Innovation Fund (Grant No. 2016-1007-06).

REFERENCES

Abd-Elrahman, I., Kosuge, H., Wises Sadan, T., Ben-Nun, Y., Meir, K., Rubinstein, C., et al. (2016). Cathepsin activity-based probes and inhibitor for preclinical atherosclerosis imaging and macrophage depletion. *PLoS One* 11:e0160522. doi: 10.1371/journal.pone.0160522

Abo, M., Li, C., and Weerapana, E. (2017). Isotopically-labeled iodoacetamide-alkyne probes for quantitative cysteine-reactivity profiling. *Mol. Pharm.* 15, 743–749. doi: 10.1021/acs.molpharmaceut.7b00832

Abo, M., and Weerapana, E. (2015). A caged electrophilic probe for global analysis of cysteine reactivity in living cells. *J. Am. Chem. Soc.* 137, 7087–7090. doi: 10.1021/jacs.5b04350

Agard, N. J., Prescher, J. A., and Bertozzi, C. R. (2004). A strain-promoted [3 + 2] azide-alkyne cycloaddition for covalent modification of biomolecules in living systems. *J. Am. Chem. Soc.* 126, 15046–15047. doi: 10.1021/ja044996f

Anderson, K. E., To, M., Olzmann, J. A., and Nomura, D. K. (2017). Chemoproteomics-Enabled covalent ligand screening reveals a thioredoxin-caspase 3 interaction disruptor that impairs breast cancer pathogenicity. *ACS Chem. Biol.* 12, 2522–2528. doi: 10.1021/acschembio.7b00711

Bachovchin, D. A., Brown, S. J., Rosen, H., and Cravatt, B. F. (2009). Substrate-free high-throughput screening identifies selective inhibitors for uncharacterized enzymes. *Nat. Biotechnol.* 27, 387–394. doi: 10.1038/nbt.1531

Bachovchin, D. A., and Cravatt, B. F. (2012). The pharmacological landscape and therapeutic potential of serine hydrolases. *Nat. Rev. Drug Discov.* 11, 52–68. doi: 10.1038/nrd3620

Bachovchin, D. A., Speersa, A. E., Wang, C., Berlin, J. M., Spicer, T. P., Fernandez-Vega, I., et al. (2011a). Academic cross-fertilization by public screening yields a remarkable class of protein phosphatase methylesterase-1 inhibitors. *Proc. Natl. Acad. Sci. U.S.A.* 108, 6811–6816. doi: 10.1073/pnas.1015248108

Bachovchin, D. A., Wolfe, M. R., Masuda, K., Brown, S. J., Spicer, T. P., Fernandez-Vega, V., et al. (2010). Oxime esters as selective, covalent inhibitors of the serine hydrolase retinoblastoma-binding protein 9 (RBBP9). *Bioorg. Med. Chem. Lett.* 20, 2254–2258. doi: 10.1016/j.bmcl.2010.02.011

Bachovchin, D. A., Zuhl, A. M., Speers, A. E., Wolfe, M. R., Weerapana, E., Brown, S. J., et al. (2011b). Discovery and optimization of sulfonyl acrylonitriles as selective, covalent inhibitors of protein phosphatase methylesterase-1. *J. Med. Chem.* 54, 5229–5236. doi: 10.1021/jm200502u

Backus, K. M., Correia, B. E., Lum, K. M., Forli, S., Horning, B. D., Gonzalez-Paez, G. E., et al. (2016). Proteome-wide covalent ligand discovery in native biological systems. *Nature* 534, 570–574. doi: 10.1038/nature18002

Bateman, L. A., Nguyen, T. B., Roberts, A. M., Miyamoto, D. K., Ku, W. M., Huffman, T. R., et al. (2017). Chemoproteomics-enabled covalent ligand screen reveals a cysteine hotspot in reticulon 4 that impairs ER morphology and cancer pathogenicity. *Chem. Commun.* 53, 7234–7237. doi: 10.1039/c7cc01480e

Bauer, R. A. (2015). Covalent inhibitors in drug discovery: from accidental discoveries to avoided liabilities and designed therapies. *Drug Discov. Today* 20, 1061–1073. doi: 10.1016/j.drudis.2015.05.005

Blum, G., Mullins, S. R., Keren, K., Fonovic, M., Jedeszko, C., Rice, M. J., et al. (2005). Dynamic imaging of protease activity with fluorescently quenched activity-based probes. *Nat. Chem. Biol.* 1, 203–209. doi: 10.1038/nchembio728

Blum, G., von Degenfeld, G., Merchant, M. J., Blau, H. M., and Bogyo, M. (2007). Noninvasive optical imaging of cysteine protease activity using fluorescently quenched activity-based probes. *Nat. Chem. Biol.* 3, 668–677. doi: 10.1038/nchembio.2007.26

Blumberg, P. M., and Strominger, J. L. (1972). Five Penicillin-binding components occur in *Bacillus subtilis* membranes. *J. Biol. Chem.* 247, 8107–8113.

Bottcher, T., and Sieber, S. A. (2008). Beta-lactones as privileged structures for the active-site labeling of versatile bacterial enzyme classes. *Angew. Chem. Int. Ed. Engl.* 47, 4600–4603. doi: 10.1002/anie.200705768

Cassiano, C., Margarucci, L., Esposito, R., Riccio, R., Tosco, A., Casapullo, A., et al. (2014). In cell scalaradial interactome profiling using a bio-orthogonal clickable probe. *Chem. Commun.* 50, 6043–6045. doi: 10.1039/c4cc00989d

Chang, P. V., Prescher, J. A., Sletten, E. M., Baskin, J. M., Miller, I. A., Agard, N. J., et al. (2010). Copper-free click chemistry in living animals. *Proc. Natl. Acad. Sci. U.S.A.* 107, 1821–1826. doi: 10.1073/pnas.0911116107

Charron, G., Zhang, M. M., Yount, J. S., Wilson, J., Raghavan, A. S., Shamir, E., et al. (2009). Robust fluorescent detection of protein fatty-acylation with chemical reporters. *J. Am. Chem. Soc.* 131, 4967–4975. doi: 10.1021/ja810122f

Chen, X., Wong, Y. K., Wang, J., Zhang, J., Lee, Y. M., Shen, H. M., et al. (2017). Target identification with quantitative activity based protein profiling (ABPP). *Proteomics* 17, 1–15. doi: 10.1002/pmic.201600212

Cravatt, B. F., Wright, A. T., and Kozarich, J. W. (2008). Activity-based protein profiling: from enzyme chemistry to proteomic chemistry. *Annu. Rev. Biochem.* 77, 383–414. doi: 10.1146/annurev.biochem.75.101304.124125

Edgington, L. E., Berger, A. B., Blum, G., Albrow, V. E., Paulick, M. G., Lineberry, N., et al. (2009). Noninvasive optical imaging of apoptosis by caspase-targeted activity-based probes. *Nat. Med.* 15, 967–973. doi: 10.1038/nm.1938

Garland, M., Yim, J. J., and Bogyo, M. (2016). A bright future for precision medicine: advances in fluorescent chemical probe design and their clinical application. *Cell Chem. Biol.* 23, 122–136. doi: 10.1016/j.chembiol.2015.12.003

Hacker, S. M., Backus, K. M., Lazear, M. R., Forli, S., Correia, B. E., and Cravatt, B. F. (2017). Global profiling of lysine reactivity and ligandability in the human proteome. *Nat. Chem.* 9, 1181–1190. doi: 10.1038/nchem.2826

Heal, W. P., Dang, T. H., and Tate, E. W. (2011). Activity-based probes: discovering new biology and new drug targets. *Chem. Soc. Rev.* 40, 246–257. doi: 10.1039/c0cs00004c

Huber, L. A. (2003). Is proteomics heading in the wrong direction? *Nat. Rev. Mol. Cell Biol.* 4, 74–80. doi: 10.1038/nrm1007

Joyce, J. A., Baruch, A., Chehade, K., Meyer-Morse, N., Giraudo, E., Tsai, F. Y., et al. (2004). Cathepsin cysteine proteases are effectors of invasive growth and angiogenesis during multistage tumorigenesis. *Cancer Cell* 5, 443–453. doi: 10.1016/S1535-6108(04)00111-4

Knuckley, B., Jones, J. E., Bachovchin, D. A., Slack, J., Causey, C. P., Brown, S. J., et al. (2010). A fluopol-ABPP HTS assay to identify PAD inhibitors. *Chem. Commun.* 46, 7175–7177.

Kozarich, J. W. (2003). Activity-based proteomics enzyme chemistry redux. *Curr. Opin. Chem. Biol.* 7, 78–83. doi: 10.1016/S1367-5931(02)00013-3

Krysiak, J., and Breinbauer, R. (2012). Activity-based protein profiling for natural product target discovery. *Top. Curr. Chem.* 324, 43–84. doi: 10.1007/128_2011_289

Lanning, B. R., Whitby, L. R., Dix, M. M., Douhan, J., Gilbert, A. M., Hett, E. C., et al. (2014). A road map to evaluate the proteome-wide selectivity of covalent kinase inhibitors. *Nat. Chem. Biol.* 10, 760–767. doi: 10.1038/nchembio.1582

Lee, S., Nam, Y., Koo, J. Y., Lim, D., Park, J., Ock, J., et al. (2014). A small molecule binding HMGB1 and HMGB2 inhibits microglia-mediated neuroinflammation. *Nat. Chem. Biol.* 10, 1055–1060. doi: 10.1038/nchembio.1669

Leriche, G., Chisholm, L., and Wagner, A. (2012). Cleavable linkers in chemical biology. *Bioorg. Med. Chem.* 20, 571–582. doi: 10.1016/j.bmc.2011.07.048

Leung, D., Hardouin, C., Boger, D. L., and Cravatt, B. F. (2003). Discovering potent and selective reversible inhibitors of enzymes in complex proteomes. *Nat. Biotechnol.* 21, 687–691. doi: 10.1038/nbt826

Li, N., Overkleeft, H. S., and Florea, B. I. (2012). Activity-based protein profiling: an enabling technology in chemical biology research. *Curr. Opin. Chem. Biol.* 16, 227–233. doi: 10.1016/j.cbpa.2012.01.008

Liao, L. X., Song, X. M., Wang, L. C., Lv, H. N., Chen, J. F., Liu, D., et al. (2017). Highly selective inhibition of IMPDH2 provides the basis of antineuroinflammation therapy. *Proc. Natl. Acad. Sci. U.S.A.* 114, E5986–E5994. doi: 10.1073/pnas.1706778114

Liu, Y., Patricelli, M. P., and Cravatt, B. F. (1999). Activity-based protein profiling The serine hydrolases. *Proc. Natl. Acad. Sci. U.S.A.* 96, 14694–14699. doi: 10.1073/pnas.96.26.14694

Lone, A. M., Bachovchin, D. A., Westwood, D. B., Speers, A. E., Spicer, T. P., Fernandez-Vega, V., et al. (2011). A substrate-free activity-based protein profiling screen for the discovery of selective PREPL inhibitors. *J. Am. Chem. Soc.* 133, 11665–11674. doi: 10.1021/ja2036095

Martell, J., and Weerapana, E. (2014). Applications of copper-catalyzed click chemistry in activity-based protein profiling. *Molecules* 19, 1378–1393. doi: 10.3390/molecules19021378

Molina, D. M., Jafari, R., Ignatushchenko, M., Seki, T., Larsson, E. A., Dan, C., et al. (2013). Monitoring Drug target engagement in cells and tissues using the cellular thermal shift assay. *Science* 341, 84–87. doi: 10.1126/science.1233606

Nasheri, N., Joyce, M., Rouleau, Y., Yang, P., Yao, S., Tyrrell, D. L., et al. (2013). Modulation of fatty acid synthase enzyme activity and expression during hepatitis c virus replication. *Chem. Biol.* 20, 570–582. doi: 10.1016/j.chembiol.2013.03.014

Niphakis, M. J., and Cravatt, B. F. (2014). Enzyme inhibitor discovery by activity-based protein profiling. *Annu. Rev. Biochem.* 83, 341–377. doi: 10.1146/annurev-biochem-060713-035708

Park, J., Oh, S., and Park, S. B. (2012). Discovery and target identification of an antiproliferative agent in live cells using fluorescence difference in two-dimensional gel electrophoresis. *Angew. Chem. Int. Ed. Engl.* 51, 5447–5451. doi: 10.1002/anie.201200609

Pichler, C. M., Krysiak, J., and Breinbauer, R. (2016). Target identification of covalently binding drugs by activity-based protein profiling (ABPP). *Bioorg. Med. Chem.* 24, 3291–3303. doi: 10.1016/j.bmc.2016.03.050

Presolski, S. I., Hong, V. P., and Finn, M. G. (2011). Copper-Catalyzed Azide-Alkyne Click Chemistry for Bioconjugation. *Curr. Protoc. Chem. Biol.* 3, 153–162. doi: 10.1002/9780470559277.ch110148

Roberts, A. M., Miyamoto, D. K., Huffman, T. R., Bateman, L. A., Ives, A. N., Akopian, D., et al. (2017). Chemoproteomic screening of covalent ligands reveals UBA5 As a novel pancreatic cancer target. *ACS Chem. Biol.* 12, 899–904. doi: 10.1021/acschembio.7b00020

Rosenthal, E. L., Warram, J. M., de Boer, E., Basilion, J. P., Biel, M. A., Bogyo, M., et al. (2015). Successful translation of fluorescence navigation during oncologic surgery: a consensus report. *J. Nucl. Med.* 57, 144–150. doi: 10.2967/jnumed.115.158915

Rudolf, G. C., Heydenreuter, W., and Sieber, S. A. (2013). Chemical proteomics: ligation and cleavage of protein modifications. *Curr. Opin. Chem. Biol.* 17, 110–117. doi: 10.1016/j.cbpa.2012.11.007

Samsdodd, F. (2005). Target-based drug discovery: is something wrong? *Drug Discov. Today* 10, 139–147. doi: 10.1016/s1359-6446(04)03316-1

Schenone, M., Dancik, V., Wagner, B. K., and Clemons, P. A. (2013). Target identification and mechanism of action in chemical biology and drug discovery. *Nat. Chem. Biol.* 9, 232–240. doi: 10.1038/nchembio.1199

Singh, J., Petter, R. C., Baillie, T. A., and Whitty, A. (2011). The resurgence of covalent drugs. *Nat. Rev. Drug Discov.* 10, 307–317. doi: 10.1038/nrd3410

Speers, A. E., and Cravatt, B. F. (2009). Activity-based protein profiling (ABPP) and click chemistry (CC)-ABPP by MudPIT mass spectrometry. *Curr. Protoc. Chem. Biol.* 1, 29–41. doi: 10.1002/9780470559277.ch090138

Suginaka, H., Blumberg, P. M., and Strominger, J. L. (1972). Multiple penicillin-binding components in *Bacillus subtilis, Bacillus cereus, Staphylococcus aureus,* and *Escherichia coli. J. Biol. Chem.* 247, 5279–5288.

Tsuboi, K., Bachovchin, D. A., Speers, A. E., Spicer, T. P., Fernandez-Vega, V., Hodder, P., et al. (2011). Potent and selective inhibitors of glutathione S-transferase omega 1 that impair cancer drug resistance. *J. Am. Chem. Soc.* 133, 16605–16616. doi: 10.1021/ja2066972

Verdoes, M., Oresic Bender, K., Segal, E., van der Linden, W. A., Syed, S., Withana, N. P., et al. (2013). Improved quenched fluorescent probe for imaging of cysteine cathepsin activity. *J. Am. Chem. Soc.* 135, 14726–14730. doi: 10.1021/ja4056068

Wang, C., Weerapana, E., Blewett, M. M., and Cravatt, B. F. (2014). A chemoproteomic platform to quantitatively map targets of lipid-derived electrophiles. *Nat. Methods* 11, 79–85. doi: 10.1038/nmeth.2759

Wang, J., Zhang, C. J., Chia, W. N., Loh, C. C., Li, Z., Lee, Y. M., et al. (2015). Haem-activated promiscuous targeting of artemisinin in *Plasmodium falciparum*. *Nat. Commun.* 6:10111. doi: 10.1038/ncomms10111

Wang, J., Zhang, J., Zhang, C. J., Wong, Y. K., Lim, T. K., Hua, Z. C., et al. (2016). In situ proteomic profiling of curcumin targets in HCT116 colon cancer cell line. *Sci. Rep.* 6:22146. doi: 10.1038/srep22146

Weerapana, E., Wang, C., Simon, G. M., Richter, F., Khare, S., Dillon, M. B., et al. (2010). Quantitative reactivity profiling predicts functional cysteines in proteomes. *Nature* 468, 790–795. doi: 10.1038/nature09472

Wilkins, M. R., Sanchez, J. C., Williams, K. L., and Hochstrasser, D. F. (1996). Current challenges and future applications for protein maps and post-translational vector maps in proteome projects. *Electrophoresis* 17, 830–838. doi: 10.1002/elps.1150170504

Willems, L. I., Overkleeft, H. S., and van Kasteren, S. I. (2014). Current developments in activity-based protein profiling. *Bioconjug. Chem.* 25, 1181–1191. doi: 10.1021/bc500208y

Wright, M. H., and Sieber, S. A. (2016). Chemical proteomics approaches for identifying the cellular targets of natural products. *Nat. Prod. Rep.* 33, 681–708. doi: 10.1039/c6np00001k

Yu, W. L., Guizzunti, G., Foley, T. L., Burkart, M. D., and La Clair, J. J. (2010). An optimized immunoaffinity fluorescent method for natural product target elucidation. *J. Nat. Prod.* 73, 1659–1666. doi: 10.1021/np100371k

Yue, R., Shan, L., Yang, X., and Zhang, W. (2012). Approaches to target profiling of natural products. *Curr. Med. Chem.* 19, 3841–3855. doi: 10.2174/092986712801661068

12

Exploring G Protein-Coupled Receptors (GPCRs) Ligand Space via Cheminformatics Approaches: Impact on Rational Drug Design

Shaherin Basith†, Minghua Cui†, Stephani J. Y. Macalino, Jongmi Park, Nina A. B. Clavio, Soosung Kang and Sun Choi**

College of Pharmacy and Graduate School of Pharmaceutical Sciences, Ewha Womans University, Seoul, South Korea

***Correspondence:**
Soosung Kang
sskang@ewha.ac.kr
Sun Choi
sunchoi@ewha.ac.kr

†These authors have contributed equally to this work.

The primary goal of rational drug discovery is the identification of selective ligands which act on single or multiple drug targets to achieve the desired clinical outcome through the exploration of total chemical space. To identify such desired compounds, computational approaches are necessary in predicting their drug-like properties. G Protein-Coupled Receptors (GPCRs) represent one of the largest and most important integral membrane protein families. These receptors serve as increasingly attractive drug targets due to their relevance in the treatment of various diseases, such as inflammatory disorders, metabolic imbalances, cardiac disorders, cancer, monogenic disorders, etc. In the last decade, multitudes of three-dimensional (3D) structures were solved for diverse GPCRs, thus referring to this period as the "golden age for GPCR structural biology." Moreover, accumulation of data about the chemical properties of GPCR ligands has garnered much interest toward the exploration of GPCR chemical space. Due to the steady increase in the structural, ligand, and functional data of GPCRs, several cheminformatics approaches have been implemented in its drug discovery pipeline. In this review, we mainly focus on the cheminformatics-based paradigms in GPCR drug discovery. We provide a comprehensive view on the ligand– and structure-based cheminformatics approaches which are best illustrated *via* GPCR case studies. Furthermore, an appropriate combination of ligand-based knowledge with structure-based ones, i.e., integrated approach, which is emerging as a promising strategy for cheminformatics-based GPCR drug design is also discussed.

Keywords: GPCR, cheminformatics, drug discovery, ligand-based drug design, structure-based drug design

INTRODUCTION

Rational drug design is the inventive process of identifying pharmaceutically-relevant drug candidates based on the information garnered from a biological target (Jazayeri et al., 2015). Discovery of ligands that modulate a target's activity has contributed largely to the understanding of both physiological and pathological processes (Wacker et al., 2017a). Navigating vast chemical space to identify such ligands seems a daunting task (Oprea and Gottfries, 2001; Lipinski and Hopkins, 2004). Techniques including medicinal chemistry, combinatorial chemistry, and high-throughput screening (HTS) are helpful in the identification of ligands, which can serve as effective modulators for pharmaceutically attractive targets. However, considering the astronomical number of possible drug-like candidates ($\sim 10^{23}$-10^{60}), chemical space assessed by experimental techniques is still limited (Rodríguez et al., 2016; Mullard, 2017). In such a scenario, cheminformatics, which belongs to a part of the *in silico* realm, dominates in the exploration of a larger fraction of the chemical space.

Cheminformatics was defined by Brown (1998) as the combination of all available information that can be used in the optimization of a ligand to a potential drug candidate (Bajorath, 2004). This method aids in storing, searching, managing, and analyzing huge amount of chemical data, thereby expediting the development of novel ligand phenotypes (Bajorath, 2004; Valerio and Choudhuri, 2012). Additionally, the extraction of information and knowledge from chemical data could be helpful in the modeling of relationships between chemical structures and biological activities, and in the bioactivity prediction of other compounds from their structures (Schuffenhauer et al., 2006; Humbeck and Koch, 2017). Interestingly, cheminformatics fuses both chemical and biological data from drug candidates and drug targets, respectively, for the identification of new chemical entities (NCEs) and improvement of the reliability of data outcomes.

In the drug discovery pipeline, several cheminformatics approaches play a potent role in the identification of drug target and lead compounds, as well as in the prediction of ADMET properties (**Figure 1**). Chemogenomics-based databases, as well as computational polypharmacological analyses, have increased in popularity over the last several years as a supplementary method in the identification and validation of potential drug targets (Xie et al., 2014). Once a drug target is identified, the lead candidates with desirable properties are screened out of huge chemical compound libraries, thus underscoring the importance of cheminformatics tools in virtual screening (VS) (Varnek and Tropsha, 2008). Another potent cheminformatics approach, machine-learning is employed for the identification of novel drug candidates from lead compounds *via* generation of computational models (Lee et al., 2010, 2017; Varnek and Baskin, 2012; Mitchell, 2014). Other cheminformatics approaches including similarity and substructure searching could be utilized for the identification of novel scaffolds from large compounds repositories (Vass et al., 2016). The candidate compounds retrieved could be further docked onto the target protein to propose their possible binding affinities toward the target (Lenselink et al., 2016b). Upon identification of the drug-like candidates, these could be further evaluated for ADMET properties using computational models, thus helping in the elimination of undesired compounds at an early stage of drug discovery, and minimizing the time and costs involved.

G protein-coupled receptors (GPCRs) belong to a large family of signaling proteins that mediate cellular responses to most hormones, metabolites, cytokines, and neurotransmitters, and therefore serve as "fruitful targets" for drug discovery (Shoichet and Kobilka, 2012). More than 800 genes comprise this receptor family, which modulate several signaling processes involved in behavior, blood pressure regulation, cognition, immune response, mood, smell, and taste (Thomsen et al., 2005). GPCRs are categorized into six classes based on sequence and function, namely Class A—rhodopsin-like receptors, Class B—secretin family, Class C—metabotropic glutamate receptors, Class D—fungal mating pheromone receptors, Class E—cAMP receptors, and Class F—frizzled (FZD) and smoothened (SMO) receptors (Lee et al., 2018). All GPCR members share a common seven transmembrane (7TM) architecture linked by three extracellular (ECL) and three intracellular (ICL) loops (Ciancetta et al., 2015). However, they have low sequence identity and possess different extracellular N-terminal domains and diverse ligand-binding pockets (**Figure 2**). In case of class A GPCRs, the endogenous ligand is recognized by a ligand-binding site in the 7TM region. For class B GPCRs, the ligand is recognized by both extracellular and 7TM domains. For class C GPCRs, the ligand-binding pocket is found in the extracellular domain (ECD) that contains a Venus flytrap (VFT) module. In case of class F GPCRs, both SMO and FZD receptors possess an ECD that is comprised of an extracellular cysteine-rich domain (CRD) and an ECD linker domain. The endogenous lipoglycoprotein ligand, Wnt binds to the CRD of the FZD receptors (Wang et al., 2013; Wu et al., 2014). Upon ligand binding, GPCRs activate at least one of the two signaling partners, namely heterotrimeric GTP-binding proteins (G-proteins) or β-arrestins, and mediate signal flow *via* modulation of various downstream effectors.

GPCR drug discovery has been successful and many of the world's top-selling drugs have targeted this receptor family (Sriram and Insel, 2018). Class A GPCRs are the most immensely investigated GPCR drug target within the drug market due to their centrality in diseases, structural availability, and relative ease of accessibility. The high druggability of GPCRs and its central role in diseases (including alzheimer's disease, cancer, diabetes, obesity, and psychiatric disorders) provide a strong spearhead for its continuous efforts in drug discovery and development (Tautermann, 2016). A recent study of all GPCR drugs and agents currently in clinical trials revealed that 475 drugs (i.e., ~34% of all drugs approved by Food and Drug administration [FDA]) mediate their effects through 108 unique GPCRs (Hauser et al., 2017). Additionally, the success rates for GPCR-targeted agents in the last 5 years were 78% (phase I), 39% (phase II), and 29% (phase III) (Hauser et al., 2017). The most recently FDA approved GPCR-targeted drug is Zilretta (triamcinolone acetonide extended-release injectable suspension), a glucocorticoid receptor agonist, which is used for the pain management of knee osteoarthritis (https://www.drugs.com/history/zilretta.html).

To utilize cheminformatics approaches in GPCR drug design, understanding the nature of the ligands, structural intricacies of the receptor, ligand-receptor interactions, and interaction of the receptors with downstream signaling complexes or other signaling partners is essential. Additionally, unveiling the relationships among ligand, receptor, and effector is necessary to investigate positive and negative allosterism, inverse agonism, biased signaling, and multimeric receptor pharmacology (Lane et al., 2017). Recent upsurge in the crystal structures of GPCRs provides a robust, 3D structural framework for identification of pharmaceutically-relevant ligands using ligand– and structure-based computational approaches, including molecular modeling

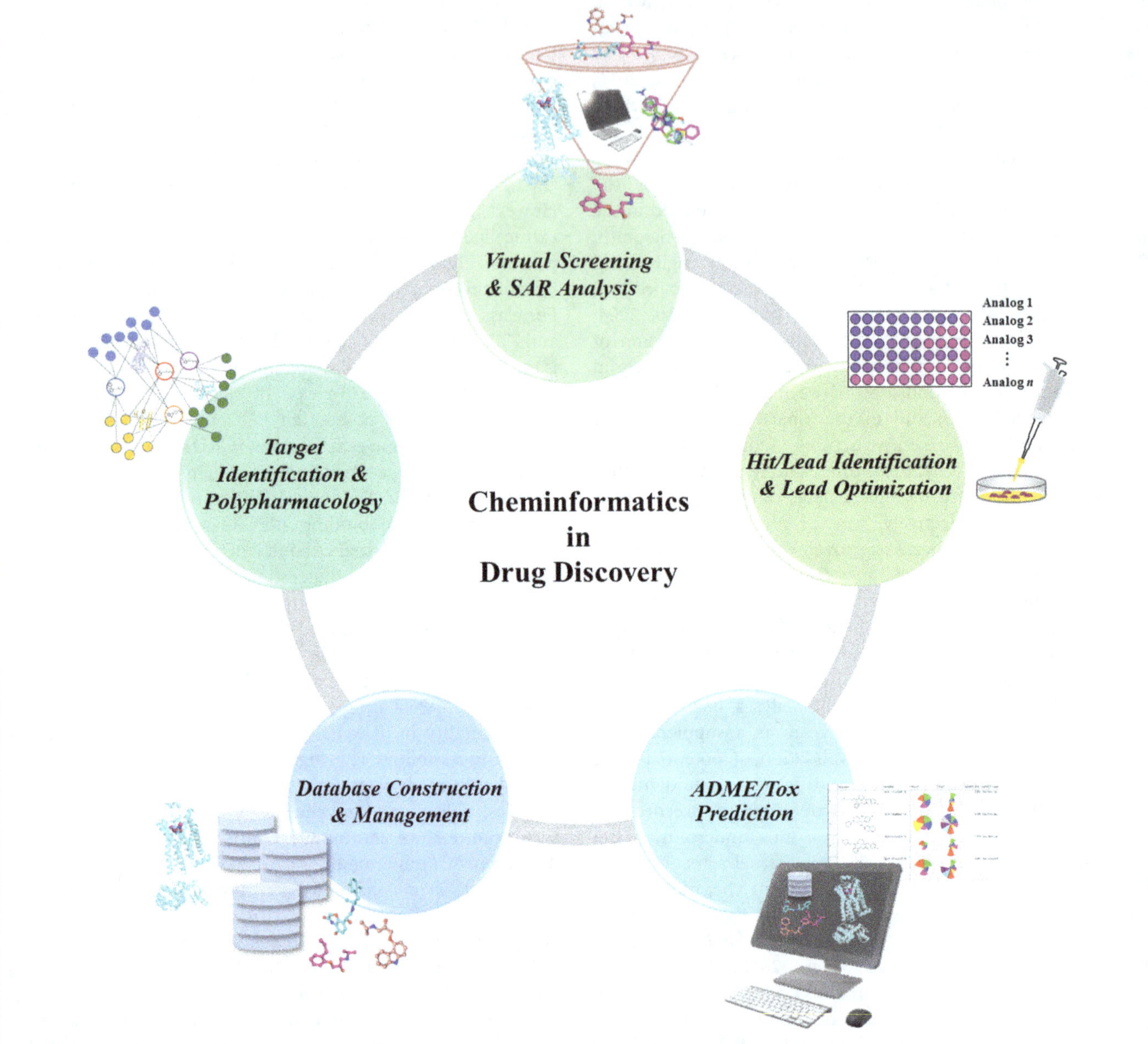

FIGURE 1 | Role of Cheminformatics in the drug discovery process. Cheminformatics is involved in almost every step of the drug discovery pipeline due to the employment and analysis of available data to translate into valuable knowledge, which can in turn be used as a data for further studies.

of receptor dynamics, ligand docking, and virtual ligand screening (VLS) (Coudrat et al., 2017a). Following the successful application of VLS approaches in targets such as kinases, proteases, and other enzyme families, it is also becoming a popular ligand screening tool for GPCRs (Heifetz, 2018). The success of structure-based VLS could be visualized by the encouragingly high hit-rates ranging from 20 to 70% in the identification of novel ligands for several class A GPCRs (**Table 1**).

In this review, we deliver a comprehensive assessment on the state-of-the-art cheminformatics approaches for GPCR drug discovery with successful models from literature. Firstly, insights on GPCR ligand space and its recent structural advances are summarized. Subsequently, the key principles and boundaries of ligand–, structure-based, and integrated cheminformatics approaches in GPCR drug discovery are discussed in the main text. We also shed some light on the contemporary cheminformatics tools utilized in GPCR drug discovery. Additionally, the limitations associated with cheminformatics approaches have been discussed, which could assist the reader to rationale the best *in silico* tool during their research. Lastly, we conclude with a summary of the review contents and prospects of the cheminformatics approaches in GPCR drug discovery.

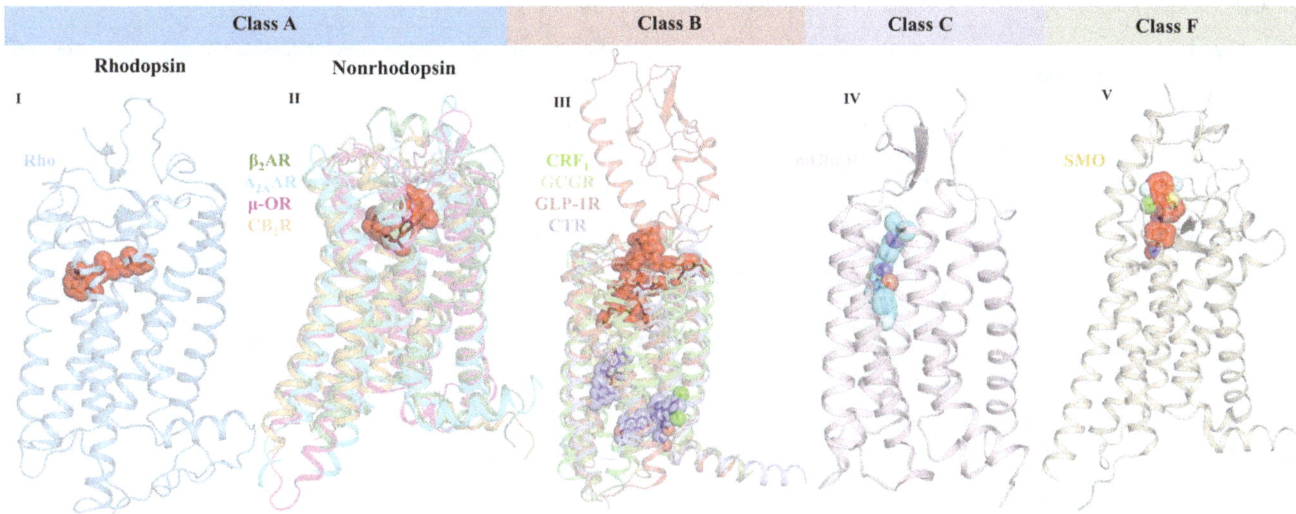

FIGURE 2 | Crystal structures of representative GPCR-ligand complexes from classes A, B, C, and F presenting diverse ligand-binding sites. Class A GPCRs are classified into rhodopsin (bRho, PDB ID: 2HPY) and nonrhodopsin GPCRs. The representative structures of class A nonrhodopsin GPCRs which are further subdivided into aminergic-like (β_2AR, PDB ID: 3P0G), nucleotide-like (A_{2A}AR, PDB ID: 3QAK), peptide-like (μ-OR, PDB ID: 5C1M), and lipid-like receptors (CB_1R, PDB ID: 5XRA) along with their bound ligands are shown. Similarly, representative structures for class B (CRF_1 [PDB ID: 4K5Y], GCGR [PDB ID: 5EE7], full-length GLP-1R [PDB ID: 5NX2], and CTR [5UZ7]), class C ($mGlu_1$R [PDB ID: 4OR2]), and class F (SMO [PDB ID: 4QIN] bound to negative allosteric modulator) are shown. Receptors are shown in cartoon representation and the ligands are shown as stick models with transparent surfaces. Agonists are represented as red sticks, antagonists are shown as purple sticks, and negative allosteric modulator is shown as blue stick model.

BOOMING AGE OF GPCR STRUCTURAL BIOLOGY

The pioneering study of two-dimensional (2D) structure for bovine rhodopsin (bRho) in 1983 marked the beginning of GPCR structural biology (Hargrave et al., 1983). A decade later, 2D projection map was calculated from the solved 2D crystals of bRho using electron cryomicroscopy, which served as the basis for the construction of the receptor molecular model (Baldwin, 1993; Schertler et al., 1993). However, the first three-dimensional (3D) structure of bRho in its inactive state was released only in 2000 (Palczewski et al., 2000). Despite relentless efforts, elucidation of GPCR structures remained challenging due to several factors, including maintenance of structural integrity of the receptors by embedding in a membrane-like environment, presence of flexible ECLs and ICLs, low expression level of the receptor, and displaying basal signaling activity even in the absence of a ligand. However, all the aforementioned problems have been circumvented with the advances in GPCR crystallography, protein engineering, and innovations in biotechnology. Introduction of small, stable fusion proteins (T4 lysozyme and b562RIL) decreased the flexibility of the receptor regions (ICL3, ICL2, and N-terminal regions), and improved the crystal contacts. Likewise, antibody fragments or nanobodies improved the conformational stability of the receptors. Insertion of mutations (stabilized receptor (StaR) approach) enhanced the receptor thermostability in a particular conformational state and increased the protein expression levels.

The first structural breakthrough of a human GPCR, i.e., β_2-adrenergic receptor (β_2AR with a diffusible ligand), using different crystallization techniques came in 2007 (Cherezov et al., 2007). Moreover, the first crystal structures for GPCR classes B, C, and F have been solved (Hollenstein et al., 2013; Wang et al., 2013; Wu et al., 2014). So far, experimental structures of 44 distinct GPCRs and ~205 ligand-receptor complexes covering all the four classes, A–C, and F are available, of which most belong to the Class A subfamily (Hauser et al., 2017). It is to be noted that most of the existing GPCR structures are inactive ones, bound to an inhibitor. In the last year (2017) alone, more than 40 GPCR crystal structures have been determined which are listed in **Table 2**. GPCR structural studies have revealed the arrangement of the TM domains, location of the orthosteric, allosteric, bitopic, and biased ligand binding sites, homo- or heterooligomerization of receptors, and structural rearrangements involved in conformational changes upon GPCR activation or inactivation (Manglik and Kruse, 2017; Schrage and Kostenis, 2017). Besides garnering these 3D structural insights, the molecular basis of GPCR signal transduction coupled to G-proteins or β-arrestins were elucidated through X-ray crystallography and electron cryomicroscopy techniques. Oligomeric complex structures of bRho coupled to G-protein peptide (Rho/GαCT) (Scheerer et al., 2008), human Rho coupled to visual arrestins (Kang et al., 2015; Zhou et al., 2017), β_2AR coupled to Gs-protein (Rasmussen et al., 2011) and β-arrestin 1 (Shukla et al., 2014), A_{2A} adenosine receptor (A_{2A}AR) in complex with a mini-G_s protein (Carpenter et al., 2016), glucagon-like peptide 1 receptor (GLP-1R) in complex with a Gs-protein (Zhang et al., 2017), and calcitonin receptor (CTR) coupled to Gs-protein (Liang et al., 2017) have been elucidated. These complex structures provide full mechanistic insights into

TABLE 1 | Key details of GPCR virtual screening campaigns reported in the last 5 years (2013–2017).

GPCR class and classification type	Receptor type	VS library and size	Hits/hit rate	Structure of notable hits	References
A, nonrhodopsin (aminergic)	β_2AR	ZINC database: (a) 2.7 million lead-like subset (b) 400k fragment-like subset	6 hits (27.3%)	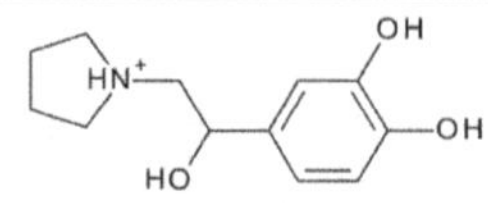 pKi = 3.9	Weiss et al., 2013
A, nonrhodopsin (aminergic)	D_2R	ZINC database: (a) 2.7 million lead-like subset (b) 400k fragment-like subset	3 hits (20%)	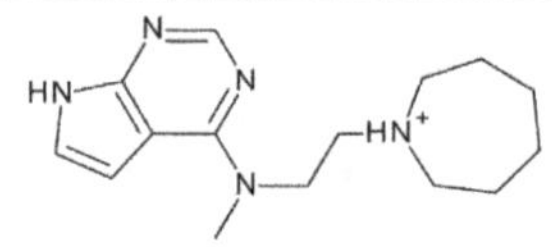 $pEC_{50} = 4$	Weiss et al., 2013
A, nonrhodopsin (aminergic)	M_2R	ZINC database: 3.1 million compounds	11 of 19 (57.9%)	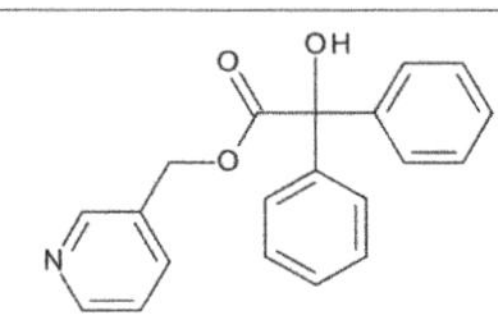 Ki = 1.2 uM	Kruse et al., 2013
A, nonrhodopsin (aminergic)	M_3R	ZINC database: 3.1 million compounds	8 of 16 (50%)	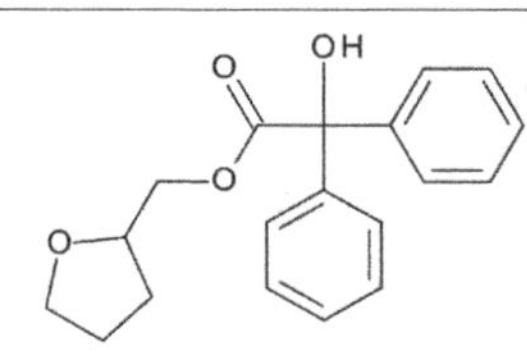 Ki = 1.2 uM	Kruse et al., 2013
A, nonrhodopsin (lipid-like)	CB_2R	Enamine, Otava, ChemBridge, ChemDiv, Vitasm, IBS, LifeChemicals, Specs, and TimTec: 5,613,820 compounds	13 hits $\geq$ 50% inhibition at 10 uM (13.4%)	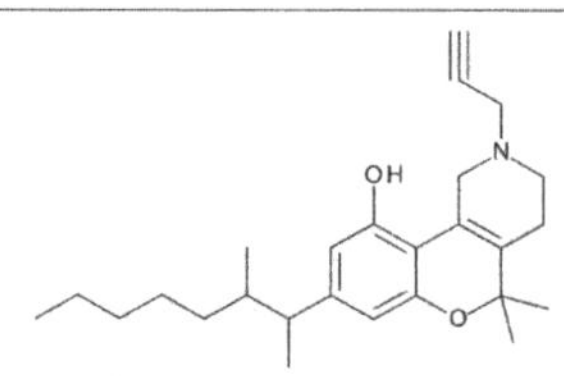 Ki = 2.3 nM	Renault et al., 2013
A, nonrhodopsin (aminergic)	AgOAR45B	ZINC drug-like subset: 12 million compounds	45 hits (64.3%)	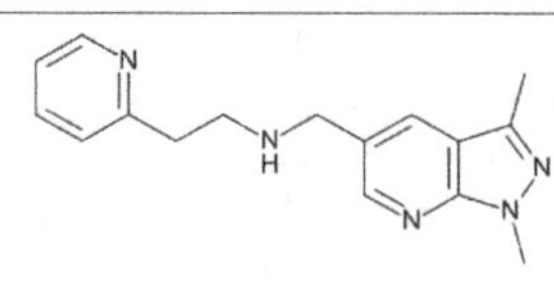 Ki = 2.7 uM	Kastner et al., 2014
A, nonrhodopsin (aminergic)	5-HT_{1A}R	WDI, PCL, TimTec, and ASINEX: 80,800 compounds	9 hits $\geq$ 50% inhibition at 10 uM (60%)	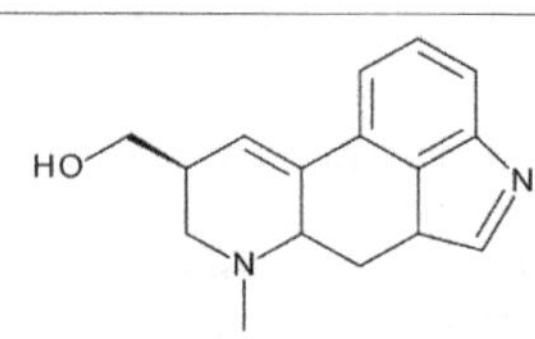 $IC_{50} = 2.3$ nM	Luo et al., 2014
A, nonrhodopsin (peptide-like)	NOP receptor	ZINC database CNS Permeable subset: 400,000 compounds	6 hits $\geq$ 50% inhibition at 300 uM (30%)	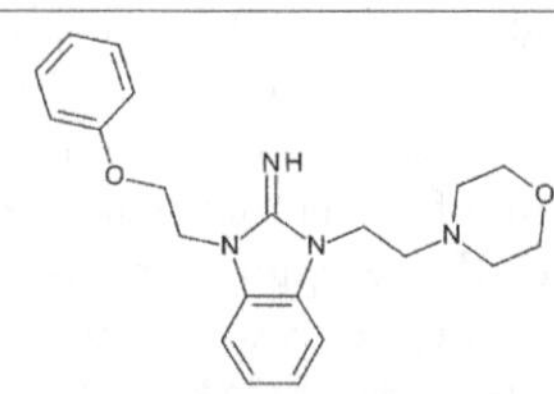 $K_i = 1.42$	Daga et al., 2014

(Continued)

TABLE 1 | Continued

GPCR class and classification type	Receptor type	VS library and size	Hits/hit rate	Structure of notable hits	References
A, nonrhodopsin (peptide-like)	PAR2	FDA-approved drugs: 1,216 compounds	4 hits ≥ 50% inhibition at 30 uM	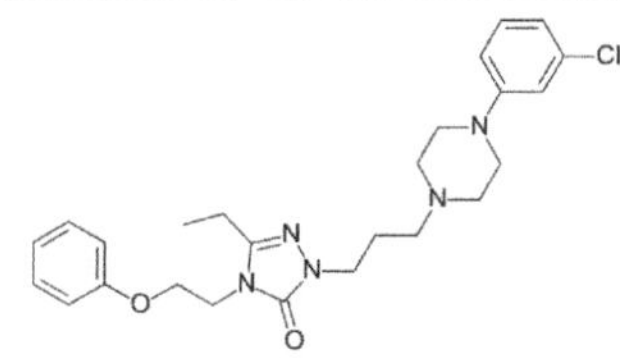 IC_{50} = 10 uM	Xu et al., 2015
A, nonrhodopsin (aminergic)	5-HT_6R	ChEMBL: 12,608 compounds	6 hits (16.7%)	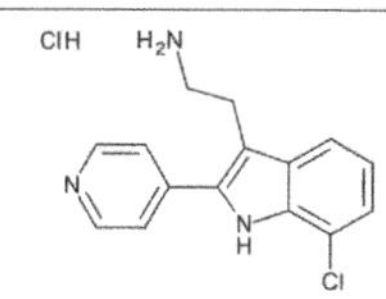 IC_{50} = 0.1 uM	Kelemen et al., 2016
A, nonrhodopsin (aminergic)	H_1R	ChEMBL: 108,790 compounds	19 hits (73.1%)	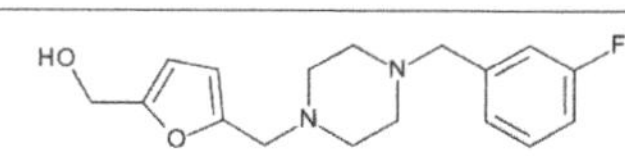 pK_i = 4.72	Kooistra et al., 2016
A, nonrhodopsin (aminergic)	β_2AR	ChEMBL: 108,790 compounds	18 hits (52.9%)	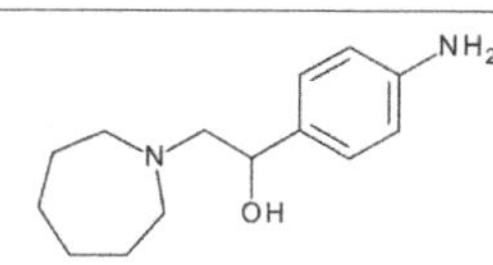 pEC_{50} = 4.52	Kooistra et al., 2016
C, metabotropic glutamate	$mGlu_1$R	Asinex: 695,855 compounds	5 hits (14.3%)	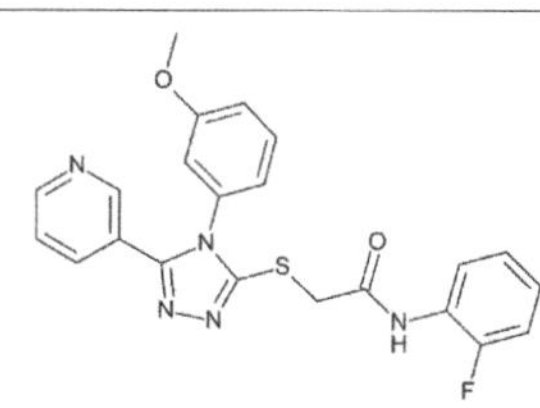 IC_{50} = 10.22 uM	Jang et al., 2016
	FGSG_02655 (Class I, pheromone receptor)	Life Chemicals GPCR Targeted Libraries: 11,571 compounds	10 VS hits	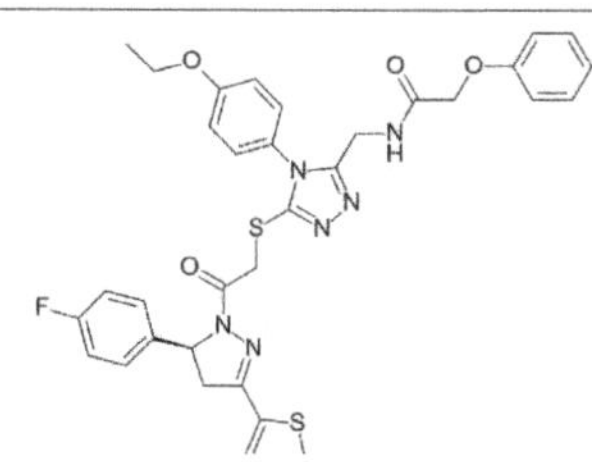	Bresso et al., 2016
A, nonrhodopsin (peptide-like)	PAR2	(a) Asinex: 433,973 compounds (b) ChemDiv: 1,213,470 compounds	3 hits ≥ 30% inhibition at 10 uM (6.4%)	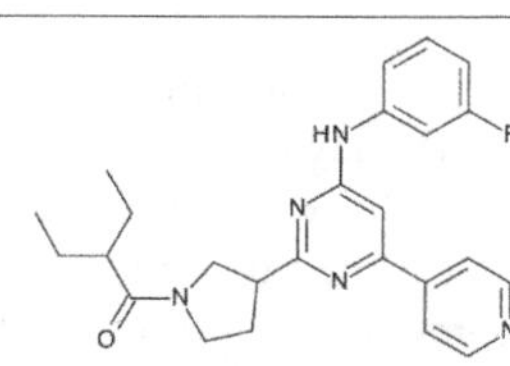 IC_{50} = 8.22 uM	Cho et al., 2016

(Continued)

TABLE 1 | Continued

GPCR class and classification type	Receptor type	VS library and size	Hits/hit rate	Structure of notable hits	References
A, nonrhodopsin (peptide-like)	NTSR1	ZINC, ChemBridge, and J&K: 1,000,000 compounds	4 hits (9.1%)	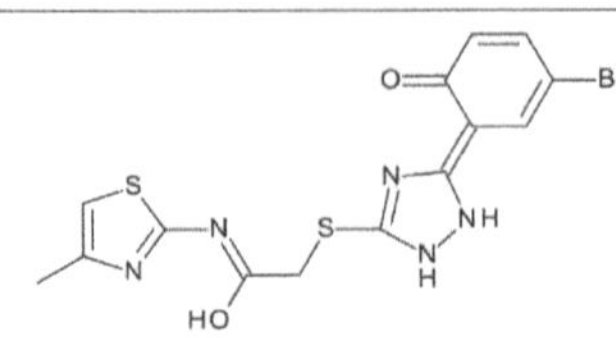 IC_{50} = 14.47 uM	Zhang et al., 2016
A, nonrhodopsin (aminergic)	5-HT_{2A}R	ZINC Clean Lead-like subset: 140,809 compounds	15 VS hits	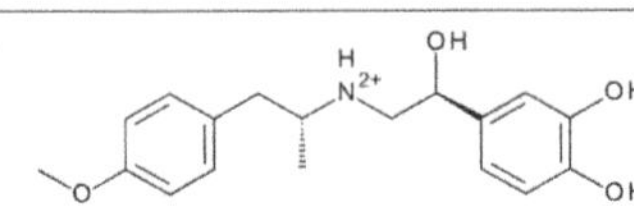	Gandhimathi and Sowdhamini, 2016
A, nonrhodopsin (aminergic)	D_2R	6,500,000 compounds	10 hits (47.6%)	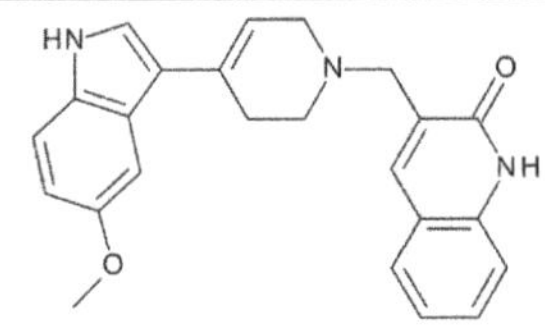 Ki = 58.1	Kaczor et al., 2016
A, nonrhodopsin (aminergic)	M_2R	NCI Diversity Set: 1,600 compounds	19 hits (50%)	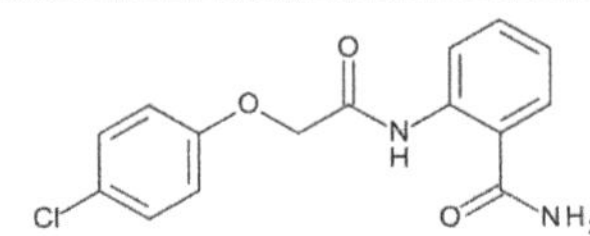 pKi = 3.8	Miao et al., 2016
A, nonrhodopsin (aminergic)	H_3R	Phase database	6 hits (8%)	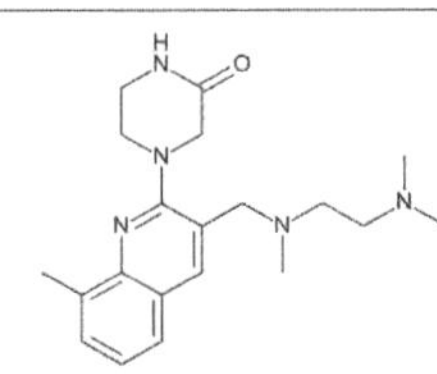 pKi = 6.1	Frandsen et al., 2017
A, rhodopsin	GPR91	ZINC In-Stock subset: 12,782,590 compounds	12 hits (10.8%)	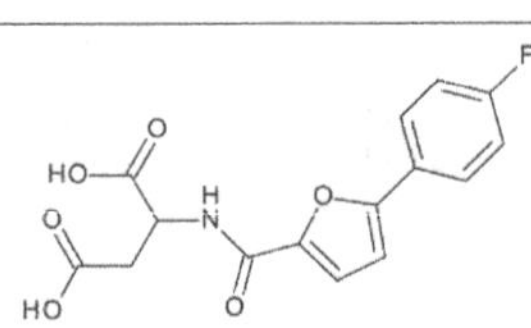 EC_{50} = 1.9 uM	Trauelsen et al., 2017

GPCR and biased signaling, thus underpinning their functional significance and pharmacological targeting.

GPCRs are known to exist or function as monomers, dimers, and/or higher order oligomers, including homo- or hetero- dimers/oligomers (Guo et al., 2017). In addition to the accumulated experimental data through biochemical and biophysical techniques, the structural information on GPCR dimers or higher order oligomers were provided by X-ray crystallography. The first reported higher-order crystal structure of Rho and opsin in native membranes were reported in 2003 (Liang et al., 2003). Consequently, several structures including rhodopsin and nonrhodopsin class A GPCRs were elucidated (Lee et al., 2018). The oligomeric structures of GPCRs are essential for modulation of receptor function, mediation of cross-talk between GPCRs or other signaling pathways, and cellular trafficking, hence they have been associated with specific functional effects. Moreover, targeting these oligomeric structures as drug candidates could provide a new arena for drug development and specificity. The wealth of information supporting the existence of homo- and heterooligomers of GPCRs can be retrieved from the RCSB PDB (https://www.rcsb.org/pdb/home/home.do) or GPCR Oligomerization Knowledge

TABLE 2 | Summary of GPCR solved structures released in the past 1 year (Dec '16-Nov '17).

Class type, classification	Receptor type	Species	Ligand	Ligand type	Released year	Resolution	PDB ID
A, rhodopsin	Rhodopsin[a]	Human	N/A	N/A	2017	3.0	5W0P
	Rhodopsin[b]	Bovine	N/A	N/A	2017	2.7	5TE3
	Rhodopsin	Bovine	10,20-Methanoretinal	Agonist	2017	4.0	5TE5
A, nonrhodopsin (aminergic receptors)	β_2AR	Human	Carazolol; 4-carbamoyl-N-[(2R)-2-cyclohexyl-2-phenylacetyl]-L-phenylalanyl-3-bromo-N-methyl-L-phenylalaninamide	Inverse agonist; Allosteric antagonist	2017	2.7	5X7D
	D_4R	Human	Nemonapride	Antagonist	2017	2.0	5WIU
	D_4R	Human	Nemonapride	Antagonist	2017	2.1	5WIV
	5-HT_{2B}	Human	Lysergic acid diethylamide	Agonist	2017	2.9	5TVN
	5-HT_{2B}	Human	Ergotamine	Agonist	2017	3.0	5TUD
A, nonrhodopsin (nucleotide-like receptors)	A_1AR	Human	DU172	Covalent antagonist	2017	3.2	5UEN
	A_1AR	Human	PSB36	Antagonist	2017	3.3	5N2S
	A_{2A}AR	Human	ZM241385	Inverse agonist	2017	1.7	5NM4
	A_{2A}AR	Human	ZM241385	Inverse agonist	2017	2.0	5NM2
	A_{2A}AR	Human	ZM241385	Inverse agonist	2017	2.1	5NLX
	A_{2A}AR	Human	Theophylline	Antagonist	2017	2.0	5MZJ
	A_{2A}AR	Human	PSB36	Antagonist	2017	2.8	5N2R
	A_{2A}AR	Human	Caffeine	Neutral antagonist	2017	2.1	5MZP
	A_{2A}AR	Human	ZM241385	Inverse agonist	2017	2.8	5JTB
	A_{2A}AR	Human	ZM241385	Inverse agonist	2017	3.2	5UVI
	A_{2A}AR	Human	5-Amino-N-[(2-Methoxyphenyl)methyl]-2-(3-Methylphenyl)-2h-1,2,3-Triazole-4-Carboximidamide	Bitopic antagonist	2017	3.5	5UIG
A, nonrhodopsin (peptide-like receptors)	CCR2	Human	BMS-681; CCR2-RA-[R]	Orthosteric antagonist; Allosteric antagonist	2016	2.8	5T1A
	CCR5	Human	5P7-CCL5	Antagonist	2017	2.2	5UIW
	CCR9	Human	Vercirnon	Allosteric antagonist	2016	2.8	5LWE
	NTSR1	Rat	NTS_{8-13}	Agonist	2016	3.3	5T04
	APJR	Human	AMG3054	Agonist	2017	2.6	5VBL
	PAR2	Human	AZ3451	Allosteric antagonist	2017	3.6	5NDZ
	PAR2	Human	AZ8838	Antagonist	2017	2.8	5NDD
	PAR2	Human	AZ7188	Antagonist	2017	4.0	5NJ6
	AT_2R	Human	N-benzyl-N-(2-ethyl-4-oxo-3-{[2′-(2H-tetrazol-5-yl)[1,1′-biphenyl]-4-yl]methyl}-3,4-dihydroquinazolin-6-yl)thiophene-2-carboxamide	Antagonist	2017	2.8	5UNG
	AT_2R	Human	N-[(furan-2-yl)methyl]-N-(4-oxo-2-propyl-3-{[2′-(2H-tetrazol-5-yl)[1,1′-biphenyl]-4-yl]methyl}-3,4-dihydroquinazolin-6-yl)benzamide	Dual antagonist	2017	2.9	5UNH

(Continued)

TABLE 2 | Continued

Class type, classification	Receptor type	Species	Ligand	Ligand type	Released year	Resolution	PDB ID
	AT_2R	Human	N-benzyl-N-(2-ethyl-4-oxo-3-{[2′-(2H-tetrazol-5-yl)[1,1′-biphenyl]-4-yl]	Antagonist	2017	2.8	5UNF
	ET_BR	Human	Bosentan	Dual antagonist	2017	3.6	5XPR
	ET_BR	Human	K-8794	Antagonist	2017	2.2	5X93
A, nonrhodopsin (lipid-like receptors)	FFAR1	Human	MK-8666; AP8	Partial agonist; Full allosteric agonist	2017	3.2	5TZY
	FFAR1	Human	MK-8666	Partial agonist	2017	2.2	5TZR
	LPA_6R[b]	Zebrafish	N/A	N/A	2017	3.2	5XSZ
	CB_1R	Human	AM11542	Full agonist	2017	2.8	5XRA
	CB_1R	Human	AM841	Full agonist	2017	3.0	5XR8
	CB_1R	Human	Taranabant	Inverse Agonist	2016	2.6	5U09
B, secretin-like receptors	GLP-1R	Human	Truncated peptide	Agonist	2017	3.7	5NX2
	GLP-1R	Human	PF-06372222	Negative allosteric modulator	2017	2.7	5VEW
	GLP-1R	Human	NNC0640	Negative allosteric modulator	2017	3.0	5VEX
	GLP-1R[c]	Rabbit	GLP-1	Agonist	2017	4.1	5VAI
	GCGR	Human	NNC0640	Negative allosteric modulator	2017	3.0	5XEZ
	GCGR	Human	NNC0640	Negative allosteric modulator	2017	3.2	5XF1
	CTR[c]	Human	sCT	Agonist	2017	4.1	5UZ7

[a]*Arrestin-bound state of the receptor.*
[b]*Ligand-free basal state of the receptor.*
[c]*Fully-active receptor complexed with a G protein.*

Base (Khelashvili et al., 2010). In addition to these structural intricacies, GPCR signaling is also modulated by the presence of ligands other than orthosteric, which will be discussed in the following sections. Furthermore, adding details like GPCR dynamics to the structural information would provide a bigger picture to the biomedical researchers in this field. Such dynamic events triggered upon receptor activation or inhibition mechanisms could be covered by powerful methodologies including, bottom-up Hydrogen Deuterium eXchange Mass Spectrometry (HDX-MS) and resonance energy transfer (RET) (Li et al., 2015; Zhang, 2017). These important structural tools aid in better GPCR drug design by adding valuable information to our understanding of GPCR function, dynamics, protein-protein interactions, and receptor-ligand interactions (Vilardaga, 2011; Kauk and Hoffmann, 2017). Collectively, all the structural studies provide unprecedented insights into the structural and functional diversity of this receptor family. The wealth of structural information on all GPCRs is invaluable for ligand-based drug design (LBDD), structure-based drug design (SBDD), and integrated paradigms which complement traditional drug discovery efforts.

INSIGHTS INTO GPCR LIGAND SPACE

Various signaling pathways involve several GPCRs whose activities are mediated by ligand binding. Based on activation intensity, GPCR modulators can be divided into agonists, partial agonists, antagonists, and inverse agonists. Full agonists can stimulate maximal GPCR activity leading to recruitment of downstream proteins for signal transduction. Partial agonists, on the other hand, cannot induce 100% activation of receptors and acts as a type of antagonist while in the presence of full agonists. However, it can act as full agonists when there are excess receptors and in the absence of actual full agonists. Antagonists act as agonist blockers and can be divided into neutral antagonists and inverse agonists. Neutral antagonists can bind to GPCRs but do not affect the receptor's constitutive activity, whereas inverse agonists can block agonist effects. These modulators can directly interact with the orthosteric binding site of GPCRs (Wacker et al., 2017a).

While structural architecture of the TM region is largely conserved, the remarkable diversity in GPCR sequences are most notable in the ECL and ICL regions. This leads credence to the capacity of the GPCR family to interact with a wide range of ligands that vary in size, shape, and physicochemical properties, most of which bind to the orthosteric site to modulate receptor activity. In the ECL region, ECL2 plays a critical role in ligand recognition, access, and selectivity (Dror et al., 2011; Kruse et al., 2012; Zhang H. T. et al., 2015). For Class A GPCRs, lipophilic ligands often come from the lipid membrane and access the orthosteric site through the "lid" formed by the N-terminus and ECL2. In the case of hydrophilic ligands, ECL2 of different receptors only partially covers the ECL region through a variety of structures that shapes the entrance to the binding pocket (Venkatakrishnan et al., 2013). On the other hand, modulators of class B GPCRs are frequently peptide ligands, which possess large volume and high flexibility, requiring a more solvent-accessible orthosteric binding pocket (Liang et al., 2017).

Increase in static GPCR structures and advances in MD facilities have assisted in the elucidation of GPCR-ligand binding interaction. A thorough investigation of the ligand binding pocket of several GPCRs indicated the presence of multiple topologically equivalent residues that forms a consensus ligand binding network in almost all Class A receptors, providing an explanation for cross-reactivity and polypharmacology. Moreover, deviations from these consensus binding residues can account for ligand specificity in different GPCR members, and can thus be exploited in the design of specific and potent ligands (Venkatakrishnan et al., 2013). Regardless of the upsurge in information in the last few decades, it is still difficult to understand the differences in ligand binding requirements for agonists, antagonists, and inverse agonists of a given receptor, despite having almost identical structures (**Figure 3**). This calls for more studies focused on identifying key residues for agonism and antagonism, not only ligand binding specificity. Along with this, it is important to scrutinize activity cliffs of ligands as significant shifts in modulation type could be observed through small changes in ligand structures.

Besides the orthosteric site, GPCR ligands can also bind to allosteric pockets and indirectly modulate receptor activity. Allosteric modulators can be divided into two types: (a) positive allosteric modulators (PAMs), which increases agonist affinity, and (b) negative allosteric modulators (NAMs), which acts as an allosteric antagonist or inverse agonist to decrease agonist affinity (Christopher et al., 2013, 2015; Kenakin, 2016). Additionally, there are some molecules that can both interact with orthosteric and allosteric sites, known as bitopic modulators (Dror et al., 2013; Fronik et al., 2017). Allosteric modulators can be either endogenous molecules, like sodium and cholesterol (Katritch et al., 2014), or exogenous molecules like natural products and synthetic compounds. Since allosteric modulators bind to sites other than the orthosteric site, they can co-bind with the putative ligand on the receptor to alter conformation and activity, thus affecting downstream signaling.

In case of CC chemokine receptor type 9 (CCR9), vercirnon (antagonist) was co-crystallized and unexpectedly found to interact with the intracellular binding site, blocking G-protein coupling (Oswald et al., 2016). Another example of an allosteric modulator is 1-(2-(2-(tert-butyl)phenoxy)pyridin-3-yl)-3-(4-(trifluoromethoxy)phenyl)urea (BPTU), which binds outside the purinergic $P2Y_1$ receptor, flanking the TM bundle inside the lipid bilayer. While BPTU shows lower potency than known orthosteric antagonist, MRS2500, its allosteric interactions allow higher selectivity for the $P2Y_1$ receptor (Zhang D. et al., 2015). Apart from small molecule compounds, ions can also function as an allosteric modulator, as illustrated by the discovery of the conserved allosteric binding pocket for Na^+ in Class A GPCRs (Katritch et al., 2014).

The current rising star in GPCR research is biased signaling. Previously, GPCRs were presumed to exist as a simple two-state receptor model ["on" (activation) and "off" (inactivation)]. However, extensive analyses of different signaling pathways paved way to an exciting discovery that GPCRs have multiple conformations, each tailored to a specific response and downstream effect. Different ligands induce different receptor conformations, and each conformational state could initiate a specific downstream signal. While this finding increases the difficulty in drug discovery and design, there is also an opportunity to selectively block pathways implicated in various pathologies, while leaving normal homeostatic processes intact (Bologna et al., 2017). Typically, G protein signaling occurs upon agonist binding, whereas arrestin-mediated signaling occurs through arrestin binding. In this instance, GPCR drug design strategy could be dependent on identifying agonists biased for either G protein or arrestin signaling, leading to higher drug efficacy and diminished adverse effects (DeWire and Violin, 2011). Some excellent examples of biased ligands include lysergic acid diethylamide (LSD) (Wacker et al., 2017b), a well-known hallucinogen which appears to display bias toward β-arrestin signaling, and synthetic opioids TRV-130 (DeWire et al., 2013) and PZM-21 (Manglik et al., 2016), which are biased toward G protein signaling. Altogether, these accumulated data may provide extremely beneficial hints in the discovery and design of GPCR ligands based on the intended activity and targeted pathology. **Figure 4** depicts some of the common GPCR modulators that are distinguished by activity types.

CHEMINFORMATICS-BASED PARADIGMS IN GPCR DRUG DISCOVERY

Cheminformatics Approaches Based on the Knowledge Derived From GPCR Ligands

Cheminformatics tools are frequently utilized in GPCR research due to the enormous amount of GPCR ligand data. Difficulties in

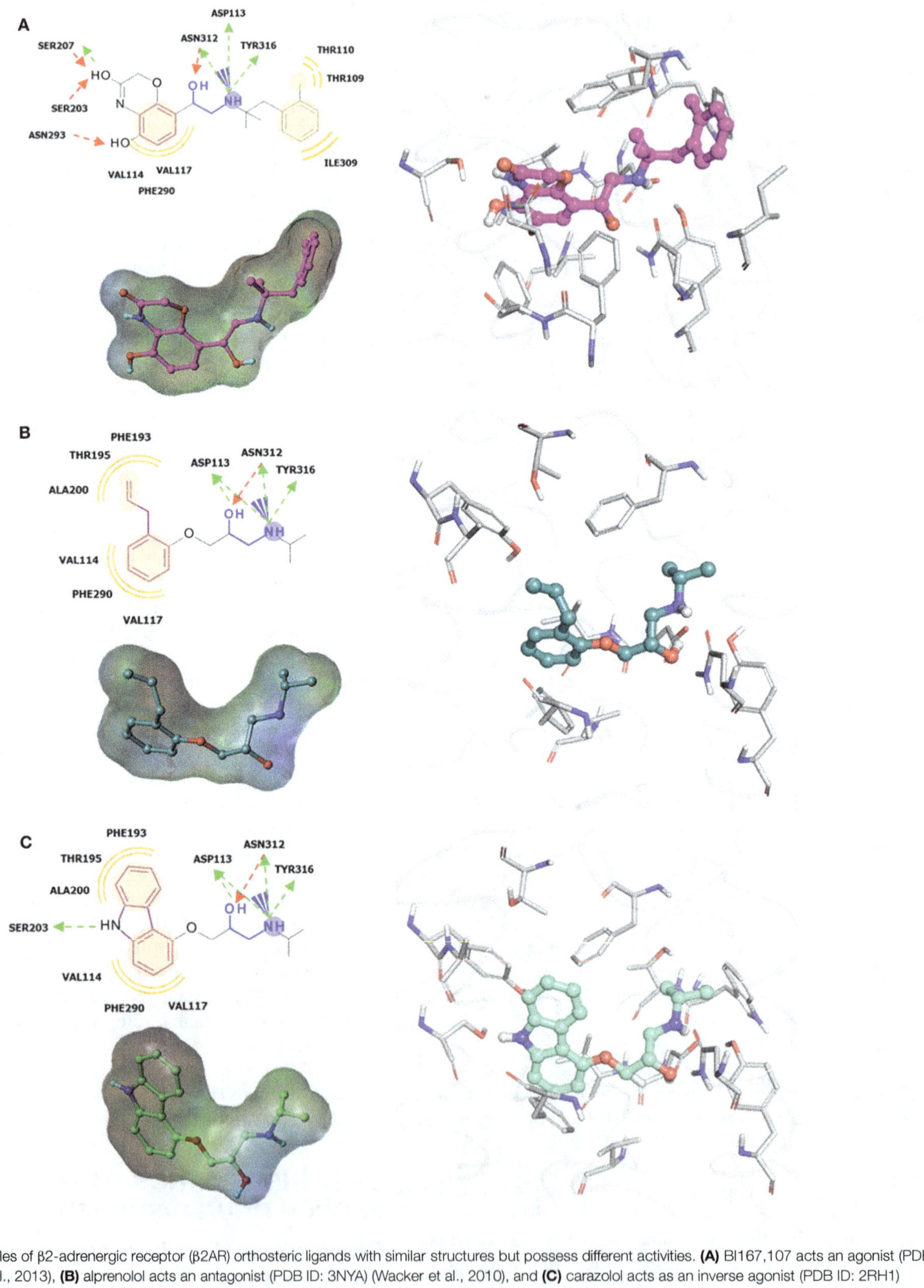

FIGURE 3 | Examples of β2-adrenergic receptor (β2AR) orthosteric ligands with similar structures but possess different activities. **(A)** BI167,107 acts an agonist (PDB ID: 4LDE) (Ring et al., 2013), **(B)** alprenolol acts an antagonist (PDB ID: 3NYA) (Wacker et al., 2010), and **(C)** carazolol acts as an inverse agonist (PDB ID: 2RH1) (Cherezov et al., 2007).

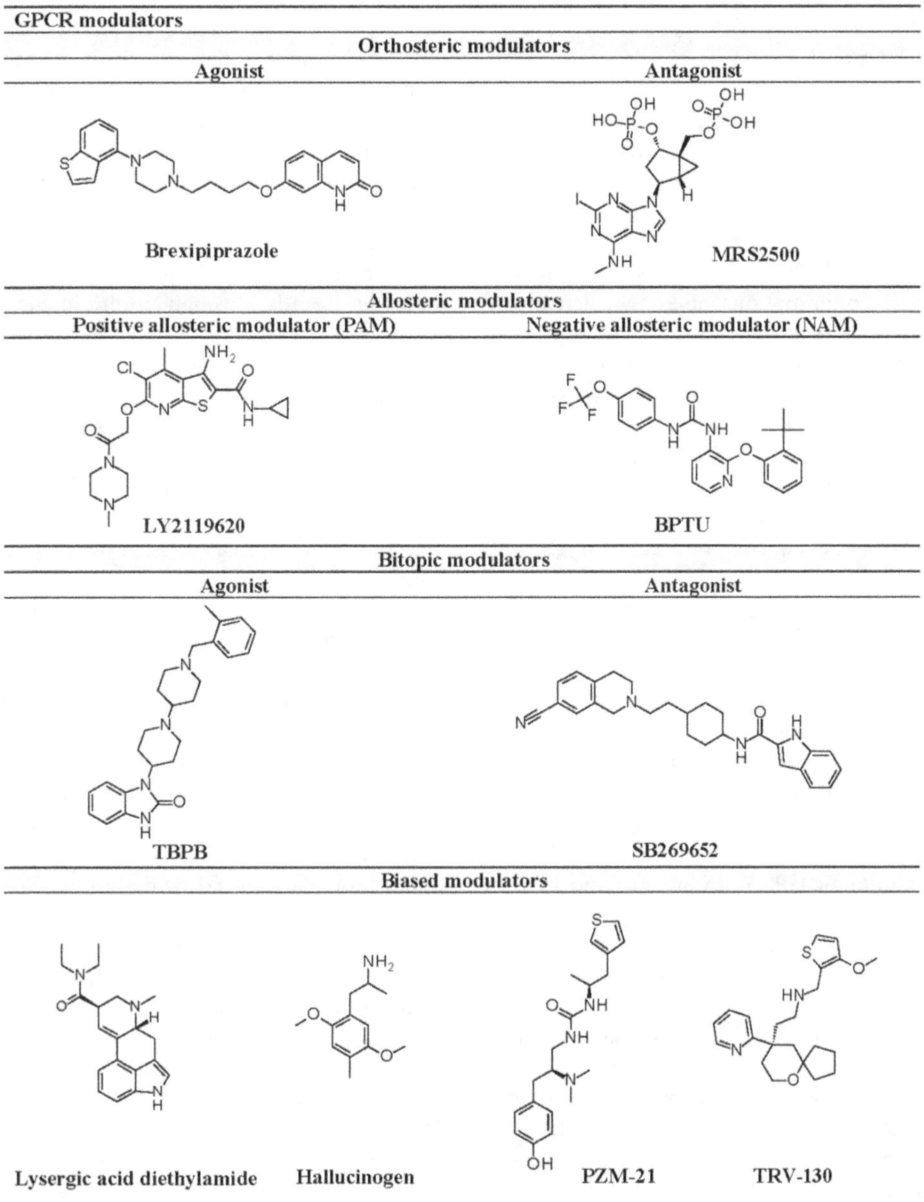

FIGURE 4 | Representative chemical structures of various GPCR modulators.

crystallizing membrane proteins and receptor flexibility hindered structural elucidation and drug discovery research for this receptor. Due to these shortcomings, ligand-based approaches started to thrive in order to provide a better understanding of GPCR function and pharmacology. Some of the major ligand-based cheminformatics approaches are detailed below.

Cheminformatics and Virtual Screening

In silico screening method started to become popularly used after the integration of high throughput screening (HTS) and information technology (Coudrat et al., 2017b). Several computational and VS methods are frequently utilized in different stages of drug discovery and development, but some of the earliest and most commonly used ones are similarity- and QSAR-based strategies due to their efficiency and capability in analyzing simple 2D structures. These strategies are dependent on the principle that similar structures are predicted to display similar activities. Similarity-based methods need at least one established hit whose chemical structure is used to calculate pertinent molecular fingerprints, which is then employed to screen chemical libraries for compounds containing similar structure or fragments. On the other hand, QSAR-based strategies rely on the developed mathematical models which require an adequate number of biologically active compounds with activities covering a wide span of concentration. In this case, screening is dependent on the quality of the dataset used and the accuracy of the developed model (Luo et al., 2016).

Similarity-based VS was applied in a recent study for the discovery of a novel series of cannabinoid receptor 2 (CB_2R) agonists (Gianella-Borradori et al., 2015). CB_2R is a class A, lipid-like GPCR that regulates the effects of endogenously produced cannabinoid receptor ligands and has been implicated in several inflammatory diseases. In this study, an in-house database containing around 25,000 compounds was screened based on 40 low-energy conformations of known active and selective compound HU-308. Compounds were ranked based on their similarity with any of the 40 conformers of HU-308, and the top 94 were selected for biochemical screening based on the combined color score, which refers to chemistry alignment akin to pharmacophore features, and shape Tanimoto score, which accounts for 3D conformer overlay. From the initial hits, the top 16 active compounds displayed 6 new core scaffolds. Upon combined inspection of bioactivity, molecular weight, and lipophilicity, DIAS1 was chosen and used for further mining of the in-house library with the help of the newly identified scaffold. The second VS led to the discovery of DIAS2, which exhibited better activity and reduced lipophilicity as compared to DIAS1. Further structure-activity relationship (SAR) studies were performed for the optimization of the lead compound to improve potency, selectivity, and pharmacokinetic properties, resulting in candidate compounds that show nanomolar activity and selectivity for CB_2R.

Another study used the US EPA's ToxCast database to develop QSAR models for 18 aminergic GPCRs (Mansouri and Judson, 2016). While the ToxCast program can screen hundreds of compounds *in vitro* to determine toxicity, the chemical space covered by their database is not enough to include all compounds of interest. However, the database can be employed in the development of predictive QSAR models. Two QSAR models were developed during the study, a qualitative (active vs. non-active) and a quantitative (potency value prediction) model. Various descriptors were calculated from the 2D structures of the compounds in the database and were subjected to genetic algorithms (GAs) to identify the best and most predictive descriptors. Several model-fitting methods, including PLSDA (partial least square discriminant analysis), SVMs (support vector machines), kNNs (k-nearest neighbors), and PLSs (partial least squares), were used to generate the QSAR models, which were later evaluated for accuracy and predictability. As a result, they were able to produce suitable models for aminergic GPCR assays and demonstrate the reliability of QSAR-based methods for analysis.

Cheminformatics and *de Novo* Ligand Design

Typically, ligand-based *de novo* drug design utilizes approved drugs or known inhibitors as reference structures or a source of pharmacophores that are relevant for bioactivity to build new chemical structures. While novelty and potency are always favored in drug discovery research, *de novo* structures should also have desirable pharmacokinetic properties (Kawashita et al., 2015). The combination of *de novo* drug design and computer-aided VS, along with the application of ADME/Tox models for the prediction of pharmacokinetic properties, has the capability of more effectively identifying NCEs with the desirable pharmacological activity profiles. In this sense, *de novo* drug design approach has become the forerunner of the long-envisioned personalized medicine where patients can be given custom-tailored drugs with increased efficacy and reduced adverse effects.

Rodrigues et al. worked on 5-hydroxytryptamine receptor subtype 2B ($5\text{-}HT_{2B}$) drug discovery and were able to identify selective ligands through multidimensional *de novo* design (Rodrigues et al., 2015). In the Molecular Ant Algorithm (MAntA) software (Reutlinger et al., 2014), chemically advanced template search version 2 (CATS2), pharmacophores, and Morgan substructure fingerprints were employed to generate $5\text{-}HT_{2B}$ selective ligands via reductive amination, resulting in over 5,000 new compound structures from which 4 were selected based on calculated $5\text{-}HT_{2B}$ selectivity. To further improve selectivity and increase the scaffold diversity, *de novo* design software DOGS (Hartenfeller et al., 2012) and FDA-approved drug molecule structures were utilized to produce NCEs. The resulting compounds were screened with PAINS (Baell and Holloway, 2010) and ADMET filters (Lagorce et al., 2008) to remove undesirable molecules before performing experimental validation assays. Finally, four more compounds were obtained and among them, one compound showed promising selectivity for the $5\text{-}HT_{2B}$ receptor. Even though the newly designed compound was not comparable in potency with the most potent existing antagonists, this study still provides an excellent application of *de novo* drug design in GPCR drug discovery field.

Cheminformatics and Chemical Genomics

While the number of currently available GPCR structures is increasing, it only covers a small portion of this protein superfamily and several other pharmaceutically relevant members are not yet elucidated. Chemical genomics can be applied to overcome the difficulty of target and drug identification by screening small molecule libraries and measuring their effects on entire biological systems or a specific group of targets, such as GPCRs. This combines the strength of traditional pharmaceutical techniques and genomics to facilitate discovery and validation of therapeutic targets, as well as identification of potential drug candidates for optimization (Hauser et al., 2018). Moreover, application of this strategy provides information concerning activated signaling pathways and biological effects through measurable gene expressions, leading to relevant data about target specificity and noninteraction pairs. In this sense, chemical genomics works on mining huge chemical data with the help of structural bioinformatics to rapidly identify target structure-function relationships (Valerio and Choudhuri, 2012). One of the most popular chemical genomics-based database found online is GLIDA (GPCR-Ligand Database), a publicly available Chemical Genomics database that can be used for GPCR drug discovery (Okuno et al., 2008). It contains GPCR biological and ligand information, as well as GPCR-ligand binding data. Therefore, it can be utilized for LBDD with the help of techniques such as machine learning-based classification and similarity-based search.

Shiraishi et al. reported an interesting research wherein chemical genomics approach was employed to predict GPCR-ligand interaction for class A GPCRs (Shiraishi et al., 2013). GPCR-ligand interaction data was collected from GVK Biosciences database and kernel methods were applied to evaluate compound-protein interaction (CPI) pair similarities based on Extended Connectivity Fingerprint (ECFP) and Dragon software descriptors generated for the ligands, along with target specific regions, such as full structure, loop region, and TM region. The results showed that compared to kernels accounting for the full structure and loop regions, kernels for the TM region showed significantly improved performance, which agrees with experimental findings that the TM region of class A GPCRs plays a critical role in ligand binding. Reliability of the machine learning model was improved with the addition of negative noninteraction pairs. Careful investigation of GPCR-ligand pairs revealed that high co-occurrence of residue-fragment pairs may be indicative of importance in ligand binding and specificity, as well as conservation of binding modes among Class A GPCRs. Key interactions identified in their study can be used for future VS and lead optimization studies and is beneficial when employed in combination with structure-based studies.

Cheminformatics, Polypharmacology, Drug Repositioning, and Repurposing

Recently, pharmaceutical research focuses not only on the discovery of novel compounds for a known target but also on the discovery of new indications for currently approved drugs. Polypharmacology has quickly emerged as a critical part of drug discovery research with the knowledge of how interconnected pathways in biological systems are. Though this field is most often used to investigate adverse effects and toxicity, information garnered from possible off-target effects can also offer information about new drug indications or cross-reactivity leading to higher drug efficacy (Jacobson et al., 2014). With the upsurge of polypharmacological information, it is no surprise that it is now frequently combined with cheminformatics strategies to predict off-target effects ahead of extensive biochemical analyses in order to save time and resources.

Xie et al. reported an interesting chemical genomics-based polypharmacology study focusing on GPCR-related drug abuse problem (Xie et al., 2014). Initially, a drug-abuse domain specific chemogenomics knowledgebase (DA-KB) was built to consolidate chemogenomics data regarding drug abuse and CNS diseases. This database was later used to investigate molecular interaction networks that encompass both drug abuse and GPCR modulation. Upon identifying 85 drug abuse-related GPCRs, distribution information of these receptors was collected and studied from the MetaCore database (Ekins et al., 2006). Using HTDocking (https://omictools.com/htdocking-tool) and GPCRDocking programs, polypharmacology and polydrug addiction analyses were performed to investigate the interactions between drug abuse-related receptors and ligands, along with cross-reactivities. As a result, the DA-KB became a powerful tool that has the capability of transforming data to useable polypharmacology knowledge. Moreover, TargetHunter server was also developed and can be used for target or off-target discovery.

Cheminformatics Approaches Based on the GPCR Structural Data

SBDD is one of the potent tools in lead discovery and optimization (Andrews et al., 2014). The application of SBDD is proven to be more efficient than traditional methods due to its working principle, which includes understanding the molecular basis of the disease and utilizing the 3D structural data of the target protein in the drug discovery pipeline (Cavasotto and Palomba, 2015). It has played a valuable role in several drug discovery projects involving enzyme targets (Wlodawer and Vondrasek, 1998; Varghese, 1999). Due to the difficulties in the expression and crystallography of GPCRs, there was only limited information available for SBDD of such targets. However, methodological advances in GPCR crystallography have paved way for the elucidation of several GPCR structures in the recent past. The availability of GPCR structures led to increased application of structure-based approaches in GPCR drug design, an area which has long been dominated by ligand-based ones. Breakthroughs in GPCR structural biology provide invaluable insights into the GPCR structure, function, and polypharmacology. The abundance of ligand-bound GPCR structures unveils the intricacies of ligand-receptor interactions, thus triggering a shift from conventional HTS techniques to less cost and highly efficient SBDD approaches for the design and discovery of potent ligands with improved pharmacological profiles. The main drawback of SBDD approaches lies on the scoring functions used by docking algorithms, wherein numerous approximations and restraints to protein flexibility are applied to expedite the process (Kim and Cho, 2016). In the following section, we briefly discuss the structure-based cheminformatics approaches for identifying novel GPCR ligands targeting ligand- and/or allosteric binding sites with few thriving models from the literature.

Identification of GPCR Novel Chemotypes via Structure-Based Virtual Screening

Utilizing crystal structures or homology models of target proteins in rational drug design is considered as the most powerful and popular method of choice in the design and/or screening of new lead compounds. In the early phase of drug discovery pipeline, structure-based virtual screening (SBVS) or docking-based VS has been utilized for the prediction of novel bioactive compounds from large and chemically diverse libraries (Cheng et al., 2012). In general, SBVS requires knowledge about the target's (protein or receptor) 3D structural information determined through experimental (X-ray or NMR) or *in silico* methods (homology modeling). Procedure involves docking of large chemical libraries of small compounds into crystal structure or homology model of the receptor. The selection criteria of small compounds for further experimental testings are based on the docking score, which assesses the binding affinity of protein-ligand complexes, predicted binding poses, chemical diversity, interactions with key residues, etc. (Ngo et al., 2016). The small compounds that cause a biological response are known as hits, which act as new chemical scaffolds for hit-to-lead development. The general VS workflow applied in several GPCR VS studies is shown in **Figure 5**.

SBVS studies for the first crystal structures of GPCRs, including β_2AR, A_{2A}AR, dopamine D_3R, and histamine (H_1R) have shown high hit rates. The pioneering study of SBVS for a druggable GPCR using the β_2AR crystal structure was reported (Cherezov et al., 2007). In another SBVS, the authors utilized the inactive structure of β_2AR/carazolol (PDB code: 2RH1) (Sabio et al., 2008) and screened proprietary and public databases for the identification of β_2AR ligands. The hit rates obtained were 36 and 12%, respectively. Similarly, Kolb et al. (2009) docked $\sim 1 \times 10^6$ commercially available compounds onto the same crystal structure and the top 25 virtual hits were selected based on their commercial availability, chemical diversity, and complementarity to the binding sites, and subjected for biological testings. Among them, six compounds had detectable binding affinities with the best one showing a Ki of 9 nM. All six hit molecules had novel chemotypes, and five of them were confirmed as inverse agonists. Apart from the reported VS studies using crystal structures, there were also few reports using receptor homology models. Langmead et al. identified highly potent and novel chemotype 1,3,5-triazine derivatives using A_{2A}AR homology models (Langmead et al., 2012). A virtual library of 5.45×10^5 compounds was screened and the initial hits were selected based on the shape geometry and electrostatic properties of the orthosteric site. A hit rate of 9% was obtained and the structures were modified and optimized using X-ray crystallography and structure-based optimization techniques. This series of optimization led to the successful identification of AZD4635 (HTL-1071), which is in phase 1 clinical trials for immunooncology (Jazayeri et al., 2017).

Interestingly, a large-scale VS study was carried out by Lane et al. (2013) for the identification of both orthosteric and allosteric ligands of D_3R. Based on the crystal structure of D_3R, two optimized D_3R models were prepared. To account for protein flexibility, conformers of D_3R models were generated and subsequently evaluated by VS performance, i.e., conformers that can separate D_3R actives from decoys were selected for the following analyses. The Molsoft Screen Pub database, which contains 4.1×10^6 compounds, was virtually screened using

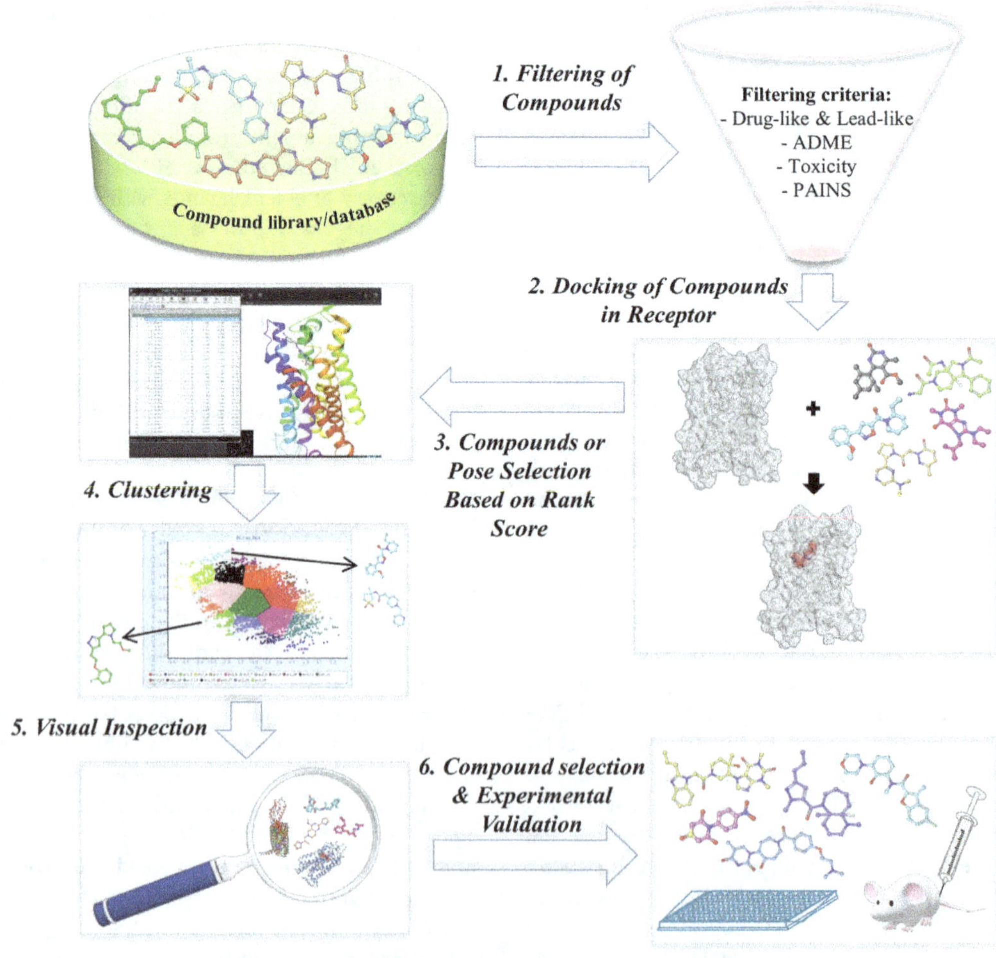

FIGURE 5 | Overview of the typical workflow of structure-based virtual screening (SBVS).

docking calculations. Top 300 hits in each model were selected and clustered by chemical similarity (0.3 Tanimoto distance). The top 25 compounds selected did not have a positively charged amine forming a conserved salt bridge to $D110^{3.32}$, which is contrary to D_3R apo model, but has interactions with TM1, 2, 3, and 7 as well as ECL1 and ECL2. These hits also reach dopamine and $D110^{3.32}$ at the end of the orthosteric pocket. Finally, the predicted novel allosteric ligands were experimentally validated, showing distinct functional profiles on dopamine-signaling efficiency. Another SBVS approach identified nanomolar lead compounds for the melanin-concentrating hormone-1 receptor (MCH-1R) (Lionta et al., 2014). This approach combines GPCR molecular modeling, antagonist binding site prediction, design, synthesis, and a focused library screening. A primary hit compound from a pyranose-based VAST library was initially used for the construction of a high quality MCH-1R model. Furthermore, the model validation was performed using a virtual enrichment experiment, along with the model-driven structure-based expansion of the initial hit, for identification of potent interactions in the binding site. A SBVS of a library with ≤0.7 Tanimoto similarity to existing MCH-1R ligands provided a 14% hit rate and 10 unique chemotypes of potent MCH-1R inhibitors, including two nanomolar leads (Lionta et al., 2014).

In silico screening territory for classes B, C, and F largely remains uncharted due to the limited number of crystal structures available. Using SBVS approach, noncompetitive ligands (allosteric modulators) of related class B GPCRs, namely glucagon receptor (GLR) and glucagon-like peptide 1 receptor (GLP-1R), were identified (de Graaf et al., 2011b). Based on the crystal structure of corticotropin-releasing factor 1 receptor (CRF_1R), a homology model for GLR was constructed. A database containing 1.9×10^6 compounds was assessed for chemical similarity to the current GLR noncompetitive inhibitors and docked onto the TM cavity of GLR. Based on the protein-ligand interaction fingerprints (IFPs), 23 compounds were selected and subjected for *in vitro* evaluations. Only two compounds were found to dose-dependently inhibit the effect of glucagon. One hit that was predicted as inactive for GLR bound to GLP-1R and potentiated a response similar to the endogenous GLP-1 ligand. For class C GPCRs, successful *in silico* VS studies were carried out against the VFT crystal structures (orthosteric N-terminal domain) of metabotropic glutamate receptor subtypes, $mGlu_3R$ and $mGlu_4R$ (Selvam et al., 2010). Besides the above-mentioned studies of VS campaigns, there are several computational works reported in the literature to discover novel orthosteric ligands for various GPCRs (which is well summarized in several review articles; Andrews et al., 2014; Cavasotto and Palomba, 2015; Shonberg et al., 2015; Ngo et al., 2016; Lee et al., 2018). Since SBVS on GPCRs is too broad to cover in this section, we have summarized representative case studies reported in the last 5 years (2013–2017) in **Table 1**.

Relevance of Fragment-Based Drug Discovery (FBDD) on GPCR Targets

Sequential piecing of fragments together to develop a novel lead compound is known as fragment-based drug discovery (FBDD) or fragment-based lead discovery (FBLD). FBDD is a potent scaffold-hopping and lead structure optimization tool for drug discovery projects and serves as an alternative to HTS (Matricon et al., 2017). The success of this approach in drug discovery campaign could be visualized by the increase in the number of compounds (originated from virtual fragment screens) entering clinical trials. A remarkable example of drugs identified *via* FBDD approach is vemurafenib, which was approved for the treatment of metastatic melanoma in 2011 (Baker, 2013). FBDD uses small molecules comprising ≤20 heavy atoms as a starting fragment for effective hit optimization. The main concept of this approach is to discover ligands that are smaller than a regular drug compound. The enlarged coverage of uncharted chemical space in fragment databases provides an exciting opportunity to find ligands after screening only a few thousand compounds (Chen et al., 2013). A fragment library can be designed and screened using molecular docking studies (Lee et al., 2018). The retrieved fragments could be further optimized using other computational approaches for growing, linking, or both.

Strategies utilized in the development of fragments into a lead compound include fragment growing, fragment linking, sequential docking, and group-based QSAR techniques. Fragment growth strategy initially begins with a fragment in the receptor' active site and allows extension of the fragment to maximize its interaction with the residues in the binding pocket. Fragment linking refers to the covalent linking of two or more fragments to form a single molecule which provides a new chemical scaffold in the active site. The application of FBDD to SBVS increases the structural space of hit-to-lead compounds. Even though ligands retrieved from fragment libraries lack selectivity and exhibit low affinity, they can be used as starting points for novel lead discovery. Despite its numerous advantages, there are still limitations associated with this approach, such as low accuracy prediction of fragment binding modes and rapid accumulation of errors. However, this approach proves to be useful when complemented with experimental techniques. Fragment screening of GPCR ligands *via* experimental methods (NMR, SPR, and X-ray crystallography) is challenging due to the difficulties in obtaining substantial amounts of functional protein, inherent conformational flexibility of the receptors outside the membrane, and low expression of the receptors (Lee et al., 2018). Therefore, *in silico* FBDD approaches could be utilized for GPCRs and other therapeutic targets. In the following paragraphs, we discuss the successful application of FBDD on GPCR drug discovery from literature.

The importance of *in silico* screening against GPCR protein structures or homology models to investigate novel fragment-like ligand chemical space is applicable for several GPCR targets. One of the first successful virtual fragment screening was developed by de Graaf et al. against doxepin bound human H_1R crystal structure (de Graaf et al., 2011a; Shimamura et al., 2011). In this approach, molecular docking and receptor-ligand IFP protocols were combined to discover a chemically diverse set of new fragment-like H_1R ligands. Out of 26 fragment-like compounds, 19 showed high binding affinity at the receptor level (hit rate 73%). Similarly, another structure-based virtual fragment screening (SBVFS) was performed against two GPCR targets, namely dopamine (D_3R) crystal structure and H_4R homology model structure, and an in-house fragment library of 12,905 fragments (Vass et al., 2014b). Additionally, molecular dynamics (MD) simulations were performed to represent different conformational states of the receptor orthosteric site (Vass et al., 2014b). Single structure- and ensemble docking screens were carried out for both receptors. The resulting 50 virtual hits were subjected for *in vitro* studies. Both the single and ensemble structures were found to be suitable for docking-based VS of fragments against GPCR targets. Chen et al. complemented *in silico* SBVFS with experimental biophysical screening to test the efficiency of their developed method (Chen et al., 2013). Initially, a set of 500 fragments were docked onto the orthosteric pocket of antagonist-bound $A_{2A}AR$ crystal structure (Jaakola et al., 2008) and ranked by affinity prior to target immobilized NMR screening of the same library (TINS). TINS resulted in 94 hits, where five fragments were identified to exceed the threshold affinity for the GPCR target. In the *in silico* screening, four out of five compounds were found in the top 50 fragments. Apart from these four fragments, the remaining 46 fragments also showed high binding affinities. Thus, a second computational screening approach using commercially available fragments (3.28×10^5) was performed and the 22 top-ranked compounds were tested experimentally. Among them, 14 fragments were identified as $A_{2A}AR$ ligands. Furthermore, QSAR studies were performed for three potent $A_{2A}AR$ ligands followed by optimization of the fragments by MD simulations and free-energy calculations. Similarly, another successful application of fragment-based screening and lead optimization using both biophysical and *in silico* techniques was shown in β_1AR target leading to the discovery of novel high affinity leads (Christopher et al., 2013).

Verheij et al. studied target selectivity against histamine subtype H_4R and 5-HT_{3A} (ion channel) homology models using SBVFS approach (Verheij et al., 2011). The results of fragment-based screening showed that both receptors yielded a common pool of hit fragments, thus underlining remarkable similarities in ligand recognition. This knowledge could assist in efficiently navigating chemical space during hit optimization. Besides the orthosteric binding site (primary), allosteric sites (secondary) have also been targeted for identification of novel compounds by SBVFS approach. Vass et al. applied a sequential docking protocol to predict starting points for fragment linking using D_3R crystal structure and D_2R homology model to identify subtype selectivity (Vass et al., 2014a). Two in-house focused fragment libraries (196 fragments function as primary binding site ligands for D_2 and D_3 receptors and 266 fragments function as secondary binding site ligands for D_3R) were docked in the orthosteric and allosteric binding sites and the best fragment combinations were listed. Similar top-scoring fragments were identified for the orthosteric site, whereas allosteric site fragments showed subtype selectivity. Three fragment-linked compounds that showed 9-, 39-, and 55-fold selectivity for D_3R were synthesized, and docking results were validated by the experimental data.

In tandem with SBDD, FBDD has also been successfully applied to other GPCR classes. Novel $mGlu_5R$ NAMs were identified through combination of fragment-based screening and medicinal chemistry approaches (Christopher et al., 2015). In addition, the binding modes of NAMs with the receptor were crystallographically solved. Recently, an *in silico* fragment-based approach was applied on the crystal structures of $mGlu_5R$ (Doré et al., 2014; Christopher et al., 2015) for the design of novel allosteric modulators (Bian et al., 2017). Initially, a fragment library for reported GPCR allosteric modulators was constructed using the data from Allosteric Database (ASD). Subsequently, the novel compounds were generated and analyzed using retrosynthetic combinatorial analysis procedure (RECAP). Molecular docking was applied to screen the hits for the target by docking the *in silico* generated compounds into the binding pocket. Additionally, other computational methodologies, such as benchmark dataset verification, docking, QSAR model simulations, etc., were performed to assess validation of the hits. Twenty structurally diverse hits were predicted as potential $mGlu_5$ allosteric modulators based on the binding energies and docking scores. This study highlights the importance of purely computational FBDD approach for facilitating the design of novel compounds for other targets as well. In addition to the above-mentioned GPCR case studies on SBVFS campaigns, there are several other *in silico* reports available regarding the discovery of novel ligands which are summarized elsewhere (Hubbard and Murray, 2011; Murray et al., 2012; Shoichet and Kobilka, 2012; Visegrády and Keseru, 2013; Andrews et al., 2014; Lee et al., 2018).

Integration of Ligand- and Structure-Based Cheminformatics Approaches

The use of cheminformatics in drug discovery provides an excellent foundation for the integration of structure- and ligand-based strategies due to its application in different stages of drug discovery. With the rising number of available structures, biological databases, and *in silico* techniques for cheminformatics and modern drug discovery, it is not surprising that ligand- and structure-based approaches are used in combination to take advantage of the abundant GPCR ligand information while employing recently elucidated crucial protein structural information to aid in increasing success in GPCR drug discovery research. Furthermore, integration of LBDD and SBDD complements strengths and weaknesses of each method, leading to better insights in critical ligand functionalities and receptor-ligand interaction information. Researchers are now able to use 3D protein structures to predict binding modes and study the pharmacology of known drugs and their analogs through docking, providing rationalization of ligand activity and useful SAR information for the design and optimization of new agonists and antagonists (Munk et al., 2016). In addition, rapid innovation of hardware and computing power allows the use of MD simulations for more in-depth study of GPCR ligand binding and activity modulation (McRobb et al., 2016; Clark, 2017).

An excellent case of ligand- and structure-based integration in GPCR drug discovery is shown in studies involving $A_{2A}AR$, an attractive drug target for the treatment of Parkinson's disease. Since $A_{2A}AR$ receptor was one among the first GPCRs to be crystallized, it has become one of the most extensively studied drug target. The later release of a high-resolution $A_{2A}AR$ structure, which revealed the presence of water in the binding site, further increased the efforts for drug design and optimization. Over the years, most of $A_{2A}AR$ antagonists, such as istradefylline (Jenner, 2005) and preladenant (Neustadt et al., 2007), have been designed based on the purine scaffold and other related heterocycles. Although the abundance in ligand information for $A_{2A}AR$ helps in the elucidation of important chemical fingerprints and ligand binding interactions, it has become difficult to discover novel entities for drug development. In a study by Lenselink et al. (2016a), they performed VS using an ensemble of A_{2A} receptor structures split into a structure-based decision tree (Lenselink et al., 2014). Ligands were docked to each protein structure and proceeded to the next receptor docking based on a GlideScore cut-off of the previous procedure. The resulting ligands were filtered using Rapid Elimination of Swill (REOS) (Walters and Namchuk, 2003) and re-scored using MM-GBSA. Consequently, similarity-based analysis (against compounds tested for $A_{2A}AR$ activity recorded in ChEMBL) was performed to determine the structural novelty of the remaining hits and select the most unique compounds to be tested experimentally. Out of 71 novel ligands, only 2 compounds displayed suitable $A_{2A}AR$ binding affinity. They also performed a retrospective analysis of the current $A_{2A}AR$ ligands to determine novelty in structure and its relation to observed $A_{2A}AR$ activity. Decades of research efforts for this target left little room for discovery of new ligand scaffolds, as seen in previous VS studies showing ligand Tanimoto similarity in the range of 0.19–0.68 (Carlsson et al., 2010; Katritch et al., 2010; Langmead et al., 2012; Rodriguez et al., 2015), with the lowest similarity showing the least activity. While most of the virtual hits were found to be similar in structure to experimentally validated compounds from ChEMBL, it should be noted that several of the tested compounds or scaffold structures were also discovered using computational methods, highlighting the value of *in silico* approaches in drug discovery and design.

Aside from combining known structure- and ligand-based methods, hybrid tools that assimilate features from both approaches have been developed to afford computational chemists other strategies which can compensate current individual limitations of SBDD and LBDD. One of the hybrid methods that has gained popularity in recent years is proteochemometric (PCM) modeling. PCM modeling is similar to traditional QSAR studies since both methods require descriptors, bioactivity data, and machine learning functions for model development (Qiu et al., 2017). However, a cross-term descriptor is also required in PCM modeling to consider amino acids and ligand functional groups that are crucial for binding interaction of the complex (Lapinsh et al., 2001; van Westen et al., 2011; Qiu et al., 2017). This method has been found to be useful on polypharmacological studies as it can provide information on target selectivity (Cortes-Ciriano et al., 2015), especially in large protein families like GPCRs. In a recent study by Gao et al. (2013), 24 PCM models were developed for amine GPCRs and their corresponding ligands using machine learning methods, support vector regression (SVR), and Gaussian processes (GP). Two typical descriptors were generated per receptor: z-scale and transmembrane identity descriptors, and two typical descriptors were generated for each ligand: general (atomic contributions, logP, etc.,) and drug-like index descriptors. These descriptors were first used to build 24 PCM models, which were validated using a test-set. Although, most of the models showed strong goodness-of-fit (R^2) and predictivity (Q^2), the addition of cross-terms led to a lower predictive capability of the PCM models. This may be because it is still difficult to fully translate receptor-ligand interfaces to a descriptor value. Despite this, their PCM models showed great potential in predicting cross interactions between GPCRs and ligands.

SUMMARY OF CHEMINFORMATICS SOFTWARES/TOOLS UTILIZED IN GPCR DRUG DISCOVERY

HTS has undergone technological advances and innovations that has rendered it as the principal method of drug discovery for years. However, it did not necessarily lead to a great leap forward in the discovery of NCEs as the hit rate for this method is frequently low, in addition to the enormous costs and efforts involved. In turn, computer-aided drug design (CADD) have been recognized and continuously receives increase in interest and usage such that most of GPCR drug discovery research efforts make use of one or more computational tools, especially in the initial stages of drug design. Due to the complexities of experimental GPCR research, it is of no surprise that CADD has emerged as a method of choice to expedite GPCR drug discovery and design. Furthermore, increasing knowledge of GPCR systems has led to the rising popularity of cheminformatics and chemogenomics as evidenced by the growing number of publicly available databases, which can provide structural or interaction information regarding receptor and its associated ligands.

There are several cheminformatics softwares and web servers available to identify lead compounds targeting GPCRs (Khan et al., 2011; Yadav et al., 2016). As mentioned previously, *in silico* approaches are classified into two approaches: SBDD and LBDD. If there are already known NMR and X-ray crystal structures or reliable homology models available, computational methods based on target protein structures can be exploited (Lyne, 2002). These tools are related with several computational approaches, including molecular docking, VS, pharmacophore generation, and binding pocket detection. As shown in **Table 3**, several *in silico* cheminformatics methods have been applied for GPCR targeted drug discovery. In cases where no protein structures are available, ligand-based virtual screening (LBVS) can be utilized. LBVS can be further sub-classified into three: pharmacophore-, similarity-, and machine learning-based VS (Basith et al., 2016). As shown in **Table 4**, several *in silico* cheminformatics methods could be exploited for generation of pharmacophores, searching 3D similarity, and identifying targets (polypharmacology). Moreover, commercially available chemical libraries for VS are shown in **Table 5**.

TABLE 3 | Cheminformatics tools for structure-based drug discovery.

Tools	Description				Availability	References
	VS	Docking	Pharmacophore generation	Cavity detection		
AutoDock 4	Y	Y			Public	Morris et al., 2009
AutoDock Vina	Y	Y			Public	Trott and Olson, 2010
FlexX	Y	Y			Commercial	Kramer et al., 1999
OEDocking (FRED, HYBRID)	Y	Y			Commercial	McGann, 2012
Galaxy7TM		Y			Public	Lee and Seok, 2016
Glide (HTVS, SP, XP)	Y	Y			Commercial	Friesner et al., 2006
GOLD	Y	Y			Commercial	Jones et al., 1997
GOMoDo	Y	Y		Y	Public	Sandal et al., 2013
GPCR automodel		Y			Public	Launay et al., 2012
ICM-Pro	Y	Y			Commercial	Neves et al., 2012
MOE	Y	Y		Y	Commercial	Roy and Luck, 2007
Snooker	Y		Y			Sanders et al., 2011
Surflex-Dock		Y			Commercial	Jain, 2007
fPocket	Y			Y	Public	Le Guilloux et al., 2009
Pocketome				Y	Public	Kufareva et al., 2012
UCSF DOCK		Y	Y		Commercial	http://dock.compbio.ucsf.edu/
MOLS		Y			Public	Paul and Gautham, 2016
iScreen	Y	Y		Y	Public	Tsai et al., 2011

TABLE 4 | Cheminformatics tools for ligand-based drug discovery.

Tools	Description				Availability	References
	VS	Pharmacophore generation	3D similarity searching	Poly pharmacology		
Discovery studio	Y	Y			Commercial	
FlexS			Y		Commercial	Lemmen et al., 1998
ICM-Pro	Y	Y	Y	Y	Commercial	Grigoryan et al., 2010
LigandScout	Y	Y			Commercial	Wolber and Langer, 2005
PharmaGist	Y	Y			Commercial	Schneidman-Duhovny et al., 2008
QSARPro	Y		Y		Commercial	http://www.vlifesciences.com
ROCS			Y		Commercial	Hawkins et al., 2007
Surflex-Sim			Y		Commercial	Spitzer and Jain, 2012
Swiss similarity			Y		Public	Zoete et al., 2016
Topomer CoMFA	Y		Y		Commercial	Cramer, 2003

LIMITATIONS OF CHEMINFORMATICS APPROACHES IN GPCR DRUG DISCOVERY

In the last several years, the increasing number of high resolution GPCR structures has unlocked new avenues for structure-based GPCR drug discovery and design. However, several obstacles remain, including rapid identification of novel fragment-like compounds and structure-based elucidation of GPCR ligand function to name a few.

With the recent innovations in high-throughput, computer, and software technologies, as well as the upsurge of publicly available data, cheminformatics methodologies has no doubt become an essential part of most drug discovery efforts to date. However, a major flaw is seen during cheminformatics model development, wherein the experimental data used is assumed to be correct. In contrast to this assumption, databases can contain errors for ligand structures, bioactivity, activity types, and other information, which often results in ambiguous models leading to erroneous findings. Several recent articles (Fourches et al., 2010, 2016; Williams and Ekins, 2011; Williams et al., 2012) have discussed this topic at length and how it can have a negative effect on model development and performance. A study by Olah et al. (2005) mentioned that there were two molecules with incorrect structures on average for each medicinal chemistry journal, indicating a total error percentage of 8% in the WOMBAT database. Another more recent study by Tiikkainen et al. (2013), estimated the ligand error rates in ChEMBL, Liceptor, and WOMBAT databases to be 5, 7, and 6%, respectively. Error values for activity values in the three databases

TABLE 5 | Available chemical database for high-throughput virtual screening.

Database	Number of compounds	Containing GPCR focused library	References
AnalytiCon	35,000		https://ac-discovery.com
Asinex	600,000	Y	http://www.asinex.com
Bionet	80,700		https://www.keyorganics.net
ChemBridge	1,100,000	Y	http://www.chembridge.com
ChemDiv	1,500,000	Y	http://www.chemdiv.com
CoCoCo	6,981,500		http://cococo.isof.cnr.it/cococo
eMolecules	5,900,000		https://www.emolecules.com
Enamine	2,300,000	Y	http://www.enamine.net
InterBioScreen	550,000		https://www.ibscreen.com
Life Chemicals	1,292,000	Y	http://www.lifechemicals.com/
Maybridge	53,000		http://www.maybridge.com/
NCI	260,000		https://cactus.nci.nih.gov/
OCTVAchemicals	260,000	Y	http://www.otavachemicals.com
Prestwick Chemical	1,280		http://www.prestwickchemical.com
Selleck Chemicals	482	Y	http://www.selleckchem.com
SuperDrug2	3,900		http://cheminfo.charite.de/superdrug2/downloads.html
TCM Database	32,300		http://tcm.cmu.edu.tw/
Timtec	2,300	Y	http://www.timtec.net/
Vitas-M	1,500,000		http://www.vitasmlab.com
ZINC	35,000,000		Irwin et al., 2012

ranged from 1 to 2%. It is therefore important to carefully and manually curate chemical and biological databases, since even minor errors can cause a substantial decrease in the predictive capability of generated models. Moreover, while the increasing sophistication of computer programs has allowed researchers an atomistic view of several GPCR systems, approximations of crucial energy terms that cannot be computationally explored at present has greatly limited the accuracy in the perception of these systems. Because of these, researchers should constantly gauge findings against their own scientific knowledge to see whether the results are significant or not. It should always be remembered that computational tools are created and continuously developed to assist in making the drug discovery process more efficient, but nothing can replace a researcher's own knowledge and experience.

Moreover, insights about GPCR structure, function, and binding partners have increased significantly compared to a few decades ago. Despite this, a great deal of information is still beyond our fingertips, such as protein structures of hundreds of unique GPCRs and ligand information for orphan GPCRs. It is imperative not lose fervor in gathering new knowledge to further enhance our understanding of GPCR structures and functions.

CONCLUSIONS

In the nineteenth century, chemical space exploration was initiated as a counting game to estimate its size (Reymond, 2015). However, the advent of cheminformatics field and powerful *in silico* technologies assisted in the exploration of uncharted ligand space from large chemical libraries. The availability of large public and commercial chemical databases, as well as ligand chemical space exploration tools, provide researchers the ease of accessibility to handle and explore huge chemical data. Cheminformatics is a complex field of study that translates large data into useful knowledge for drug design and optimization protocols. The expansion of GPCR structures and ligands over the past decade is mainly due to the progress in its structural biology and theoretical advancements. These structural and *in silico* breakthroughs have led to the implementation of cheminformatics approaches in GPCR drug discovery pipeline. In the GPCR drug discovery protocol, ligand- and structure-based approaches are the most commonly applied ones. LBDD is known as a fast and simple technique for the identification of vital chemical functionalities required for biological activity. However, absence of binding pocket information limits its ability in incorporating several important factors, such as receptor flexibility and ligand bioactive conformation, thereby restricting the discovery of candidate leads to only the ligand classes used in model development (Saxena et al., 2017). But due to the prolonged absence of GPCR structures, researchers relied heavily on ligand-based methods for drug discovery and lead optimization, leading to copious ligand structural information for these targets. Following the crystallization of bRho in 2000 (Palczewski et al., 2000) and β_2AR in 2007 (Rasmussen et al., 2007), a striking increase in GPCR structural information have been observed in the last several years. While the current available structures are unable to cover the structural diversity of GPCR protein family members, there is enough that can be used as templates for homology modeling to perform SBDD. In contrast to ligand-based techniques, SBDD can be used to predict ligand bioactive conformation, thus providing a better understanding of receptor-ligand interactions and allowing the discovery of

NCEs. Furthermore, recent researches underpin the significance of emerging integrated approaches in GPCR drug design and discovery. Assimilating LBDD and SBDD methods, as well as the use of integrated approaches, has proven to increase the success rate of finding promising leads, especially for well-studied targets such as GPCRs. All the cheminformatics approaches discussed in this review are focused toward the identification of novel ligands for GPCR targets based on the structural and ligand data, where several case studies signify the importance of VS. The evolution of cheminformatics techniques and their synergy in GPCR drug discovery pipeline is the driving force that will facilitate cost-effective and prolific outcomes in the exploration of uncharted GPCR ligand space. Yet, an expert human touch is entailed to authenticate and tame the computer-generated outcome.

AUTHOR CONTRIBUTIONS

SB and MC summarized the literature, wrote the manuscript, and prepared the figures. SM wrote part of the manuscript, prepared the figures, and revised the manuscript. JP and NC prepared the tables. SK and SC supervised all the works, provided critical comments, and wrote the manuscript.

ACKNOWLEDGMENTS

This work was supported by the Mid-career Researcher Program (NRF-2017R1A2B4010084) funded by the Ministry of Science and ICT (MSIT) through the National Research Foundation of Korea (NRF).

REFERENCES

Andrews, S. P., Brown, G. A., and Christopher, J. A. (2014). Structure-based and fragment-based GPCR drug discovery. *ChemMedChem* 9, 256–275. doi: 10.1002/cmdc.201300382

Baell, J. B., and Holloway, G. A. (2010). New substructure filters for removal of pan assay interference compounds (PAINS) from screening libraries and for their exclusion in bioassays. *J. Med. Chem.* 53, 2719–2740. doi: 10.1021/jm901137j

Bajorath, J. (2004). *Chemoinformatics: Concepts, Methods, and Tools for Drug Discovery.* New Jersey, NJ: Humana Press.

Baker, M. (2013). Fragment-based lead discovery grows up. *Nat. Rev. Drug Discov.* 12, 5–7. doi: 10.1038/nrd3926

Baldwin, J. M. (1993). The probable arrangement of the helices in G protein-coupled receptors. *EMBO J.* 12, 1693–1703.

Basith, S., Cui, M., Macalino, S. J. Y., and Choi, S. (2016). Expediting the design, discovery, and development of anticancer drugs using computational approaches. *Curr. Med. Chem.* 24, 4753–4778. doi: 10.2174/0929867323666160902160535

Bian, Y., Feng, Z., Yang, P., and Xie, X. Q. (2017). Integrated *in silico* fragment-based drug design: case study with allosteric modulators on metabotropic glutamate receptor 5. *AAPS J.* 19, 1235–1248. doi: 10.1208/s12248-017-0093-5

Bologna, Z., Teoh, J. P., Bayoumi, A. S., Tang, Y., and Kim, I. M. (2017). Biased G protein-coupled receptor signaling: new player in modulating physiology and pathology. *Biomol. Ther.* 25, 12–25. doi: 10.4062/biomolther.2016.165

Bresso, E., Togawa, R., Hammond-Kosack, K., Urban, M., Maigret, B., and Martins, N. F. (2016). GPCRs from fusarium graminearum detection, modeling and virtual screening - the search for new routes to control head blight disease. *BMC Bioinform.* 17:463. doi: 10.1186/s12859-016-1342-9

Brown, F. K. (1998). Chemoinformatics: what is it and how does it impact drug discovery. *Ann. Rep. Med. Chem.* 33, 375–384. doi: 10.1002/0471250953.bi1401s18

Carlsson, J., Yoo, L., Gao, Z. G., Irwin, J. J., Shoichet, B. K., and Jacobson, K. A. (2010). Structure-based discovery of A2A adenosine receptor ligands. *J. Med. Chem.* 53, 3748–3755. doi: 10.1021/jm100240h

Carpenter, B., Nehmé, R., Warne, T., Leslie, A. G., and Tate, C. G. (2016). Structure of the adenosine A(2A) receptor bound to an engineered G protein. *Nature* 536, 104–107. doi: 10.1038/nature18966

Cavasotto, C. N., and Palomba, D. (2015). Expanding the horizons of G protein-coupled receptor structure-based ligand discovery and optimization using homology models. *Chem. Commun.* 51, 13576–13594. doi: 10.1039/C5CC05050B

Chen, D., Ranganathan, A., Ijzerman, A. P., Siegal, G., and Carlsson, J. (2013). Complementarity between *in silico* and biophysical screening approaches in fragment-based lead discovery against the A(2A) adenosine receptor. *J. Chem. Inf. Model.* 53, 2701–2714. doi: 10.1021/ci4003156

Cheng, T., Li, Q., Zhou, Z., Wang, Y., and Bryant, S. H. (2012). Structure-based virtual screening for drug discovery: a problem-centric review. *AAPS J.* 14, 133–141. doi: 10.1208/s12248-012-9322-0

Cherezov, V., Rosenbaum, D. M., Hanson, M. A., Rasmussen, S. G., Thian, F. S., Kobilka, T. S., et al. (2007). High-resolution crystal structure of an engineered human beta2-adrenergic G protein-coupled receptor. *Science* 318, 1258–1265. doi: 10.1126/science.1150577

Cho, N. C., Seo, S. H., Kim, D., Shin, J. S., Ju, J., Seong, J., et al. (2016). Pharmacophore-based virtual screening, biological evaluation and binding mode analysis of a novel protease-activated receptor 2 antagonist. *J. Comput. Aided Mol. Des.* 30, 625–637. doi: 10.1007/s10822-016-9937-9

Christopher, J. A., Aves, S. J., Bennett, K. A., Doré, A. S., Errey, J. C., Jazayeri, A., et al. (2015). Fragment and structure-based drug discovery for a class C GPCR: discovery of the mGlu5 negative allosteric modulator HTL14242 (3-Chloro-5-[6-(5-fluoropyridin-2-yl)pyrimidin-4-yl]benzonitrile). *J. Med. Chem.* 58, 6653–6664. doi: 10.1021/acs.jmedchem.5b00892

Christopher, J. A., Brown, J., Doré, A. S., Errey, J. C., Koglin, M., Marshall, F. H., et al. (2013). Biophysical fragment screening of the beta1-adrenergic receptor: identification of high affinity arylpiperazine leads using structure-based drug design. *J. Med. Chem.* 56, 3446–3455. doi: 10.1021/jm400140q

Ciancetta, A., Sabbadin, D., Federico, S., Spalluto, G., and Moro, S. (2015). Advances in Computational techniques to study GPCR-ligand recognition. *Trends Pharmacol. Sci.* 36, 878–890. doi: 10.1016/j.tips.2015.08.006

Clark, T. (2017). G-Protein coupled receptors: answers from simulations. *Beilstein J. Org. Chem.* 13, 1071–1078. doi: 10.3762/bjoc.13.106

Cortes-Ciriano, I., Ul Ain, Q., Subramanian, V., Lenselink, E. B., Mendez-Lucio, O., IJzerman, A. P., et al. (2015). Polypharmacology modelling using proteochemometrics (PCM): recent methodological developments, applications to target families, and future prospects. *MedChemComm* 6, 24–50. doi: 10.1039/C4MD00216D

Coudrat, T., Christopoulos, A., Sexton, P. M., and Wootten, D. (2017a). Structural features embedded in G protein-coupled receptor co-crystal structures are key to their success in virtual screening. *PLoS ONE* 12:e0174719. doi: 10.1371/journal.pone.0174719

Coudrat, T., Simms, J., Christopoulos, A., Wootten, D., and Sexton, P. M. (2017b). Improving virtual screening of G protein-coupled receptors via ligand-directed modeling. *PLoS Comput. Biol.* 13:e1005819. doi: 10.1371/journal.pcbi.1005819

Cramer, R. D. (2003). Topomer CoMFA: a design methodology for rapid lead optimization. *J. Med. Chem.* 46, 374–388. doi: 10.1021/jm020194o

Daga, P. R., Polgar, W. E., and Zaveri, N. T. (2014). Structure-based virtual screening of the nociceptin receptor: hybrid docking and shape-based approaches for improved hit identification. *J. Chem. Inf. Model.* 54, 2732–2743. doi: 10.1021/ci500291a

de Graaf, C., Kooistra, A. J., Vischer, H. F., Katritch, V., Kuijer, M., Shiroishi, M., et al. (2011a). Crystal structure-based virtual screening for fragment-like ligands of the human histamine H(1) receptor. *J. Med. Chem.* 54, 8195–8206. doi: 10.1021/jm2011589

de Graaf, C., Rein, C., Piwnica, D., Giordanetto, F., and Rognan, D. (2011b). Structure-based discovery of allosteric modulators of two related class B G-protein-coupled receptors. *ChemMedChem* 6, 2159–2169. doi: 10.1002/cmdc.201100317

DeWire, S. M., and Violin, J. D. (2011). Biased ligands for better cardiovascular drugs: dissecting G-protein-coupled receptor pharmacology. *Circ. Res.* 109, 205–216. doi: 10.1161/CIRCRESAHA.110.231308

DeWire, S. M., Yamashita, D. S., Rominger, D. H., Liu, G., Cowan, C. L., Graczyk, T. M., et al. (2013). A G protein-biased ligand at the mu-opioid receptor is potently analgesic with reduced gastrointestinal and respiratory dysfunction compared with morphine. *J. Pharmacol. Exp. Ther.* 344, 708–717. doi: 10.1124/jpet.112.201616

Doré, A. S., Okrasa, K., Patel, J. C., Serrano-Vega, M., Bennett, K., Cooke, R. M., et al. (2014). Structure of class C GPCR metabotropic glutamate receptor 5 transmembrane domain. *Nature* 511, 557–562. doi: 10.1038/nature 13396

Dror, R. O., Green, H. F., Valant, C., Borhani, D. W., Valcourt, J. R., Pan, A. C., et al. (2013). Structural basis for modulation of a G-protein-coupled receptor by allosteric drugs. *Nature* 503, 295–299. doi: 10.1038/nature 12595

Dror, R. O., Pan, A. C., Arlow, D. H., Borhani, D. W., Maragakis, P., Shan, Y., et al. (2011). Pathway and mechanism of drug binding to G-protein-coupled receptors. *Proc. Natl. Acad. Sci. U.S.A.* 108, 13118–13123. doi: 10.1073/pnas.1104614108

Ekins, S., Bugrim, A., Brovold, L., Kirillov, E., Nikolsky, Y., Rakhmatulin, E., et al. (2006). Algorithms for network analysis in systems-ADME/Tox using the MetaCore and MetaDrug platforms. *Xenobiotica* 36, 877–901. doi: 10.1080/00498250600861660

Fourches, D., Muratov, E., and Tropsha, A. (2010). Trust, but verify: on the importance of chemical structure curation in cheminformatics and QSAR modeling research. *J. Chem. Inf. Model.* 50, 1189–1204. doi: 10.1021/ci100176x

Fourches, D., Muratov, E., and Tropsha, A. (2016). Trust, but verify II: a practical guide to chemogenomics data curation. *J. Chem. Inf. Model.* 56, 1243–1252. doi: 10.1021/acs.jcim.6b00129

Frandsen, I. O., Boesgaard, M. W., Fidom, K., Hauser, A. S., Isberg, V., Bräuner-Osborne, H., et al. (2017). Identification of histamine H3 receptor ligands using a new crystal structure fragment-based method. *Sci. Rep.* 7:4829. doi: 10.1038/s41598-017-05058-w

Friesner, R. A., Murphy, R. B., Repasky, M. P., Frye, L. L., Greenwood, J. R., Halgren, T. A., et al. (2006). Extra precision glide: docking and scoring incorporating a model of hydrophobic enclosure for protein-ligand complexes. *J. Med. Chem.* 49, 6177–6196. doi: 10.1021/jm051256o

Fronik, P., Gaiser, B. I., and Sejer Pedersen, D. (2017). Bitopic ligands and metastable binding sites: opportunities for G protein-coupled receptor (GPCR) medicinal chemistry. *J. Med. Chem.* 60, 4126–4134. doi: 10.1021/acs.jmedchem.6b01601

Gandhimathi, A., and Sowdhamini, R. (2016). Molecular modelling of human 5-hydroxytryptamine receptor (5-HT2A) and virtual screening studies towards the identification of agonist and antagonist molecules. *J. Biomol. Struct. Dyn.* 34, 952–970. doi: 10.1080/07391102.2015.1062802

Gao, J., Huang, Q., Wu, D., Zhang, Q., Zhang, Y., Chen, T., et al. (2013). Study on human GPCR-inhibitor interactions by proteochemometric modeling. *Gene* 518, 124–131. doi: 10.1016/j.gene.2012.11.061

Gianella-Borradori, M., Christou, I., Bataille, C. J., Cross, R. L., Wynne, G. M., Greaves, D. R., et al. (2015). Ligand-based virtual screening identifies a family of selective cannabinoid receptor 2 agonists. *Bioorg. Med. Chem.* 23, 241–263. doi: 10.1016/j.bmc.2014.11.002

Grigoryan, A. V., Kufareva, I., Totrov, M., and Abagyan, R. A. (2010). Spatial chemical distance based on atomic property fields. *J. Comput. Aided Mol. Des.* 24, 173–182. doi: 10.1007/s10822-009-9316-x

Guo, H., An, S., Ward, R., Yang, Y., Liu, Y., Guo, X. X., et al. (2017). Methods used to study the oligomeric structure of G-protein-coupled receptors. *Biosci. Rep.* 37:BSR20160547. doi: 10.1042/BSR20160547

Hargrave, P. A., McDowell, J. H., Curtis, D. R., Wang, J. K., Juszczak, E., Fong, S. L., et al. (1983). The structure of bovine rhodopsin. *Biophys. Struct. Mech.* 9, 235–244. doi: 10.1007/BF00535659

Hartenfeller, M., Zettl, H., Walter, M., Rupp, M., Reisen, F., Proschak, E., et al. (2012). DOGS: reaction-driven *de novo* design of bioactive compounds. *PLoS Comput. Biol.* 8:e1002380. doi: 10.1371/journal.pcbi.1002380

Hauser, A. S., Attwood, M. M., Rask-Andersen, M., Schiöth, H. B., and Gloriam, D. E. (2017). Trends in GPCR drug discovery: new agents, targets and indications. *Nat. Rev. Drug Discov.* 16, 829–842. doi: 10.1038/nrd.2017.178

Hauser, A. S., Chavali, S., Masuho, I., Jahn, L. J., Martemyanov, K. A., Gloriam, D. E., et al. (2018). Pharmacogenomics of GPCR drug targets. *Cell* 172, 41–54. doi: 10.1016/j.cell.2017.11.033

Hawkins, P. C., Skillman, A. G., and Nicholls, A. (2007). Comparison of shape-matching and docking as virtual screening tools. *J. Med. Chem.* 50, 74–82. doi: 10.1021/jm0603365

Heifetz, A. (2018). *Computational Methods for GPCR Drug Discovery*. New Jersey, NJ: Humana Press.

Hollenstein, K., Kean, J., Bortolato, A., Cheng, R. K., Doré, A. S., Jazayeri, A., et al. (2013). Structure of class B GPCR corticotropin-releasing factor receptor 1. *Nature* 499, 438–443. doi: 10.1038/nature12357

Hubbard, R. E., and Murray, J. B. (2011). Experiences in fragment-based lead discovery. *Methods Enzymol.* 493, 509–531. doi: 10.1016/B978-0-12-381274-2.00020-0

Humbeck, L., and Koch, O. (2017). What can we learn from bioactivity data? Chemoinformatics tools and applications in chemical biology research. *ACS Chem. Biol.* 12, 23–35. doi: 10.1021/acschembio.6b00706

Irwin, J. J., Sterling, T., Mysinger, M. M., Bolstad, E. S., and Coleman, R. G. (2012). ZINC: a free tool to discover chemistry for biology. *J. Chem. Inf. Model.* 52, 1757–1768. doi: 10.1021/ci3001277

Jaakola, V. P., Griffith, M. T., Hanson, M. A., Cherezov, V., Chien, E. Y., Lane, J. R., et al. (2008). The 2.6 angstrom crystal structure of a human A2A adenosine receptor bound to an antagonist. *Science* 322, 1211–1217. doi: 10.1126/science.1164772

Jacobson, K. A., Costanzi, S., and Paoletta, S. (2014). Computational studies to predict or explain G protein coupled receptor polypharmacology. *Trends Pharmacol. Sci.* 35, 658–663. doi: 10.1016/j.tips.2014.10.009

Jain, A. N. (2007). Surflex-Dock 2.1: robust performance from ligand energetic modeling, ring flexibility, and knowledge-based search. *J. Comput. Aided Mol. Des.* 21, 281–306. doi: 10.1007/s10822-007-9114-2

Jang, J. W., Cho, N. C., Min, S. J., Cho, Y. S., Park, K. D., Seo, S. H., et al. (2016). Novel scaffold identification of mGlu1 receptor negative allosteric modulators using a hierarchical virtual screening approach. *Chem. Biol. Drug Des.* 87, 239–256. doi: 10.1111/cbdd.12654

Jazayeri, A., Andrews, S. P., and Marshall, F. H. (2017). Structurally enabled discovery of adenosine A2A receptor antagonists. *Chem. Rev.* 117, 21–37. doi: 10.1021/acs.chemrev.6b00119

Jazayeri, A., Dias, J. M., and Marshall, F. H. (2015). From G protein-coupled receptor structure resolution to rational drug design. *J. Biol. Chem.* 290, 19489–19495. doi: 10.1074/jbc.R115.668251

Jenner, P. (2005). Istradefylline, a novel adenosine A2A receptor antagonist, for the treatment of Parkinson's disease. *Expert Opin. Investig. Drugs* 14, 729–738. doi: 10.1517/13543784.14.6.729

Jones, G., Willett, P., Glen, R. C., Leach, A. R., and Taylor, R. (1997). Development and validation of a genetic algorithm for flexible docking. *J. Mol. Biol.* 267, 727–748. doi: 10.1006/jmbi.1996.0897

Kaczor, A. A., Silva, A. G., Loza, M. I., Kolb, P., Castro, M., and Poso, A. (2016). Structure-based virtual screening for dopamine D2 receptor ligands as potential antipsychotics. *ChemMedChem* 11, 718–729. doi: 10.1002/cmdc.2015 00599

Kang, Y., Zhou, X. E., Gao, X., He, Y., Liu, W., Ishchenko, A., et al. (2015). Crystal structure of rhodopsin bound to arrestin by femtosecond X-ray laser. *Nature* 523, 561–567. doi: 10.1038/nature14656

Kastner, K. W., Shoue, D. A., Estiu, G. L., Wolford, J., Fuerst, M. F., Markley, L. D., et al. (2014). Characterization of the Anopheles gambiae octopamine receptor and discovery of potential agonists and antagonists using a combined computational-experimental approach. *Malar. J.* 13:434. doi: 10.1186/1475-2875-13-434

Katritch, V., Fenalti, G., Abola, E. E., Roth, B. L., Cherezov, V., and Stevens, R. C. (2014). Allosteric sodium in class A GPCR signaling. *Trends Biochem. Sci.* 39, 233–244. doi: 10.1016/j.tibs.2014.03.002

Katritch, V., Jaakola, V. P., Lane, J. R., Lin, J., Ijzerman, A. P., Yeager, M., et al. (2010). Structure-based discovery of novel chemotypes for adenosine A(2A) receptor antagonists. *J. Med. Chem.* 53, 1799–1809. doi: 10.1021/jm901647p

Kauk, M., and Hoffmann, C. (2017). Intramolecular and intermolecular FRET sensors for GPCRs - monitoring conformational changes and beyond. *Trends Pharmacol. Sci.* 39, 123–135. doi: 10.1016/j.tips.2017.10.011

Kawashita, N., Yamasaki, H., Miyao, T., Kawai, K., Sakae, Y., Ishikawa, T., et al. (2015). A mini-review on chemoinformatics approaches for drug discovery. *J. Comput. Aided Chem.* 16, 15–29. doi: 10.2751/jcac.16.15

Kelemen, Á. A., Kiss, R., Ferenczy, G. G., Kovács, L., Flachner, B., Lorincz, Z., et al. (2016). Structure-based consensus scoring scheme for selecting class A aminergic GPCR fragments. *J. Chem. Inf. Model.* 56, 412–422. doi: 10.1021/acs.jcim.5b00598

Kenakin, T. P. (2016). *Pharmacology in Drug Discovery and Development: Understanding Drug Response.* Boston, MA: Elsevier; Academic Press.

Khan, F., Yadav, D. K., Maurya, A., Sonia, and Srivastava, S. K. (2011). Modern methods & web resources in drug design & discovery. *Lett. Drug Des. Discov.* 8, 469–490. doi: 10.2174/157018011795514249

Khelashvili, G., Dorff, K., Shan, J., Camacho-Artacho, M., Skrabanek, L., Vroling, B., et al. (2010). GPCR-OKB: the G protein coupled receptor oligomer knowledge base. *Bioinformatics* 26, 1804–1805. doi: 10.1093/bioinformatics/btq264

Kim, M., and Cho, A. E. (2016). Incorporating, QM and solvation into docking for applications to GPCR targets. *Phys. Chem. Chem. Phys.* 18, 28281–28289. doi: 10.1039/C6CP04742D

Kolb, P., Rosenbaum, D. M., Irwin, J. J., Fung, J. J., Kobilka, B. K., and Shoichet, B. K. (2009). Structure-based discovery of beta2-adrenergic receptor ligands. *Proc. Natl. Acad. Sci. U.S.A.* 106, 6843–6848. doi: 10.1073/pnas.0812657106

Kooistra, A. J., Vischer, H. F., McNaught-Flores, D., Leurs, R., de Esch, I. J. P., and de Graaf, C. (2016). Function-specific virtual screening for GPCR ligands using a combined scoring method. *Sci. Rep.* 6:28288. doi: 10.1038/srep28288

Kramer, B., Rarey, M., and Lengauer, T. (1999). Evaluation of the FLEXX incremental construction algorithm for protein-ligand docking. *Proteins* 37, 228–241. doi: 10.1002/(SICI)1097-0134(19991101)37:2<228::AID-PROT8>3.0.CO;2-8

Kruse, A. C., Hu, J., Pan, A. C., Arlow, D. H., Rosenbaum, D. M., Rosemond, E., et al. (2012). Structure and dynamics of the M3 muscarinic acetylcholine receptor. *Nature* 482, 552–556. doi: 10.1038/nature10867

Kruse, A. C., Weiss, D. R., Rossi, M., Hu, J., Hu, K., Eitel, K., et al. (2013). Muscarinic receptors as model targets and antitargets for structure-based ligand discovery. *Mol. Pharmacol.* 84, 528–540. doi: 10.1124/mol.113.087551

Kufareva, I., Ilatovskiy, A. V., and Abagyan, R. (2012). Pocketome: an encyclopedia of small-molecule binding sites in 4D. *Nucleic Acids Res.* 40, D535–D540. doi: 10.1093/nar/gkr825

Lagorce, D., Sperandio, O., Galons, H., Miteva, M. A., and Villoutreix, B. O. (2008). FAF-Drugs2: free ADME/tox filtering tool to assist drug discovery and chemical biology projects. *BMC Bioinformatics* 9:396. doi: 10.1186/1471-2105-9-396

Lane, J. R., Chubukov, P., Liu, W., Canals, M., Cherezov, V., Abagyan, R., et al. (2013). Structure-based ligand discovery targeting orthosteric and allosteric pockets of dopamine receptors. *Mol. Pharmacol.* 84, 794–807. doi: 10.1124/mol.113.088054

Lane, J. R., May, L. T., Parton, R. G., Sexton, P. M., and Christopoulos, A. (2017). A kinetic view of GPCR allostery and biased agonism. *Nat. Chem. Biol.* 13, 929–937. doi: 10.1038/nchembio.2431

Langmead, C. J., Andrews, S. P., Congreve, M., Errey, J. C., Hurrell, E., Marshall, F. H., et al. (2012). Identification of novel adenosine A(2A) receptor antagonists by virtual screening. *J. Med. Chem.* 55, 1904–1909. doi: 10.1021/jm201455y

Lapinsh, M., Prusis, P., Gutcaits, A., Lundstedt, T., and Wikberg, J. E. (2001). Development of proteo-chemometrics: a novel technology for the analysis of drug-receptor interactions. *Biochim. Biophys. Acta* 1525, 180–190. doi: 10.1016/S0304-4165(00)00187-2

Launay, G., Téletchéa, S., Wade, F., Pajot-Augy, E., Gibrat, J. F., and Sanz, G. (2012). Automatic modeling of mammalian olfactory receptors and docking of odorants. *Protein Eng. Des. Sel.* 25, 377–386. doi: 10.1093/protein/gzs037

Lee, G. R., and Seok, C. (2016). Galaxy7TM: flexible GPCR-ligand docking by structure refinement. *Nucleic Acids Res.* 44, W502–W506. doi: 10.1093/nar/gkw360

Lee, J. H., Basith, S., Cui, M., Kim, B., and Choi, S. (2017). *In silico* prediction of multiple-category classification model for cytochrome P450 inhibitors and non-inhibitors using machine-learning method. *SAR QSAR Environ. Res.* 28, 863–874. doi: 10.1080/1062936X.2017.1399925

Lee, J. H., Lee, S., and Choi, S. (2010). *in silico* classification of adenosine receptor antagonists using Laplacian-modified naive Bayesian, support vector machine, and recursive partitioning. *J. Mol. Graph. Model.* 28, 883–890. doi: 10.1016/j.jmgm.2010.03.008

Lee, Y., Basith, S., and Choi, S. (2018). Recent advances in structure-based drug design targeting class A G protein-coupled receptors utilizing crystal structures and computational simulations. *J. Med. Chem.* 61, 1–46. doi: 10.1021/acs.jmedchem.6b01453

Le Guilloux, V., Schmidtke, P., and Tuffery, P. (2009). Fpocket: an open source platform for ligand pocket detection. *BMC Bioinformatics* 10:168. doi: 10.1186/1471-2105-10-168

Lemmen, C., Lengauer, T., and Klebe, G. (1998). FLEXS: a method for fast flexible ligand superposition. *J. Med. Chem.* 41, 4502–4520. doi: 10.1021/jm981037l

Lenselink, E. B., Beuming, T., Sherman, W., van Vlijmen, H. W., and IJzerman, A. P. (2014). Selecting an optimal number of binding site waters to improve virtual screening enrichments against the adenosine A2A receptor. *J. Chem. Inf. Model.* 54, 1737–1746. doi: 10.1021/ci5000455

Lenselink, E. B., Beuming, T., van Veen, C., Massink, A., Sherman, W., van Vlijmen, H. W., et al. (2016a). In search of novel ligands using a structure-based approach: a case study on the adenosine A2A receptor. *J. Comput. Aided Mol. Des.* 30, 863–874. doi: 10.1007/s10822-016-9963-7

Lenselink, E. B., Louvel, J., Forti, A. F., van Veldhoven, J. P. D., de Vries, H., Mulder-Krieger, T., et al. (2016b). Predicting binding affinities for GPCR ligands using free-energy perturbation. *ACS Omega* 1, 293–304. doi: 10.1021/acsomega.6b00086

Li, S., Lee, S. Y., and Chung, K. Y. (2015). Conformational analysis of g protein-coupled receptor signaling by hydrogen/deuterium exchange mass spectrometry. *Methods Enzymol.* 557, 261–278. doi: 10.1016/bs.mie.2014.12.004

Liang, Y., Fotiadis, D., Filipek, S., Saperstein, D. A., Palczewski, K., and Engel, A. (2003). Organization of the G protein-coupled receptors rhodopsin and opsin in native membranes. *J. Biol. Chem.* 278, 21655–21662. doi: 10.1074/jbc.M302536200

Liang, Y. L., Khoshouei, M., Radjainia, M., Zhang, Y., Glukhova, A., Tarrasch, J., et al. (2017). Phase-plate cryo-EM structure of a class B GPCR-G-protein complex. *Nature* 546, 118–123. doi: 10.1038/nature22327

Lionta, E., Spyrou, G., Vassilatis, D. K., and Cournia, Z. (2014). Structure-based virtual screening for drug discovery: principles, applications and recent advances. *Curr. Top. Med. Chem.* 14, 1923–1938. doi: 10.2174/1568026614666140929124445

Lipinski, C., and Hopkins, A. (2004). Navigating chemical space for biology and medicine. *Nature* 432, 855–861. doi: 10.1038/nature03193

Luo, M., Wang, X. S., Roth, B. L., Golbraikh, A., and Tropsha, A. (2014). Application of quantitative structure-activity relationship models of 5-HT1A receptor binding to virtual screening identifies novel and potent 5-HT1A ligands. *J. Chem. Inf. Model.* 54, 634–647. doi: 10.1021/ci400460q

Luo, M., Wang, X. S., and Tropsha, A. (2016). Comparative analysis of QSAR-based vs. chemical similarity based predictors of GPCRs binding affinity. *Mol. Inform.* 35, 36–41. doi: 10.1002/minf.201500038

Lyne, P. D. (2002). Structure-based virtual screening: an overview. *Drug Discov. Today* 7, 1047–1055. doi: 10.1016/S1359-6446(02)02483-2

Manglik, A., and Kruse, A. C. (2017). Structural basis for G protein-coupled receptor activation. *Biochemistry* 56, 5628–5634. doi: 10.1021/acs.biochem.7b00747

Manglik, A., Lin, H., Aryal, D. K., McCorvy, J. D., Dengler, D., Corder, G., et al. (2016). Structure-based discovery of opioid analgesics with reduced side effects. *Nature* 537, 185–190. doi: 10.1038/nature19112

Mansouri, K., and Judson, R. S. (2016). *in silico* study of *in vitro* GPCR assays by QSAR modeling. *Methods Mol. Biol.* 1425, 361–381. doi: 10.1007/978-1-4939-3609-0_16

Matricon, P., Ranganathan, A., Warnick, E., Gao, Z. G., Rudling, A., Lambertucci, C., et al. (2017). Fragment optimization for GPCRs by molecular dynamics free energy calculations: probing druggable subpockets of the A 2A adenosine receptor binding site. *Sci. Rep.* 7:6398. doi: 10.1038/s41598-017-04905-0

McGann, M. (2012). FRED and HYBRID docking performance on standardized datasets. *J. Comput. Aided Mol. Des.* 26, 897–906. doi: 10.1007/s10822-012-9584-8

McRobb, F. M., Negri, A., Beuming, T., and Sherman, W. (2016). Molecular dynamics techniques for modeling G protein-coupled receptors. *Curr. Opin. Pharmacol.* 30, 69–75. doi: 10.1016/j.coph.2016.07.001

Miao, Y., Goldfeld, D. A., Moo, E. V., Sexton, P. M., Christopoulos, A., McCammon, J. A., et al. (2016). Accelerated structure-based design of chemically diverse allosteric modulators of a muscarinic G protein-coupled receptor. *Proc. Natl. Acad. Sci. U.S.A.* 113, E5675–E5684. doi: 10.1073/pnas.1612353113

Mitchell, J. B. (2014). Machine learning methods in chemoinformatics. *Wiley Interdiscip. Rev. Comput. Mol. Sci.* 4, 468–481. doi: 10.1002/wcms.1183

Morris, G. M., Huey, R., Lindstrom, W., Sanner, M. F., Belew, R. K., Goodsell, D. S., et al. (2009). AutoDock4 and AutoDockTools4: automated docking with selective receptor flexibility. *J. Comput. Chem.* 30, 2785–2791. doi: 10.1002/jcc.21256

Mullard, A. (2017). The drug-maker's guide to the galaxy. *Nature* 549, 445–447. doi: 10.1038/549445a

Munk, C., Harpsøe, K., Hauser, A. S., Isberg, V., and Gloriam, D. E. (2016). Integrating structural and mutagenesis data to elucidate GPCR ligand binding. *Curr. Opin. Pharmacol.* 30, 51–58. doi: 10.1016/j.coph.2016.07.003

Murray, C. W., Verdonk, M. L., and Rees, D. C. (2012). Experiences in fragment-based drug discovery. *Trends Pharmacol. Sci.* 33, 224–232. doi: 10.1016/j.tips.2012.02.006

Neustadt, B. R., Hao, J., Lindo, N., Greenlee, W. J., Stamford, A. W., Tulshian, D., et al. (2007). Potent, selective, and orally active adenosine A2A receptor antagonists: arylpiperazine derivatives of pyrazolo[4,3-e]-1,2,4-triazolo[1,5-c]pyrimidines. *Bioorg. Med. Chem. Lett.* 17, 1376–1380. doi: 10.1016/j.bmcl.2006.11.083

Neves, M. A., Totrov, M., and Abagyan, R. (2012). Docking and scoring with ICM: the benchmarking results and strategies for improvement. *J. Comput. Aided Mol. Des.* 26, 675–686. doi: 10.1007/s10822-012-9547-0

Ngo, T., Kufareva, I., Coleman, J. L. J., Graham, R. M., Abagyan, R., and Smith, N. J. (2016). Identifying ligands at orphan GPCRs: current status using structure-based approaches. *Br. J. Pharmacol.* 173, 2934–2951. doi: 10.1111/bph.13452

Okuno, Y., Tamon, A., Yabuuchi, H., Niijima, S., Minowa, Y., Tonomura, K., et al. (2008). GLIDA: GPCR–ligand database for chemical genomics drug discovery–database and tools update. *Nucleic Acids Res.* 36, D907–D912. doi: 10.1093/nar/gkm948

Olah, M., Mracec, M., Ostopovici, L., Rad, R., Bora, A., Hadaruga, N., et al. (2005). "9. WOMBAT: world of molecular bioactivity," in *Chemoinformatics in Drug Discovery*, ed T. I. Oprea (Weinheim: WILEY-VCH Verlag GmbH & Co.), 221–239.

Oprea, T. I., and Gottfries, J. (2001). Chemography: the art of navigating in chemical space. *J. Comb. Chem.* 3, 157–166. doi: 10.1021/cc0000388

Oswald, C., Rappas, M., Kean, J., Doré, A. S., Errey, J. C., Bennett, K., et al. (2016). Intracellular allosteric antagonism of the CCR9 receptor. *Nature* 540, 462–465. doi: 10.1038/nature20606

Palczewski, K., Kumasaka, T., Hori, T., Behnke, C. A., Motoshima, H., Fox, B. A., et al. (2000). Crystal structure of rhodopsin: a G protein-coupled receptor. *Science* 289, 739–745. doi: 10.1126/science.289.5480.739

Paul, D. S., and Gautham, N. (2016). MOLS 2.0: software package for peptide modeling and protein-ligand docking. *J. Mol. Model.* 22, 239. doi: 10.1007/s00894-016-3106-x

Qiu, T., Qiu, J., Feng, J., Wu, D., Yang, Y., Tang, K., et al. (2017). The recent progress in proteochemometric modelling: focusing on target descriptors, cross-term descriptors and application scope. *Brief. Bioinform.* 18, 125–136. doi: 10.1093/bib/bbw004

Rasmussen, S. G., Choi, H. J., Rosenbaum, D. M., Kobilka, T. S., Thian, F. S., Edwards, P. C., et al. (2007). Crystal structure of the human beta2 adrenergic G-protein-coupled receptor. *Nature* 450, 383–387. doi: 10.1038/nature06325

Rasmussen, S. G., DeVree, B. T., Zou, Y., Kruse, A. C., Chung, K. Y., Kobilka, T. S., et al. (2011). Crystal structure of the beta2 adrenergic receptor-Gs protein complex. *Nature* 477, 549–555. doi: 10.1038/nature10361

Renault, N., Laurent, X., Farce, A., El Bakali, J., Mansouri, R., Gervois, P., et al. (2013). Virtual screening of CB(2) receptor agonists from bayesian network and high-throughput docking: structural insights into agonist-modulated GPCR features. *Chem. Biol. Drug Des.* 81, 442–454. doi: 10.1111/cbdd.12095

Reutlinger, M., Rodrigues, T., Schneider, P., and Schneider, G. (2014). Multi-objective molecular *de novo* design by adaptive fragment prioritization. *Angew. Chem. Int. Ed. Engl.* 53, 4244–4248. doi: 10.1002/anie.201310864

Reymond, J. L. (2015). The chemical space project. *Acc. Chem. Res.* 48, 722–730. doi: 10.1021/ar500432k

Ring, A. M., Manglik, A., Kruse, A. C., Enos, M. D., Weis, W. I., Garcia, K. C., et al. (2013). Adrenaline-activated structure of β(2)-adrenoceptor stabilized by an engineered nanobody. *Nature* 502, 575–579. doi: 10.1038/nature12572

Rodrigues, T., Hauser, N., Reker, D., Reutlinger, M., Wunderlin, T., Hamon, J., et al. (2015). Multidimensional *de novo* design reveals 5-HT2B receptor-selective ligands. *Angew. Chem. Int. Ed. Engl.* 54, 1551–1555. doi: 10.1002/anie.201410201

Rodríguez, D., Chakraborty, S., Warnick, E., Crane, S., Gao, Z. G., O'Connor, R., et al. (2016). Structure-based screening of uncharted chemical space for atypical adenosine receptor agonists. *ACS Chem. Biol.* 11, 2763–2772. doi: 10.1021/acschembio.6b00357

Rodriguez, D., Gao, Z. G., Moss, S. M., Jacobson, K. A., and Carlsson, J. (2015). Molecular docking screening using agonist-bound GPCR structures: probing the A(2A) adenosine receptor. *J. Chem. Inf. Model.* 55, 550–563. doi: 10.1021/ci500639g

Roy, U., and Luck, L. A. (2007). Molecular modeling of estrogen receptor using molecular operating environment. *Biochem. Mol. Biol. Educ.* 35, 238–243. doi: 10.1002/bmb.65

Sabio, M., Jones, K., and Topiol, S. (2008). Use of the X-ray structure of the beta2-adrenergic receptor for drug discovery. Part 2: identification of active compounds. *Bioorg. Med. Chem. Lett.* 18, 5391–5395. doi: 10.1016/j.bmcl.2008.09.046

Sandal, M., Duy, T. P., Cona, M., Zung, H., Carloni, P., Musiani, F., et al. (2013). GOMoDo: a GPCRs online modeling and docking webserver. *PLoS ONE* 8:e74092. doi: 10.1371/journal.pone.0074092

Sanders, M. P., Verhoeven, S., de Graaf, C., Roumen, L., Vroling, B., Nabuurs, S. B., et al. (2011). Snooker: a structure-based pharmacophore generation tool applied to class A GPCRs. *J. Chem. Inf. Model.* 51, 2277–2292. doi: 10.1021/ci200088d

Saxena, A. K., Bhunia, S. S., and Saxena, M. (2017). "Integration on ligand and structure based approaches in GPCRs," in *Topics in Medicinal Chemistry*, eds P. R. Bernstein, G. I. Georg, T. Keller, T. Kobayashi, J. A. Lowe, N. A. Meanwell, A. K. Saxena, U. Stilz, C. T. Supuran, and A. Zhang (Berlin; Heidelberg: Springer), 1–61.

Scheerer, P., Park, J. H., Hildebrand, P. W., Kim, Y. J., Krauss, N., Choe, H. W., et al. (2008). Crystal structure of opsin in its G-protein-interacting conformation. *Nature* 455, 497–502. doi: 10.1038/nature07330

Schertler, G. F., Villa, C., and Henderson, R. (1993). Projection structure of rhodopsin. *Nature* 362, 770–772. doi: 10.1038/362770a0

Schneidman-Duhovny, D., Dror, O., Inbar, Y., Nussinov, R., and Wolfson, H. J. (2008). Deterministic pharmacophore detection via multiple flexible alignment of drug-like molecules. *J. Comput. Biol.* 15, 737–754. doi: 10.1089/cmb.2007.0130

Schrage, R., and Kostenis, E. (2017). Functional selectivity and dualsteric/bitopic GPCR targeting. *Curr. Opin. Pharmacol.* 32, 85–90. doi: 10.1016/j.coph.2016.12.001

Schuffenhauer, A., Brown, N., Selzer, P., Ertl, P., and Jacoby, E. (2006). Relationships between molecular complexity, biological activity, and structural diversity. *J. Chem. Inf. Model.* 46, 525–535. doi: 10.1021/ci0503558

Selvam, C., Oueslati, N., Lemasson, I. A., Brabet, I., Rigault, D., Courtiol, T., et al. (2010). A virtual screening hit reveals new possibilities for developing group III metabotropic glutamate receptor agonists. *J. Med. Chem.* 53, 2797–2813. doi: 10.1021/jm901523t

Shimamura, T., Shiroishi, M., Weyand, S., Tsujimoto, H., Winter, G., Katritch, V., et al. (2011). Structure of the human histamine H1 receptor complex with doxepin. *Nature* 475, 65–70. doi: 10.1038/nature10236

Shiraishi, A., Niijima, S., Brown, J. B., Nakatsui, M., and Okuno, Y. (2013). Chemical genomics approach for GPCR-ligand interaction prediction and extraction of ligand binding determinants. *J. Chem. Inf. Model.* 53, 1253–1262. doi: 10.1021/ci300515z

Shoichet, B. K., and Kobilka, B. K. (2012). Structure-based drug screening for G-protein-coupled receptors. *Trends Pharmacol. Sci.* 33, 268–272. doi: 10.1016/j.tips.2012.03.007

Shonberg, J., Kling, R. C., Gmeiner, P., and Löber, S. (2015). GPCR crystal structures: medicinal chemistry in the pocket. *Bioorg. Med. Chem.* 23, 3880–3906. doi: 10.1016/j.bmc.2014.12.034

Shukla, A. K., Westfield, G. H., Xiao, K. H., Reis, R. I., Huang, L. Y., Tripathi-Shukla, P., et al. (2014). Visualization of arrestin recruitment by a G-protein-coupled receptor. *Nature* 512, 218–222. doi: 10.1038/nature 13430

Spitzer, R., and Jain, A. N. (2012). Surflex-dock: docking benchmarks and real-world application. *J. Comput. Aided Mol. Des.* 26, 687–699. doi: 10.1007/s10822-011-9533-y

Sriram, K., and Insel, P. A. (2018). GPCRs as targets for approved drugs: how many targets and how many drugs? *Mol. Pharmacol.* 93, 251–258. doi: 10.1124/mol.117.111062

Tautermann, C. S. (2016). Impact, determination and prediction of drug-receptor residence times for GPCRs. *Curr. Opin. Pharmacol.* 30, 22–26. doi: 10.1016/j.coph.2016.07.004

Thomsen, W., Frazer, J., and Unett, D. (2005). Functional assays for screening GPCR targets. *Curr. Opin. Biotechnol.* 16, 655–665. doi: 10.1016/j.copbio.2005.10.008

Tiikkainen, P., Bellis, L., Light, Y., and Franke, L. (2013). Estimating error rates in bioactivity databases. *J. Chem. Inf. Model.* 53, 2499–2505. doi: 10.1021/ci400099q

Trauelsen, M., Rexen Ulven, E., Hjorth, S. A., Brvar, M., Monaco, C., Frimurer, T. M., et al. (2017). Receptor structure-based discovery of non-metabolite agonists for the succinate receptor GPR91. *Mol. Metab.* 6, 1585–1596. doi: 10.1016/j.molmet.2017.09.005

Trott, O., and Olson, A. J. (2010). AutoDock Vina: improving the speed and accuracy of docking with a new scoring function, efficient optimization, and multithreading. *J. Comput. Chem.* 31, 455–461. doi: 10.1002/jcc.21334

Tsai, T. Y., Chang, K. W., and Chen, C. Y. (2011). iScreen: world's first cloud-computing web server for virtual screening and *de novo* drug design based on TCM database@Taiwan. *J. Comput. Aided Mol. Des.* 25, 525–531. doi: 10.1007/s10822-011-9438-9

Valerio, L. G. Jr., and Choudhuri, S. (2012). Chemoinformatics and chemical genomics: potential utility of *in silico* methods. *J. Appl. Toxicol.* 32, 880–889. doi: 10.1002/jat.2804

van Westen, G. J. P., Wegner, J. K., Geluykens, P., Kwanten, L., Vereycken, I., Peeters, A., et al. (2011). Which compound to select in lead optimization? Prospectively validated proteochemometric models guide preclinical development. *PLoS ONE* 6:e27518. doi: 10.1371/journal.pone.0027518

Varghese, J. N. (1999). Development of neuraminidase inhibitors as anti-influenza virus drugs. *Drug Dev. Res.* 46, 176–196. doi: 10.1002/(SICI)1098-2299(199903/04)46:3/4<176::AID-DDR4>3.0.CO;2-6

Varnek, A., and Baskin, I. (2012). Machine learning methods for property prediction in chemoinformatics: Quo Vadis? *J. Chem. Inf. Model.* 52, 1413–1437. doi: 10.1021/ci200409x

Varnek, A., and Tropsha, A. (2008). *Chemoinformatics Approaches to Virtual Screening*. Cambridge: RSC Publishing.

Vass, M., Agai-Csongor, E., Horti, F., and Keseru, G. M. (2014a). Multiple fragment docking and linking in primary and secondary pockets of dopamine receptors. *ACS Med. Chem. Lett.* 5, 1010–1014. doi: 10.1021/ml500201u

Vass, M., Kooistra, A. J., Ritschel, T., Leurs, R., de Esch, I. J., and de Graaf, C. (2016). Molecular interaction fingerprint approaches for GPCR drug discovery. *Curr. Opin. Pharmacol.* 30, 59–68. doi: 10.1016/j.coph.2016.07.007

Vass, M., Schmidt, É., Horti, F., and Keseru, G. M. (2014b). Virtual fragment screening on GPCRs: a case study on dopamine D3 and histamine H4 receptors. *Eur. J. Med. Chem.* 77, 38–46. doi: 10.1016/j.ejmech.2014.02.034

Venkatakrishnan, A. J., Deupi, X., Lebon, G., Tate, C. G., Schertler, G. F., and Babu, M. M. (2013). Molecular signatures of G-protein-coupled receptors. *Nature* 494, 185–194. doi: 10.1038/nature11896

Verheij, M. H., de Graaf, C., de Kloe, G. E., Nijmeijer, S., Vischer, H. F., Smits, R. A., et al. (2011). Fragment library screening reveals remarkable similarities between the G protein-coupled receptor histamine H(4) and the ion channel serotonin 5-HT(3)A. *Bioorg. Med. Chem. Lett.* 21, 5460–5464. doi: 10.1016/j.bmcl.2011.06.123

Vilardaga, J. P. (2011). Studying ligand efficacy at G protein-coupled receptors using FRET. *Methods Mol. Biol.* 756, 133–148. doi: 10.1007/978-1-61779-160-4_6

Visegrády, A., and Keseru, G. M. (2013). Fragment-based lead discovery on G-protein-coupled receptors. *Expert Opin. Drug. Discov.* 8, 811–820. doi: 10.1517/17460441.2013.794135

Wacker, D., Fenalti, G., Brown, M. A., Katritch, V., Abagyan, R., Cherezov, V., et al. (2010). Conserved binding mode of human β(2) adrenergic receptor inverse agonists and antagonist revealed by X-ray crystallography. *J. Am. Chem. Soc.* 132, 11443–11445. doi: 10.1021/ja105108q

Wacker, D., Stevens, R. C., and Roth, B. L. (2017a). How ligands illuminate GPCR molecular pharmacology. *Cell* 170, 414–427. doi: 10.1016/j.cell.2017.07.009

Wacker, D., Wang, S., McCorvy, J. D., Betz, R. M., Venkatakrishnan, A. J., Levit, A., et al. (2017b). Crystal structure of an LSD-bound human serotonin receptor. *Cell* 168, 377 e312–389 e312. doi: 10.1016/j.cell.2016.12.033.

Walters, W. P., and Namchuk, M. (2003). Designing screens: how to make your hits a hit. *Nat. Rev. Drug Discov.* 2, 259–266. doi: 10.1038/nrd1063

Wang, C., Wu, H., Katritch, V., Han, G. W., Huang, X. P., Liu, W., et al. (2013). Structure of the human smoothened receptor bound to an antitumour agent. *Nature* 497, 338–343. doi: 10.1038/nature12167

Weiss, D. R., Ahn, S., Sassano, M. F., Kleist, A., Zhu, X., Strachan, R., et al. (2013). Conformation guides molecular efficacy in docking screens of activated beta-2 adrenergic G protein coupled receptor. *ACS Chem. Biol.* 8, 1018–1026. doi: 10.1021/cb400103f

Williams, A. J., and Ekins, S. (2011). A quality alert and call for improved curation of public chemistry databases. *Drug Discov. Today* 16, 747–750. doi: 10.1016/j.drudis.2011.07.007

Williams, A. J., Ekins, S., and Tkachenko, V. (2012). Towards a gold standard: regarding quality in public domain chemistry databases and approaches to improving the situation. *Drug Discov. Today* 17, 685–701. doi: 10.1016/j.drudis.2012.02.013

Wlodawer, A., and Vondrasek, J. (1998). Inhibitors of HIV-1 protease: a major success of structure-assisted drug design. *Annu. Rev. Biophys. Biomol. Struct.* 27, 249–284. doi: 10.1146/annurev.biophys.27.1.249

Wolber, G., and Langer, T. (2005). LigandScout: 3-D pharmacophores derived from protein-bound ligands and their use as virtual screening filters. *J. Chem. Inf. Model.* 45, 160–169. doi: 10.1021/ci049885e

Wu, H., Wang, C., Gregory, K. J., Han, G. W., Cho, H. P., Xia, Y., et al. (2014). Structure of a class C GPCR metabotropic glutamate receptor 1 bound to an allosteric modulator. *Science* 344, 58–64. doi: 10.1126/science.1249489

Xie, X. Q., Wang, L., Liu, H., Ouyang, Q., Fang, C., and Su, W. (2014). Chemogenomics knowledgebased polypharmacology analyses of drug abuse related G-protein coupled receptors and their ligands. *Front. Pharmacol.* 5:3. doi: 10.3389/fphar.2014.00003

Xu, W., Lim, J., Goh, C. Y., Suen, J. Y., Jiang, Y., Yau, M. K., et al. (2015). Repurposing registered drugs as antagonists for protease-activated receptor 2. *J. Chem. Inf. Model.* 55, 2079–2084. doi: 10.1021/acs.jcim.5b00500

Yadav, D. K., Rai, P., Pratap, R., and Singh, H. (2016). "Software and web resources for computer-aided molecular modeling and drug discovery," in *Chemometrics Applications and Research: QSAR in Medicinal Chemistry*, eds A. G. Mercader, P. R. Duchowicz, and P. M. Sivakumar (Oakville, ON: Apple Academic Press), 33–99.

Zhang, D., Gao, Z. G., Zhang, K., Kiselev, E., Crane, S., Wang, J., et al. (2015). Two disparate ligand-binding sites in the human P2Y1 receptor. *Nature* 520, 317–321. doi: 10.1038/nature14287

Zhang, G., Wang, K., Li, X. D., Zhang, D. L., and Xu, F. (2016). Discovery of novel antagonists of human neurotensin receptor 1 on the basis of ligand and protein structure. *Biomed. Pharmacother.* 84, 147–157. doi: 10.1016/j.biopha.2016.09.025

Zhang, H., Unal, H., Desnoyer, R., Han, G. W., Patel, N., Katritch, V., et al. (2015). Structural basis for ligand recognition and functional selectivity at angiotensin receptor. *J. Biol. Chem.* 290, 29127–29139. doi: 10.1074/jbc.M115.689000

Zhang, X. (2017). Seven perspectives on GPCR H/D-exchange proteomics methods. *F1000Res* 6:89. doi: 10.12688/f1000research.10667.1

Zhang, Y., Sun, B., Feng, D., Hu, H., Chu, M., Qu, Q., et al. (2017). Cryo-EM structure of the activated GLP-1 receptor in complex with a G protein. *Nature* 546, 248–253. doi: 10.1038/nature22394

Zhou, X. E., He, Y., de Waal, P. W., Gao, X., Kang, Y., Van Eps, N., et al. (2017). Identification of phosphorylation codes for arrestin recruitment by G protein-coupled receptors. *Cell* 170, 457 e413–469 doi: 10.1016/j.cell.2017.07.002

Zoete, V., Daina, A., Bovigny, C., and Michielin, O. (2016). SwissSimilarity: a web tool for low to ultra high throughput ligand-based virtual screening. *J. Chem. Inf. Model.* 56, 1399–1404. doi: 10.1021/acs.jcim.6b00174

13

LeadOp+R: Structure-Based Lead Optimization with Synthetic Accessibility

*Fang-Yu Lin [1], Emilio Xavier Esposito [2] and Yufeng J. Tseng [1,3]**

[1] Graduate Institute of Biomedical Electronics and Bioinformatics, National Taiwan University, Taipei, Taiwan, [2] exeResearch, LLC, East Lansing, MI, United States, [3] Department of Computer Science and Information Engineering, National Taiwan University, Taipei, Taiwan

***Correspondence:**
Yufeng J. Tseng
yjtseng@csie.ntu.edu.tw

We previously described a structure-based fragment hopping for lead optimization using a pre-docked fragment database, "LeadOp," that conceptually replaced "bad" fragments of a ligand with "good" fragments while leaving the core of the ligand intact thus improving the compound's activity. LeadOp was proven to optimize the query molecules and systematically developed improved analogs for each of our example systems. However, even with the fragment-based design from common building blocks, it is still a challenge for synthesis. In this work, "LeadOp+R" was developed based on 198 classical chemical reactions to consider the synthetic accessibility while optimizing leads. LeadOp+R first allows user to identify a preserved space defined by the volume occupied by a fragment of the query molecule to be preserved. Then LeadOp+R searches for building blocks with the same preserved space as initial reactants and grows molecules toward the preferred receptor-ligand interactions according to reaction rules from reaction database in LeadOp+R. Multiple conformers of each intermediate product were considered and evaluated at each step. The conformer with the best group efficiency score would be selected as the initial conformer of the next building block until the program finished optimization for all selected receptor-ligand interactions. The LeadOp+R method was tested with two biomolecular systems: Tie-2 kinase and human 5-lipoxygenase. The LeadOp+R methodology was able to optimize the query molecules and systematically developed improved analogs for each of our example systems. The suggested synthetic routes for compounds proposed by LeadOp+R were the same as the published synthetic routes devised by the synthetic/organic chemists.

Keywords: fragment-based, lead optimization, structure-based drug design, computer-assisted synthesis, human 5-lipoxygenase, tie-2 kinase

INTRODUCTION

We recently reported a new structure-based fragment hopping method in lead optimization, LeadOp, (Lin and Tseng, 2011). Our lead optimization method works by decomposing a chemical structure into fragments of different parts, either by chemical or user-defined rules. The fragments are evaluated in a pre-docked fragment database and ranked according to specific fragment-receptor binding interactions. The ranked fragments provide the ability to replace fragments possessing less favorable contributions to binding. With optimal fragments selected, LeadOp reassembles the fragments to form the new drug-like compound. LeadOp is an algorithm that can automatically optimize a query molecule by searching and replacing fragments from a pre-docked fragment database in the active site to generate structures with better binding without prior knowledge of better fragments. Additionally, users can specify parts of structures to be optimized based on known interactions or the user's preference. However, the proposed compounds are not always easy to synthesize. In this study, we demonstrate lead optimization with synthetic accessibility, LeadOp+R, an advanced approach for lead optimization with synthetic accessibility.

A basic difficulty in most applications of computer-aided drug design is that designed (suggested) molecules are often of uncertain synthetic accessibility, leading to a slow feedback-improvement loop between the experimental syntheses and modeling design (Hopkins et al., 2004). Various synthetic planning software, WODCA (Ihlenfeldt and Gasteiger, 1996), SYNGEN (Hendrickson and Toczko, 1988), and ROBIA, 4 (Socorro and Goodman, 2006) were developed to provide the synthetic route generation, that involves either searching a database of chemical reactions or transformation rules for reaction centers that match the target compound to propose analogous transformations. Tools in route generation, mostly retrosynthetic software, can suggest routes based on encoded generalized reaction rules to identify those bond disconnections most apt to lead to synthetically accessible precursor structures (Corey et al., 1975; Corey and Jorgensen, 1976) while Hendrickson's group (Hendrickson et al., 1985) developed a logic-based synthesis design method with formalized reaction constraints. A good example of route generation is Route Designer (Law et al., 2009), that use rules describing retrosynthetic transformations automatically generated from reaction database and generates complete synthetic routes for target molecules starting from available reactants. Applications combining the synthetic route designing and de-novo design for the target binding sites have also been developed, such as SPROUT (Mata et al., 1995), which starts from generation of a skeleton followed by atom substitution to convert the solution skeletons to molecules and rank the output from SPROUT according to ease of synthesis. However, the molecules are generated from the ease of synthesis, the desired core of potential inhibitors could not be easily preserved.

To make the synthetic-modeling feedback loop more straightforward, we develop and implement "LeadOp+R"—**Lead Op**timization with synthetic accessibility based on chemical **R**eaction route. LeadOp+R is an algorithm that performs structure-based lead optimization while considering the synthetic reactions from reactants to products according to reaction rules. It takes into consideration the chemical reaction environment; this information is based on known chemical synthesis. The synthetic routes suggested by LeadOp+R are examined to ensure the validity of transformation from one starting reactant into the final product through the use of the LeadOp+R reaction database. The extracted reaction rules in LeadOp+R reaction database do not take into account temporarily or unwanted chemical reactions; on the contrary, these extracted reaction rules consider direct chemical reactions that transform the starting reactants into products. LeadOp+R's algorithm consists of the following five steps: (i) identify a preserved space (defined by the volume occupied by a fragment of the query molecule to be preserved by the user) and searches for building blocks with the same preserved space as initial reactants, (ii) search the reaction rules for each reactants identified, (iii) generate reaction products based on reaction rules, (iv) evaluate the conformations of each products of each reaction, and (v) select the conformer from previous steps that would be selected as the reactant to grow molecules until optimizations are fulfilled for each selected inhibitor–receptor interactions by users. Multiple conformers of each product for each step were considered and evaluated. The conformer with the best group efficiency score would be selected as the next reactant, wherein the group efficiency score is calculated based on binding energy divided by the number of heavy atoms. Thus, this evaluation would favor the conformers with stronger binding toward the specified receptor-ligand interactions with less heavy atoms (Hopkins et al., 2004; Ciulli et al., 2006; Alex and Flocco, 2007; Saxty et al., 2007; Congreve et al., 2008; Orita et al., 2009). Compounds passing the molecular property filters comprised the final list of proposed compounds. The compounds were then energy-minimized and ranked on the basis of the overall ligand–receptor binding energy. To investigate the interactions between the newly assembled molecules and their receptor, molecular dynamics simulations were performed to explore the compounds' poses and interactions with the solved crystal structure of the receptor.

To demonstrate the LeadOp+R algorithm, we selected the Tie-2 kinase (Hodous et al., 2007) and human 5-lipoxygenase (5-LOX) (Ducharme et al., 2010) protein systems and their associated inhibitors as model systems. The endothelium-specific receptor tyrosine kinase Tie-2 (tyrosine kinase containing Ig and EGF homology domains) is primarily expressed in the vascular endothelium and is involved in vessel branching, sprouting, remodeling, maturation, and stability (Yu, 2005). The role of tyrosine kinases in angiogenesis and in the vascularization of solid tumors has drawn considerable interest (Hasegawa et al., 2007) and is considered to be angiogenesis-dependent in cancer. Interference with the Tie-2 pathway by diverse blocking agents has been shown to suppress tumor growth in xenograft studies (Oliner et al., 2004). The development of Tie-2 kinase inhibitors may block the beneficial anti-inflammatory and vascular stabilizing effects, thus the discovery of potent Tie-2 kinase inhibitors has advanced into clinical studies (Huang et al., 2010). Lipoxygenases are a family of iron-containing enzymes found in a large variety of organisms, including bacteria and animals. It catalyzes the dioxygenation of polyunsaturated fatty acids containing a *cis*-1,4-pentadiene structure—the first committed structure in a metabolic pathway cascade—and involved in the initiation of signaling molecule synthesis and inducing structural or metabolic changes (Steele et al., 1999). Four major isozymes of lipoxygenases have been identified (Ivanov et al., 2010), including 5-, 8-, 12-, and 15-LOX, that are key enzymes in the metabolism of prostaglandins and leukotrienes. In particular, leukotrienes are produced through the 5-LOX pathway and the increased activity of the 5-LOX pathway is strongly associated with atherosclerosis

(Woods et al., 1993). As the 5-LOX biological pathways and byproducts lead to inflammation, discovering a 5-lipoxygenase inhibitor is important to the fields of inflammatory and allergic diseases (Shaffer and Mansmann, 1997).

MATERIALS AND METHODS

Overall Procedure

The general protocol for LeadOp+R is illustrated in **Figure 1** and the details of each step are described in the following sections. Prior to applying the LeadOp+R optimization procedure, a reaction rule database is constructed, containing reaction rules for the reactant moiety, the product moiety, and the building blocks of each reaction. Thus, participants involved in each reaction are known for synthetic assessment in LeadOp+R. The initial step of LeadOp+R requires the user to select the favored inhibitor-receptor interaction positions for optimization. The inhibitor-receptor interaction positions determine the "direction" for virtual synthesis and optimizations. LeadOp+R will systematically optimize and grow a structure until all the user-defined directions are processed. LeadOp+R initiates the analysis with the inhibitor-receptor complex from docking studies or crystal structures. The user can determine which fragment(s) in the query inhibitor (initial compound) to preserve during optimization. To ensure that the initial synthesis is accessible, the starting building block—containing the preserved fragment—is used as the initial building block. LeadOp+R then searches the reaction rule database with this building block to identify associated reactions rules. Once the reactions rules and associated participants are identified, the products of each reaction rule are generated virtually. The best binding conformation of the proposed compound is selected from an ensemble of conformers are constructed of each compound. The conformer of each compound with the lowest group efficiency value is selected as the initial conformer of the next building block until the program reaches the termination condition. By evaluating the contribution of each product upon binding with group efficiency, LeadOp+R selects compounds that bind stronger yet possess less heavy atoms. The compounds passing a set of molecular property filters comprised the final list of proposed compounds. Following a short molecular dynamics simulation, the compounds are energy-minimized and ranked on the basis of the overall ligand–receptor binding (interaction) energy. This provides a series of new and more potent compounds that are chemical accessibility.

Example Systems

Tie-2 kinase (PDB: 2p4i), an endothelium-specific receptor tyrosine kinase (Hodous et al., 2007) and human 5-LOX enzyme (Charlier et al., 2006) a key enzyme in leukotriene biosynthesis, were selected as model systems to examine the LeadOp+R approach. One Tie-2 kinase inhibitor, compound 46 in reference 16 (denoted as compound rA in this study) and a human 5-LOX inhibitor, compound 7 (substituted coumarins) in reference 17 (denoted as compound rB in this study), were selected as the LeadOp+R optimization examples.

Construction of the LeadOp+R Reaction Database

LeadOp+R collects chemical reactions, building blocks, and reaction rules with reactant moieties and product moieties of each reaction to construct the LeadOp+R reaction database. LeadOp+R includes 198 classic chemical reactions from the Reaxy Database and 2,091 organic building blocks from the commercially available Sigma-Alderich Co[1]. product library. These building blocks include the typical building blocks in a chemical synthesis such as various nitrogen compounds (amines, isocyanides) and carbonyl compounds (amides, aldehydes, and ketones). A reaction rule in LeadOp+R includes the reactant moieties and product moieties extracted from the full structure of reactants and products of each reaction collected. In LeadOp+R, the reaction moieties were defined and extracted from a chemical reaction according the following steps (see **Figure 2** for the illustration of the steps):

(1) Identification of reaction core. A collection of atoms that take part in the chemical transformation (reaction) have their atom type changed (element, number and type of bonds, and number of neighboring atoms) are considered the reaction core. These atoms are determined by comparing the atoms of the starting compound and product to those within the LeadOp+R reaction database; atoms that differ are part of the reaction core. Since the reaction core does not contain enough chemical information to accurately describe the reaction, additional information is gathered from atoms bound to the reaction core.

(2) Extraction of the reactant and product moieties for a reaction. The initial reaction cores typically do not include enough atoms and thus their "chemical environment" is expanded. The reaction core is increased to bonded (neighboring) atoms until the minimum reactant and product substructures are included to fully represent the reaction. Within a reaction, the reactant portion is denoted as the "reactant moiety" and as expected the product portion is denoted as "product moiety." The extension step is performed by traversing the atom types within the reaction core, as discussed in Step 1, until a single sp^3 carbon is found and the atoms searched during the extension step are considered part of the same moiety. For cases where the searched atoms are in an aromatic ring, the extension was terminated when all the atoms in the aromatic ring are included in the moiety, thus all the atoms in the aromatic ring are considered part of the moiety.

Finally, the building blocks with the same reactant moiety for each reaction rule are collected (through a JChem application-programming interface; JChem API) and classified by the reaction. Building blocks for each reaction rule are recorded and used for virtual synthesis in the LeadOp+R algorithm.

Identify Reactant

LeadOp+R initiates the analysis of a complexed structure (inhibitor-receptor) taken from a docking study or crystal

[1]"Sigma-Aldrich Chemie GmbH." (Steinheim, Germany).

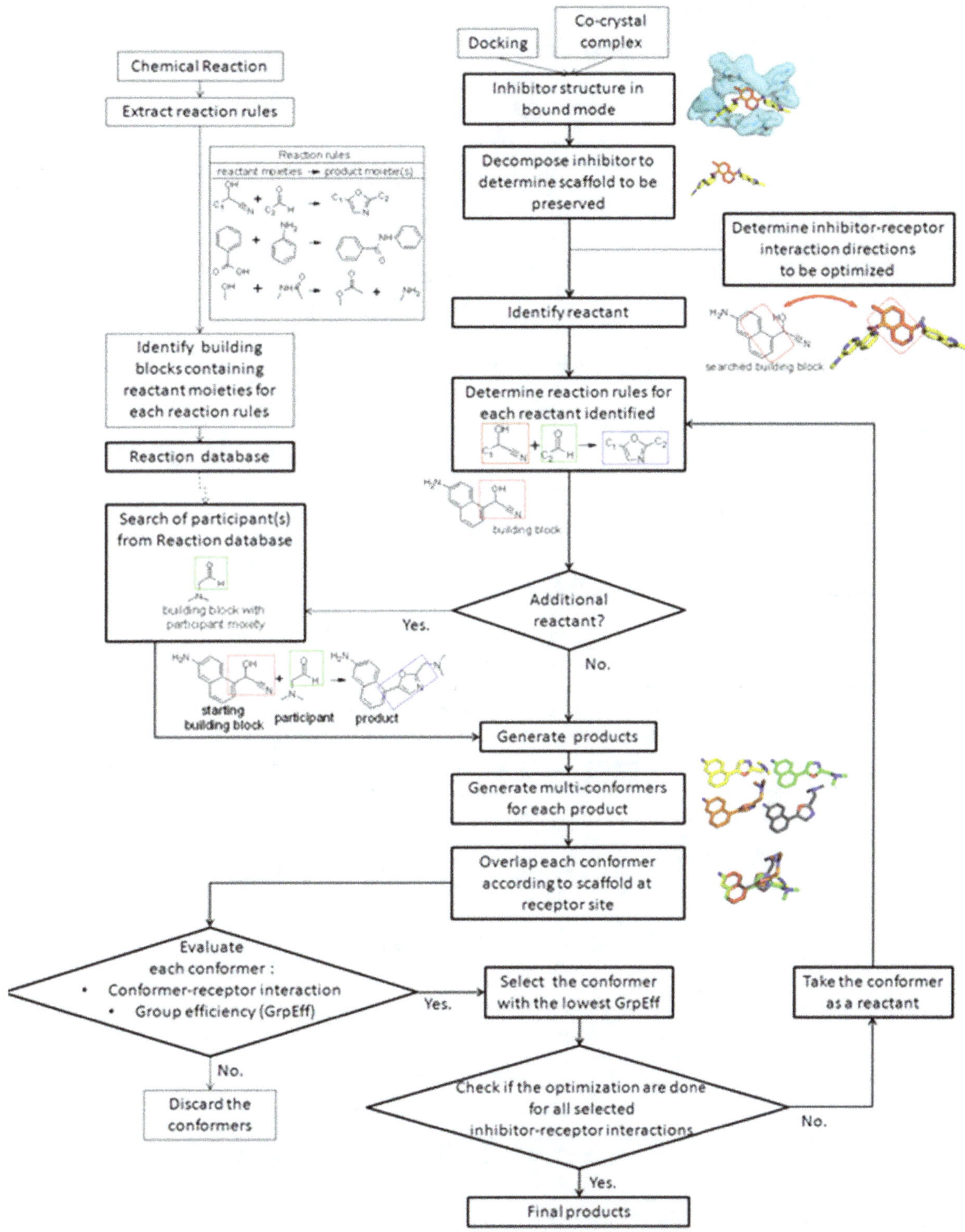

FIGURE 1 | Illustration of the LeadOp+R optimization workflow.

structure. Initially, the user identifies and preserves the "fragment space" of a query molecule defined by a fragment's volume. LeadOp+R then searches for building blocks with the same volume as the potential initial reactants. Products of each potential initial reactant are virtually synthesized according to the steps below. For each product molecule that passes the evaluation

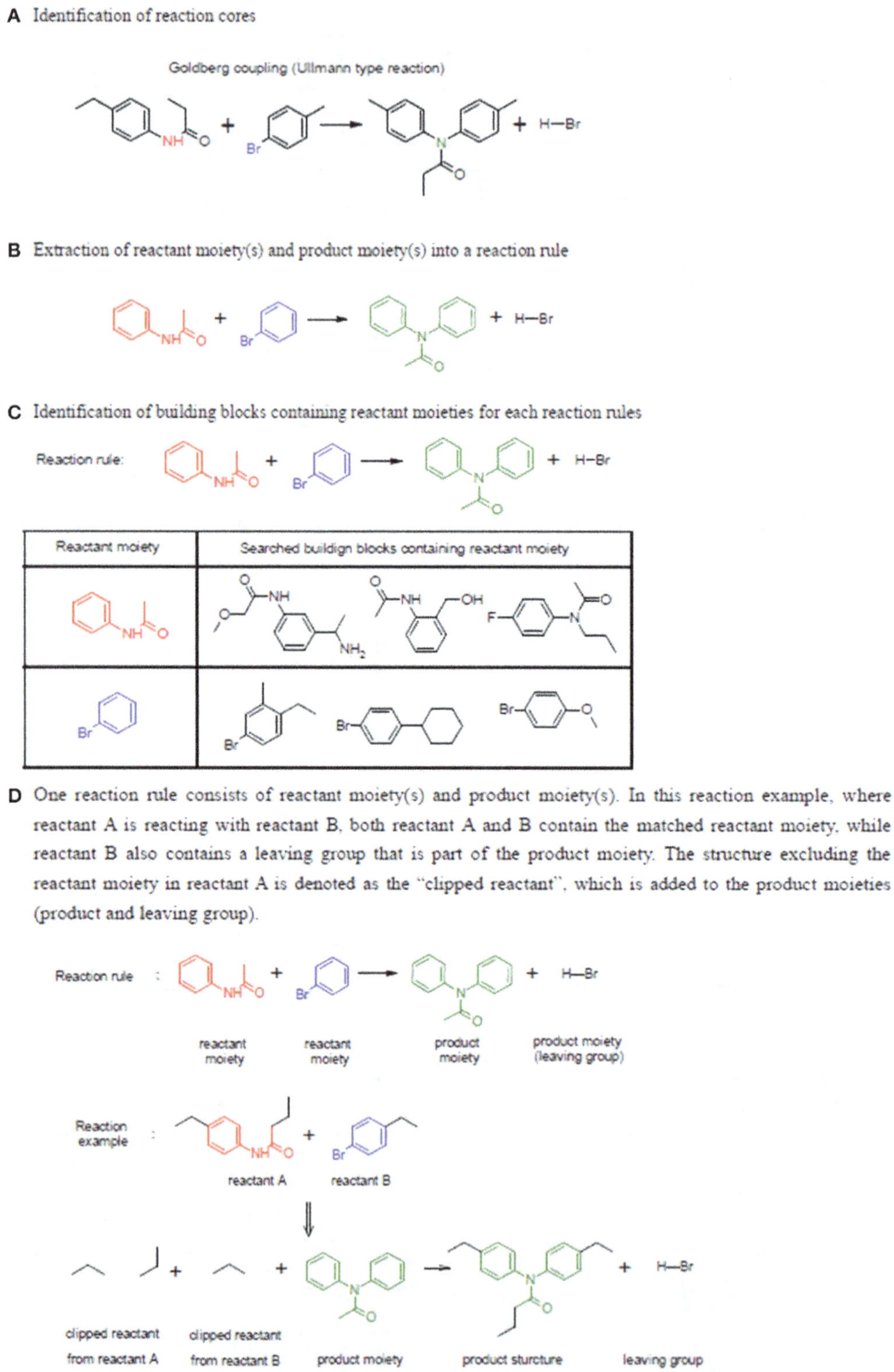

FIGURE 2 | Example of three steps used to construct the table of reaction rules. **(A)** Identification of reaction cores. The atoms with changed atom attributes are highlighted in red and blue within the two reactants. **(B)** Extraction of the moieties. **(C)** Identification of building blocks containing the reactant moieties. **(D)** Illustration of the steps in generating products.

step, that product molecule becomes the next reactant in the next synthesis step.

Determine Reaction Rules for Each Reactant Identified

When a reactant is identified in the previous step, there are many potential reactant moieties and reactions associated with this reactant. Each reactant is subjected to sub-structure searching[2] to identify atom arrangements (moieties) that are part of a chemical reaction rule within the LeadOP+R reaction database. This is done to determine potential chemical reactions for this specific reactant.

Generation of Reaction Products Based on Reaction Rules

Once all the potential reaction rules of a reactant are identified, the corresponding products are generated by "reacting" the reactant moieties and participant reactants (**Figure 2D**). In LeadOp+R, each reactant has two parts: one structure matches the reactant moiety and the other structure—excluding the reactant moiety—is denoted as the "clipped reactant." The same definition is used for other building blocks (participants) involved in a reaction. Each product is generated by combining the clipped portion of the reactant and the clipped portion of the participants as well as the product moiety based on the search of the reaction rule.

Evaluation of the Products for Each Reaction

Thirty conformers of each product are generated using the Java and JChem application-programming interface (Imre et al., 2006). Each conformer is aligned with the preserved space of the query molecule, while maximizing the overlap volumes, using the flexible 3D alignment tool of Marvin[3] (see **Figure 3**). A conformer for each product was selected for the next step if the following criteria are met: (1) the binding mode of each conformer, aligned with the query molecule within the receptor site, has the same inhibitor-receptor interaction direction, and (2) the new moiety has a group efficiency value <−0.1.

Final Selection by Structure-Based Analysis

The selected conformer for each product is the reactants for the next reaction in the selected inhibitor-receptor interaction direction. The molecule continues to grow until all the inhibitor-receptor interaction directions are exhausted. The collection of potential new compounds is reduced using the following criteria: molecular weight <600 g mol^{-1} and a calculated lipophilicity (cLogP) <5, which is taken into account based on the Lipinski's Rule-of-Five (Lipinski et al., 2001). The compounds that pass the molecular property filters comprised the final list of proposed compounds. These compounds are then energy-minimized within the binding site and ranked based on the overall ligand-receptor binding energy.

[2]"JChem." 5.4.1.1 ed. (Budapest, Hungary: ChemAxon Ltd).
[3]"Marvin." 5.4.0.1 ed., (Budapest, Hungary: ChemAxon Ltd).

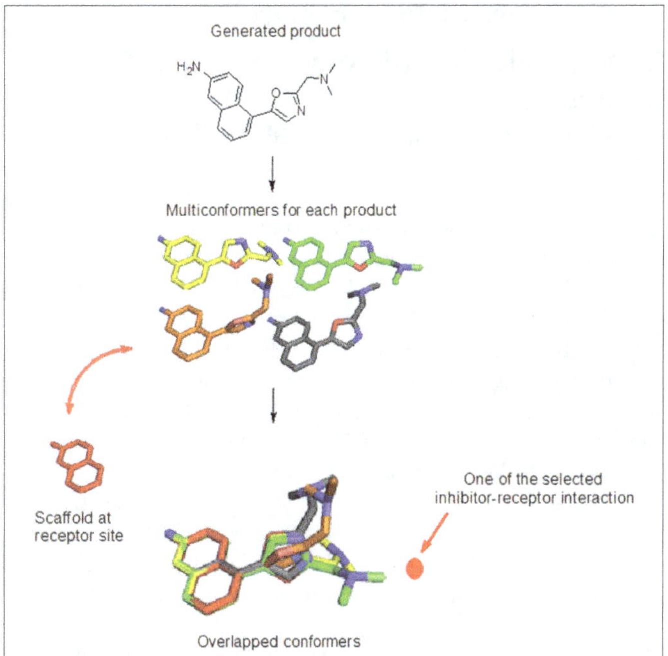

FIGURE 3 | Evaluation of each product for each reaction. Thirty conformers are generated (colored in yellow, green, orange, and gray sticks) and overlaid with the reactant within the binding site (colored in red stick). The user-defined inhibitor-receptor interaction direction (location) is indicated by the dotted red line.

Molecular Dynamics Simulations

The bound pose of the newly "constructed" compound, as determined with AutoDock Vina (Trott and Olson, 2010), is refined from the lowest binding free energy and the largest number of favorable ligand-receptor interactions within the binding site. The unfavorable contacts between the docked pose of the energy minimized "constructed" compound (fragments connected to the initial core of the compound) and the residues within the binding site are alleviated using molecular dynamics simulations; allowing the ligand-receptor complex to explore the local energy landscape. The best complex pose (ligand-receptor interaction) was selected and molecular dynamics was performed using GROMACS version 4.03 (Hess et al., 2008) and the GROMOS 53A6 force field (Oostenbrink et al., 2005). The complexes are placed in a simple cubic periodic box of SPC216 type water molecules (Berendsen et al., 1981), and the distance between the protein and each edge of the box was set to 0.9 nm. To maintain overall electrostatic neutrality and isotonic conditions, Na^+ and Cl^- ions were randomly positioned within the solvation box. To maintain the proper structure and remove unfavorable van der Waals contacts, a 1,000-step steepest descent energy minimization was employed and terminated when the convergence criteria of an energy difference between subsequent steps differ <1,000 kJ mol^{-1} nm^{-1}. Following the energy minimization, the system is subjected to a 1,200 ps molecular dynamics simulation at constant temperature (300 K), pressure (1 atm), and a time step of 0.002 ps (2 fs) with the coordinates of the system recorded every ps.

RESULT AND DISCUSSION

LeadOp+R Optimization for Tie-2 Kinase Inhibitors

Structure-Based Lead Optimization With Synthetic Routes

From the literature (Bridges, 2001), it is known that a good kinase inhibitors should possess a hydrogen-bond donor/acceptor/donor motif to best interact with the backbone carbonyl/NH(amide)/carbonyl presented in the ATP-binding cleft. In the case of Tie-2 kinase, the residues in the active site of the ATP-binding cleft are Ala905 (carbonyl and amide NH) and Glu903 (carbonyl). Additionally, two hydrophobic pockets are part of the active site in the Tie-2 receptor and are designated as the first hydrophobic pocket (HP) and the extended hydrophobic pocket (EHP). We selected a series of Tie-2 inhibitors from the literature (Hodous et al., 2007) containing a co-crystal structure of inhibitor compound 47 with Tie-2 receptor (PDB code: 2p4i). In this co-crystal structure, the 2-(methylamino)pyrimidine ring of inhibitor compound 47 interacts with residue Ala905 via two hydrogen bonds and the pyrimidine is also within van der Waals contact of the Glu903. The central methyl-substituted aryl ring of compound 47 resides in the first hydrophobic pocket (HP), while the pyridine ring forms an edge-to-face π-stacking interaction with Phe983 of the DFG-motif. The carbonyl oxygen makes a hydrogen bond with the backbone NH of Asp982 (DFG motif) and the aryl amide moiety directs the terminal CF_3-substituted aromatic ring into the EHP. **Figure 4A** illustrates the ligand-protein interaction of this co-crystal structure.

To demonstrate how LeadOp+R optimizes a compound automatically while considering the potential synthetic route, compound 46 is the query molecule for lead optimization (denoted as compound rA in this study) with a biologically determined IC_{50} value of 399 nM (Hodous et al., 2007). Compound rA was docked into the Tie-2 binding site and the lowest energy conformation was selected. The selected conformation possessed similar molecular interactions, as discussed earlier, with the Tie-2 active site (**Figure 4A**). The amide functional group of compound rA forms a hydrogen bond with the backbone amide of Asp982, while the pyridine and benzene rings extend into the hydrophobic pocket (HP) and EHP, respectively. The aminobenzoic fragment was designated as the preserved space in this example of LeadOp+R due to the important hydrogen bonding.

To evaluate our algorithm, we compared all of the LeadOp+R generated compounds to Tie-2 kinase inhibitor from the literature and found nine of the LeadOp+R compounds have also been synthesized and their ability to inhibit Tie-2 kinase measured. The inclusive synthesis of proposed products in each LeadOp+R step combined with systematically examining the proposed ligand-receptor interactions resulted in nine compounds with more potent IC_{50} values than the original compound (compound rA). All the LeadOp+R generated compounds were energy minimized in the active site of Tie-2, and then ranked on the basis of the overall ligand–receptor interaction energy. Among all LeadOp+R suggested compounds, nine compounds were previously studied in the literature (Hodous et al., 2007), and the priority suggested by the calculated binding energy had same trend as the experimentally determined IC_{50} values. In this study of Tie-2 kinase inhibitor design—three compounds, denoted as compounds rA1, rA2, and rA3 of the nine LeadOp+R generated compounds—were selected for further investigation. For these three compounds we found detailed synthetic route information (Hodous et al., 2007) and inhibition potency in the literature. These three compound rA1-rA3, have a higher potency than the query compound rA and the suggested priority of the new compounds with the calculated binding energy have a similar IC_{50} potency trend. Depicted representations of compounds rA1-rA3, as well as the corresponding inhibition data from the biological experiments and their predicted binding energy are provided in **Table 1.**

Molecular dynamics simulations were performed with three LeadOp+R generated compounds, rA1–rA3, to further analyze the ligand-protein interactions within the Tie-2 kinase active site. Following geometry optimization of the compounds with respect to Tie-2, molecular dynamics simulation studies were performed and the unique low-energy conformations of the complexes, from the final 50 ps of the MDS (50 configurations), are shown in **Figures 4B–D.**

In the generated compounds (rA1, rA2, and rA3) both amide arrangements are engaged in strong hydrogen bonds with Asp982 of the DFG-motif (first three residues of the activation loop). The pyrimidine ring in compounds rA1 and rA2 makes key hydrogen bonds with the backbone amide of the linker residue Ala905, situating the pyridine rings in alignment and within edge-to-face π-stacking distance of Phe983 of the DFG-motif. Additionally, the central and terminal aryl rings overlap with only slight differences in orientation for compounds rA1, rA2, and rA3. The additional a hydrogen bond forms between the methoxy group of compound rA1 and residue Asp982, while the CF_3-groups are placed in essentially the same location within the EHP for compounds rA2 and rA3. These optimized results indicate the hydrogen-bonding and hydrophobic interactions are important for ligands binding to and inhibiting Tie-2, as previously reported (Hodous et al., 2007).

Synthetic Routes Suggested by LeadOp+R

For Tie-2 kinase inhibitors, favorable interactions occur between the ligand and the specific receptor residues Glu 872, Asp 982, Phe983, Ala905, and Glu903 (see **Figure 4A**). In this example, these interactions are selected as preferred inhibitor-receptor interactions for LeadOp+R to optimize based on the provided query molecule in a selective and systematic process. Experimental synthetic routes from the literature (Hodous et al., 2007; **Figures 5A, 6A, 7A**) and the reaction routes suggested by LeadOp+R (**Figures 5B, 6B, 7B**) to generate compound rA1, rA2, and rA3 are summarized below to demonstrate how LeadOP+R suggests the synthetic reaction routes that are similar to those proposed by organic and medicinal chemists. Matched reaction rules are listed to the right of **Figures 4C, 5C, 6C** with details of each synthetic step identified by LeadOp+R, for each product, described below.

Figure 5A illustrates the experimental reactions required to synthesize compound rA1 (compound **7**) by reacting **5** (which

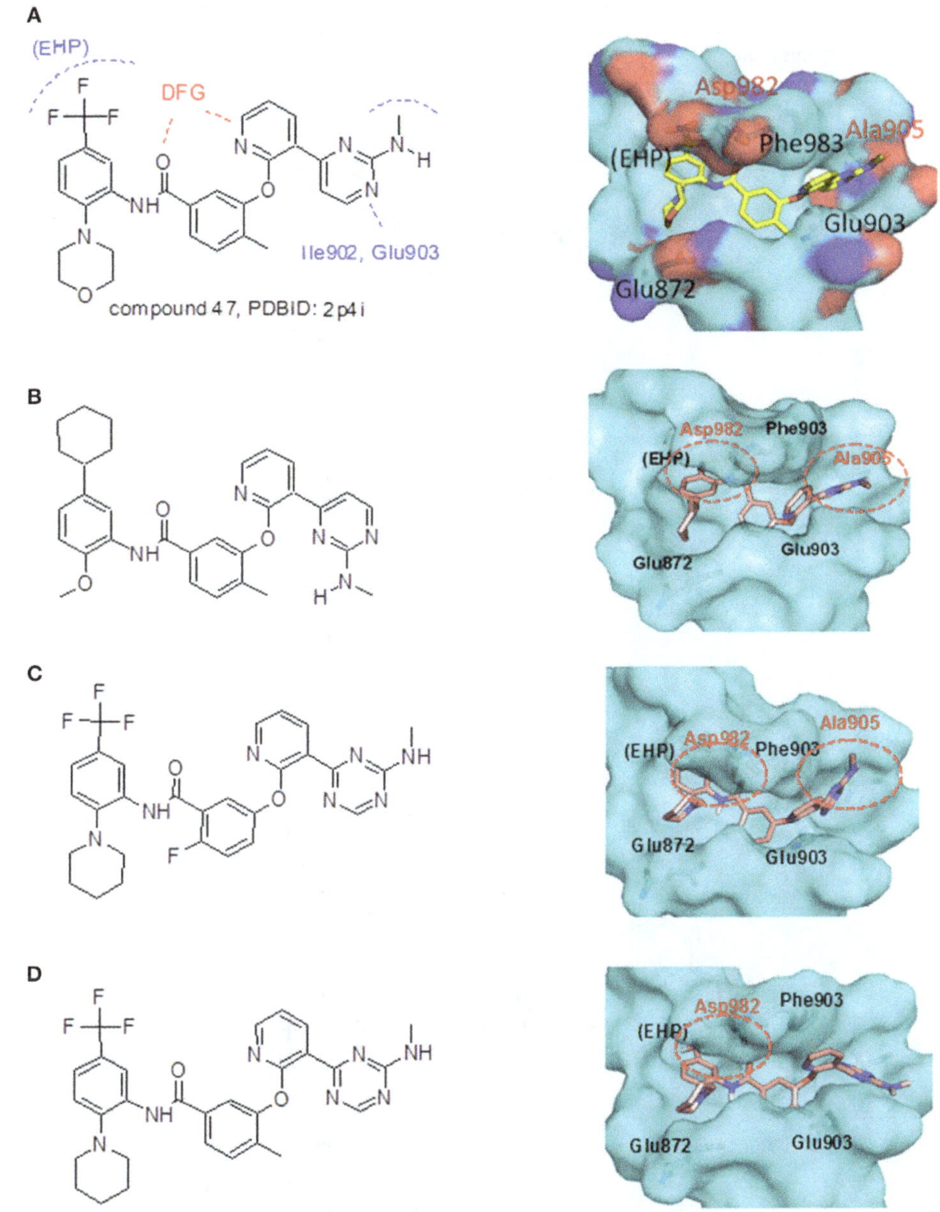

FIGURE 4 | LeadOp+R result for the Tie-2 model system. **(A)** Chemical characteristic of each residue and interaction within the complex of compound 47 from the co-crystal structure (PDB code: 2p4i). **(B–D)** Chemical structure (left) and MDS result (right) of the generated compound rA1 **(B)**, the generated compound rA2 **(C)**, and the generated compound rA3 **(D)**. Carbon atoms are colored pink. Amino acid residues that participate in hydrogen-bonding interactions (labeled red) with the proposed compound at the binding site are depicted with cyan molecular surface.

was generated through transforming **2** into **4**) followed by reacting **1** with **6**. To compare LeadOp+R's suggested virtual synthesis of compound rA1 to proven synthetic routes; we compared the key reaction rules from experimental synthetic steps in the literature.

Figure 5B shows the LeadOp+R suggested synthetic routes to generate compound rA1 using the selected and preferred inhibitor-receptor interactions that allowed LeadOp+R to selectively and systematically optimize the query molecule. Initially, compound **1** was identified as the first reactant by searching all building blocks with the preserved fragment. LeadOp+R then proceed to produce product **8** by coupling **1** with **6** with the reaction rule (i) that conserves the preferred interaction with Glu872 specified. The reaction rule suggested by LeadOp+R matched the synthetic steps in the literature that forms compound **7** by combining compound **5** and fragment **6**. Next, product **8** was considered as the reactant to interact with compound **2** to generate product **9** by growing molecules

TABLE 1 | Rank of the proposed LeadOp+R compounds based on the calculated binding energy, inhibition concentration (IC_{50}) of Tie-2 from the literature (Hodous et al., 2007).

Rank	Structure	Inhibition IC_{50} (nM)
Query	*rA* 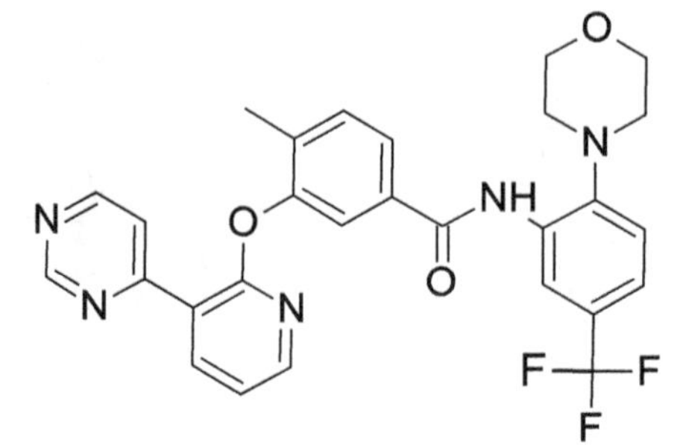	399
38	*rA1* 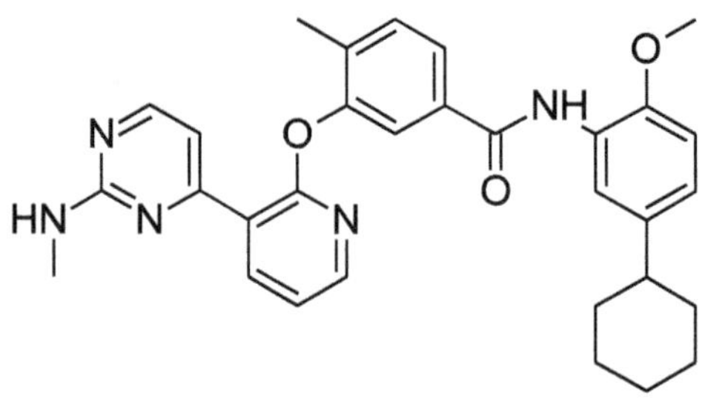	4
113	*rA2* 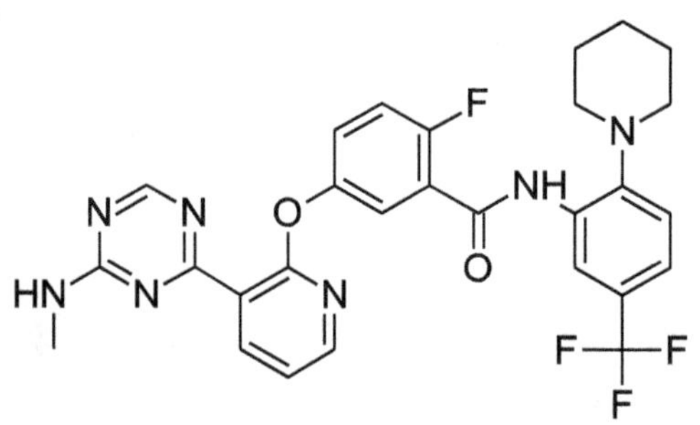	30
292	*rA3* 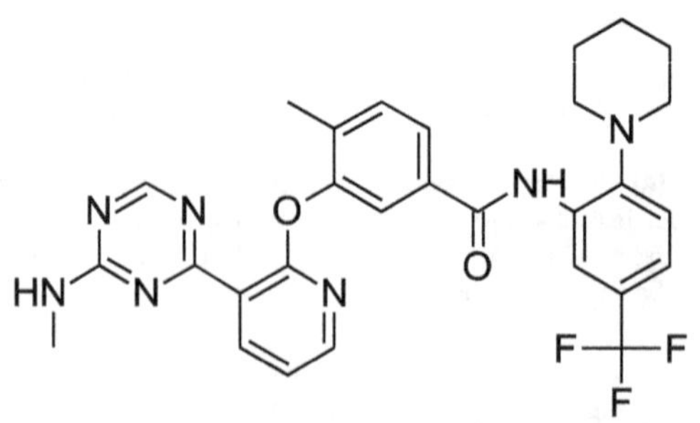	108

All proposed compounds have a lower IC_{50} value than the query compound and the suggested priority of the three new compounds (out of 631) have a similar trend as the IC_{50} potency values.

with preferred interaction toward Phe983. The second reaction rule (ii) suggested by LeadOp+R lead to product **9** that matched the same synthetic steps as those in the literature to synthesize compound **5** by reacting **1** with **4**. It is interesting to note that at this step, the structure marked in red is the current structure **9**, the same partial structure highlighted in red within the final product **7** (compound rA1) in the experimental synthesis. LeadOp+R continued the recursive optimization toward the

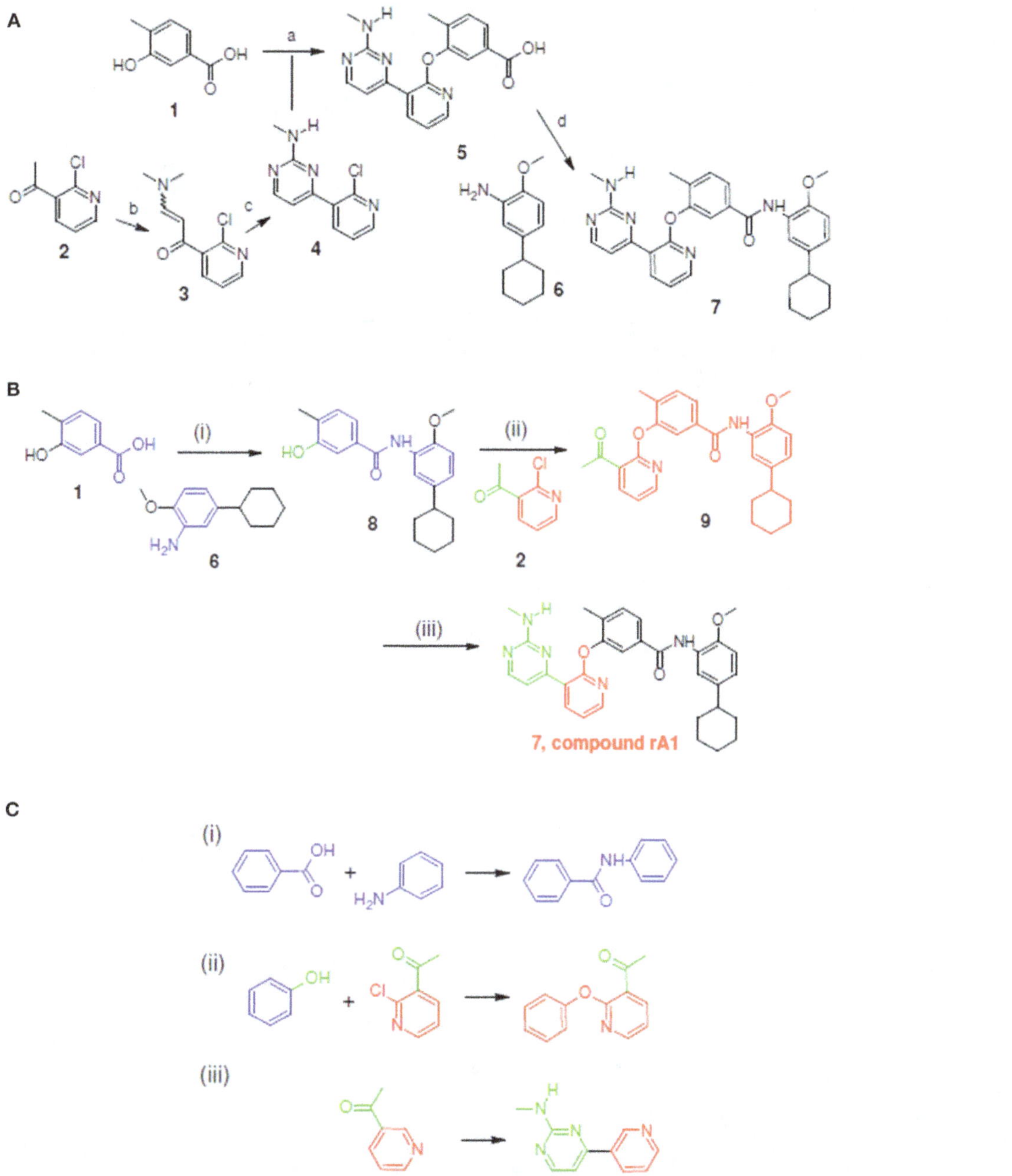

FIGURE 5 | Synthetic routes for compound rA1 and sub-structure searching to identify atom arrangements (moieties) that are part of a chemical reaction rule within the LeadOp+R reaction database. **(A)** Synthetic routes with reagents and condition (a–d) from experimental studies (Hodous et al., 2007). **(B)** Synthetic routes and **(C)** matched reaction rules provided by LeadOp+R.

cavity near Phe983 and Ala905 to transform **9** to **7** (compound rA1) with the third reaction rule, **Figure 5C**. This reaction route suggested by LeadOp+R also matches the experimental synthetic route in the literature to transform **2** into **4**. To this end, LeadOp+R has successfully optimized the query compound rA to compound rA1 and suggested corresponding synthetic routes. In this example, we demonstrated how LeadOp+R controls the synthetic flow by extending the molecules with preferred interactions, available building blocks and associated reactions rules to reach fragment based optimization and synthetic accessible. Thus, the sequence of reactions to "grow" molecules may not be the same as those verified in experimental synthesis.

Figure 6A shows the experimental reaction to synthesize compound rA2 (compound **19**) by reacting **18** (which was generated through the transformation of **13–18**) with **12** (which was generated through the reaction of **10** with **11**). To compare

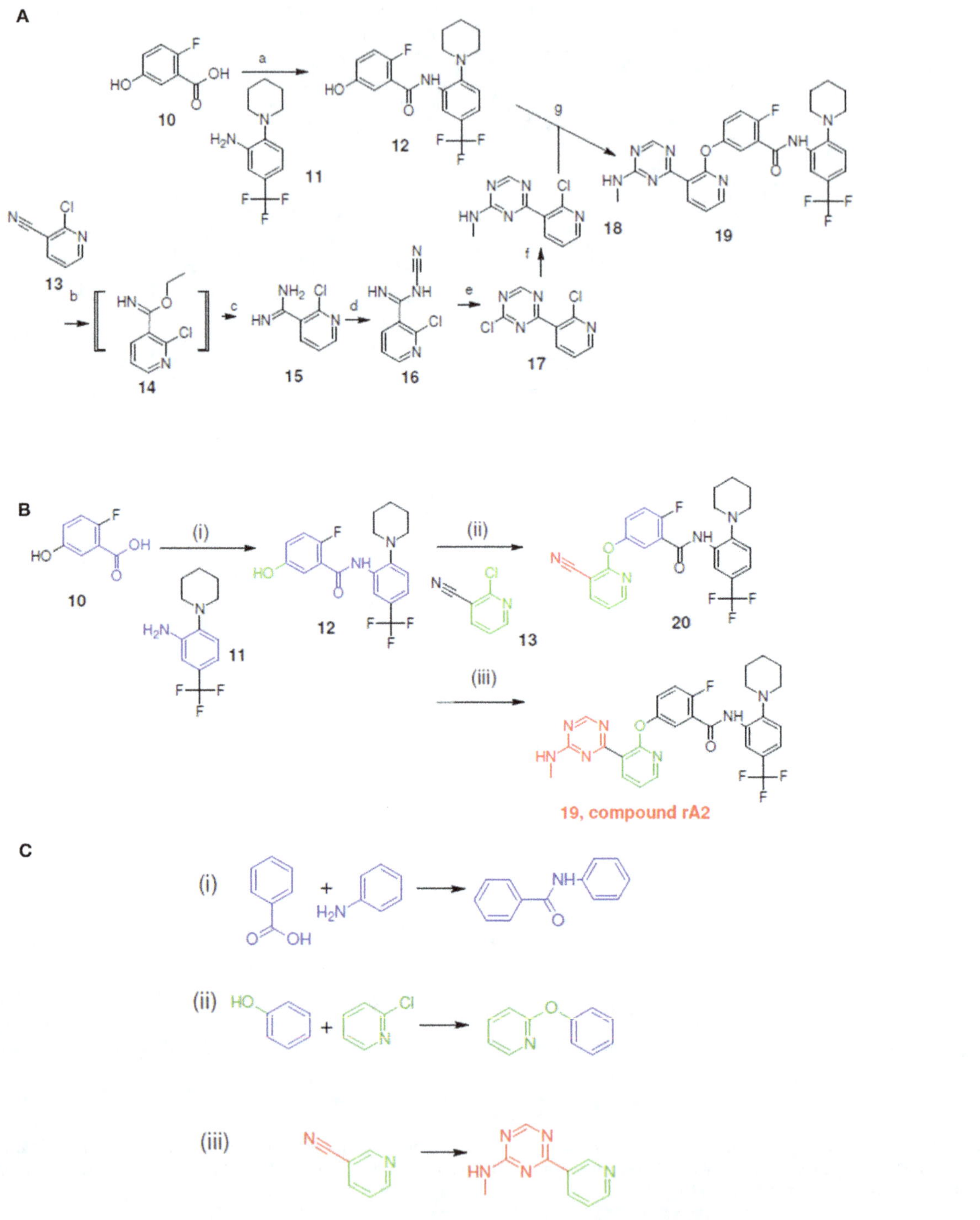

FIGURE 6 | Synthetic routes for compound rA2 and sub-structure searching to identify atom arrangements (moieties) that are part of a chemical reaction rule within the LeadOp+R reaction database. **(A)** Synthetic routes with reagents and condition (a–g) from experimental studies (Hodous et al., 2007). **(B)** Synthetic routes and **(C)** matched reaction rules provided by LeadOp+R.

the LeadOp+R suggested virtual synthesis route for compound rA2 with the experimental synthetic route, we compared the key reaction rules from the experimental synthetic steps in the literature with the LeadOp+R suggested synthetic routes.

Figure 6B shows the LeadOp+R suggested synthetic routes for compound rA2, using the selected and preferred inhibitor-receptor interactions to optimize the query molecule in a selective and systematic manner. Initially, a hydroxy benzoic acid of **10**

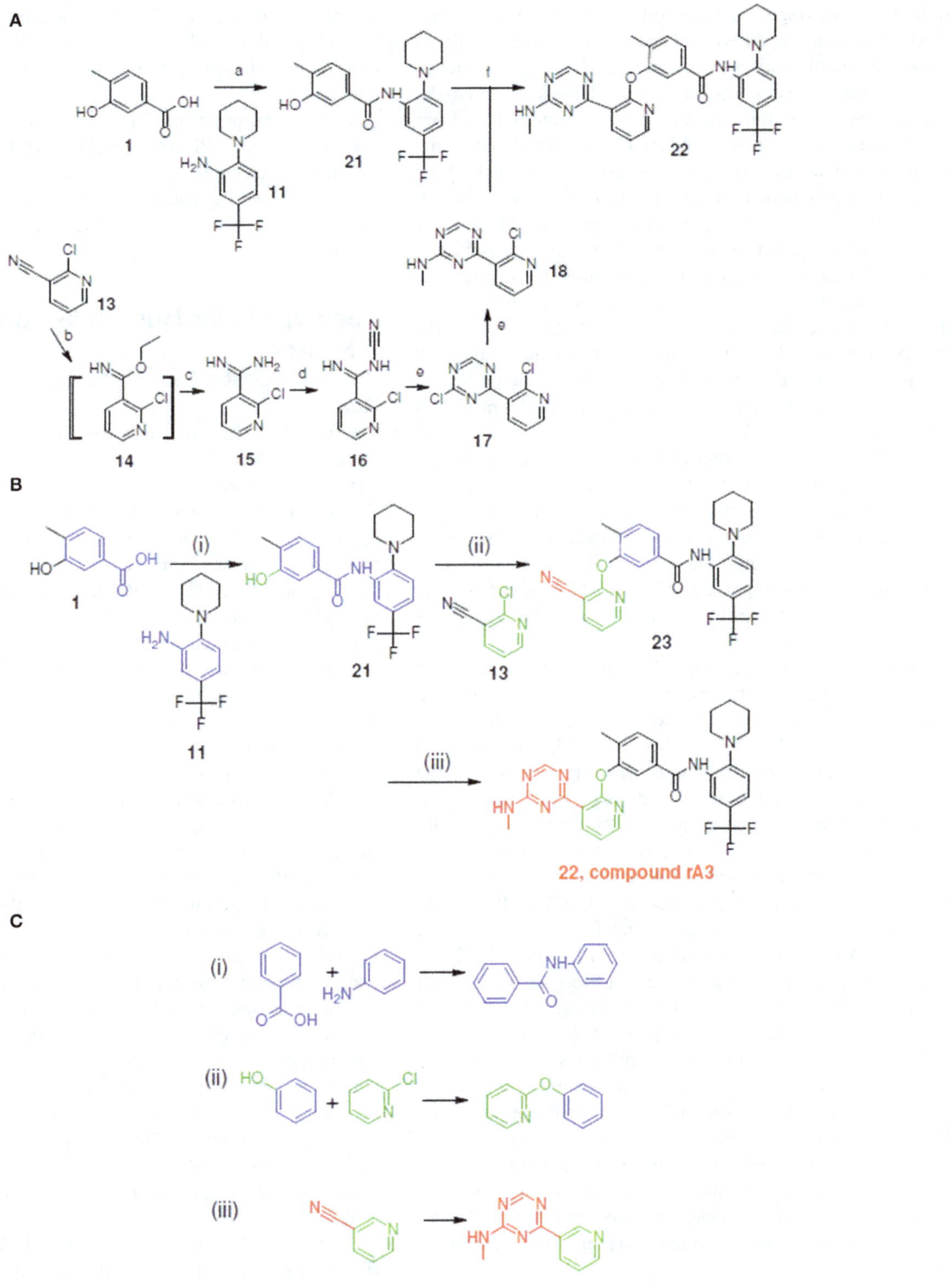

FIGURE 7 | Synthetic routes for compound rA3 and sub-structure searching to identify atom arrangements (moieties) that are part of a chemical reaction rule within the LeadOp+R reaction database. **(A)** Synthetic routes with reagents and condition (a–f) from experimental studies (Hodous et al., 2007). **(B)** Synthetic routes and **(C)** matched reaction rules provided by LeadOp+R.

was identified as the first reactant by searching all building blocks with the preserved fragment. LeadOp+R then proceed to suggest product **12** by reacting **10** with **11** via the first reaction rule (i) that preserves the ligand's interaction with Glu972 of the active site. The reaction rule suggested by LeadOp+R matched the synthetic steps in the literature that forms compound **12** from compounds **10** and **11**. Next, product **12** was considered as the reactant to react with compound **13** to generate product **20**, by growing molecules with preferred interaction toward Phe983. The second reaction rule (ii) generates product **20** and the reaction route suggested by LeadOp+R matches the synthetic steps in the literature to synthesize compound **19** through the reaction of **12** with **18**. LeadOp+R's recursive optimization continues toward the cavity near Phe983 and Ala905 to transform **20** to **19** (compound rA2) via the third reaction rule (iii), **Figure 6C**. This reaction route suggested by LeadOp+R also matched the experimental synthetic step in the literature to transform compound **13–18.**

Figure 7A shows the experimental reaction to synthesize compound rA3 (compound **22**) by reacting **21** (which was generated through the reaction of **1** with **11**) with **18** (which was synthesized from **13**). To compare LeadOp+R's suggested synthesis route for compound rA3 with the experimental synthetic routes, we compared the key reaction rules from the experimental synthetic steps in the literature with the LeadOp+R suggested synthetic routes.

Figure 7B depicts the LeadOp+R suggested synthetic routes to generate compound rA3, using the selected and preferred inhibitor-receptor interactions to optimize the query molecule. Initially, compound **1**, a hydroxybenzoic acid, was identified as the first reactant by searching all building blocks with the preserved fragment indicated in red, **Figure 7B**. LeadOp+R then proceeded to produce compound **21** by reacting **1** with **11** via the first reaction rule (i) directing the growth of the compound (inhibitor) toward the preferred ligand interaction with Glu972. The reaction rule suggested by LeadOp+R matched the synthetic steps in the literature that forms compound **21** via the transformation of compound **1** with fragment **11**. Next, product **21** was reacted with compound **13** to generate product **23**, growing the transformed molecule toward Phe983. The second reaction rule (ii) generated product **22** as suggested by LeadOp+R and matches the same synthetic steps as those in the literature to synthesize compound **22** through the reaction of compound **21** with fragment **18**. The recursive optimization of the initial query compound toward the cavity near Phe983 and Ala905 by LeadOp+R transformed compound **23** to **22** (compound rA3) with the third reaction rule (iii) as illustrated in **Figure 7C**. This reaction rule, suggested by LeadOp+R, also matches the experimental synthetic step in the literature to transform **13–18.**

LeadOp+R has successfully optimized the query compound rA to compounds rA1, rA2, and rA3 with synthetic routes that match experimental synthetic routes for each compound. Through the systematic synthesis and constant evaluation of intermediate products via group efficiency, LeadOp+R searched each product and discovered higher binding inhibitors. Increased hydrophobic interactions between compound rA1 and the receptor were observed between the compound's aromatic group that resides in the EHP pocket (**Figure 4B**) and the methylpyrimidine. This corresponds to the experimental results and rA1 exhibits stronger inhibitor potency than compounds rA2 and rA3.

In the example of Tie-2 inhibitor design, LeadOp+R demonstrates its ability to control the synthetic flow by extending the query molecules to optimize the preferred ligand-receptor interactions while using the available building blocks and associated reactions rules to find the most feasible synthetic accessibility.

LeadOp+R for Human 5-Lipoxygenase Inhibitor

Structure-Based Lead Optimization With Synthetic Routes

The human 5-Lipoxygenase (5-LOX) enzyme with the well-known 5-LOX inhibitors was selected as the second LeadOp+R test case. To design better 5-LOX inhibitors, structural insight of the 5-LOX active site and its associated interactions with ligands would be helpful; therefore we selected a theoretical model (comparative/homology protein structure/model) of 5-LOX (Charlier et al., 2006) that has good agreement with mutagenesis studies (Hammarberg et al., 1995; Schwarz et al., 2001). The proposed active site of 5-LOX forms a deep and bent cleft (channel) that extends from Phe177 and Tyr181 at the top of the cleft to the Trp599 and Leu420 amino acid residues at the bottom of the cleft (shown in **Figure 8A**). Most of the residues lining the cleft are hydrophobic with several *key* polar residues (Gln363, Asn425, Gln557, Ser608, and Arg411) distributed along the channel with the ability to interact with the ligand during the binding process. A small side pocket off of the main channel is composed of hydrophobic residues (Phe421, Gln363, and Lue368) and it is postulated that the lipophilic interactions between the ligand and receptor may enhance activity. The purported major pharmacophore interactions needed for a ligand to bind to 5-LOX includes: (i) two hydrophobic groups, (ii) a hydrogen bond acceptor, (iii) an aromatic ring, and (iv) two secondary interactions. The two secondary interactions are between the ligand and an acidic moiety (amino acid residue) and a hydrogen bond acceptor within the binding pocket of the receptor. The hydrogen bond acceptor of the ligand most likely interacts with the key anchoring points of the receptor (Tyr181, Asn425, and Arg411) to form hydrogen bonds, while Leu414 and Phe421 form a hydrophobic interaction between the ligand and the binding cavity (Charlier et al., 2006).

The 5-LOX inhibitor, compound 7 in the literature (Ducharme et al., 2010), was selected as our initial query molecule (denoted as compound rB in this study), which had a biologically determined IC_{50} value of 145 nM. Compound rB was docked into the 5-LOX computationally derived binding site and the lowest energy conformation was submitted to LeadOp+R. This selected pose (conformation) possesses similar ligand-receptor interactions as previously reported (Charlier et al., 2006). The oxochromen ring favorably interacts with the hydrophobic

A
B
C
D
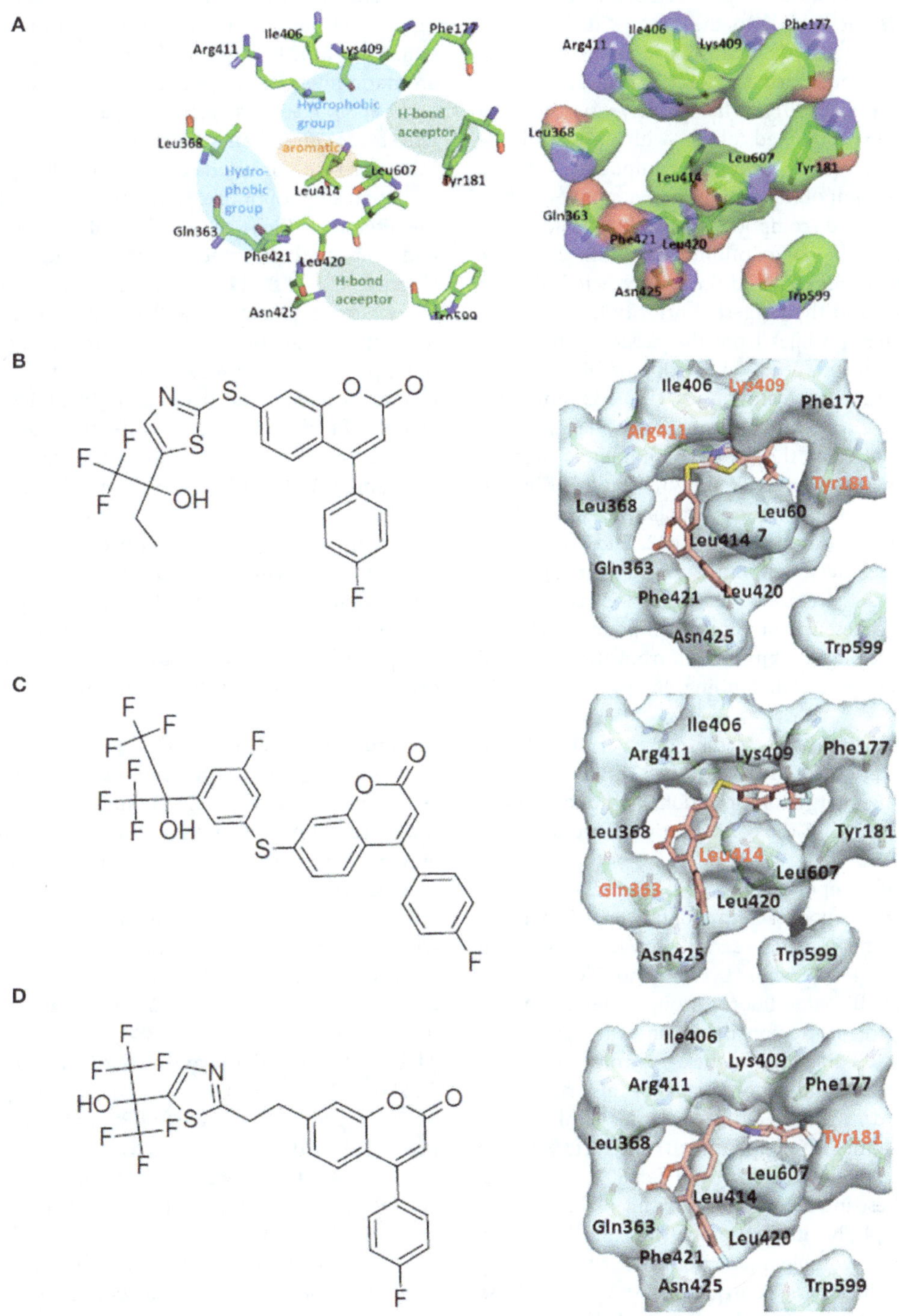

FIGURE 8 | LeadOp+R result for the 5-LOX kinase model system. **(A)** Schematic representation of the human 5-LOX active site (left) and the binding pocket (right). The purported pharmacophores of the binding site of 5-LOX involving two hydrophobic groups (blue ovals), two hydrogen bond acceptors (green ovals), and an aromatic ring (orange oval) for ligand binding at the binding cavity. **(B–D)** Chemical structure (left) and MDS result (right) of the generated compound rB1 **(B)**, the generated compound rB2 **(C)**, and the generated compound rB3 **(D)**. Carbon atoms are colored pink. Amino acid residues that participate in hydrogen-bonding interactions (labeled red) with the proposed compound within the binding site are depicted with gray molecular surfaces.

residue Leu414 (CH-π interaction) in the middle of the cavity, while the fluoro phenyl group extends into the hydrogen-bond acceptor region in the lower cleft of the active site. The docked conformation of compound rB was selected as the reference inhibitor with the oxochromen ring serving as the template structure.

To evaluate our algorithm, we compared all of the LeadOp+R generated compounds for 5-LOX to the analogs described in the literature and found that six of the LeadOp+R proposed compounds have been synthesized and their biological activities measured (Schwarz et al., 2001). The inclusive synthesis of products at each step combined along with systematically examining the interactions of the proposed compounds with the receptor generated six compounds with more potent IC_{50} values than the original compound (compound rB). All the LeadOp+R generated compounds were energy minimized within the active site of 5-LOX and then ranked based on the predicted binding energy of the complex and the suggested priority has the same trend as the IC_{50} potency values from the experimental study (Schwarz et al., 2001). In this study of 5-LOX inhibitor design, three compounds (denoted as compounds rB1, rB2, and rB3) of the nine LeadOp+R generated compounds, were selected for further investigation. For these three compounds detailed synthetic information (Ducharme et al., 2010) and inhibition potency is available from the literature (Ducharme et al., 2010). Additionally, these three compound rB1, rB2, and rB3 have a higher potency than the query compound rB and their suggested priority, based on predicted binding energy, as well as a similar IC_{50} trend. Depicted representations of the compounds rB1, rB2, and rB3, the corresponding inhibition data from the biological experiments, and their predicted binding energy are listed in **Table 2.**

Molecular dynamics simulation studies were performed with the final poses of compounds rB1, rB2, and rB3 with respect to 5-LOX. The unique low-energy conformations of the complexes, from the last 50 ps of the MDS (50 configurations), are shown in **Figures 8B–D**.

The interactions of compounds rB1, rB2, and rB3 all reside within the hydrophobic pocket and contain participate in hydrogen bonding interactions between the oxygen or nitrogen atoms of the thiazol group with Lys409 and Tyr181. For compounds rB1 and B3, the fluoro group extends to the hydrogen-bond acceptor in the upper domain of the active site and interacts with Lys409. In addition, the oxochromen ring is in close proximity to Leu414 and is potentially an important CH-π contact as indicated in the literature (Charlier et al., 2006). Also, the thiazole structure of compound rB1 interacts with the 5-LOX hydrophobic residues Leu420 and Leu607 and it has been suggested that these interactions improve ligand binding via complementary hydrophobic interaction between the ligand and receptor. Additionally, favorable interactions occur between the fluoro group and residues Lys409, Arg411, and Tyr181. These contributions to the ligand-protein binding probably accounts for compound rB1's better inhibition compared to compounds rB, rB2, and rB3. These optimized results indicate that hydrogen bonding and hydrophobic interactions are important for ligands binding to and inhibiting, 5-LOX as previous report (Hodous et al., 2007).

Synthetic Routes Suggested by LeadOp+R

The favorable interactions between inhibitors and 5-LOX, as stated in the literature, are two hydrogen-bond acceptor interactions within the binding pocket (including ligand interactions with Asn425 and Tyr181), two hydrophobic interaction pockets (including ligand interactions with Leu368, Gln363, Phe421, Arg411, Ile406, Lys409, and Phe177), and aromatic interactions (between the ligand and residues Leu414 and Leu607). In this example, ligand interactions with Asn425, Leu414, Leu607, and Tyr181 are indicated as "preferred" inhibitor-receptor interactions for LeadOp+R to selectively and systematically optimize. Experimental synthetic routes from the literature (Schwarz et al., 2001) (**Figures 9A, 10A, 11A**) and the synthetic reaction routes suggested by LeadOp+R (**Figures 9B, 10B, 11B**) to generate compound rB1, rB2, and rB3 are summarized below. To demonstrate LeadOp+R's ability to suggest reaction routes similar—or exactly the same—to those proposed and executed by synthetic chemists, the matched reaction rules are listed to the right of **Figures 9C, 10C, 11C**. Details of each synthetic step, identified by LeadOp+R for each product (proposed compounds/inhibitor), are described below.

Figure 9A shows the experimental reaction route (Schwarz et al., 2001) to synthesize compound rB1 (compound **30**) by reacting compound **26** (which was generated through the reaction of **24** with **25**) with **29** (which was generated through the reaction of **27** with **28**). To compare the LeadOp+R suggested synthesis with the experimental synthetic route for compound rB1, we compared the key reaction rules for the experimental synthetic steps in the literature with those suggested by LeadOp+R.

Figure 9B shows the LeadOp+R suggested synthetic routes to generate compound rB1 using the selected preferred inhibitor-receptor interactions. Compound **24** was identified as the initial reactant by searching all the available building blocks and preserving the molecular fragment. LeadOp+R suggested product **26** by reacting **24** with **25** with the first reaction rule (i) "growing" the compound toward the preferred interaction with Asn425. The reaction rule suggested by LeadOp+R matches the synthetic steps in the literature that yields compounds **26, 24,** and **25**. Next, product **26** was considered as the reactant to interact with compound **28** to generate product compound **31** by extending the ligand toward preferred interactions with Leu414. The second reaction rule (ii) to generate compound **31**, as suggested by LeadOp+R, matches the synthetic routes presented in the literature to synthesize the thioether bond in compound **30** through the reaction of **26** with **29**. It should be indicated that in this step, the structure marked in red is compound **31** and it is the same as the partial structure denoted in red for the final product **30** (compound rB1) in the experimental synthesis. The recursive optimization continues via LeadOp+R toward the cavity near Ile406 and the synthesis of compound **30** (compound rB1) by reacting **31** with **27** and the third reaction rule (iii) in **Figure 9C**. The LeadOp+R suggested reaction route also matches the experimental synthetic step in the literature to synthesize compound **29** through the reaction of **27** with **28**. To this end, LeadOp+R has successfully optimized the query compound rB to compound rB1 and suggested feasible synthetic routes. In this example, we demonstrated LeadOp+R's control of the synthetic flow by extending the molecules to exploit preferred interactions, available building blocks, and associated reactions rules to achieve fragment based optimization and synthetic

TABLE 2 | Rank of the proposed LeadOp+R compounds based on the calculated binding energy, inhibition contraction (IC_{50}) of 5-LOX from the literature (Ducharme et al., 2010).

Rank	Structure	Inhibition IC_{50} (nM)
Query	*rB* 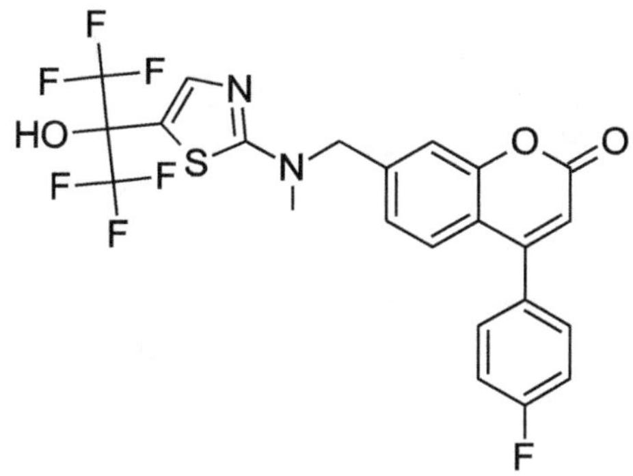	145
52	*rB1* 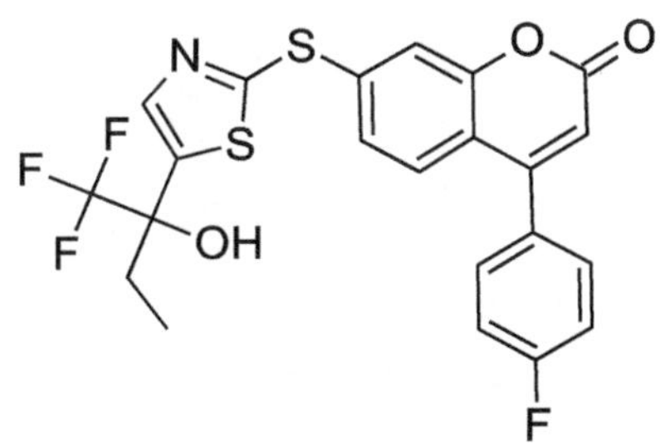	7 ± 2
107	*rB2* 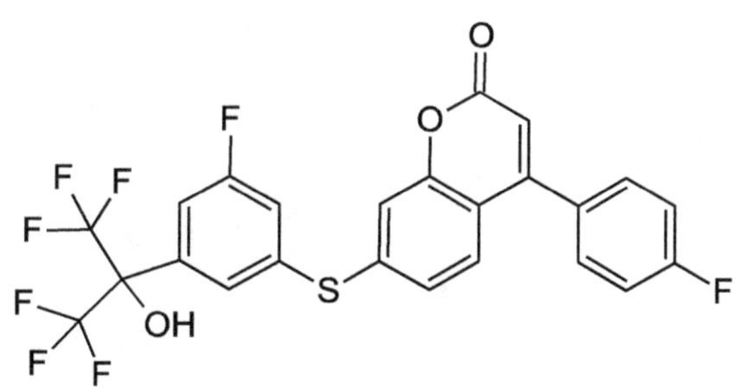	27 ± 16
297	*rB3* 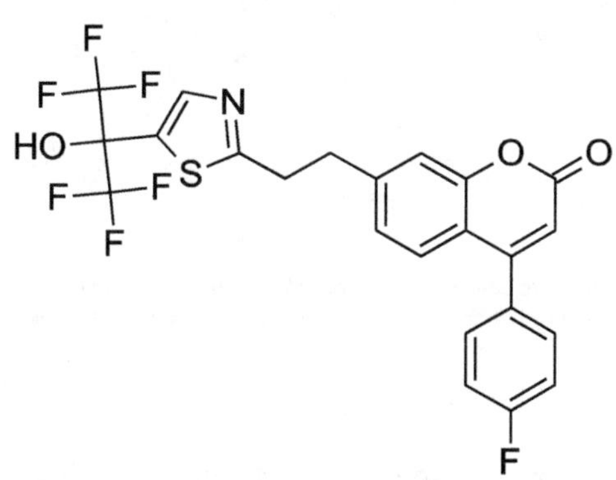	64 ± 3

All proposed compounds have a higher IC_{50} value than the query compound and the suggested priority of the three new compounds (out of 419) have a similar trend as the IC_{50} potency values.

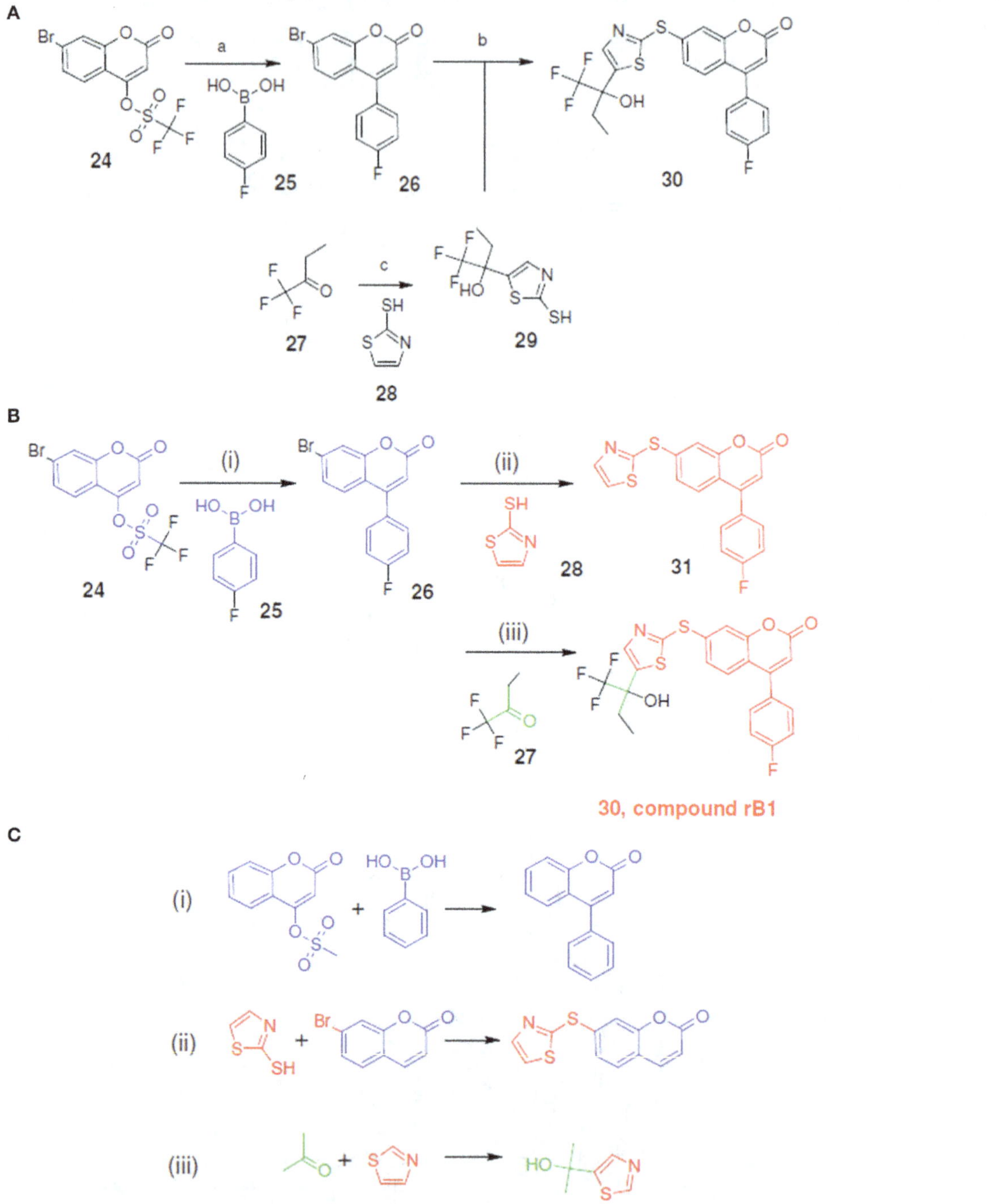

FIGURE 9 | Synthetic routes for compound rB1 and sub-structure searching to identify atom arrangements (moieties) that are part of a chemical reaction rule within the LeadOp+R reaction database. **(A)** Synthetic routes with reagents and condition (a–c) from experimental studies (Ducharme et al., 2010). **(B)** Synthetic routes and **(C)** matched reaction rules provided by LeadOp+R.

accessibility. For these reasons, the sequence of steps to "grow" molecules may not be the same as the published experimental synthesis.

Figure 10A depicts the experimental reaction scheme (Schwarz et al., 2001) to synthesize compound rB2 (compound **38**) by reacting **26** (which was generated through the reaction of **24** with **25**) with **37** (which was synthesized through a series of reaction starting with compound **32** to formed **37**). To compare LeadOp+R's suggested synthesis of compound rB2 to the experimental synthetic routes, we explored the key reaction rules of the experimental synthetic steps in the literature for the proposed compound.

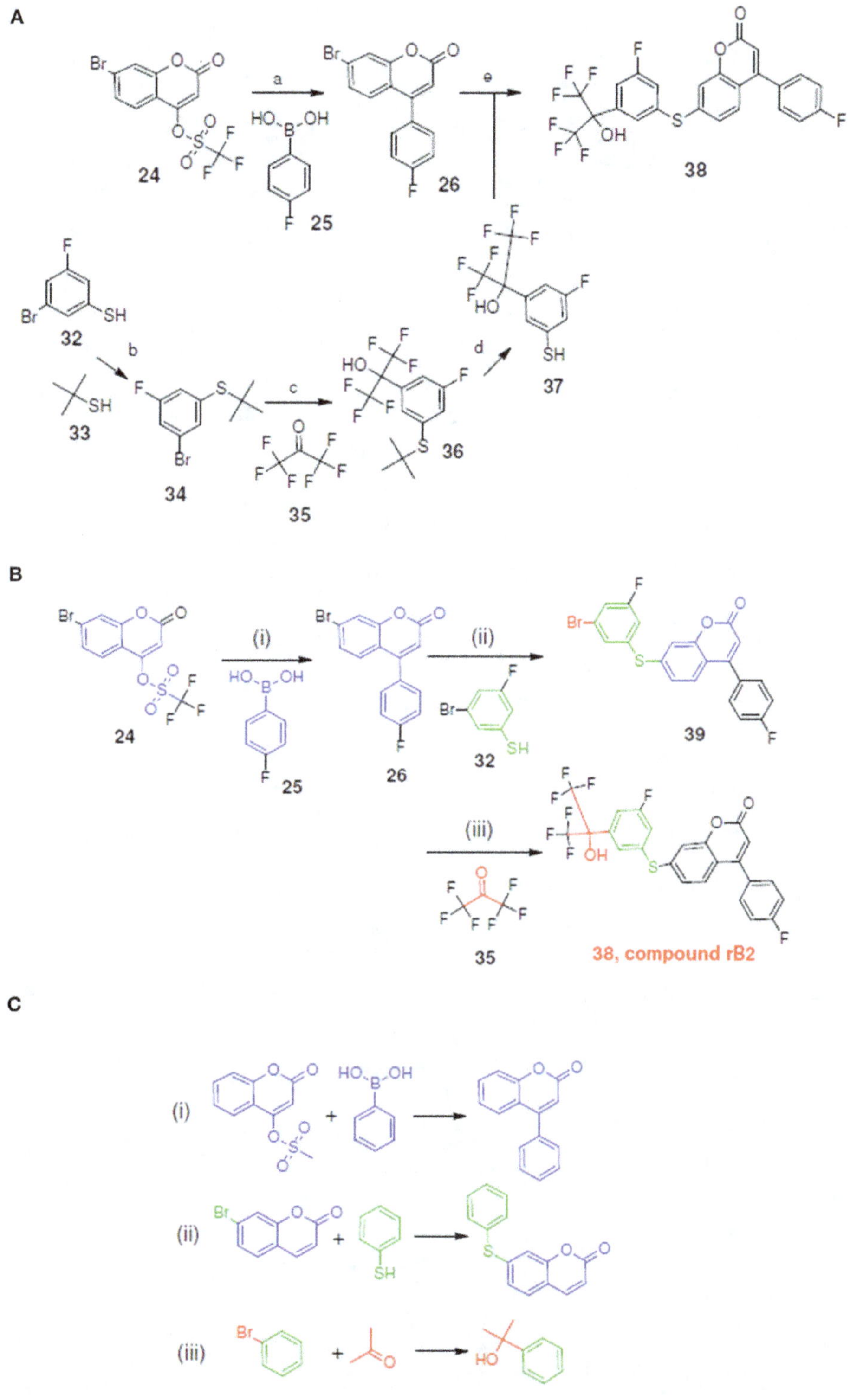

FIGURE 10 | Synthetic routes for compound rB2 and sub-structure searching to identify atom arrangements (moieties) that are part of a chemical reaction rule within the LeadOp+R reaction database. **(A)** Synthetic routes with reagents and condition (a–e) from experimental studies (Ducharme et al., 2010). **(B)** Synthetic routes and **(C)** matched reaction rules provided by LeadOp+R.

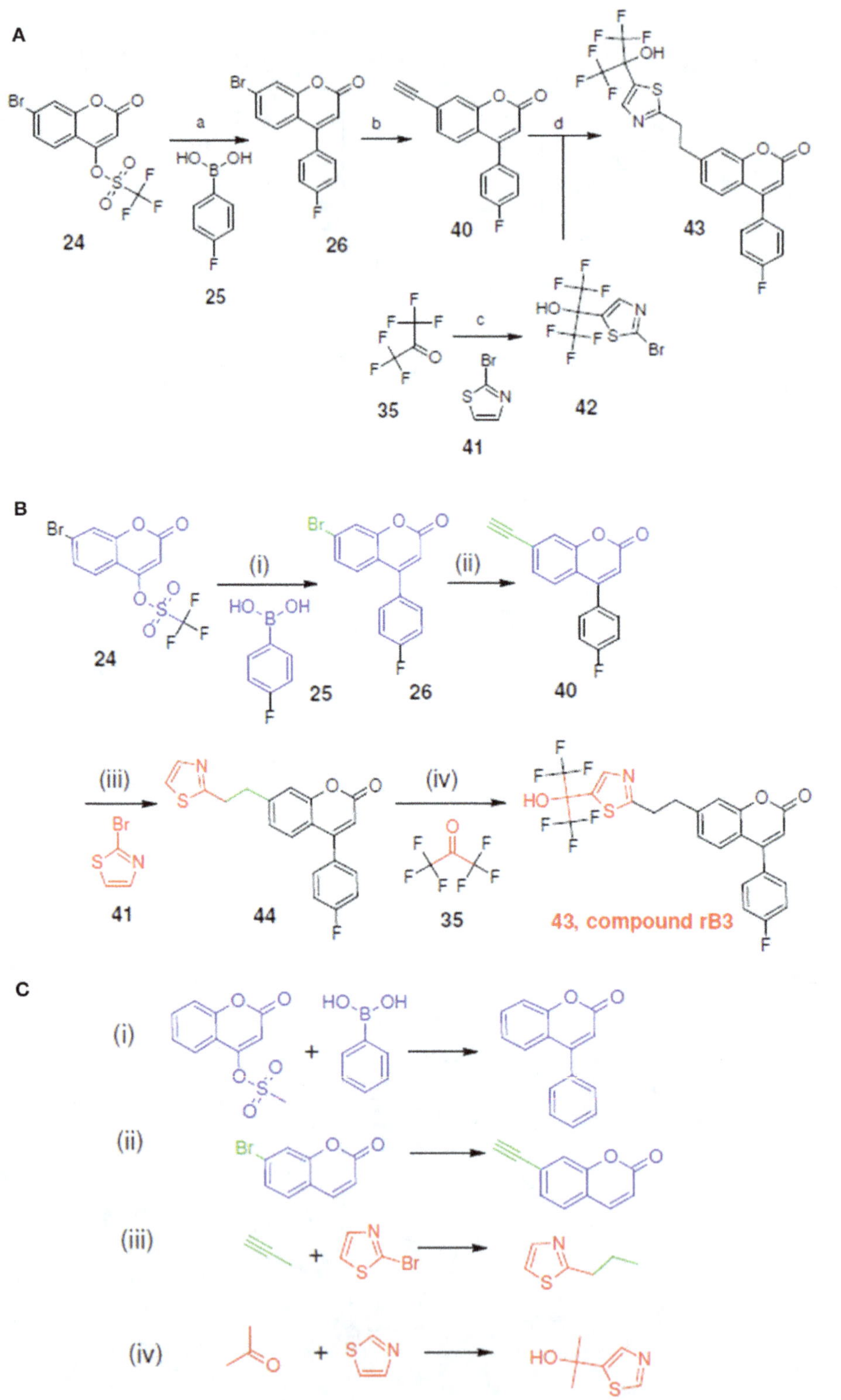

FIGURE 11 | Synthetic routes for compound rB3 and sub-structure searching to identify atom arrangements (moieties) that are part of a chemical reaction rule within the LeadOp+R reaction database. **(A)** Synthetic routes with reagents and condition (a–d) from experimental studies (Ducharme et al., 2010). **(B)** Synthetic routes and **(C)** matched reaction rules provided by LeadOp+R.

Figure 10B shows the LeadOp+R selective and systematically suggested synthetic routes to generate compound rB2 based on the user specified preferred inhibitor-receptor interactions. Initially, compound **24** was identified as the first reactant by searching all building blocks with the preserved fragment. LeadOp+R then proceed to produce compound **26** by reacting **24** with **25** via the first reaction rule (i) that directs the suggested compound toward the preferred interaction with Leu414. The reaction rule suggested by LeadOp+R matches the synthetic steps in the literature for the synthesis of compound **26** from compound **24** and **25**. Next, product **26** was considered as the reactant to react with compound **32** to generate product **39**; again by growing the molecule toward the preferred interaction with Leu414. The second reaction rule (ii) to generate product **39** suggests the same synthetic steps as the literature to synthesize compound **38** by reacting **26** and **27**. The recursive optimization continues to explore the potential ligand interactions with Leu414 and Ile406 to generate compound **38** (compound rB2) by reacting **39** with **35** via the third reaction rule (iii) to synthesize compound **36** by the reaction of **34** and **35**, resulting in the final product compound rB2.

Figure 11A shows the experimental synthesis route (Schwarz et al., 2001) to synthesize compound rB3 (compound **43**) by reacting **40** with **42** (which was generated through the reaction of **35** with **41**). To compare the LeadOp+R suggested route to the experimental route for rB3, we look at the key reaction rules in the literature.

Figure 11B shows the LeadOp+R suggested synthetic routes for compound rB3 using the selected preferred inhibitor-receptor interactions. Initially, compound **24** was identified as the first reactant by searching all building blocks with the preserved fragment that is indicated in **Figure 11B** as the red structure. LeadOp+R proceeded to generate compound **26** by reacting **24** with **25** via the first reaction rule (i) suggested by LeadOp+R. Again, this methodology directs the growth of the new ligand toward the preferred interaction of the ligand interacting with Leu414. The synthetic reactions suggested by LeadOp+R match the synthetic steps presented in the literature that forms compound **26**. Next, product **26** was considered the reactant and transformed into product **40** by growing the ligand toward Ile406 of 5-LOX. The second reaction rule (ii) generates compound **40** and matches the synthetic steps discussed in the literature; compound **40** is identified as the same product that is discussed in the literature to synthesize compound **44**. Continuing the recursive optimization to initiate the ligand's interaction with Ile 406 and Tyr181 results in the third reaction rule (iii), **Figure 11C**, and leads to compound **43**. Compound **44** was identified as the reactant and reacted with **35** based on the fourth reaction rule (iv), generating compound **42** by reacting **35** with **41**.

LeadOp+R has successfully optimized the query compound rB into compounds rB1, rB2, and rB3 and has suggested corresponding synthetic route for each compound. Through systematic synthesis and evaluation of intermediates using group efficiency, LeadOp+R searches for "products" with higher calculated binding affinities and improved interactions with the receptor. The more hydrogen-bonding interactions between compound rB1's oxygen or nitrogen atoms of the thiazol group and the receptor (shown in **Figure 8B**) corresponds to the experimental results of stronger inhibitor potency then the proposed compounds rB2 and rB3. In the example of 5-LOX inhibitor design, we demonstrate LeadOp+R's ability to controls the synthetic flow by extending the ligands with preferred interactions, available building blocks, and associated reactions rules.

LIMITATION

LeadOp+R is an optimization algorithm that starts with a query reactant (compound) and better lead optimization occurs when starting the optimization process with a good binder that is advantageously positioned in the binding site. The LeadOp+R algorithm does not consider experimental product yield rate, reaction rate, and reaction conditions of a chemical synthesis but does propose potential synthetic routes purely based on the chemical reaction rules contained in the chemical reaction database. However, incompatibility of the reaction with specific substituents in the core may happen, the proposed synthetic routes are meant to provide a fast, systematic, and preliminary suggestion based on general reaction—synthesis—rules and structure-based (receptor) ligand optimization. The diversity of the reactant database is a critical factor when searching for the participant reactants along with the number of different poses sampled at each reaction site. The greater the number and diversity of reaction rules and reactant available for LeadOp+R to explore—for the system of interest—the greater the possibility to identify and generate new compounds.

CONCLUSION

In this work, we have implemented a structure-based lead optimization with synthetic accessibility algorithm called "LeadOp+R." Two model systems, Tie-2 kinase and human 5-LOX enzyme with their associated inhibitors, were selected to demonstrate the abilities of the LeadOp+R algorithm. We demonstrated how a query molecule was enhanced through structured-based optimization and a potential synthetic route was proposed based on reaction rules extracted from in-house synthetic database. In the case of Tie-2, co-crystalized structure is available, while the human 5-LOX example was performed using a theoretical 5-LOX receptor model (comparative or homology protein model) and a known inhibitor. LeadOp+R generates a set of potential compounds that exhibit better-calculated inhibition, possess better efficiency score(s), along with providing synthesis routes based on published reaction mechanisms (contained in an in-house reaction and reactants database). The molecular dynamic simulation analysis further demonstrates that the generated structures preserve the important ligand-protein interactions as seen in the crystal structures or reported in the literature. For the proposed compounds with biological inhibition values (IC_{50}) obtained from the literature, LeadOp+R calculated inhibition values corresponding (based on rankings) to the literature values. The interactions between the inhibitor and protein, as noted in the literature, were observed in the entire molecular dynamic simulation. Moreover, we identified fragments that created and retained ligand-receptor interactions that were stronger and more consistent than the original query compound; these fragments were selected based on reaction rules and discovered in our reactant database.

In short, LeadOp+R is an algorithm that can automatically optimize a query molecule based on reaction routes by searching and selecting reactants that can undergo chemical synthesis thus generating compounds with better binding affinity for the biological system (receptor) of interest. Additionally, users can indicate specific parts of the query compound to be optimized and assign the predicted binding space (portion of the binding site) for the generated products based on known ligand-receptor interactions or preference. LeadOp+R is an algorithm that cannot only optimize the lead compounds but also design favorable and practical synthetic routes based on known reaction mechanisms, leading to faster data feedback between experimental and computer-aided molecular design.

AUTHOR CONTRIBUTIONS

YT: Initiated the concepts; F-YL and YT: Drafted, programmed, and performed the analysis on the projects; EE: Edited and gave comments on the work.

ACKNOWLEDGMENTS

This work was funded by the Taiwan National Science Council, grants number 98-2323-B-002-011-, 106-2622-B-002-008-, 105-3011-F-002-010-, 106-2911-I-002-533, 106-2321-B-002-041-, and 106-3114-B-038-001-. Resources of the Laboratory of Computational Molecular Design and Metabolomics and the Department of Computer Science and Information Engineering of National Taiwan University were used in performing these studies.

REFERENCES

Alex, A. A., and Flocco, M. M. (2007). Fragment-based drug discovery: what has it achieved so far? *Curr. Top. Med. Chem.* 7, 1544–1567. doi: 10.2174/156802607782341082

Berendsen, H. J. C., Postma, J. P. M., van Gunsteren, W. F., and Hermans, J. (1981). "Interaction models for water in relation to protein hydration," in *Intermolecular Forces. The Jerusalem Symposia on Quantum Chemistry and Biochemistry, Vol. 14*, ed B. Pullman (Dordrecht: Springer), 331–342. doi: 10.1007/978-94-015-7658-1_21

Bridges, A. J. (2001). Chemical inhibitors of protein kinases. *Chem. Rev.* 101, 2541–2572. doi: 10.1021/cr000250y

Charlier, C., Hénichart, J. P., Durant, F., and Wouters, J. (2006). Structural insights into human 5-lipoxygenase inhibition: combined ligand-based and target-based approach. *J. Med. Chem.* 49, 186–195. doi: 10.1021/jm050870x

Ciulli, A., Williams, G., Smith, A. G., Blundell, T. L., and Abell, C. (2006). Probing hot spots at protein-ligand binding sites: a fragment-based approach using biophysical methods. *J. Med. Chem.* 49, 4992–5000. doi: 10.1021/jm060490r

Congreve, M., Chessari, G., Tisi, D., and Woodhead, A. J. (2008). Recent developments in fragment-based drug discovery. *J. Med. Chem.* 51, 3661–3680. doi: 10.1021/jm8000373

Corey, E. J., Howe, W. J., Orf, H. W., Pensak, D. A., and Petersson, G. J. (1975). General methods of synthetic analysis. Strategic bond disconnections for bridged polycyclic structures. *J. Am. Chem. Soc.* 97, 6116–6124.

Corey, E. J., and Jorgensen, W. L. (1976). Computer-assisted synthetic analysis. Synthetic strategies based on appendages and the use of reconnective transforms. *J. Am. Chem. Soc.* 98, 189–203.

Ducharme, Y., Blouin, M., Brideau, C., Châteauneuf, A., Gareau, Y., Grimm, E. L., et al. (2010). The discovery of setileuton, a potent and selective 5-lipoxygenase inhibitor. *ACS Med. Chem. Lett.* 1, 170–174. doi: 10.1021/ml100029k

Hammarberg, T., Zhang, Y. Y., Lind, B., Radmark, O., and Samuelsson, B. (1995). Mutations at the C-terminal isoleucine and other potential iron ligands of 5-lipoxygenase. *Eur. J. Biochem.* 230, 401–407. doi: 10.1111/j.1432-1033.1995.0401h.x

Hasegawa, M., Nishigaki, N., Washio, Y., Kano, K., Harris, P. A., Sato, H., et al. (2007). Discovery of novel benzimidazoles as potent inhibitors of TIE-2 and VEGFR-2 tyrosine kinase receptors. *J. Med. Chem.* 50, 4453–4470. doi: 10.1021/jm0611051

Hendrickson, J. B., Grier, D. L., and Toczko, A. G. (1985). A logic-based program for synthesis design. *J. Am. Chem. Soc.* 107, 5228–5238. doi: 10.1021/ja00304a033

Hendrickson, J. B., and Toczko, A. G. (1988). Synthesis design logic and the SYNGEN (synthesis generation) program. *Pure Appl. Chem.* 60, 1563–1572. doi: 10.1351/pac198860111563

Hess, B., Kutzner, C., van der Spoel, D., and Lindahl, E. (2008). GROMACS 4: algorithms for highly efficient, load-balanced, and scalable molecular simulation. *J. Chem. Theory Comput.* 4, 435–447. doi: 10.1021/ct700301q

Hodous, B. L., Geuns-Meyer, S. D., Hughes, P. E., Albrecht, B. K., Bellon, S., Bready, J., et al. (2007). Evolution of a highly selective and potent 2-(pyridin-2-yl)-1,3,5-triazine Tie-2 kinase inhibitor. *J. Med. Chem.* 50, 611–626. doi: 10.1021/jm061107l

Hopkins, A. L., Groom, C. R., and Alex, A. (2004). Ligand efficiency: a useful metric for lead selection. *Drug Discov. Today* 9, 430–431. doi: 10.1016/S1359-6446(04)03069-7

Huang, H., Bhat, A., Woodnutt, G., and Lappe, R. (2010). Targeting the ANGPT-TIE2 pathway in malignancy. *Nat. Rev. Cancer* 10, 575–585. doi: 10.1038/nrc2894

Ihlenfeldt, W.-D., and Gasteiger, J. (1996). Computer-assisted planning of organic syntheses: the second generation of programs. *Angew. Chem. Int. Ed.* 34, 2613–2615.

Imre, G., Kalszi, A., Jkli, I., and Farkas, Ö. (2006). "Advanced automatic generation of 3d molecular structures," in *1st European Chemistry Congress* (Budapest).

Ivanov, I., Heydeck, D., Hofheinz, K., Roffeis, J., O'Donnell, V. B., Kuhn, H., et al. (2010). Molecular enzymology of lipoxygenases. *Arch. Biochem. Biophys.* 503, 161–174. doi: 10.1016/j.abb.2010.08.016

Law, J., Zsoldos, Z., Simon, A., Reid, D., Liu, Y., Khew, S. Y., et al. (2009). Route Designer: a retrosynthetic analysis tool utilizing automated retrosynthetic rule generation. *J. Chem. Inf. Model.* 49, 593–602. doi: 10.1021/ci800228y

Lin, F. Y., and Tseng, Y. J. (2011). Structure-based fragment hopping for lead optimization using predocked fragment database. *J. Chem. Inf. Model.* 51, 1703–1715. doi: 10.1021/ci200136j

Lipinski, C. A., Lombardo, F., Dominy, B. W., and Feeney, P. J. (2001). Experimental and computational approaches to estimate solubility and permeability in drug discovery and development settings. *Adv. Drug Deliv. Rev.* 46, 3–26. doi: 10.1016/S0169-409X(00)00129-0

Mata, P., Gillet, V. J., Johnson, A. P., Lampreia, J., Myatt. G. J., Sike, S., et al. (1995). Sprout: 3d structure generation using templates. *J. Chem. Inf. Model.* 15, 479–493. doi: 10.1021/ci00025a016

Oliner, J., Min, H., Leal, J., Yu, D., Rao, S., You, E., et al. (2004). Suppression of angiogenesis and tumor growth by selective inhibition of angiopoietin-2. *Cancer Cell* 6, 507–516. doi: 10.1016/j.ccr.2004.09.030

Oostenbrink, C., Soares, T. A., van der Vegt, N. F., and van Gunsteren, W. F. (2005). Validation of the 53A6 GROMOS force field. *Eur. Biophys. J.* 34, 273–284. doi: 10.1007/s00249-004-0448-6

Orita, M., Ohno, K., and Niimi, T. (2009). Two "golden ratio" indices in fragment-based drug discovery. *Drug Discov. Today* 14, 321–328. doi: 10.1016/j.drudis.2008.10.006

Saxty, G., Woodhead, S. J., Berdini, V., Davies, T. G., Verdonk, M. L., Wyatt, P. G., et al. (2007). Identification of inhibitors of protein kinase B using fragment-based lead discovery. *J. Med. Chem.* 50, 2293–2296. doi: 10.1021/jm070091b

Schwarz, K., Walther, M., Anton, M., Gerth, C., Feussner, I., and Kuhn, H. (2001). Structural basis for lipoxygenase specificity : conversion of the human leukocyte 5-lipoxygenase to a 15-lipoxygenating enzyme species by site-directed mutagenesis. *J. Biol. Chem.* 276, 773–779. doi: 10.1074/jbc.M0051 14200

Shaffer, D. N., and Mansmann, P. T. (1997). Leukotriene inhibition and advances in the treatment of asthma: a pharmacological review. *Pediatr. Allergy Immunol.* 11, 171–179. doi: 10.1089/pai.1997.11.171

Socorro, I. M., and Goodman, J. M. (2006). The ROBIA program for predicting organic reactivity. *J. Chem. Inf. Model.* 46, 606–614. doi: 10.1021/ci05 0379e

Steele, V. E., Holmes, C. A., Hawk, E. T., Kopelovich, L., Lubet, R. A., Crowell, J. A., et al. (1999). Lipoxygenase inhibitors as potential cancer chemopreventives. *Cancer Epidem. Biomar.* 8, 467–483.

Trott, O., and Olson, A. J. (2010). AutoDock Vina: improving the speed and accuracy of docking with a new scoring function, efficient optimization, and multithreading. *J. Comput. Chem.* 31, 455–461. doi: 10.1002/jcc. 21334

Woods, J. W., Evans, J. F., Ethier, D., Scott, S., Vickers, P. J., Hearn, L., et al. (1993). 5-lipoxygenase and 5-lipoxygenase-activating protein are localized in the nuclear envelope of activated human leukocytes. *J. Exp. Med.* 178, 1935–1946. doi: 10.1084/jem.178.6.1935

Yu, Q. (2005). The dynamic roles of angiopoietins in tumor angiogenesis. *Future Oncol.* 1, 475–484. doi: 10.2217/14796694.1.4.475

14

Metabolomic Analysis of the Effects of Adipose-Derived Mesenchymal Stem Cell Treatment on Rats with Sepsis-Induced Acute Lung Injury

Yuqing Cui[1†], Shaohua Liu[1†], Xiaojuan Zhang[1], Xianfei Ding[1], Xiaoguang Duan[1], Zijia Zhu[2], Ji Zhang[2], Huoyan Liang[1], Dong Wang[1], Guojun Zhang[3], Zujiang Yu[4], Jianjun Yang[5] and Tongwen Sun[1]*

[1] General ICU, The First Affiliated Hospital of Zhengzhou University, Henan Key Laboratory of Critical Care Medicine, Zhengzhou Key Laboratory of Sepsis, Zhengzhou, China, [2] Department of Pharmacy, The First Affiliated Hospital of Zhengzhou University, Zhengzhou, China, [3] Department of Respiratory, The First Affiliated Hospital of Zhengzhou University, Zhengzhou, China, [4] Department of Infectious Diseases, The First Affiliated Hospital of Zhengzhou University, Zhengzhou, China, [5] Department of Anesthesiology, The First Affiliated Hospital of Zhengzhou University, Zhengzhou, China

***Correspondence:**
Tongwen Sun
suntongwen@163.com

†These authors have contributed equally to this work

Given the high mortality associated with sepsis, there is an urgent need for a full understanding of sepsis pathophysiology and finding new therapeutic regimens. Adipose-derived mesenchymal stem cells (ADMSCs) has been proven to have anti-inflammatory effects and could be used to treat cecal ligation and puncture (CLP) induced lung and liver injury in septic rat models. In this study, we used metabolomics to investigate small molecule metabolites between CLP and ADMSCs treatment groups. Sixty SD rats were randomly assigned to the sham operation group (SC group), the CLP group, and the CLP+ADMSCs group (CLP-ADMSCs group). We used liquid mass spectrometry-chromatography to detect metabolic changes in plasma and lung tissues. Compared with the SC group, the metabolic profile of plasma and lung tissues changed significantly 24 h after CLP. Moreover, 22 and 11 main differential metabolites involved in amino acid and glycerophospholipid metabolism were found in plasma and lung tissues, respectively. After the rats were injected with ADMSCs, these differential metabolites were reverse-regulated both in plasma and lung tissues. Besides, ADMSCs improved the survival rate and down-regulated the concentration of TNF-α and IL-6 at 24 h after CLP. The correlational analysis between plasma of IL-6/TNF-α and metabolites suggested that acetylcholine, spermine, phenylalanine, threonine of plasma and phosphatidylcholine (36:4) of lung tissues were significantly associated with IL-6/TNF-α in CLP and CLP-ADMSCs groups. ADMSCs might reverse abnormal metabolic pathways by reducing anti-inflammatory factors in sepsis-induced ALI. Our findings may provide novel metabolic mechanism of ADMSCs therapy for sepsis.

Keywords: adipose-derived mesenchymal stem cells, metabolomics, acute lung injury, sepsis, inflammation

INTRODUCTION

Sepsis has been defined as a life-threatening organ dysfunction attributed to the host's dysregulated response to infection (Singer et al., 2016). Many pro-inflammatory cytokines, such as TNF-α and IL-6, reportedly triggered in sepsis, which caused an overwhelming immune response against the infection (Cecconi et al., 2018; Nowill et al., 2019). The treatment strategy for sepsis is a comprehensive treatment that mainly entails anti-microbial treatment, fluid resuscitation, application of glucocorticoids and vasoactive drugs, and mechanical ventilation (Rhodes et al., 2017). However, the mortality of acute lung injury (ALI) caused by sepsis continues to be high (Keeley et al., 2017). Therefore, it was very important to achieve a rapid diagnosis and therapeutic regimen for sepsis.

Fortunately, adipose-derived mesenchymal stem cells (ADMSCs) treatment has shown a lot of beneficial effects on sepsis. ADMSCs promote macrophage-mediated phagocytosis and secrete antibacterial peptides (Mei et al., 2010). Some studies reported mesenchymal stem cells (MSCs) could alleviate immune response and reduce mortality by down-regulating pro-inflammatory and up-regulating anti-inflammatory cytokines in sepsis (Condor et al., 2016; Ou et al., 2016). Besides, our previous research has suggested that ADMSCs secrete a large amount of sTNFR1 to block the activity of TNF-α, thereby reducing the expression of NF-κB, AP-1, and P38 MAPK in sepsis induced ALI (Ding et al., 2019). In addition, transforming growth factor-β (TGF-β) secreted by MSCs might reduce inflammatory response and improve phagocytosis (Liu et al., 2019). However, the mechanism of ADMSCs treatment still needs lot of experiments to explore.

As a branch of systematic biology, metabolomics analyzes changes in low-molecular-weight metabolites, including substances that may be continuously generated during disease development. Metabolomics data can accurately reflect the state of biological systems and promote our understanding of sepsis pathophysiology. A previous study (Su et al., 2015) have indicated that sepsis is comorbid with metabolic disorders, including abnormalities in amino acids, fatty acids, and bile acids. However, there has been no study on the metabolic effect of ADMSCs on sepsis. Thus, for the first time, we report metabolic changes caused by ADMSCs treatment of sepsis, and explore potential metabolic mechanism of ADMSCs treatment.

MATERIALS AND METHODS

Instruments and Reagents

Exion LC AD series liquid chromatograph (SCIEX, USA), an X500R QTOF-MS mass spectrometer (SCIEX, Framingham, MA USA), and the high-speed refrigerated centrifuge 5810R (Eppendorf, Germany). Chromatography grade acetonitrile (Thermo Fisher Scientific, Waltham, MA USA), methanol (Sigma-Aldrich, St. Louis, MO USA), and pure water (Wahaha Company, China) were used. Rat TNF-α and IL-6 ELISA kits were acquired from CUSABIO (Wuhan, China). The Sprague-Dawley rat-derived ADMSCs originating from the inguinal fat were supplied by Cyagen Biotechnology (Yangzhou, China). Flow cytometry was used to assess ADMSCs that were positive for CD44, CD90, and CD29, but negative for CD34, CD11b, and CD45. ADMSCs were grown to the fourth generation based on the supplier's instructions.

Animals, Grouping, and Experimental Procedure

Adult male Sprague-Dawley (SD) rats (180–250 g, 6–8 weeks old) were bought from Charles River (Beijing, China). All the experimental rats had access to food and water *ad libitum* and were housed in a room with a 12 h/12 h of day/night cycle for one week before the experiment. The temperature of the room was maintained at 20°C–25°C, and the relative humidity at 40% to 60%. Sixty SD rats were randomly assigned to the sham operation group (SC group), the cecal ligation, and the puncture model group (CLP group), and the CLP+ADMSCs group (CLP-ADMSCs group). One million ADMSCs were injected through the tail vein 1 h after the surgery in the CLP-ADMSCs group. The same volume of saline was injected in SC and CLP groups. The experiments were conducted in accordance with the guidelines developed by the National Institutes of Health (http://grants1.nih.gov/grants/olaw/) and approved by the Animal Care and Use Committee of the Zhengzhou University.

The CLP rat model was conducted as previously reported (Rittirsch et al., 2009). Briefly, 10% chloral hydrate was used to anesthetize the rats (350 mg/kg of body weight, intraperitoneally). The hair of the abdomen was shaved and the skin was disinfected with iodophor, prior to the operation, which was conducted under a sterile sheet. An abdominal midline incision of 1–2 cm was made, and the cecum was tightly ligated. The position of ligation was below the ileocecal valve to ensure intestine continuity. The middle and lower third of the cecum were ligated uniformly. Subsequently, 18-gauge needles were used to puncture two holes in the middle of ligated cecum. The cecum was squeezed gently and feces were exteriorized, and the cecum was returned to the abdomen. Sterile 5-0 and 3-0 needles were used to suture the muscle and skin layer, respectively. The SC group underwent the same procedure, but without ligation or puncture. For resuscitation after operation, saline (3mL/100 g) pre-heated to 37°C was injected subcutaneously. At the same time, a lamp was used to warm the rats for 30 min. For CLP-ADMSCs group, ADMSCs (1×10^6) were injected through the tail vein 1 h after the operation. Then, the rats were placed in cages with access to food and water. Six rats of each group were anesthetized again 24 h after the surgery. Blood was collected from the abdominal aorta and centrifuged (2,500 rpm, 15 min) after 30 min standing at room temperature, to collect serum, which was then stored in liquid nitrogen. The chest was opened to expose the heart and inferior vena cava was cut. A perfusion needle was inserted into the apex of heart. Cold saline (100 mL–200 mL) was pushed rapidly into the left ventricle and aorta. The lungs became white, and one of the two lungs were extracted and placed in 4% paraformaldehyde overnight for histological analysis. The other lung was snap-frozen in liquid nitrogen. The lung tissues were embedded in paraffin and cut into 3- to 5-mm sections using a microtome. Sections were stained with hematoxylin and eosin and observed under a microscope (magnification: 100×) (Olympus, Japan).

Plasma and Lung Samples Pretreatment

Plasma and lung samples were thawed on ice at 4°C. The plasma (50 μl) was transferred to an Eppendorf (EP) tube and 150 μl methanol and 10 μl the internal standard (0.5 μM/L cholic acid (CA-d4) and 0.5 μM/L chenodeoxycholic acid (CDCA-d4)) were added. The mixture was vortexed for 30 s and centrifuged for 10 min at 14,000 rpm. The supernatant was collected and injected into an auto-sampler container. Then, 20 mg lung samples and 200 μl pure water were added to an EP tube and vortexed for 2 min. 800 μl of pre-cooled methanol/acetonitrile (1:1) was added to the EP tube, which was then vortexed for 30 s and centrifuged (14,000 rpm, 10 min). The supernatant (900 μl) was collected and evaporated for 2.5 h, and 120 μl of 50% acetonitrile was added to dissolve it. The solution was vortexed for 30 s, centrifuged twice (14,000 rpm, 10 min) and vortexed three times (1500 rpm, 30 s). Finally, 100 μl supernatant was collected for injection. The quality control (QC) sample was mixed with 20 μl of each sample, and 200 μl of this mixture was used for QC analysis.

Chromatography Conditions

The chromatographic column (ACQUITY UPLC HSS T3 C18, 2.1 mm × 100 mm, 1.7 μm; Waters, Milford, MA) was maintained at 30℃. The positive ion consisted of 0.1% formic acid in water (A phase) and acetonitrile (B phase), and the negative ion consisted of 5mM ammonium acetate in water (A phase) and 5 mM acetonitrile (B phase). A 14-min gradient elution method was used with a flow rate of 0.4 mL/min. The elution linear gradient started at 5% B phase, increased linearly to 30% in 1 min, 60% in the next 2 min, then increased linearly to 95% in 7 min, and remained constant for 2 min. Then, the B phase was recovered to 5% in 0.1 min and kept for 1.9 min. The injection volume was 3.0 μl.

Mass Spectrometry

Data collection and processing were performed using the SCIEX OS 1.2 software (AB, Milford, MA). The ion source of the positive and negative ion scanning modes was electrospray ionization. The temperature and spray voltage of the ion source were set at 600°C, 5500 V (positive ion mode), and 600°C, -4500 V (negative ion mode), respectively. Declustering potential, auxiliary gas 1, auxiliary gas 2, and curtain gas were set at 80 V, 60, 60, and 35 psi, respectively. Collision energy was 20, 40, and 40 eV. The quality scanning range was *m/z* 50–1000 Da. Further, dynamic background subtraction and information-dependent acquisition were used for triggering low-level components to gather MS/MS.

Multivariate Data Analysis and Identification of Potential Biomarkers

Data extraction, retention time correction, peak recognition, peak extraction, peak integration, peak alignment, and other pre-processing procedures were conducted using the Software MarkerView TM (version 1.4.1, Waters Co., Milford, MA, USA). The data matrix composed of retention time (RT), mass spectral (m/z), and peak intensity was produced after total normalization pretreatment. The Principal component analysis (PCA) was applied to draw score plots in order to evaluate the distribution of samples. The Orthogonal partial least squares discriminant analysis (OPLS-DA) was used to reduce dimension in the multi-dimensional complex data. The Variable importance projection (VIP) was computed to find differential metabolites between two groups. One-way ANOVA and the Tukey's *post hoc* test were used to analyze the data (SPSS software version 21.0, Chicago, IL). The metabolites satisfying VIP > 1.0, |FC| > 1.5, and $P < 0.05$ were considered as differential markers. Biomarkers identification and pathway enrichment analysis were investigated by combining human metabolism database (HMDB), the Kyoto Encyclopedia of genes and genomes (KEGG), MetaboAnalyst 4.0, other databases, and literature reports. Heat maps were generated with these significant metabolites by the R software (R version 3.5.3, heatmap package) to show the changes in trend. The links between plasma of IL-6/TNF-α and metabolites of plasma and lung tissues in CLP and CLP-ADMSCs groups were assessed using the R software (https://www.r-project.org/). The correlational analysis was conducted to obtain the correlation coefficient and *P* value between IL-6/TNF-α and metabolites. The correlation coefficient more than 0.75 and $P < 0.2$ were selected as differential metabolites significantly associated with IL-6/TNF-α.

RESULTS

Pathology and Inflammatory Factor Levels in Septic ALI Model

The mortality of the SC, CLP, and CLP-ADMSCs groups was 0% (0/20), 40.0% (8/20), and 25.0% (5/20) at 24 h after operation. The mortality rate in the CLP group was higher than SC group (P = 0.003) and CLP-ADMSCs group (P = 0.501). The cecum of CLP group presented adhesion and necrosis, but these manifestations were markedly attenuated in the CLP-ADMSCs group. Hematoxylin and eosin staining of the lung tissues samples was used to evaluate lung injury (**Figure 1A**). Compared with SC group, the alveolar walls of the CLP group were found to be significantly thickened, and some of the alveolar structures were destroyed. The alveolar space was reduced and infiltrated with a lot of inflammatory cells in the CLP group, but these features were ameliorated in the CLP-ADMSCs group. Our previous study had successfully proved transplanted ADMSCs engrafted into the lung at 6, 24, and 72 h after a CLP procedure (Ding et al., 2019). Moreover, we detected plasma concentration of TNF-α and IL-6 at 24 h after CLP and found levels of inflammatory factors up-regulated in the CLP group and significantly down-regulated in the CLP-ADMSCs group (**Figure 1B**).

Plasma and Lung Chromatography Analysis

The plasma and lung metabolites of the three groups were analyzed, and the total ion chromatograms of plasma and the

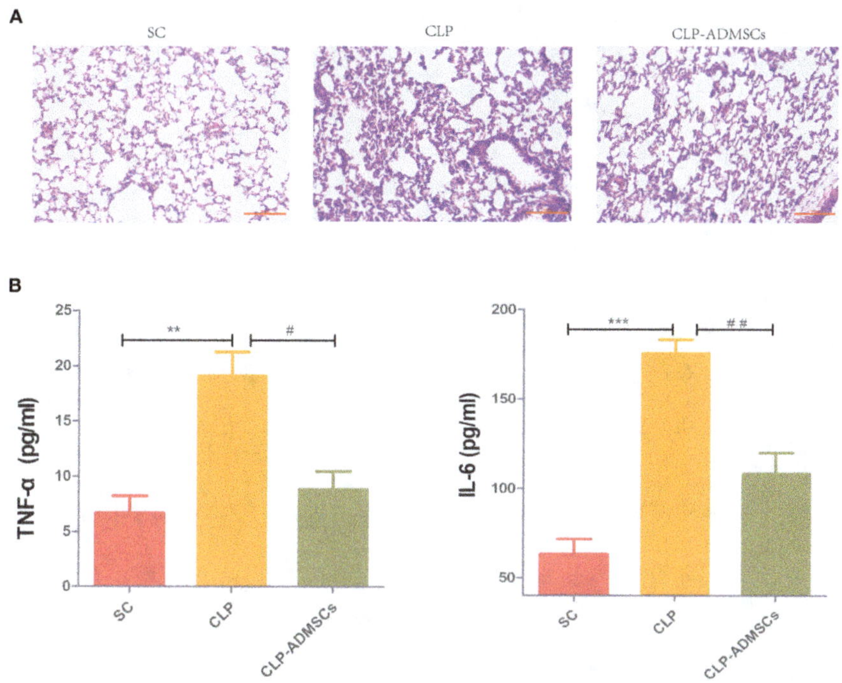

FIGURE 1 | (A) Histology of the lungs of the SC, CLP, and ADMSCs groups after CLP 24h (n = 6). Hematoxylin and eosinstaining showed significantly enhanced inflammatory infiltration, edema, and bleeding in the CLP group. ADMSCs treatment improved these abnormalities (scale bar = 100 μm). H & E: Hematoxylin and eosin. **(B)** Effects of ADMSCs treatment on the systemic inflammatory response in CLP rats (n = 6). ELISA was used to detect plasma IL-6 and TNF-α concentration in each group at 24 h. *Compared with the SC group, #compared with the CLP group; *, #$P < 0.05$; **, ##$P < 0.01$; ***, ###$P < 0.001$.

lung tissues samples were shown in **Supplementary Material (Supplementary Figures 1** and **2)**. Compared with the CLP group, the peak pattern of the CLP-ADMSCs group was similar to SC group. The results suggested that administration of ADMSCs may normalize the metabolism in CLP rats.

Multivariate Statistical Analysis

In order to make the analysis results more intuitive and visual, the unsupervised PCA method was applied. **Figures 2E, F** and **Supplementary Material Figures 3E, F** showed the three-dimensional score charts in plasma and lung tissues samples. The metabolite pattern changed significantly both in the positive and negative ion modes, and the CLP group was significantly different from the SC and CLP-ADMSCs groups. The CLP-ADMSCs group showed a significant callback trend both in plasma and lung tissues. Considering the overall change track of metabolites, it can be concluded that ADMSCs had a therapeutic effect on septic rats. In addition, the relative proximity of CLP-ADMSCs group and SC group indicated that ADMSCs had little effect on the metabolism of normal rats.

The OPLS-DA method was used to analyze the experimental data (**Figures 2A–D** and **Supplementary Material Figures 3A–D**). The scores of the CLP, SC, and CLP-ADMSCs groups were clearly different both in the plasma and lung samples, which showed that the metabolism profile changed significantly after ADMSCs treatment.

Identification of Differential Metabolites

The VIP, FC, and P values were included in the volcano plot to find differential metabolites and coding scripts were available in Github website (https://github.com/cuiyuqing2018/cuiyuqing). $P < 0.05$ ($-\log_{10}$ (P-value) > 1.30), $|FC| > 1.5$ or < 2/3 ($\log_2(FC) \geq 0.585$ or $\log_2(FC) \leq -0.585$) and VIP > 1.0 were considered statistically significant differences, as shown in **Supplementary Material Figures 4A–D** and **Supplementary Material Figures 5A–D**). The results of searches in the HMDB, the KEGG, and the MetaboAnalyst databases showed 22 and 11 differential metabolites in the plasma and lung tissues samples, respectively [**Table 1** and **Supplementary Material** (**Supplementary Table 1**)]. Among the main differential metabolites in the CLP group, the levels of plasma creatinine, betaine, threonine, niacinamide, thymine, creatine, homocysteine, acetylcholine, methionine, dopamine, histidine, phenylalanine, pyridoxine, tyrosine, spermine, deoxycytidine, cytidine, xanthosine, and phosphatidylcholine [PC (38: 6)] were found to be increased, and those of lysophosphatidylcholine and phenylpyruvate significantly decreased, compared with SC group. However, ADMSCs treatment regulated 22 identified metabolites to levels similar to SC group (**Figure 3**). Moreover, altered metabolic pathways mainly included biosynthesis of phenylalanine, tyrosine, and tryptophan, phenylalanine metabolism, tyrosine metabolism, cysteine, and methionine metabolism, glycerol phospholipid metabolism (**Figures 4A, B**). Compared with the SC group,

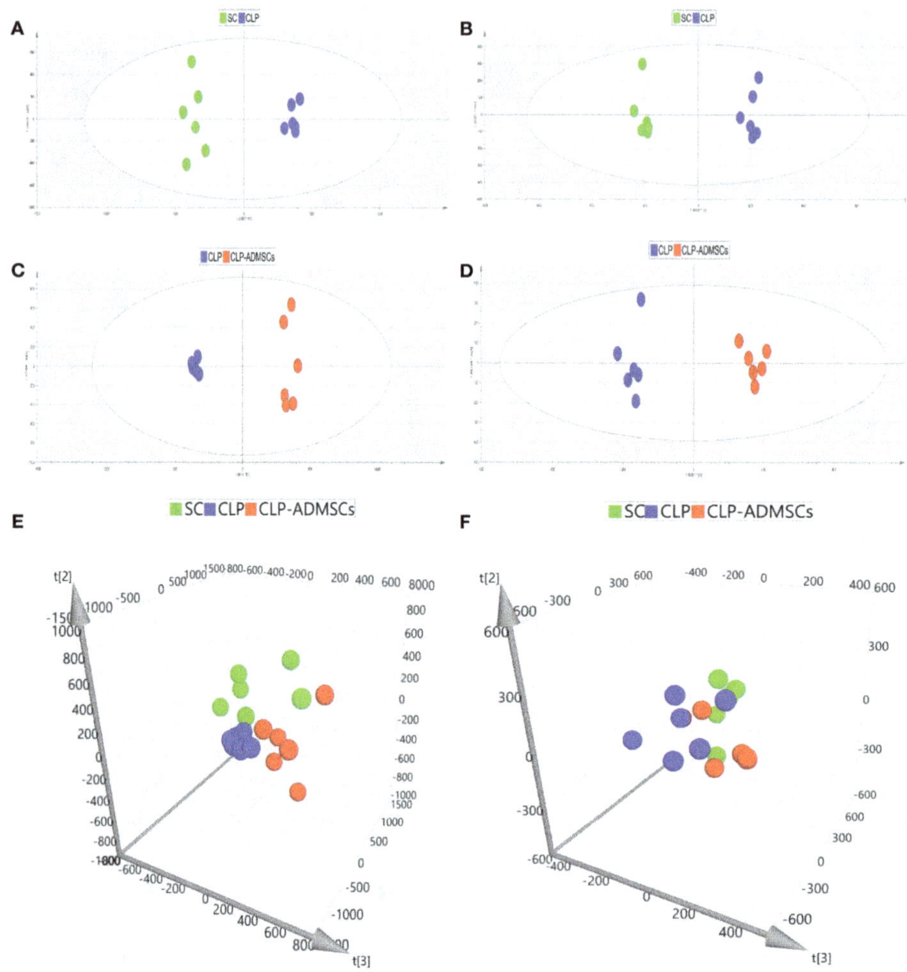

FIGURE 2 | PCA and OPLS-DA scores of plasma samples (n = 6). **(A, C, E)** Positive ion mode. **(B, D, F)** Negative ion mode.

L-valine, creatine, acetylcholine, glutamic acid, xanthine, tryptophan, cytidine, lysophosphatidylcholine [LPC (18: 3), LPC (22: 4)], and chenodeoxycholic acid (CDCA) significantly increased in the CLP group of lung tissues samples. Further, phosphatidylcholine [PC (36: 4)] was decreased (**Supplementary Material Figure 6**). Altered metabolic pathways mainly included pathways for glycerol phospholipid metabolism, arginine, and proline metabolism, D-glutamine, and D-glutamic acid metabolism (**Supplementary Material Figure 7**).

Analysis of Metabolic Data

The heat map of coding scripts have been made available at Github website (https://github.com/cuiyuqing2018/cuiyuqing). The changing tendency of metabolites is shown in **Figure 4C** and **Supplementary Material Figure 8**). Obvious demarcation lines were found in the three groups. Multiple metabolites were clearly changed in the CLP group compared with SC group, but ADMSCs injection reversibly adjusted these parameters. And we found acetylcholine, spermine, phenylalanine, threonine of plasma, and PC (36:4) of lung tissues in CLP and CLP-ADMSCs groups were significantly associated with IL-6/TNF-α (**Table 2**).

DISCUSSION

In this study, PCA and OPLS-DA were used for the discriminant analysis, and the univariate statistical analysis was used to screen important differential metabolites in untreated or ADMSCs-treated septic rats. Metabolic analysis of plasma and lung tissues revealed that amino acid and glycerol phospholipid metabolism were altered in septic rats. We found four plasma metabolites and one lung metabolite associated with IL-6/TNF-α of plasma. These results suggested that ADMSCs may reduce anti-inflammatory factors, consequently reversing abnormal metabolic pathways in sepsis induced ALI. The findings might have vital effects on elucidating the mechanism of ADMSCs treatment in sepsis.

TABLE 1 | Major differential metabolites in septic rat plasma (n = 6).

NO	Differential metabolites	m/z	RT(min)	VIP	*p* value	FC(CLP/SC)	Involved pathways
1	Creatinine	114.0675	0.85	1.89	0.00007	1.92	10
2	Betaine	118.0869	0.79	6.23	0.0004	1.90	4
3	L-Threonine	120.0813	1.85	8.17	0.0005	2.13	2,4,7
4	Niacinamide	123.0455	1.06	1.37	0.0043	1.83	Nicotinate and nicotinamide metabolism
5	Thymine	127.0376	1.07	1.08	0.0001	4.53	4
6	Creatine	132.0774	0.89	10.05	0.00001	2.77	4, 10
7	Homocysteine	136.0497	0.88	2.23	0.00007	2.31	14
8	Acetylcholine	146.119	0.91	2.06	0.0001	2.66	15
9	L-Methionine	150.0595	1.03	2.93	0.002	1.73	2, 14
10	Dopamine	154.0603	0.88	2.94	0.00007	2.48	11
11	L-Histidine	156.0783	0.76	1.22	0.004	1.98	2, 6, 12
12	L-Phenylalanine	166.087	1.85	9.5	0.0005	2.16	1, 3
13	Pyridoxine	170.0945	0.76	1.45	0.003	2.95	9
14	L-Tyrosine	182.0821	1.03	3.57	0.003	1.62	1,2, 3, 8, 11
15	Spermine	203.1524	0.9	1.02	0.029	2.10	6, 10, 13
16	Deoxycytidine	228.1005	1.04	1.19	0.006	1.76	5
17	Cytidine	244.082	1.02	1.17	0.004	1.92	5
18	Xanthosine	285.1309	0.89	1.85	0.0002	4.11	17
19	lysoPC(20:4)	544.3428	5.76	18.25	0.0005	0.57	15
20	lysoPC(22:6)	568.3436	5.73	7.72	0.003	0.55	15
21	PC(38:6)	806.5717	8.77	3.51	0.043	6.47	15
22	Phenylpyruvic acid	162.9591	0.68	1.34	0.0015	0.14	1, 3

Compared with CLP group, potential biomarker information was screened in CLP-ADMSCs group. FC, fold change; VIP, contribution rate of different substances to orthogonal partial least squares discriminant analysis (OPLS-DA) model construction. RT, retention time. Involved pathways:1. Phenylalanine, tyrosine and tryptophan biosynthesis; 2. Aminoacyl-tRNA biosynthesis; 3. Phenylalanine metabolism; 4. Glycine, serine and threonine metabolism; 5. Pyrimidine metabolism; 6. beta-Alanine metabolism; 7. Valine, leucine and isoleucine biosynthesis; 8. Ubiquinone and other terpenoid-quinone biosynthesis; 9. Vitamin B6 metabolism; 10. Arginine and proline metabolism; 11. Tyrosine metabolism; 12. Histidine metabolism; 13. Glutathione metabolism; 14. Cysteine and methionine metabolism; 15. Glycerophospholipid metabolism; 16. Tryptophan metabolism; 17. Purine metabolism.

MSCs had been reported to attenuate ALI in animal models (Aslam et al., 2009; Su et al., 2019a). There is excessive inflammation in sepsis and ALI, and pulmonary infection is the lead site of sepsis (Hirano et al., 2018), with the lung being one of the first affected organs in sepsis patients (Abe et al., 2018). Reduced inflammatory factors could prevent pulmonary edema and neutrophil aggregation (Li et al., 2018; Yang et al., 2020). We evaluated H&E-stained lung sections and observed that ADMSCs therapy might reduce inflammatory cells infiltration and lung edema by decreasing IL-6/TNF-α in plasma. In addition, we also detected apoptotic cells in lung by terminal deoxynucleotidyl transferase dUTP nick end labeling (TUNEL) staining (Ding et al., 2019). Other studies reported IL-6, TNF-α, and H&E staining could assess the severity of ALI (Sun et al., 2011; Liu et al., 2018; Su et al., 2019b). Here, we demonstrated indicators that support ADMSCs-driven reduction of ALI induced by sepsis.

Various infection factors stimulate macrophages and neutrophils to produce IL-6, TNF-α, and other pro-inflammatory transmitters. Over expression of IL-6 and TNF-α could lead to excessive inflammatory response, which aggravate tissues damage and even systemic inflammatory response (Tanaka et al., 2016). Acetylcholine, spermine, phenylalanine, and threonine of plasma had significant association with IL-6/TNF-α in both CLP and CLP-ADMSCs groups (**Table 2**). These metabolites all had an increased tendency in CLP group, but showed decreased trend after ADMSCs injection. The vesicular acetylcholine transporter was up-regulated, accompanied by acetylcholine release in sepsis (Hoover et al., 2020). Activation of acetylcholine receptors could inhibit inflammatory response and ameliorate liver injury in sepsis (Wu et al., 2020). A previous study reported that ADMSCs expressed the M2 muscarinic receptor (Piovesana et al., 2018). Therefore, we inferred that ADMSCs might bind acetylcholine to reduce excessive inflammation. In addition, elevated phenylalanine is highly correlated with poor renal function and low albumin, which is also an independent predictor of death (Huang et al., 2019). It was reported that threonine and spermine expression are also increased in sepsis (Cui et al., 2018; Zahedi et al., 2019; Izquierdo-Garcia et al., 2019). Our findings suggested that ADMSCs might have therapeutic effect by reducing IL-6/TNF-α to lower phenylalanine, spermine, and threonine. Besides, phosphatidylcholine (36:4) (PC) of lung tissues had significant association with IL-6/TNF-α in both CLP and CLP-ADMSCs groups (**Table 2**). PC forms alveolar surfactant and cell membrane, and it is the most abundant phospholipid in human (Furse and de Kroon, 2015). Our results revealed that PC was down-regulated and LPC was up-regulated in lung tissues samples. The reduction of pulmonary surfactant had resulted in ALI of sepsis (Huang et al., 2005). Therefore, we speculated that PC and alveolar surfactants were degraded due to the release of IL-6/TNF-α in CLP group. ADMSCs treatment might restore alveolar surfactants and PC to normal, and these play a vital role on alleviating lung damage. The relationship between metabolites and inflammation markers suggested ADMSCs may reverse the altered metabolites by reducing inflammatory factors, thus playing a therapeutic role. Besides, these metabolites may be regulators of inflammatory response, and have the potential to serve as novel biomedicines for the treatment of sepsis.

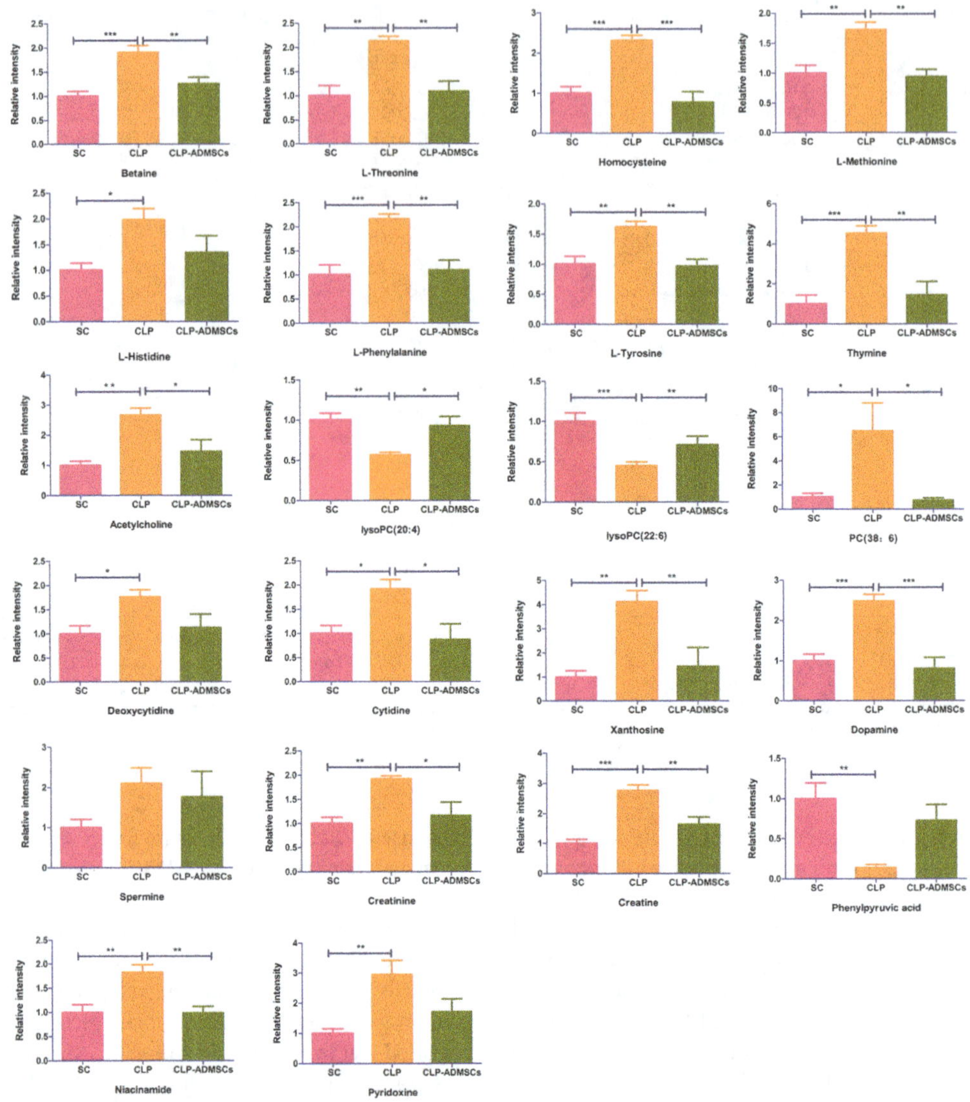

FIGURE 3 | Relative intensities of major differential metabolites in the plasma (n = 6). **P* < 0.05; ***P* < 0.01; ****P* < 0.001.

Related physiological analysis had found sepsis experienced a highly catabolic status. A lot of protein decomposed into amino acids to supply energy, which seemed to be important for the poor prognosis (Van Wyngene and Vandewalle, 2018). Thus, the concentration of amino acids demonstrated a notable upward tendency in the CLP group. However, this state was reversed and the amino acid concentration decreased in the CLP-ADMSCs group. We speculated that the tricarboxylic acid cycle may return to normal and elevated amino acids were used preferentially to provide energy after ADMSCs treatment (**Figure 5** and **Supplementary Material Figure 9**). This inference has been proved in other metabolic diseases, such as obesity and type 2 diabetes (Shree et al., 2019; Yu et al., 2019).

However, this study also had several limitations. The small number of rats used to detect the metabolic changes in each group. The finding should be validated in a larger group of models. Our experiments involved small animals; future clinical translational studies in humans would be necessary to assess the benefits of ADMSCs in clinical practice.

CONCLUSION

This study was a preliminary investigation of relevant metabolic changes in CLP and ADMSCs treatment groups. Based on metabolomics, ADMSCs restored disordered metabolic pathways, such as amino acid and glycerol phospholipid metabolism, to normal in septic rats. ADMSCs might have beneficial effect by reducing anti-inflammatory factors, reversing abnormal metabolic

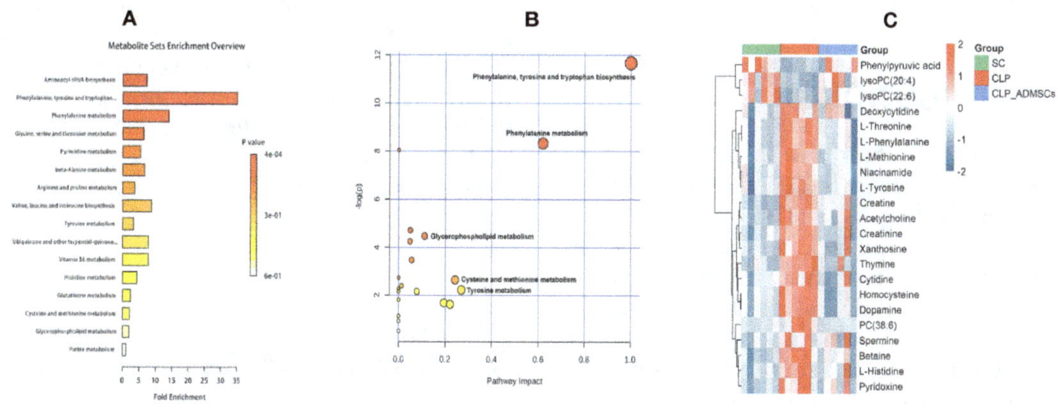

FIGURE 4 | Diagram of differential metabolic pathways and enrichment of differential metabolites in lung tissues (n = 6). **(A)** Diagram of differential metabolic pathways (n = 6). **(B)** Enrichment of differential metabolites (n = 6). **(C)** Heat map of major differential metabolites in plasma (n = 6).

TABLE 2 | The correlation analysis between plasma IL-6/TNF-α and plasma/lung metabolites (n = 6).

Metabolites	IL-6 (CLP group)	TNF-α (CLP group)	IL-6 (CLP-ADMSCs group)	TNF-α (CLP-ADMSCs group)
Acetylcholine (plasma)	−0.83 (0.04)		−0.68 (0.14)	
Spermine (plasma)		0.98 (0.001)		0.69 (0.13)
Phenylalanine (plasma)		0.76 (0.08)	−0.75 (0.09)	
Threonine (plasma)		0.75 (0.08)	−0.74 (0.09)	
PC (36:4) (lung)	0.91 (0.01)	−0.77 (0.07)	−0.46 (0.36)	0.70 (0.12)

Each cell represents the correlation coefficient and P value. The correlation coefficient≥0.75 or P ≤ 0.2 were selected as differential metabolites associated with IL-6/TNF-α. PC, phosphatidylcholine.

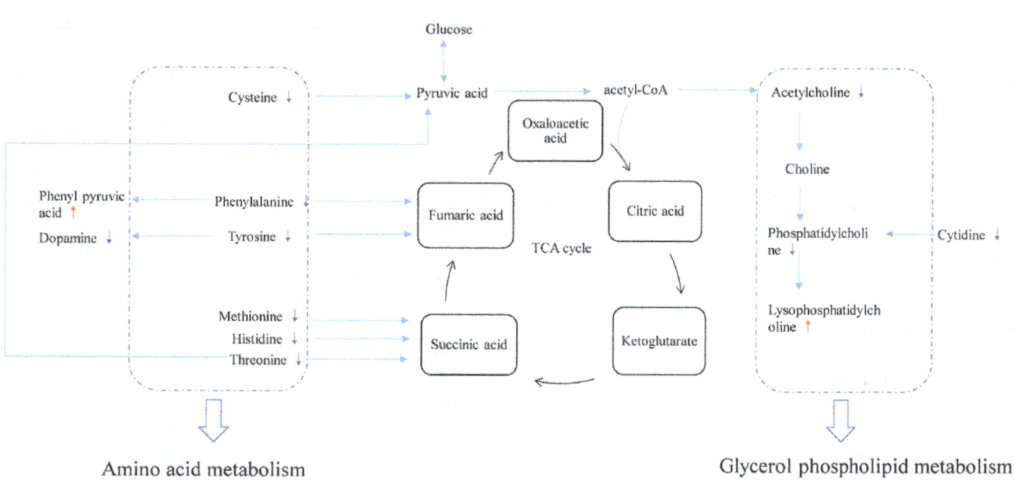

FIGURE 5 | Disturbance of various pathways in plasma and effects of ADMSCs treatment (n = 6). The red arrow indicates increase in the metabolite concentration in the CLP-ADMSCs group relative to the CLP group, and the purple arrow indicates decrease in the metabolite concentration in the CLP-ADMSCs group relative to the CLP group.

pathways in sepsis-induced ALI. This study provides new insights on ADMSCs-based strategy for sepsis treatment.

AUTHOR CONTRIBUTIONS

TS, YC, and SL conceived the study. YC, SL, XZ, XDi, and HL contributed to the animal experiments. ZZ and JZ contributed to the data processing and analysis. YC and SL contributed to the writing of the article. XDu, DW, and GZ resolved controversies. ZY, JY, and TS revised the article. All authors contributed to the article and approved the submitted version. All authors agree to be accountable for all aspects of the work in ensuring that questions related to the accuracy or integrity of any part of the work are appropriately investigated and resolved.

FUNDING

This study was supported by the Leading Talents Fund in Science and Technology Innovation in Henan Province (Grant No.194200510017), Provincial Ministry Co-construction Project from Medical Scientific and Technological Research Program of Henan Province (Grant No. SBGJ2018020), the "51282" Project Leaders of Scientific and Technological Innovative Talents from Health and Family Planning Commission in Henan Province (2016-32), and the Science and Technology people-benefit project of Zheng Zhou (2019KJHM0001).

ACKNOWLEDGMENTS

We deeply thank Sun Jun-Yi, Sun Ya-Li, Qin Xin-Tong, Li Long-Yu, and Wei Wen-Liang for their help in our animal experiments. We also thank Editage (www.editage.cn) for English language editing.

REFERENCES

Abe, T., Ogura, H., Shiraishi, A., Kushimoto, S., Saitoh, D., Fujishima, S., et al. (2018). Characteristics, management, and in-hospital mortality among patients with severe sepsis in intensive care units in Japan: the FORECAST study. *Crit. Care (London England)* 22 (1), 322. doi: 10.1186/s13054-018-2186-7

Aslam, M., Baveja, R., Liang, O. D., Fernandez-Gonzalez, A., Lee, C., Mitsialis, S. A., et al. (2009). Bone marrow stromal cells attenuate lung injury in a murine model of neonatal chronic lung disease. *Am. J. Respir. Crit. Care Med.* 180 (11), 1122–1130. doi: 10.1164/rccm.200902-0242OC

Cecconi, M., Evans, L., Levy, M., and Rhodes, A. (2018). Sepsis and septic shock. *Lancet (London England)* 392 (10141), 75–87. doi: 10.1016/s0140-6736(18)30696-2

Condor, J. M., Rodrigues, C. E., Sousa Moreira, R., Canale, D., Volpini, R. A., Shimizu, M. H., et al. (2016). Treatment With Human Wharton's Jelly-Derived Mesenchymal Stem Cells Attenuates Sepsis-Induced Kidney Injury, Liver Injury, and Endothelial Dysfunction. *Stem Cells Trans. Med.* 5 (8), 1048–1057. doi: 10.5966/sctm.2015-0138

Cui, F., Zhu, P., Ji, J., Blazenovic, I., Gholami, M., Zhang, Y., et al. (2018). Gas chromatography-mass spectrometry metabolomic study of lipopolysaccharides toxicity on rat basophilic leukemia cells. *Chemico-biol. Interact.* 281, 81–88. doi: 10.1016/j.cbi.2017.12.008

Ding, X. F., Liang, H. Y., Sun, J. Y., Liu, S. H., Kan, Q. C., Wang, L. X., et al. (2019). Adipose-derived mesenchymal stem cells ameliorate the inflammatory reaction in CLP-induced septic acute lung injury rats via sTNFR1. *J. Cell. Physiol.* 2019, 1–10. doi: 10.1002/jcp.28329

Furse, S., and de Kroon, A. I. (2015). Phosphatidylcholine's functions beyond that of a membrane brick. *Mol. Membrane Biol.* 32 (4), 117–119. doi: 10.3109/09687688.2015.1066894

Hirano, Y., Ode, Y., Ochani, M., Wang, P., and Aziz, M. (2018). Targeting junctional adhesion molecule-C ameliorates sepsis-induced acute lung injury by decreasing CXCR4(+) aged neutrophils. *J. Leukocyte Biol.* 104 (6), 1159–1171. doi: 10.1002/jlb.3a0218-050r

Hoover, D. B., Poston, M. D., Brown, S., Lawson, S. E., Bond, C. E., Downs, A. M., et al. (2020). Cholinergic leukocytes in sepsis and at the neuroimmune junction in the spleen. *Int. Immunopharmacol.* 81, 106359. doi: 10.1016/j.intimp.2020.106359

Huang, W., McCaig, L. A., Veldhuizen, R. A., Yao, L. J., and Lewis, J. F. (2005). Mechanisms responsible for surfactant changes in sepsis-induced lung injury. *Eur. Respir. J.* 26 (6), 1074–1079. doi: 10.1183/09031936.05.00085805

Huang, S. S., Lin, J. Y., Chen, W. S., Liu, M. H., Cheng, C. W., Cheng, M. L., et al. (2019). Phenylalanine- and leucine-defined metabolic types identify high mortality risk in patients with severe infection. *Int. J. Infect. Dis.: IJID : Off. Publ. Int. Soc. Infect. Dis.* 85, 143–149. doi: 10.1016/j.ijid.2019.05.030

Izquierdo-Garcia, J. L., Nin, N., Cardinal-Fernandez, P., Rojas, Y., de Paula, M., Granados, R., et al. (2019). Identification of novel metabolomic biomarkers in an experimental model of septic acute kidney injury. *Am. J. Physiol. Renal Physiol.* 316 (1), F54–f62. doi: 10.1152/ajprenal.00315.2018

Keeley, A., Hine, P., and Nsutebu, E. (2017). The recognition and management of sepsis and septic shock: a guide for non-intensivists. *Postgraduate Med. J.* 93 (1104), 626–634. doi: 10.1136/postgradmedj-2016-134519

Li, J., Zheng, Y., and Li, M. X. (2018). Tanshinone IIA alleviates lipopolysaccharide-induced acute lung injury by downregulating TRPM7 and pro-inflammatory factors. *J. Cell Mol. Med.* 22 (1), 646–654. doi: 10.1111/jcmm.13350

Liu, F. C., Yu, H. P., Lin, C. Y., Elzoghby, A. O., Hwang, T. L., and Fang, J. Y. (2018). Use of cilomilast-loaded phosphatiosomes to suppress neutrophilic inflammation for attenuating acute lung injury: the effect of nanovesicular surface charge. *J. Nanobiotechnol.* 16 (1), 35. doi: 10.1186/s12951-018-0364-z

Liu, F., Qiu, H., Xue, M., Zhang, S., Zhang, X., Xu, J., et al. (2019). MSC-secreted TGF-beta regulates lipopolysaccharide-stimulated macrophage M2-like polarization via the Akt/FoxO1 pathway. *Stem Cell Res. Ther.* 10 (1), 345. doi: 10.1186/s13287-019-1447-y

Mei, S. H., Haitsma, J. J., Dos Santos, C. C., Deng, Y., Lai, P. F., Slutsky, A. S., et al. (2010). Mesenchymal stem cells reduce inflammation while enhancing bacterial clearance and improving survival in sepsis. *Am. J. Respir. Crit. Care Med.* 182 (8), 1047–1057. doi: 10.1164/rccm.201001-0010OC

Nowill, A. E., Fornazin, M. C., Spago, M. C., and Dorgan Neto, V. (2019). Immune Response Resetting in Ongoing Sepsis. *J. Immunol.* 203 (5), 1298–1312. doi: 10.4049/jimmunol.1900104

Ou, H., Zhao, S., Peng, Y., Xiao, X., Wang, Q., Liu, H., et al. (2016). Comparison of bone marrow tissue- and adipose tissue-derived mesenchymal stem cells in the treatment of sepsis in a murine model of lipopolysaccharide-induced sepsis. *Mol. Med. Rep.* 14 (4), 3862–3870. doi: 10.3892/mmr.2016.5694

Piovesana, R., Melfi, S., Fiore, M., Magnaghi, V., and Tata, A. M. (2018). M2 muscarinic receptor activation inhibits cell proliferation and migration of rat adipose-mesenchymal stem cells. *J. Cell Physiol.* 233 (7), 5348–5360. doi: 10.1002/jcp.26350

Rhodes, A., Evans, L. E., Alhazzani, W., Levy, M. M., Antonelli, M., Ferrer, R., et al. (2017). Surviving Sepsis Campaign: International Guidelines for Management of Sepsis and Septic Shock: 2016. *Intensive Care Med.* 43 (3), 304–377. doi: 10.1007/s00134-017-4683-6

Rittirsch, D., Huber-Lang, M. S., Flierl, M. A., and Ward, P. A. (2009). Immunodesign of experimental sepsis by cecal ligation and puncture. *Nat. Protoc.* 4 (1), 31–36. doi: 10.1038/nprot.2008.214

Shree, N., Venkategowda, S., Venkatranganna, M. V., Datta, I., and Bhonde, R. R. (2019). Human adipose tissue mesenchymal stem cells as a novel treatment modality for correcting obesity induced metabolic dysregulation. *Int. J. Obesity (2005)* 43 (10), 2107–2118. doi: 10.1038/s41366-019-0438-5

Singer, M., Deutschman, C. S., Seymour, C. W., Shankar-Hari, M., Annane, D., Bauer, M., et al. (2016). The Third International Consensus Definitions for Sepsis and Septic Shock (Sepsis-3). *Jama* 315 (8), 801–810. doi: 10.1001/jama.2016.0287

Su, L., Li, H., Xie, A., Liu, D., Rao, W., Lan, L., et al. (2015). Dynamic changes in amino acid concentration profiles in patients with sepsis. *PloS One* 10 (4), e0121933. doi: 10.1371/journal.pone.0121933

Su, V. Y., Lin, C. S., Hung, S. C., and Yang, K. Y. (2019a). Mesenchymal Stem Cell-Conditioned Medium Induces Neutrophil Apoptosis Associated with Inhibition of the NF-kappaB Pathway in Endotoxin-Induced Acute Lung Injury. *Int. J. Mol. Sci.* 20 (9), 2208. doi: 10.3390/ijms20092208

Su, V. Y., Yang, K. Y., Chiou, S. H., Chen, N. J., Mo, M. H., Lin, C. S., et al. (2019b). Induced Pluripotent Stem Cells Regulate Triggering Receptor Expressed on Myeloid Cell-1 Expression and the p38 Mitogen-Activated Protein Kinase Pathway in Endotoxin-Induced Acute Lung Injury. *Stem Cells (Dayton Ohio)* 37 (5), 631–639. doi: 10.1002/stem.2980

Sun, C. K., Yen, C. H., Lin, Y. C., Tsai, T. H., Chang, L. T., Kao, Y. H., et al. (2011). Autologous transplantation of adipose-derived mesenchymal stem cells markedly reduced acute ischemia-reperfusion lung injury in a rodent model. *J. Trans. Med.* 9, 118. doi: 10.1186/1479-5876-9-118

Tanaka, T., Narazaki, M., and Kishimoto, T. (2016). Immunotherapeutic implications of IL-6 blockade for cytokine storm. *Immunotherapy* 8 (8), 959–970. doi: 10.2217/imt-2016-0020

Van Wyngene, L., and Vandewalle, J. (2018). Reprogramming of basic metabolic pathways in microbial sepsis: therapeutic targets at last? *EMBO Mol. Med.* 10 (8), e8712. doi: 10.15252/emmm.201708712

Wu, X. J., Yan, X. T., Yang, X. M., Zhang, Y., Wang, H. Y., Luo, H., et al. (2020). GTS-21 ameliorates polymicrobial sepsis-induced hepatic injury by modulating autophagy through alpha7nAchRs in mice. *Cytokine* 128, 155019. doi: 10.1016/j.cyto.2020.155019

Yang, H. H., Duan, J. X., Liu, S. K., Xiong, J. B., Guan, X. X., Zhong, W. J., et al. (2020). A COX-2/sEH dual inhibitor PTUPB alleviates lipopolysaccharide-induced acute lung injury in mice by inhibiting NLRP3 inflammasome activation. *Theranostics* 10 (11), 4749–4761. doi: 10.7150/thno.43108

Yu, S., Cheng, Y., Zhang, L., Yin, Y., Xue, J., Li, B., et al. (2019). Treatment with adipose tissue-derived mesenchymal stem cells exerts anti-diabetic effects, improves long-term complications, and attenuates inflammation in type 2 diabetic rats. *Stem Cell Res. Ther.* 10 (1), 333. doi: 10.1186/s13287-019-1474-8

Zahedi, K., Barone, S., and Soleimani, M. (2019). Polyamine Catabolism in Acute Kidney Injury. *Int. J. Mol. Sci.* 20 (19), 4790. doi: 10.3390/ijms20194790

15

Pan-Cancer Analysis and Drug Formulation for GPR139 and GPR142

Aman Chandra Kaushik[1†], Aamir Mehmood[2,3†], Xiaofeng Dai[1] and Dong-Qing Wei[2,3*]*

[1]*Wuxi School of Medicine, Jiangnan University, Wuxi, China,* [2]*School of Life Sciences and Biotechnology, Shanghai Jiao Tong University, Shanghai, China,* [3]*Peng Cheng Laboratory, Vanke Cloud City Phase I, Guangdong, China*

Correspondence:
Xiaofeng Dai
xiaofeng.daii@jiangnan.edu.cn
Dong-Qing Wei
dqwei@sjtu.edu.cn

[†]*These authors have contributed equally to this work*

GPR (G protein receptor) 139 and 142 are novel foundling GPCRs (G protein-coupled receptors) in the class "A" of the GPCRs family and are suitable targets for various biological conditions. To engage these targets, validated pharmacophores and 3D QSAR (Quantitative structure-activity relationship) models are widely used because of their direct fingerprinting capability of the target and an overall accuracy. The current work initially analyzes GPR139 and GPR142 for its genomic alteration via tumor samples. Next to that, the pharmacophore is developed to scan the 3D database for such compounds that can lead to potential agonists. As a result, several compounds have been considered, showing satisfactory performance and a strong association with the target. Additionally, it is gripping to know that the obtained compounds were observed to be responsible for triggering pan-cancer. This suggests the possible role of novel GPR139 and GPR142 as the substances for initiating a physiological response to handle the condition incurred as a result of cancer.

Keywords: GPR142, molecular modeling, pharmacophore, 3D quantitative structure-activity relationship, 7TM, pan-cancer, the cancer genome atlas

INTRODUCTION

Computational biology and immunoinformatic are the multidisciplinary fields that are progressing rapidly (Wadood et al., 2017). Besides, *in vitro*, and *in vivo* techniques are extremely demanding but still relatively challenging because of various factors such as resources, time of the experiment, experimental labor, cost, and environmental issues and safety as compared to the computational approaches. However, combining both these *in silico* and *in vitro*/*in vivo* techniques is highly essential for addressing a particular biological condition or targets such as the decryption of an immune response and vaccine design (Korber et al., 2006). The *in silico* drug designing, often referred to as Computer-Aided Drug Design is mainly grouped into two classes which are termed as structure-based and ligand-based. Thus, various techniques are practiced for this to computationally propose a drug or peptide for a particular biological condition. These techniques could either be for designing and discovering purposes or validation. For instance, to discover and recommend a drug for a unique or resistant viral infection, next to the background history and understanding the mechanism of action, a virtual screening (VS) approach is applied that scans various small compounds' databases (i.e. ZINC, PubChem, MAYBRIDGE, etc.) (Shemetulskis et al., 1995; Irwin and Shoichet, 2005; Kim et al., 2015) to discover those hits that are more likely to be engaged with the target. In the field of Computer-Aided Drug Design, the word "hits" is a term used for compounds that are hypothesized that they may have a stronger affinity with the target. Before this VS technique, a 3D ensemble of chemical and molecular features known as pharmacophore is designed (Schneider et al., 1999; Wadood et al., 2017). It is crucial because this 3D model can recognize similar ligands or macromolecules from the enormous number of drugs like compounds provided in huge databases during the VS process (Sun, 2008).

Apart from VS, molecular docking (MD) (Huang et al., 2006) is a highly acceptable and practiced technique that considers the 3D conformation of a drug and its target in real-time and scores the performance of the drug along with providing various physical and chemical properties. Additionally, it explores how a drug interacts with the target that can be visualized in a 2D or 3D plane. There exists various offline and online software that are used for VS and MD. Few of the major software and servers are GOLD (Joy et al., 2006), AutoDock (Trott and Olson, 2010), PatchDocK (Mehmood et al., 2019; Schneidman-Duhovny et al., 2005; Khan et al., 2018), Molecular Operating Environment (MOE) (Roy and Luck, 2007), Schrödinger suite (Bhachoo and Beuming, 2017), and FireDock (Andrusier et al., 2007). Drugs that perform satisfactorily are observed to be engaged with their targets are subjected to another technique that is termed as molecular dynamics simulation (MDS) which is also a real-time cellular system with an optimum human body pressure, temperature, water, and pH that is built inside a computer driven by a particular forcefield (FF) such as OPLS, AMBER96, GROMACS 431, etc. in software like AMBER (Junaid et al., 2019), GROMACS (Wang et al., 2019) or SCHRÖDINGER (Winstead and Ravaioli, 2003). Nevertheless, the successful outcomes of all these sophisticated techniques (MD and MDS) depend on the most crucial step in this whole process which is the selection of accurate compounds. This selection directly depends on the classical VS technique whose quality is dependent on the quality of the pharmacophore model. Similar to this, QSAR models also bears great importance. It is an approach of vital importance for chemistry and pharmacy that is created on the concept that the activity of a molecule can be altered by bringing amendments into its structural configuration. These structural amendments may be implemented for virtual computational operations, intentional *in vitro* projects such as synthetic research, or only meant to investigate available substances. This method involves the mapping of property and chemical spaces using modeling functions that are associated with a chemical structure to property or more simply a function that relates property to molecular descriptors. This allows us to competently design and propose new potent compounds that possess the required features and perform the desired function.

Researchers in drug designing areas frequently go for existing commercial software like the Schrodinger software suite. This package has in-built modules which are highly demanding like Phase (Dixon et al., 2006a; Dixon et al., 2006b), ConfGen (Watts et al., 2010), and MacroModel (Watts et al., 2010) for Pharmacophore hypotheses generation (Mitra et al., 2010) and 3D QSAR model development (Lee and Briggs, 2001; Kubinyi et al., 2006; Pissurlenkar et al., 2007; Jiang, 2010; Lauria et al., 2010; Puzyn et al., 2010; John et al., 2011). The G protein-coupled receptors (GPCRs) regulate a countless number of physiological signaling cascades in the body, constituting a rich source of targets for the pharmacological deterrence of various human ailments (Atanes et al., 2018). Most of the GPCRs are expressed in the pancreatic islets are still considered as "orphan" which are poorly considered functional and or still have no recommended ligands and have not been used as promising antidiabetic targets (Amisten et al., 2017). A very limited quantity of functionally characterized GPCRs in the human body is the target for greater than 30% of all the current diseases. This stresses the reputation of the rest of GPCRs that lacks a functional chart yet in this regard. Analyses of such targets could reveal innovative ways to treat several biological conditions such as metabolic syndrome, cancer, and diabetes. Concerning the current study, the GPR139 and GPR142 are vital targets for numerous conditions and are therefore targeted in this work to discover potent compounds for them using valid pharmacophore and 3D QSAR studies that may have the ability to prevent us from the situation that is likely caused by these GPCRS.

METHODOLOGY

All the steps and techniques employed here are described in detail while the overall workflow of this work is diagrammatically represented in **Figure 1**.

Genomic Modifications Summary

The GPR139 and GP142 tumor samples were used to summarize the genomic alterations. For such analysis, wide-ranging CNA (amplifications and homozygous deletions) and color tagging were considered to review alterations in the gene expression. This was an initial approach to comprehend various forms of gene signaling in the Pan-cancer. The common exclusivity and co-occurrence between GPR139 and GPR142 were examined as well. Events associated with a particular cancer are high time differing in tumor clusters i.e., only a solitary biological incident is anticipated to happen in each cancerous sample. An additional situation is the concurrent existence of changes in several genes in the same sample. This was a preliminary way to collect information linked with various gene signaling in the pan-cancer.

GPR139 and GPR142 Mutations in Pan-Cancer

The locations and frequency of all the mutations within Pfam protein domains were detailed via mutations of GPR139 and GPR142. The whole extent of GPR139 and GPR142 is represented by colored bars while the base of every bar stands for the amino acids' amount. Colored regions are representing the protein's domain and the lines and points signify the location and amount of GPR139 and GPR142. The frameshift or nonsense mutations, missense mutations, and in-frames are visually represented in **Figure 2**.

Overall Survival Inspection

To highlight changes with time for prognosis purposes, the survival analysis bears great importance. In the current work, the Kaplan-Meier plots were used to evaluate differences in the overall survival among samples that were having more or equal to one alteration as that of the query gene(s). This was applied to those samples also that exhibits no alteration.

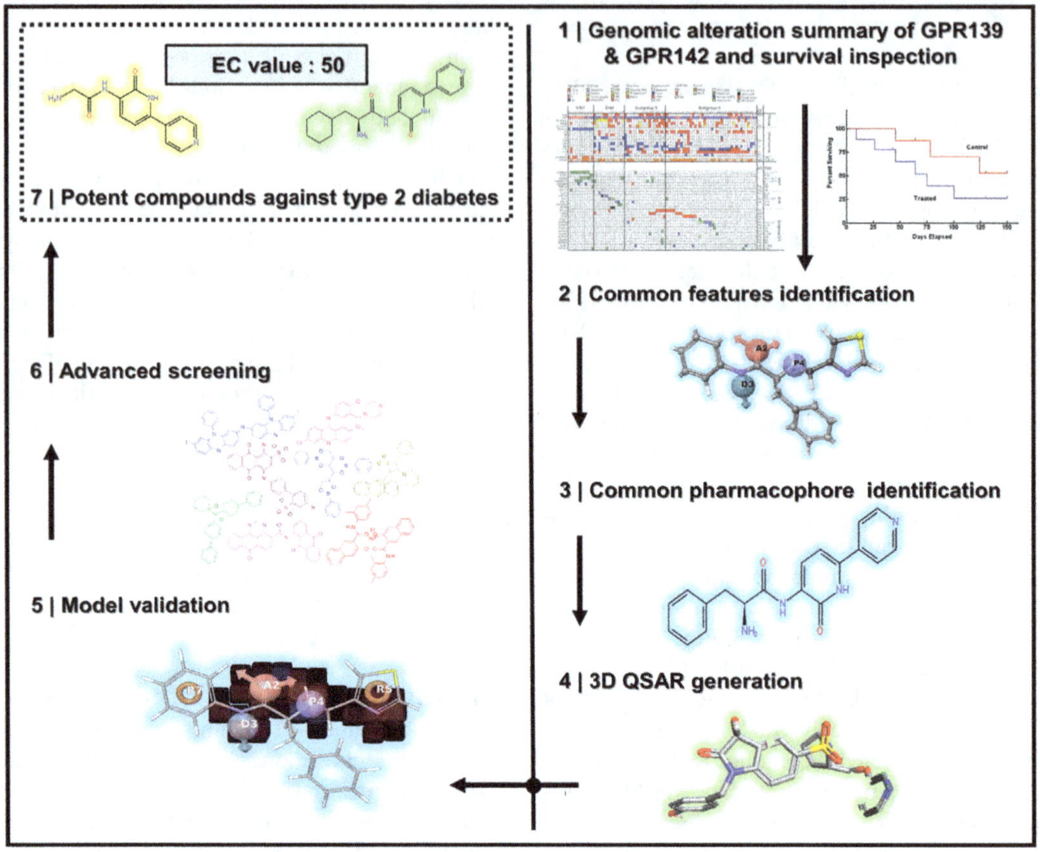

FIGURE 1 | The overall workflow of the steps taken for the successful pharmacophore's perception, 3D QSAR model development, and 3D database screening for GPR142.

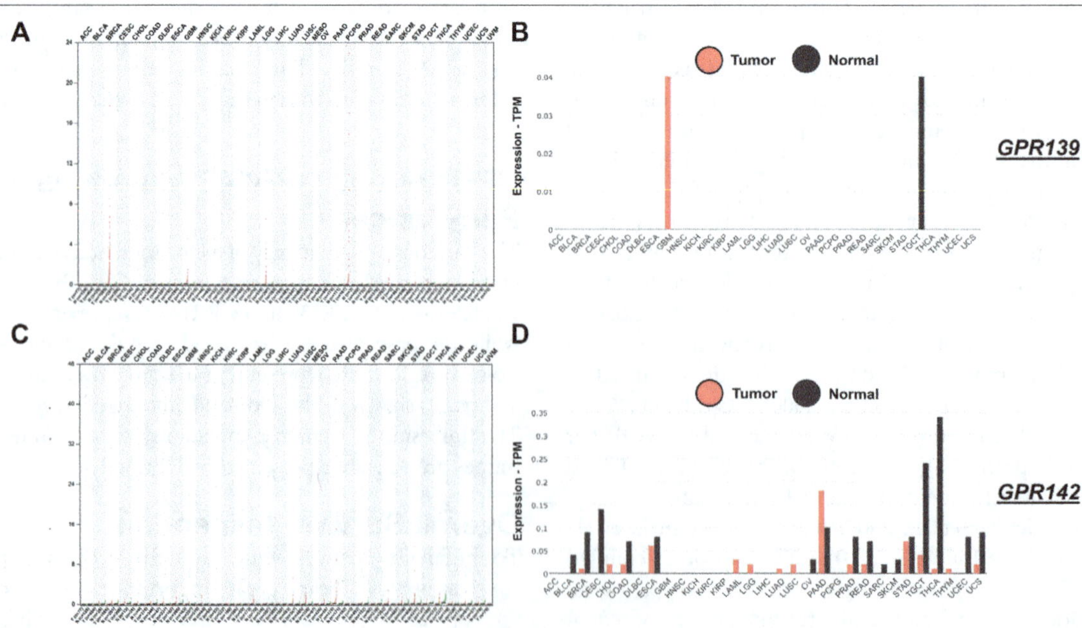

FIGURE 2 | Expression of GPR139 and GPR142 in pan-cancer from analyzed TCGA data. **Panel (A)** GPR139 expression breakdown; **Panel (B)** GPR139 tumor and normal expression breakdown; **Panel (C)** GPR142 expression study; **Panel (D)** GPR142 tumor and normal expression breakdown.

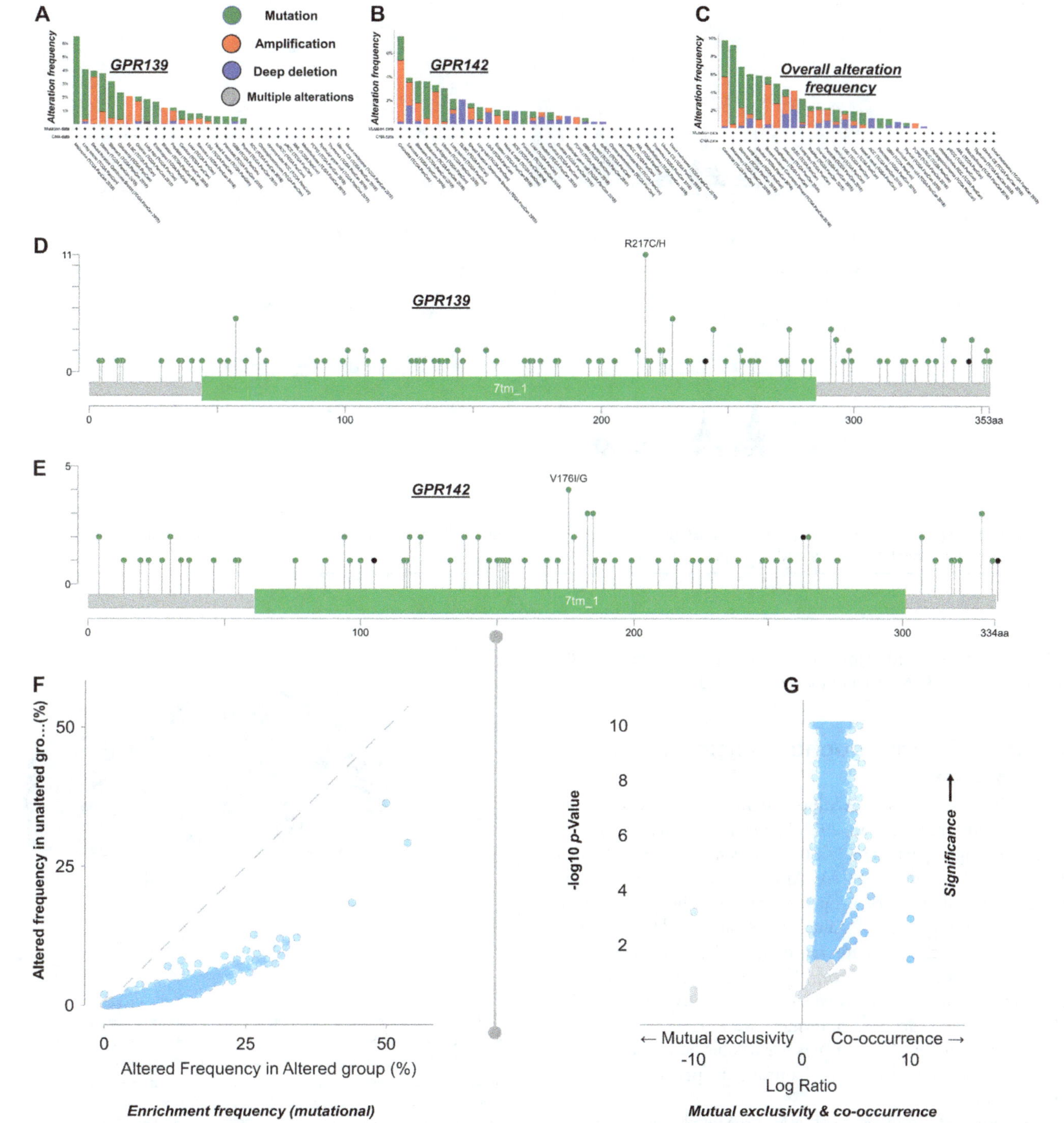

FIGURE 3 | GPR139 and GPR142 Global modification occurrence in pan-cancer based on the TCGA data **Panel (A)** GPR139 variation occurrence investigation; **Panel (B)** GPR142 variation frequency breakdown; **Panel (C)** Inclusive modification occurrence study; **Panel (D)** Ratio of the GPR139 mutations investigation; **Panel (E)**: Amount of GPR142 mutations breakdown. **Panel (F)** Amelioration rate, portraying genomic change per patient in the given samples, showing the mediation of GPR139 and GPR142 signaling in the pan-cancer. Besides, the gene signaling can be facilitated as well upon the instigation or inactivation of cell cycle control through truncating mutations. **Panel (G)** This board illustrates the amount of mutations uniqueness vs co-occurrence in the Genome.

Ligands' Preparation

First of all, ligands were prepared before the construction of pharmacophore along with the development of a 3D Database using LigPrep (Chen and Foloppe, 2010) which 3D protonates, convert the 2D structure into 3D, form stereoisomers, neutralize charged structures, balances the ionization state and pH using the

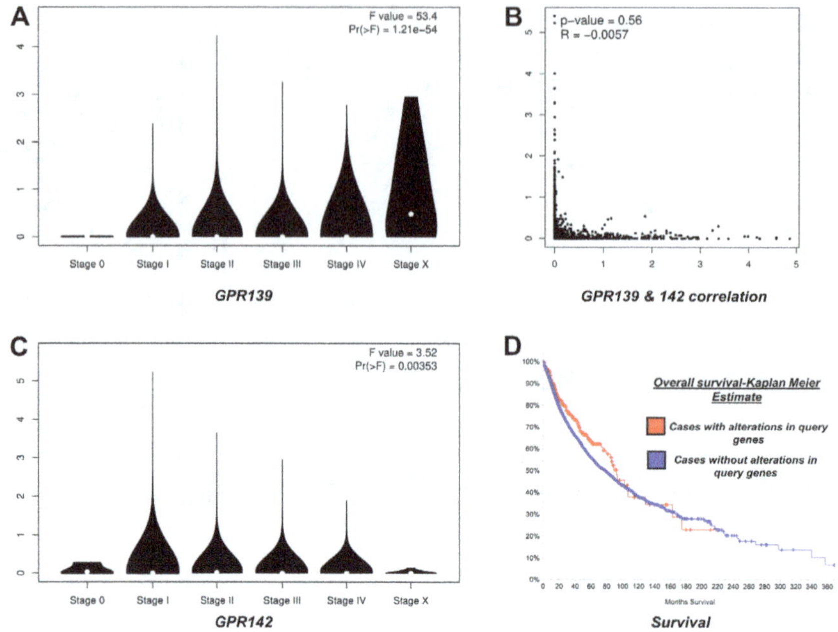

FIGURE 4 | Panel (A) Depicts stage plot of GPR139; **Panel (B)**: depicts the correlation between GPR139 and GPR142 in pan-cancer; **Panel (C)**: depicts stage plot of GPR142 and **Panel (D)**: depicts survival analysis of GPR139 and GPR142 in pan-cancer.

OPLS2005 force field (Jorgensen and Tirado-Rives, 1988; Jorgensen et al., 1996; Shivakumar et al., 2010).

Common Pharmacophore Hypotheses Development

A total of 63 compounds (see **Supplementary Table S2**) from the available literature (Du et al., 2012; Lizarzaburu et al., 2012) were chosen, having a particular EC50 value ranging from 0.036 to 33.00. Ligands were prepared; Amide activity property was selected with all primary properties' subset. The performance is given as Activity = −log[1*value]. The ligands and their various conformers were classified into sets to be used as input data (three datasets are used in this case). The ligands' conformer were generated having activity above 0.02 when Active, and activity below 0.01 when Inactive. Conformers were generated in such a way that the number of conformers per flexible bond was equal to 100. The maximum number of conformers per structure was equal to 1,000.

We employed ConfGen for the MacroModel search method that practices rapid sampling. Different conformers were used for Amide bonds which were pre-processed with a minimization step equal to 100 while the minimization step for high energy and redundant conformers was 50. The OPLS2005 force field was employed for this purpose. A maximum relative energy difference equal to 10.0 kcal/mol was maintained for the distance-dependent dielectric that eliminated redundant conformers using the RMSD of 1.0 Å. Structure cleaning- Stereoisomers retain specified chirality, meaning different chiral centers. Thus, the maximum number of stereoisomers kept was 32, and Ionization states retained the original structure using phase Schrodinger suite software (Dixon et al., 2006a).

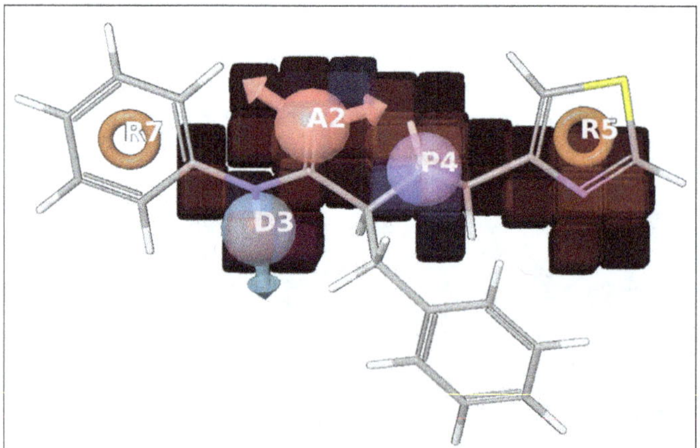

FIGURE 5 | Positive coefficient represented by dark blue color and Negative coefficient represented by the red color, Hydrogen bond donor (D), Hydrophobic/nonpolar (H), Electron-withdrawing (W) shown in the red cube, where R5 has a common pharmacophoric feature, responsible for the activity. A2 are in the negative coefficient and other R7, D3P4, and R5 are in the positive coefficient shown in the supplementary information (**Supplementary Figure S2**).

Creating Sites

For a given set of pharmacophoric features, sites of each feature in the given ligand conformations were identified and marked such as Acceptor (A), Donor (D), Hydrophobic (H), Negative (N), and

TABLE 1 | Pharmacophoric variant listing 21 out of 21 were selected, where the highest and lowest amount of positions are 7 and 4 correspondingly.

AAAADDP	AAAADDR	AAAADPR	AADPRRR	AAAADRR	DDPRRRR	AAPRRRR
AAAAPRR	AAAARRR	AAADDPR	AADDRRR	AAADDRR	ADPRRRR	ADDPRRR
AAADPRR	AAADRRR	AAAPRRR	AADDPRR	AAARRRR	ADDRRRR	AADRRRR

The selected variants were used for the generation of a maximum number of pharmacophoric hypotheses derived from a common pharmacophore model for the variants among the given active ligands. All the 7 out of 7 variants accompanying the number of maximum pharmacophoric features were selected.

Aromatic Rings (R). Features in the vector geometry were edited and a point was selected, in projected acceptor was selected, in point sp3, sp2, and sp were selected, 1 atom was used with distance.

First Dataset (High-Affinity EC50 Value)

The first dataset contained a total of sixty compounds. The activity thresholds were Active and Inactive if the compounds are above 0.036 and below 0.001 respectively. The maximum activity in the table was 0.930 while the minimum activity is observed as 0.036. The higher and lower number of sites were 7 and 3 and respectively that must resemble a minimum of 35 compounds out of 38 inactive or active's group. The hypotheses generation scoring, clustering and examined hypotheses, defining excluded volumes, selection of hypotheses for certain QSAR methods as well as search for the similarity or matches with the screened ligands were all carried out.

Second Dataset (Medium Affinity EC50 Value)

The second Dataset also contained the same number of compounds just like the first one, equal to 60. The activity threshold was Active and Inactive if the compounds are above 1.060 and below 1.000. On the other hand, the supreme movement was 6.6000 while a minimum activity of 1.060. The variants' list was defined with a total of 7 maximum sites and a minimum of 4 that must match at least 30 compounds out of 51 actives or in active's group. Score hypotheses generation scoring, clustering and examined hypotheses, defined excluded volumes, selection of hypotheses for certain QSAR methods as well as searching for similar compounds with screened ligands and identified best pharmacophoric featured compounds (Kaushik and Sahi, 2015).

Third Dataset (Low-Affinity EC50 Value)

The third Dataset was also comprised of 60 compounds, having an activity threshold of >0.036 and <0.035 for Active and Inactive respectively. The maximum activity in the table observed was 33.000 while the minimum activity score was found to be 0.036 that was maintained. Defined variants' list- the maximum number of sites was 7 and the minimum number of sites was 4 that had to resemble a minimum of twenty compounds with that of the total 60 actives or inactive set. Score hypotheses generation scoring, clustering and examined hypotheses, defining excluded volumes, selection of hypotheses for certain of QSAR methods as well as searching for matching with screened ligands were performed.

TABLE 2 | Selected and desired variants finding common pharmacophore for the variants among the given active ligands, 7 out of 7 selected variants can be seen in the variants' column.

Variant	Maximum number of hypotheses
ADRRR	1
AADPR	5
AAPRR	8
APRRR	7
DPRRR	6
ADPRR	22
AADRR	3

RESULTS

GPR139 and GPR142 Expression in Pan-Cancer

As a result of the expression analysis of GPR139, it was exposed that a substantial amount of up and down-regulation that explains the hotspots which are responsible for the activation and role in BRCA, GBM, LGG, PCPG, and SARC as shown in **Figure 2** while expression analysis of GPR142 revealed a substantial amount of up and down-regulation that explains the hotspots which are responsible for the activation and role in ESCA, LIHC, LUAD, LUSC, PAAD, STAD, TGCT, THCA, and UCS as shown in **Figure 2**.

Genomic Site and Variations Summary

Based on the obtained conclusions, most of the cases were found to be changing the GPR139 and GPR142. Upon further analysis, it was revealed that nearly all of the observed variations were missense mutations. Some deep deletions and few amplifications have also been noticed. Nevertheless, the remaining of the cases experienced alterations in GPR139 and GPR142 that are mainly exhibiting truncating and missense mutations. Examining the mutual exclusiveness suggests that events happened in GPR139 and GPR142 were responsible to occur again in pan-cancer (GPR139 exposed in BRCA, GBM, LGG, PCPG, and SARC) while GPR142 exposed in ESCA, LIHC, LUAD, LUSC, PAAD, STAD, TGCT, THCA, and UCS) as represented in **Figure 3**.

Analyzing Survival Rate

To inspect the rate of survival, the Kaplan-Meier approach was used to plot the complete survival analysis for the pan-cancer. Based on the global survival analysis, it was observed that mutations in the cell cycle control were concurrent and were not associated with the overall decreased survival (p-value =

TABLE 3 | Score hypotheses of ADPRR.18 where site, volume, and matches are listed with alignment for a hypothesis of ADPRR.18 where compound number 25 is observed to be a more valid and suitable one.

	Site	Vector	Volume	Selectivity	Match	Survival	Energy	Activity
ADPRR.18	0.71	0.913	0.611	2.273	31	3.237	0.000	3.300
Activity		**Pharm set**		**Fitness**		**Site matched**		**Relative energy**
3.300		Active		3.00		5		0.000

0.0615) as illustrated in **Figure 4**; while correlation analysis of clinical features observed GPR139 and GPR142 correlated in the progression of pathological stages.

Common Pharmacophoric Features Identification

Maintaining common features in a pharmacophore model is very important as they are the backbone of the parent molecules on which the functionality of the drug highly depends. All the common pharmacophoric features obtained from the 3D Database of GPR142 using phase Schrodinger suite software are summarized in the **Supplementary Table S1**. Out of 1,038 chemical structures from GPR142 3D Database; only 5 are chosen that are flexible chemical structures with an average reduction of up to 1.18 Å plus they are having a better common pharmacophoric match for pan-cancer target pharmacophore shown in **Figure 5**.

Common Pharmacophore Identification

To identify a common pharmacophore model, the selected and desired variants were used for the given active ligands (**Tables 1,2**).

Score Hypotheses

Score hypotheses generation was created by 30 out of 51. Apart from this, clustering and examination of the hypotheses, defining excluded volumes, and the selection of hypotheses for certain QSAR methods as well as the search for features with screened ligands were carried out. Score Actives; vector and site filtering maintained only those variants' that are having RMSD below 1.200 Å, vector score above 0.500 Å, and be the top 10%. The quantity should be in the range of 10 (minimum) and 50 (maximum). The survival score formula for vector score is 1.000, +1.000 for site score, +1.000 as volume score, −0.000 for the reference ligand relative conformational energy, +0.000 as selective score, +1.000 for the number of matches, and +0.000 in case of the reference ligand activity. All the values are listed in **Table 3**.

Building QSAR Model

In QSAR (Quantitative structure-activity relationship) model building, the predicted structure-activity relations for the matching ligands are investigated. The training set where the random seed was 0, keeping actives and inactive in the training set. The 3D QSAR model parameters were kept as standard. For example, the Grid sampling was 1.00 Å, the maximum PLS factor was 1, and the model type was atom-based (**Table 4**).

TABLE 4 | Training set where the random seed was 0, keeping actives and inactive in the training set where grid sampling is equal to 1.00 Å, maximum PLS factor was 1 and the model type is atom-based.

QSAR set (Training)	QSAR set (Test)
66, 64, 63, 62, 61, 60, 59, 58, 57, 56, 55, 53	54, 14, 13, 7, 6, 5, 4, 3, 2
51, 48, 45, 43, 42, 40, 39, 35, 34, 33, 32, 31	
30, 29, 27, 26, 24, 23, 22, 21, 20, 19, 18, 17	
16, 15, 52, 50, 49, 46, 41, 36, 28, 25, 11, 10, 9, 8, 1	

Model Validation

The model validation phase of the 3D QSAR models uses distinct training and testing sets for the cross-validation approach. The 3D QSAR models estimate outcome which is derived from the training set shown in **Figure 5**. The highly stable models are preferred as they don't rely completely on the training set. Regarding the statistical parameters for the training set, the m represents the number of PLS factors in the model, n represents the number of molecules in the training set, $df1 = m + 1$ represents the degrees of freedom in the model, $df2 = n - m - 2$ denotes the degree of freedom in the data, y represents the detected movement for a training set molecule i, $\hat{y_i}$ signifies the predicted activity for training set molecule i and $R^2 = 1-\sigma^2/\sigma^2$ is the R-squared or coefficient of determination. Test set prediction was performed by phase defined parameters, where T signifies the test set of molecules, n_T denotes the number of molecules in T, Y_j is the observed activity for molecule j ε T, $\hat{y_j}$ means the predicted activity for molecule j ε T, and $Q^2 = R^2$ (T) represents the Q-squared. The necessary parameters for the ADPRR are given in **Table 5**; **Figures 5,6**.

Screened Ligands and Known Compounds' Pharmacophore Analysis

The common pharmacophore using screened and known EC50 compounds was found along with a pharmacophore for those variants which are among the given active ligands. The variants' list was defined while the higher and the lower quantity regarding the sites were kept as 7 and 4 correspondingly, matching at least 20 compounds out of 137 active or inactive groups as shown in **Figure 7**. The variant list 269, after the identification of common pharmacophore, the ADHPRRR.35 was considered having maximum hypotheses as 16 with a survival rate of 2.960. The site score was 0.58, a vector was equal to 0.939, volume was 0.442, selectivity was 3.858 and the number of matches was 22. After the alignment of ADHPRRR.35 hypotheses, its fitness value turned out to be 2.02 and the number of site matches was 7 listed in **Table 6**; **Figures 7,8**.

TABLE 5 | 3D QSAR model parameters for ADPRR.18 pharmacophoric hypotheses, where R-squared value is 0.6478 which is considered a more favorable pharmacophoric feature in this case.

ID	SD	R-squared	F	P	Stability	RMSE	Q-squared	Pearson-R
ADPRR.18	1.0282	0.6478	90.1	1.097e-12	0.9449	26.7754	-7.674	0.0504

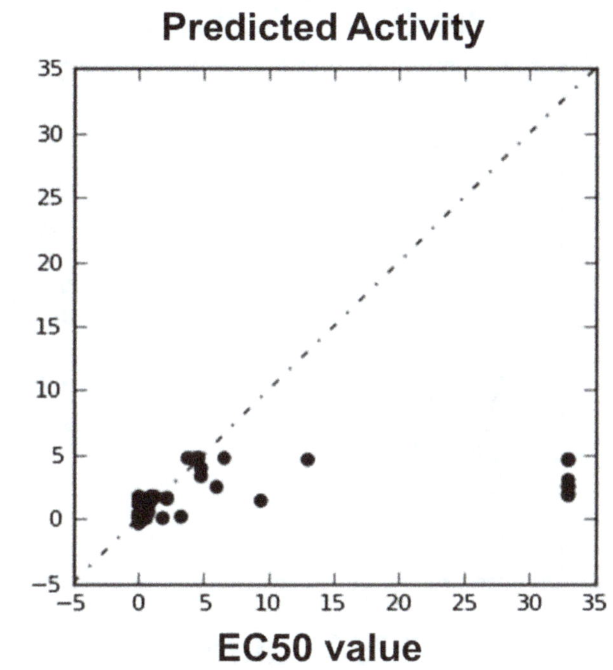

FIGURE 6 | Automatically generated regression plot of 3D QSAR EC50 value and phase predicted activity, where the *X*-axis signifies the EC50 score and *Y*-axis denotes the phase predicted activity of the chemical structure.

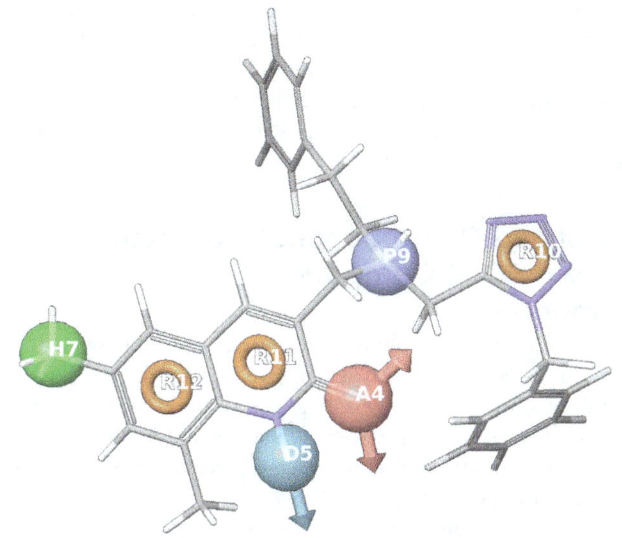

FIGURE 7 | Represents the common pharmacophore hypotheses using screened ligand and Known Compounds, where R10 has the most important common pharmacophoric feature that inhibits cancer.

New Pharmacophore Hypotheses Generation Using Glide Docking Score

The compounds were docked and scored by the newly identified common pharmacophore to find common features for the variants present among the given active ligands. Defining the variants' list and the highest and lowest number of spots as 7 and 4 correspondingly that must resemble a minimum of 95 compounds out of 137 active/inactive groups was done and maintained. After the identification of a common pharmacophore model, the variants' list was 24 where R8 is common in all pharmacophoric analysis and is observed to be responsible for the native activity of compounds, given in the supplementary information (**Supplementary Figure S1**).

Building QSAR Model

The QSAR model was build and examined for the predicted structure-activity relations concerning the matching ligands. The random seed in the training set was 0, keeping both the actives and inactive in the training set, sampled uniformly over the activity coordinates. The random training set was only 50%, 3D QSAR model parameters Grid sampling was 1.00 Å, maximum PLS factor was 1, and the model type was atom-based. After the alignment, Compound6 alignment score was observed to be 0.089967, vector score was equal to 0.996997, volume score was given as 0.428221, fitness value of 2.350246 and phase predicted score was -4.86423, Compound7 alignment score was 0.095122, vector score as 0.936649, volume score was observed to be 0.37549, fitness value was given as 2.232871 and phase predicted score was equal to −5.10154. Similarly, the Compound8 alignment score was 0.298618, vector score was 0.989711, volume score turned out to be 0.427929, fitness value as 2.168791 and phase predicted score equal to −5.16605 as shown in **Figure 9**.

Advanced Pharmacophore Screening of GPR142

Various hypotheses assisted in the identification of new matches and the conformers were generated automatically. For the conformer's generation and refinement, existing conformers were discarded, the number of structures per adjustable bond was kept as ten, the highest number of conformers per assembly was 100 with rapid sampling. The relative energy window was equal to 10.0 kcal/mol. Conformer's generation was skipped in case of rotatable bonds greater than fifteen. The matching tolerance was 2.0 Å in the inter-site and must match on at least 4 site positions out of 4. For the hit treatment purposes, hits were sorted out by decreasing fitness, that returned 1,000 hits

TABLE 6 | 3D QSAR model parameters for ADHPRRR.35 pharmacophoric hypotheses where grid sampling was 1.00 Å, maximum PLS factor was 1, and the model type was an atom-based pharmacophoric analysis.

ID	SD	R-squared	F	P	Stability	RMSE	Q-squared	Pearson-R
ADHPRRR.35	8.5856	0.3407	30	9.84e-07	0.931	7.6838	0	0

in total, i.e. 1 hit per molecule. Fitness of hit treatment was equal to 1.0 (for alignment score/1.2) + 1.0 (for vector score) and + 1.0 volume score. All hits with < −1.0 vector score and <0.0 volume score were rejected.The **Compound1, Compound2, and Compound3** were obtained after screening from the 3D database of GPR142, having the same pharmacophoric features that inhibit cancer.

Advanced Pharmacophore Screening of Known EC50 Compounds and Screened Compounds

Advanced pharmacophoric screening of known EC50 compounds and Screened Compounds was done using the default parameters. The existing conformers were discarded, the number of structures per adjustable bond was kept ten. The highest number of conformers apiece structure was kept as 100 with rapid sampling. The relative energy window was 10.0 kcal/mol, skipping conformer generation for structures with >15 rotatable bonds. Matching in inter-site distance matching tolerance was maintained at 2.0 Å and must match on at least 4 site positions out of 4. For the case of hit treatment purpose, hits by decreasing fitness turned out 1,000 in total which is equivalent to 1 hit per molecule. Fitness of the hit treatment was 1.0 (for alignment score/1.2) + 1.0 (for vector score) + 1.0 volume score. All hits with < −1.0 vector score and < 0.0 volume score were totally rejected. **Compound4 and compound5** were obtained after screening the 3D Database of GPR142, which has the same pharmacophoric features and common chemical structures that can inhibit cancer.

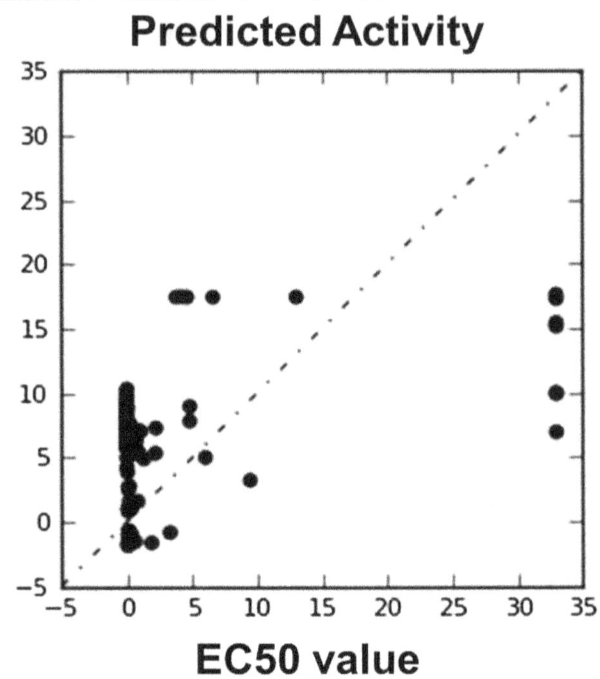

FIGURE 8 | Automatically generated regression plot of 3D QSAR known EC50 value and phase predicted activity, where *X*-axis signifies the EC50 score activity and *Y*-axis signifies the phase predicted activity of chemical structure.

Advanced Pharmacophore Screening and Analysis of New Pharmacophore Model

Advanced pharmacophoric screening of the newly identified pharmacophore model was performed by the glide docking scoring system. The number of conformers was set per rotatable bond as 10, a maximum number of conformers per structure was 100 with rapid sampling. The relative energy window was 10.0 kcal/mol. All the conformers' generation in case of structures with >15 rotatable bonds were skipped. The matching in inter-site distance matching tolerance was kept as 2.0 Å and must match on four sites position out of 4. Hits were sorted by decreasing fitness returning at its most equal to1000 hits in total that is 1 hit per molecule. The fitness of hit treatment was 1.0 (for alignment score/1.2) + 1.0 (for vector score) + 1.0 volume score. Reject hits with < −1.0 vector score and < 0.0 volume score. In all the considered compounds, **Compound6, compound7, and Compound8** were chosen after screening the 3D Database of GPR142. They all were having the same pharmacophoric features and can inhibit cancer.

Advanced Pharmacophore Screening of GPR139

The Paralog of the GPR142 gene is GPR139, and the similarity gene and protein between GPR139 and GPR142 is 50%, sharing suggested ligands. The advanced pharmacophoric screening was carried out by these protocols such as; finding matches from the generated features' search during conformers exploration that were automatically generated. All existing conformers were discarded, the conformers apiece adjustable bond was chosen to be 10. On the other hand, the maximum amount for conformers apiece structure was chosen to be 100, the relative energy window was equal to 10.0 kcal/mol. Similarly, conformers' generation for structures with greater than 15 rotatable bonds was skipped. Matching in inter-site distance matching tolerance was 2.0 Å and must match on at four site positions out of the total 4. All hits were sorted decreasing the fitness value, returning at the most given hits which are 1,000 in total that is 1 hit per molecule. Fitness of hit treatment was 1.0 (for alignment score/1.2) + 1.0 (for vector score) + 1.0 as the volume score. Hits were rejected with < −1.0 vector score and < 0.0 volume score. The **Compound9 and Compound10** were selected as a result

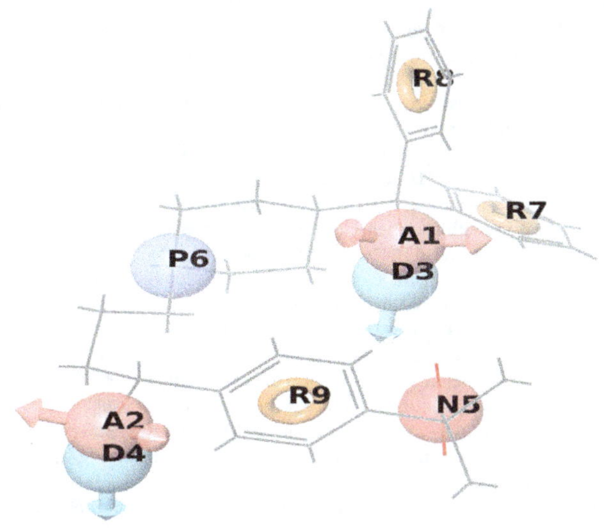

FIGURE 9 | Represents the common pharmacophore hypotheses using the docking score of screened ligands, where R8 has the most important common pharmacophoric feature that inhibits cancer.

of screening from the 3D Database of GPR139, which contains similar pharmacophoric features like GPR142 target compounds. Compound9 and Compound10 might be helpful in the proteins' dimerization activity and neuropeptide receptor activity as provided in the supplementary data (**Supplementary Table S3**).

CONCLUSION

Computational drug design mainly emphasizes structure-based techniques. The *in silico* screening of small compounds in large databases using developed pharmacophoric features is a good way to discover and identify the best chemical compounds by using common pharmacophoric hypotheses generation and 3D QSAR models. However, extra care should be taken during the development of such a model as the performance of the predicted compounds depends on the features considered. It is a more feasible, robust, and flexible way to use such models. The current study reports on genomic alterations of GPR139 and GPR142 through tumor samples, assisting in the identification of common drug compounds for GPR142 target by 3D database by scanning common pharmacophoric features and experimental EC50 value which might be useful in the inhibition of cancer. We intend to subject these compounds to explore their interactions with the target and stability in the host region via long term molecular dynamics simulation and *in vitro* analysis.

AUTHOR CONTRIBUTIONS

AC and D-QW designed the experiment, D-QW and AC performed the entire computational experiments and assisted in writing the manuscript, D-QW, AC, and AM analyzed the data and wrote the manuscript. AC, D-QW, XD, and AM read the manuscript and advised on method development. All authors have approved the final version of the manuscript.

FUNDING

This work is supported by the grants from the Key Research Area Grant 2016YFA0501703, 2018ZX10302205-004-002, and 2018ZX10302-205-004 of the Ministry of Science and Technology of China, the National Natural Science Foundation of China (Contract No. 61832019, 61503244, and BK20161130), the State Key Lab of Microbial Metabolism and Joint Research Funds for Medical and Engineering and Scientific Research at Shanghai Jiao Tong University (YG2017ZD14). The Six Talent Peaks Project in Jiangsu Province (Grant No. SWYY-128), Major Project of Science and Technology in Henan Province (Grant No.161100311400), The Technology Development Funding of Wuxi (Grant No. WX18IVJN017), Research Funds for the Medical School of Jiangnan University ESI special cultivation project (Grant No. 1286010241170320). These funding sources have no role in the writing of the manuscript or the decision to submit it for publication.

ACKNOWLEDGMENTS

The heavy-duty computational operations carried out in this work was supported by the Center for High-Performance Computing, Shanghai Jiao Tong University.

REFERENCES

Amisten, S., Atanes, P., Hawkes, R., Ruz-Maldonado, I., Liu, B., Parandeh, F., et al. (2017). A comparative analysis of human and mouse islet G-protein coupled receptor expression. *Sci. Rep.* 7, 46600. doi:10.1038/srep46600

Andrusier, N., Nussinov, R., and Wolfson, H. J. (2007). FireDock: fast interaction refinement in molecular docking. *Proteins* 69 (1), 139–159. doi:10.1002/prot.21495

Atanes, P., Ruz-Maldonado, I., Hawkes, R., Liu, B., Zhao, M., Huang, G. C., et al. (2018). Defining G protein-coupled receptor peptide ligand expressomes and signalomes in human and mouse islets. *Cell. Mol. Life Sci.* 75 (16), 3039–3050. doi:10.1007/s00018-018-2778-z

Bhachoo, J., and Beuming, T. (2017). "Investigating protein-peptide interactions using the schrödinger computational suite, *Methods molecular biology, Modeling peptide-protein interactions*, Editors O. Schueler-Furman and N. London New York, NY: Humana Press, Vol. 1561, 235–254. doi:10.1007/978-1-4939-6798-8_14

Chen, I. J., and Foloppe, N. (2010). Drug-like bioactive structures and conformational coverage with the LigPrep/ConfGen suite: comparison to programs MOE and catalyst. *J. Chem. Inf. Model.* 50 (5), 822–839. doi:10.1021/ci100026x

Dixon, S. L., Smondyrev, A. M., and Rao, S. N. (2006). PHASE: a novel approach to pharmacophore modeling and 3D database searching. *Chem. Biol. Drug Des.* 67 (5), 370–372. doi:10.1111/j.1747-0285.2006.00384.x

Dixon, S. L., Smondyrev, A. M., Knoll, E. H., Rao, S. N., Shaw, D. E., and Friesner, R. A. (2006a). PHASE: a new engine for pharmacophore perception, 3D QSAR model development, and 3D database screening: 1. Methodology and preliminary results. *J. Comput. Aided Mol. Des.* 20 (10–11), 647–671. doi:10.1007/s10822-006-9087-6

Du, X., Kim, Y. J., Lai, S., Chen, X., Lizarzaburu, M., Turcotte, S., et al. (2012). Phenylalanine derivatives as GPR142 agonists for the treatment of type II diabetes. *Bioorg. Med. Chem. Lett.* 22 (19), 6218–6223. doi:10.1016/j.bmcl.2012.08.015

Huang, N., Shoichet, B. K., and Irwin, J. J. (2006). Benchmarking sets for molecular docking. *J. Med. Chem.* 49 (23), 6789–6801. doi:10.1021/jm0608356

Irwin, J. J., and Shoichet, B. K. (2005). ZINC– a free database of commercially available compounds for virtual screening. *J. Chem. Inf. Model.* 45 (1), 177–182. doi:10.1021/ci049714

Jiang, Y.-K. (2010). Molecular docking and 3D-QSAR studies on beta-phenylalanine derivatives as dipeptidyl peptidase IV inhibitors. *J. Mol. Model.* 16 (7), 1239–1249. doi:10.1007/s00894-009-0637-4

John, S., Thangapandian, S., Arooj, M., Hong, J. C., Kim, K. D., and Lee, K. W. (2011). Development, evaluation and application of 3D QSAR Pharmacophore model in the discovery of potential human renin inhibitors. *BMC Bioinf.* 12, S4. doi:10.1186/1471-2105-12-S14-S4

Jorgensen, W. L., and Tirado-Rives, J. (1988). The OPLS [optimized potentials for liquid simulations] potential functions for proteins, energy minimizations for crystals of cyclic peptides and crambin. *J. Am. Chem. Soc.* 110 (6), 1657–1666. doi:10.1021/ja00214a001

Jorgensen, W. L., Maxwell, D. S., and Tirado-Rives, J. (1996). Development and testing of the OPLS all-atom force field on conformational energetics and properties of organic liquids. *J. Am. Chem. Soc.* 118 (45), 11225–11236. doi:10.1021/ja9621760

Joy, S., Nair, P. S., Hariharan, R., and Pillai, M. R. (2006). Detailed comparison of the protein-ligand docking efficiencies of GOLD, a commercial package and ArgusLab, a licensable freeware. *Silico Biol.* 6 (6), 601–605.

Junaid, M., Shah, M., Khan, A., Li, C.-D., Khan, M. T., Kaushik, A. C., et al. (2019). Structural-dynamic insights into the H. pylori cytotoxin-associated gene A (CagA) and its abrogation to interact with the tumor suppressor protein ASPP2 using decoy peptides. *J. Biomol. Struct. Dyn.* 37 (15), 4035–4050. doi:10.1080/07391102.2018.1537895

Kaushik, A. C., and Sahi, S. (2015). Boolean network model for GPR142 against Type 2 diabetes and relative dynamic change ratio analysis using systems and biological circuits approach. *Syst. Synth. Biol.* 9 (1–2), 45–54. doi:10.1007/s11693-015-9163-0

Khan, A., Junaid, M., Kaushik, A. C., Ali, A., Ali, S. S., Mehmood, A., et al. (2018). Computational identification, characterization and validation of potential antigenic peptide vaccines from hrHPVs E6 proteins using immunoinformatics and computational systems biology approaches. *PloS One* 13 (5), e0196484. doi:10.1371/journal.pone.0196484

Kim, S., Thiessen, P. A., Bolton, E. E., Chen, J., Fu, G., Gindulyte, A., et al. (2016). PubChem substance and compound databases. *Nucleic Acids Res.* 44 (D1), D1202–D1213. doi:10.1093/nar/gkv951

Korber, B., LaBute, M., and Yusim, K. (2006). Immunoinformatics comes of age. *PLoS Comput. Biol.* 2 (6), e71. doi:10.1371/journal.pcbi.0020071

Kubinyi, H., Folkers, G., and Martin, Y. C. (2006). *3D QSAR in drug design: recent advances*. Ludwigshafen, Germany: Springer Science & Business Media.

Lauria, A., Ippolito, M., Fazzari, M., Tutone, M., Di Blasi, F., Mingoia, F., et al. (2010). IKK-beta inhibitors: an analysis of drug-receptor interaction by using molecular docking and pharmacophore 3D-QSAR approaches. *J. Mol. Graph. Model.* 29 (1), 72–81. doi:10.1016/j.jmgm.2010.04.008

Lee, K. W., and Briggs, J. M. (2001). Comparative molecular field analysis (coMFA) study of epothilones-tubulin depolymerization inhibitors: pharmacophore development using 3D QSAR methods. *J. Comput. Aided Mol. Des.* 15 (1), 41–55. doi:10.1023/a:1011140723828

Lizarzaburu, M., Turcotte, S., Du, X., Duquette, J., Fu, A., Houze, J., et al. (2012). Discovery and optimization of a novel series of GPR142 agonists for the treatment of type 2 diabetes mellitus. *Bioorg. Med. Chem. Lett.* 22 (18), 5942–5947. doi:10.1016/j.bmcl.2012.07.063

Mehmood, A., Kaushik, A. C., and Wei, D. Q. (2019). Prediction and validation of potent peptides against Herpes Simplex Virus Type 1 (HSV-1) via immunoinformatic and systems biology approach. *Chem. Biol. Drug Des.* 94, 1868–1883. doi:10.1111/cbdd.13602

Mitra, I., Saha, A., and Roy, K. (2010). Pharmacophore mapping of arylamino-substituted benzo[b]thiophenes as free radical scavengers. *J. Mol. Model.* 16 (10), 1585–1596. doi:10.1007/s00894-010-0661-4

Pissurlenkar, R. R., Shaikh, M. S., and Coutinho, E. C. (2007). 3D-QSAR studies of Dipeptidyl peptidase IV inhibitors using a docking based alignment. *J. Mol. Model.* 13 (10), 1047–1071. doi:10.1007/s00894-007-0227-2

Puzyn, T., Gajewicz, A., Leszczynska, D., and Leszczynski, J. (2010). Nanomaterials–the next great challenge for QSAR modelers," in *Recent advances in QSAR studies* (Gdansk, Poland: Springer), 383–409.

Roy, U., and Luck, L. A. (2007). Molecular modeling of estrogen receptor using molecular operating environment. *Biochem. Mol. Biol. Educ.* 35 (4), 238–243. doi:10.1002/bmb.65

Schneider, G., Neidhart, W., Giller, T., and Schmid, G. (1999). "Scaffold-hopping" by topological pharmacophore search: a contribution to virtual screening. *Angew. Chem. Int. Ed.* 38 (19), 2894–2896. doi:10.1002/(sici)1521-3773(19991004)38:19<2894::aid-anie2894>3.0.co;2-f

Schneidman-Duhovny, D., Inbar, Y., Nussinov, R., and Wolfson, H. J. (2005). PatchDock and SymmDock: servers for rigid and symmetric docking. *Nucleic Acids Res.* 33 (Suppl. 2), W363–W367. doi:10.1093/nar/gki481

Shemetulskis, N. E., Dunbar, J. B., Dunbar, B. W., Moreland, D. W., and Humblet, C. (1995). Enhancing the diversity of a corporate database using chemical database clustering and analysis. *J. Comput. Aided Mol. Des.* 9 (5), 407–416. doi:10.1007/BF00123998

Shivakumar, D., Williams, J., Wu, Y., Damm, W., Shelley, J., and Sherman, W. (2010). Prediction of absolute solvation free energies using molecular dynamics free energy perturbation and the OPLS force field. *J. Chem. Theor. Comput.* 6 (5), 1509–1519. doi:10.1021/ct900587b

Sun, H. (2008). Pharmacophore-based virtual screening. *Curr. Med. Chem.* 15 (10), 1018–1024. doi:10.2174/092986708784049630

Trott, O., and Olson, A. J. (2010). AutoDock Vina: improving the speed and accuracy of docking with a new scoring function, efficient optimization, and multithreading. *J. Comput. Chem.* 31 (2), 455–461. doi:10.1002/jcc.21334

Wadood, A., Mehmood, A., Khan, H., Ilyas, M., Ahmad, A., Alarjah, M., et al. (2017). Epitopes based drug design for dengue virus envelope protein: a computational approach. *Comput. Biol. Chem.* 71, 152–160. doi:10.1016/j.compbiolchem.2017.10.008

Wang, Q., Mehmood, A., Wang, H., Xu, Q., Xiong, Y., and Wei, D.-Q. (2019). Computational screening and analysis of lung cancer related non-synonymous single nucleotide polymorphisms on the human Kirsten rat sarcoma gene. *Molecules* 24 (10), 1951. doi:10.3390/molecules24101951

Watts, K. S., Dalal, P., Murphy, R. B., Sherman, W., Friesner, R. A., and Shelley, J. C. (2010). ConfGen: a conformational search method for efficient generation of bioactive conformers. *J. Chem. Inf. Model.* 50 (4), 534–546. doi:10.1021/ci100015j

Winstead, B., and Ravaioli, U. (2003). A quantum correction based on Schrodinger equation applied to Monte Carlo device simulation. *IEEE Trans. Electron. Dev.* 50 (2), 440–446. doi:10.1109/TED.2003.809431

16

The Mu.Ta.Lig. Chemotheca: A Community-Populated Molecular Database for Multi-Target Ligands Identification and Compound-Repurposing

Francesco Ortuso [1], Donatella Bagetta [1], Annalisa Maruca [1], Carmine Talarico [1], Maria L. Bolognesi [2], Norbert Haider [3], Fernanda Borges [4], Sharon Bryant [5], Thierry Langer [3], Hanoch Senderowitz [6] and Stefano Alcaro [1]*

[1] Department of Health Sciences, Magna Græcia University of Catanzaro, Catanzaro, Italy, [2] Department of Pharmacy and Biotechnology, Università di Bologna, Bologna, Italy, [3] Department of Pharmaceutical Chemistry, Faculty of Life Sciences, University of Vienna, Vienna, Austria, [4] Department of Chemistry and Biochemistry, Faculty of Sciences, CIQUP, Universidade do Porto, Porto, Portugal, [5] Inte:Ligand GmbH, Vienna, Austria, [6] Department of Chemistry, Bar-Ilan University, Ramat Gan, Israel

***Correspondence:**
Francesco Ortuso
ortuso@unicz.it

For every lead compound developed in medicinal chemistry research, numerous other inactive or less active candidates are synthetized/isolated and tested. The majority of these compounds will not be selected for further development due to a sub-optimal pharmacological profile. However, some poorly active or even inactive compounds could live a second life if tested against other targets. Thus, new therapeutic opportunities could emerge and synergistic activities could be identified and exploited for existing compounds by sharing information between researchers who are working on different targets. The Mu.Ta.Lig (Multi-Target Ligand) Chemotheca database aims to offer such opportunities by facilitating information exchange among researchers worldwide. After a preliminary registration, users can (a) virtually upload structures and activity data for their compounds with corresponding, and eventually known activity data, and (b) search for other available compounds uploaded by the users community. Each piece of information about given compounds is owned by the user who initially uploaded it and multiple ownership is possible (this occurs if different users uploaded the same compounds or information pertaining to the same compounds). A web-based graphical user interface has been developed to assist compound uploading, compounds searching and data retrieval. Physico-chemical and ADME properties as well as substructure-based PAINS evaluations are computed on the fly for each uploaded compound. Samples of compounds that match a set of search criteria and additional data on these compounds could be requested directly from their owners with no mediation by the Mu.Ta.Lig Chemotheca team. Guest access provides a simplified search interface to retrieve only basic information such as compound IDs and related 2D or 3D chemical structures. Moreover, some compounds can be hidden to Guest users according to an owner's decision. In contrast, registered users have full access to all of the Chemotheca data including the permission to upload new compounds and/or update experimental/theoretical data (e.g., activities against new targets tested) related to already stored compounds. In order to facilitate scientific collaborations, all available data are connected to the corresponding owner's email address (available for registered users only). The Chemotheca web site is accessible at http://chemotheca.unicz.it.

Keywords: molecular database, multi-target drugs, drug repurposing, LAMP server, openbabel, Pybel, molecular descriptors, scientific collaboration

INTRODUCTION

The Chemotheca database was developed within the framework of the COST ACTION CA15135, "MuTaLig." It is focused on the identification of multi-target ligands and on the possibility for repurposing such bio-active compounds. These goals could be reached by stimulating new scientific collaborations among research groups involved, in various ways, in the study of drugs, and by merging their results. In fact, large numbers of molecules with a potential pharmaceutical relevance are developed in universities and in pharmaceutical industry each year. Most of these compounds will never reach the market due to some failure in pharmacology profile. Nevertheless, these chemical entities and their pharmacological profiles can be considered as a source of information evaluable against other targets. With this in mind, an information exchange platform, designed to allow for a direct connection among its users, has been developed. In contrast with already available services, such as ZINC (Irwin and Shoichet, 2005; Irwin et al., 2012), ChEMBL (Bento et al., 2014), PubChem (Kim et al., 2016), ChemSpider (www.chemspider.com), DrugBank (Wishart et al., 2006, 2018), WOMBAT (Good and Oprea, 2008), DUD (Huang et al., 2006), CSD (Groom et al., 2016), and others, which typically provide only compound download options, the Chemotheca database permits registered users to directly upload their own data. Such information immediately becomes available on the web site and contains the corresponding owner's contact details. Chemotheca software, automatically and user transparently, checks if the uploading compound structure has been designed according to chemistry rules and if it is consistent with mandatory fields required data. Additional information includable with uploaded compounds can be both experimental and theoretical and contain attributes such as molecular structures, activities, ADME/t properties, physico-chemical descriptors and references. For each new uploaded compound, 90 molecular descriptors are computed, on the fly. To safeguard intellectual property, and to facilitate collaboration among participants, the (user)name and the email address of the user who has uploaded the data are shown. To prevent abuse (such as spam), these details are disclosed to registered users only. A very detailed query form has been developed for searching deposited records. Matching query results can be exported as standard SMILES, SDF, MOL2 and HTML file formats.

MATERIALS AND METHODS

The Chemotheca was developed with open-source programming environments, its core being a web-accessible molecular database. It is hosted at the Magna Græcia University of Catanzaro (Italy) by the Medicinal Chemistry laboratory. An Intel Xeon 64 bit dual processor cluster facility, running under the Linux CentOS 7 (www.centos.org) operating system, offers the service. Apache software (www.apache.org) serves the web site, which complies with the W3C DTD HTML 4 standard (www.w3.org). Static and dynamic web pages have been written using the PHP programming language (www.php.net). The advanced search form and the compound upload user interfaces include the JSME molecular editor (Bienfait and Ertl, 2013). All Chemotheca data are stored in a MySQL database (www.mysql.com). An *ad hoc* developed Python (www.python.org) code (CDC) computes molecular descriptors for each uploaded compound, by using the OpenBabel library (O'Boyle et al., 2011) and its wrapper Pybel (O'Boyle et al., 2008).

The molecule upload process uses the isomeric SMILES code produced by the JSME applet. The CDC converts SMILES into a fingerprint. Fingerprint pattern matching prevents duplicate structures. If the compound is already available, another (new) owner will be added only. In case of a new structure entry, SMILES is converted into 2D and 3D SDF and MOL2 file formats. The 3D structure atom coordinates are optimized using the MMFF94 force field *in vacuo*. The energy minimization protocol consists of 150 steps of Steepest Descent algorithm followed by variable steps of Conjugate Gradients (50 for each rotatable bond). A convergence criterion of 0.05 kcal/mol·$Å^{-1}$ is used. Molecular descriptors, such as Lipinski rule compliance, CNS bioavailability, PAINS matching, LogBB, LogP, total polar surface area (TPSA), molecular weight, are computed using OpenBabel and Pybel built-in functions. The Central Nervous System (CNS) bioavailability and the LogBB descriptors are estimated according to Vilar et al. (2010). The Pan Assay INterference compoundS (PAINS) detection is based on the Pybel Smarts comparison between the new compound and the substructures reported by Baell and Holloway (2010). Users should carefully evaluate the application of any PAINS filtering because of the controversial opinions in the literature (Aldrich et al., 2017; Capuzzi et al., 2017). Search procedures are based on MySQL queries that are built and executed by the PHP code of the "Simple search" or "Advanced search" forms.

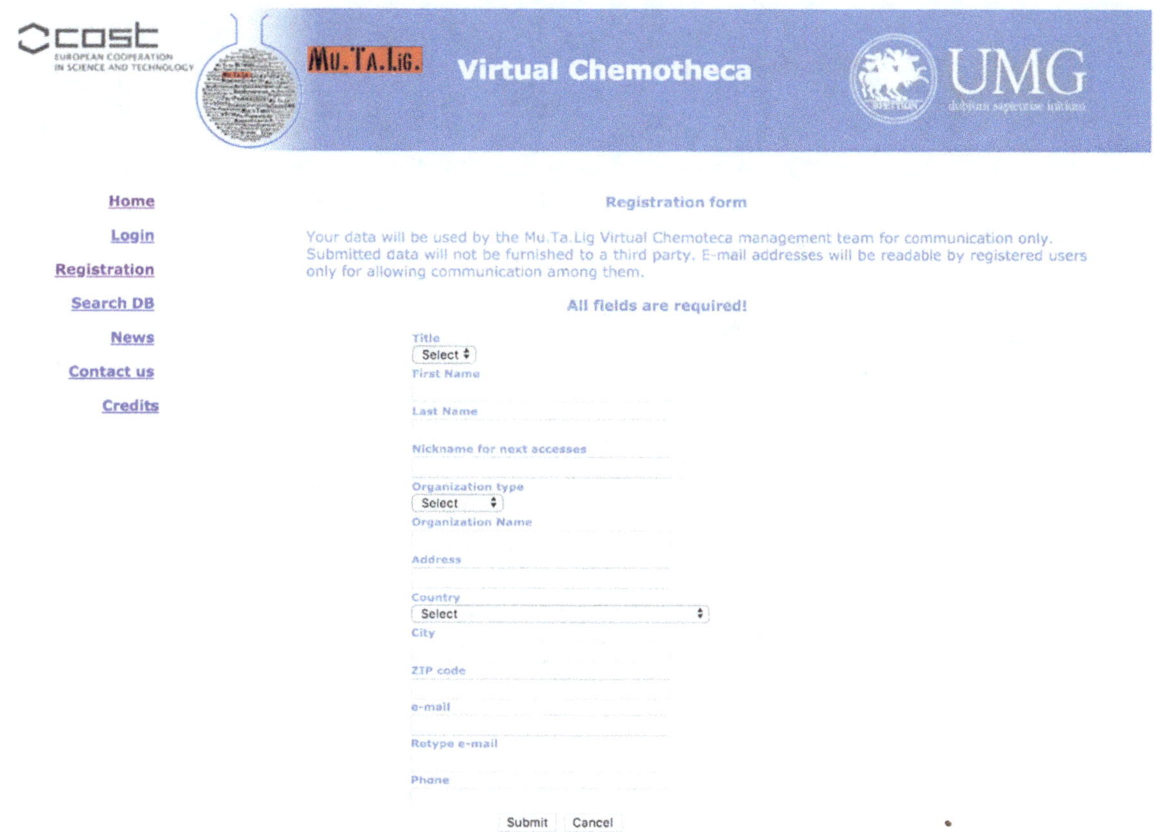

FIGURE 1 | Registration form.

DISCUSSION

The Chemotheca has been developed with the aims of (a) identifying multi-target agents and repurposing known active compounds and (b) stimulating new scientific collaborations between researchers while saving intellectual property of all involved researchers. The success of this approach will depend not only on its unique concept and the quality of its infrastructure, but mainly on its visibility to the scientific community and on its attractiveness for researchers to join.

Registration

The users' registration is crucial for the Chemotheca purposes and it is strongly encouraged. Guest access is allowed but it is very limited in terms of offered functionalities: (a) the upload of new information is not possible, (b) the advanced search form is not available, and (c) the search results consist of a list of molecular structures only. Basically, guest access should be considered for the very first visit to the web site. The registration procedure has been designed to be as easy as possible: a predefined form has to be filled with minimal personal information and, after its submission, an automatic email message will summarize the registration data and will communicate the password for the first authenticated access. After the login, the "Your Profile" menu allows the update of the personal information and the management of frequently used search queries, if they have been previously saved (**Figure 1**).

Search Facilities

All users can search for stored compounds by using the simple search query form. The advanced search interface is available for registered users only. In simple search, SMILES notation, owner username, InChI, InChIKey or, if known, the compound identity code (ID) can be, singularly, applied as query items. The advanced search interface offers many more options linked together by the Boolean operator AND. In addition to simple search criteria, the advanced query form can take into account (a) chemical substructure, (b) owner furnished compound's features such as chirality, origin (natural, organic synthesis or theoretical), purity, (c) Chemotheca computed properties, and (d) functional groups, chemical bonds and atom type. Before submitting the search, the user can save the query in the "Your Profile" menu to be reloaded for further investigation. The results detail level can be customized (**Figure 2**).

Results are displayed, as a pageable table reporting the 2D chemical structure of matching compounds, their owner(s) and properties according to the detail level previously selected. By default, 10 rows per page will be shown, but the user can

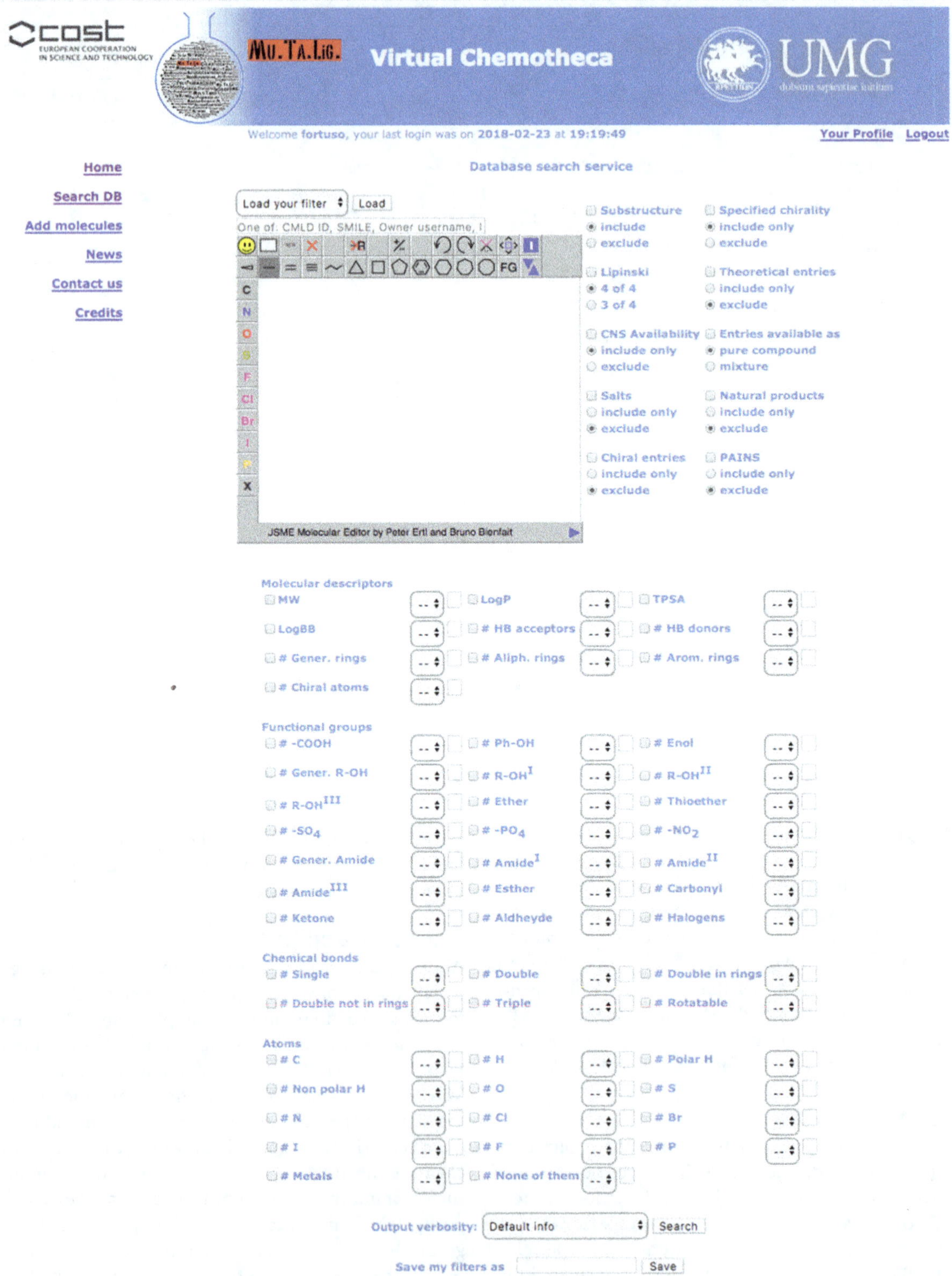

FIGURE 2 | Advanced search form.

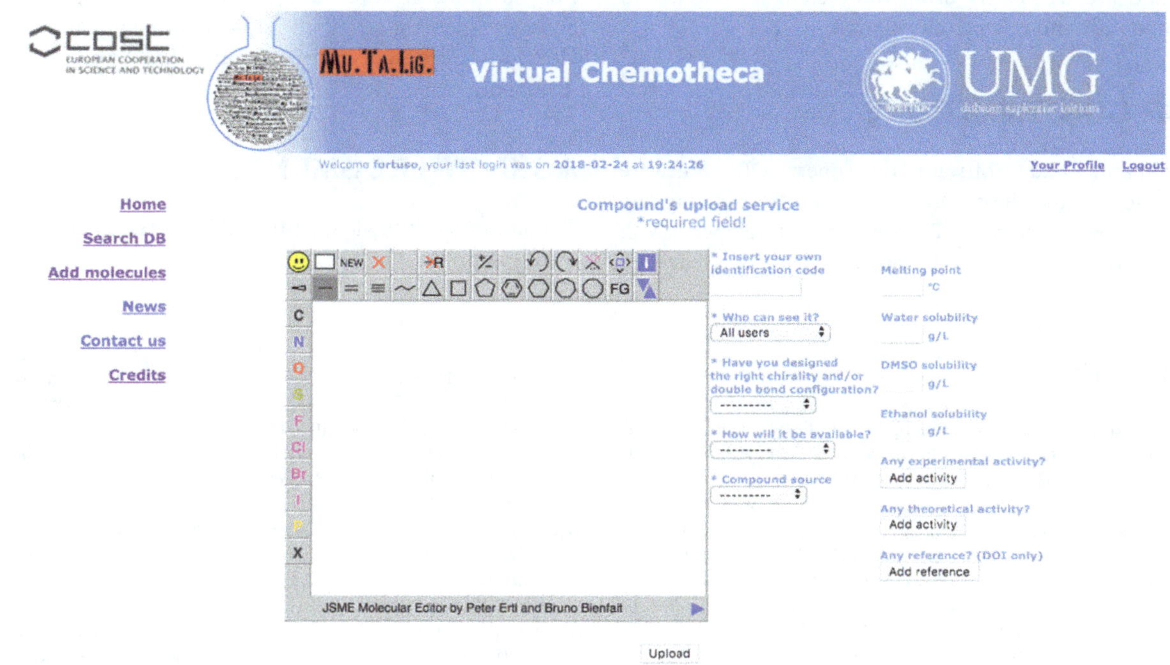

FIGURE 3 | New data upload service.

modify this parameter. By clicking on structures, these will be magnified and all related properties will be displayed in a new popup window. "Edit query" and "Re-filter hits" options are available to improve search efficacy and focus the results. The first option from the results table returns to the search form where the previous query appears. This query could be modified and used for searching again the entire database. The "Re-filter hits" appears similar but the modified query will only be applied to the previous results.

New Compound Upload

Registered users can add their own compounds and/or their own data to existing compounds. A specific form has been developed and is hidden to guest users (**Figure 3**).

Structures for uploaded compounds must be drawn with the embedded JSME editor. The user has to fill in four mandatory fields: (a) a unique molecule identification code, which will help if other researchers contact the owner, (b) whether the structure has been properly designated with respect to chirality and double bonds configuration, (c) how the molecule will be delivered, i.e., pure compound, mixture of isomers, or theoretical (of course, a theoretical entry cannot be delivered and should be considered as an inspiration source for researchers involved in chemical synthesis), and (d) the origin of the molecule, i.e., natural or synthetic. Fields (b) and (c) will be taken into account together for verifying the data coherence and to prevent low quality information: Chemotheca allows the upload of theoretical or pure compounds if their chemical structures explicitly report chirality and double bond configuration. This is not mandatory for compounds delivered as a mixture. By using the corresponding menu, both experimental and theoretical information, and references can be added. These data can be included also for already available structures, owned by different users. In this case, the new properties will be linked to the molecular structure and a new ownership, related to the corresponding information, will be added.

Further Development

The Chemotheca has reached a stable state of development. At present, the web interface allows for a single-compound upload only. This is a limitation when several/multiple structures need be added. At the moment, it is possible to overcome such a limitation by filling in a spreadsheet template furnished by the Chemotheca's developers. In the near future, a multiple compounds upload facility will be implemented. Another feature under development is the possibility, for the corresponding owner, to edit the information included in the database. For now the data editing, excluding the personal information, is possible only by contacting the developers. Finally, a new advanced search form is under development: it will allow the database search by using activities as query criteria. The Chemotheca's developer team is open to suggestions and offers to contribute.

CONCLUSION

According to the mission of COST ACTION CA15135, a computational platform has been developed for stimulating scientific collaboration among research groups worldwide, focused on multi-target ligands identification and compound-repurposing. Already about one hundred researchers are registered and are frequently using the system to search and upload compounds and related information.

AUTHOR CONTRIBUTIONS

FO: Coordinator and Software developer; DB: Software debugging and database population; AM: Software debugging and database population; CT: Software developer; MB: Software features design; NH: Software features design; FB: Software feature design and database population; SB: Software debugging; TL: Software design and debugging; HS: Software design and debugging; SA: Software design and debugging.

ACKNOWLEDGMENTS

The authors acknowledge Mu.Ta.Lig COST ACTION CA15135 for the support.

REFERENCES

Aldrich, C., Bertozzi, C., Georg, G. I., Kiessling, L., Lindsley, C., Liotta, D., et al. (2017). The ecstasy and agony of assay interference compounds. *J. Med. Chem.* 60, 2165–2168. doi: 10.1021/acs.jmedchem.7b00229

Baell, J. B., and Holloway, G. A. (2010). New substructure filters for removal of pan assay interference compounds (PAINS) from screening libraries and for their exclusion in bioassays. *J. Med. Chem.* 53, 2719–2740. doi: 10.1021/jm901137j

Bento, A. P., Gaulton, A., Hersey, A., Bellis, L. J., Chambers, J., Davies, M., et al. (2014). The ChEMBL bioactivity database: an update. *Nucleic Acids Res.* 42, 1083–1090. doi: 10.1093/nar/gkt1031

Bienfait, B., and Ertl, P. (2013). JSME: a free molecule editor in JavaScript. *J. Cheminformatics* 5:24. doi: 10.1186/1758-2946-5-24

Capuzzi, S. J., Muratov, E. N., and Tropsha, A. (2017). Phantom PAINS: problems with the utility of alerts for pan-assay interference compounds. *J. Chem. Inf. Model.* 57, 417–427. doi: 10.1021/acs.jcim.6b00465

Good, A. C., and Oprea, T. I. (2008). Optimization of CAMD techniques 3. Virtual screening enrichment studies: a help or hindrance in tool selection? *J. Comput. Aided Mol. Des.* 22, 169–178. doi: 10.1007/s10822-007-9167-2

Groom, C. R., Bruno, I. J., Lightfoot, M. P., and Ward, S. C. (2016). The cambridge structural database. *Acta Cryst. B*72, 171–179. doi: 10.1107/S2052520616003954

Huang, N., Shoichet, B. K., and Irwin, J. J. (2006). Benchmarking sets for molecular docking. *J. Med. Chem.* 23, 6789–6801. doi: 10.1021/jm0608356

Irwin, J. J., and Shoichet, B. K. (2005). ZINC – a free database of commercially available compounds for virtual screening. *J. Chem. Inf. Model.* 1:177–182. doi: 10.1021/ci049714

Irwin, J. J., Sterling, T., Mysinger, M. M., Bolstad, E. S., and Coleman, R. G. (2012). ZINC: a free tool to discover chemistry for biology. *J. Chem. Inf. Model.* 7, 1757–1768. doi: 10.1021/ci3001277

Kim, S., Thiessen, P. A., Bolton, E. E., Chen, J., Fu, G., Gindulyte, A., et al. (2016). PubChem substance and compound databases. *Nucleic Acids Res.* 44, D1202–D1213. doi: 10.1093/nar/gkv951

O'Boyle, N. M., Banck, M., James, C. A., Morley, C., Vandermeersch, T., and Hutchison, G. R. (2011). Open babel: an open chemical toolbox. *J. Cheminformatics* 3:33. doi: 10.1186/1758-2946-3-33

O'Boyle, N. M., Morley, C., and Hutchison, G. R. (2008). Pybel: a Python wrapper for the openbabel cheminformatics toolkit. *Chem. Cent. J.* 2:5. doi: 10.1186/1752-153X-2-5

Vilar, S., Chakrabarti, M., and Costanzi, S. (2010). Prediction of passive blood-brain partitioning: straightforward and effective classification models based on *in silico* derived physicochemical descriptors. *J. Mol. Graph. Model.* 8, 899–903. doi: 10.1016/j.jmgm.2010.03.010

Wishart, D. S., Feunang, Y. D., Guo, A. C., Lo, E. J., Marcu, A., Grant, J. R., et al. (2018). DrugBank 5.0: a major update to the DrugBank database for 2018. *Nucleic Acids Res.* 46, D1074–D1082. doi: 10.1093/nar/gkx1037

Wishart, D. S., Knox, C., Guo, A. C., Shrivastava, S., Hassanali, M., Stothard, P., et al. (2006). DrugBank: a comprehensive resource for *in silico* drug discovery and exploration. *Nucleic Acids Res.* 34, D668–D672. doi: 10.1093/nar/gkj067

17

Data Mining and Machine Learning Models for Predicting Drug Likeness and their Disease or Organ Category

Abraham Yosipof[1]*, Rita C. Guedes*[2] *and Alfonso T. García-Sosa*[3*]

[1] *Department of Information Systems and Department of Business Administration, College of Law & Business, Ramat-Gan, Israel,* [2] *Department of Medicinal Chemistry, Faculty of Pharmacy, Research Institute for Medicines (iMed.ULisboa), Universidade de Lisboa, Lisbon, Portugal,* [3] *Department of Molecular Technology, Institute of Chemistry, University of Tartu, Tartu, Estonia*

Correspondence:
Alfonso T. García-Sosa
alfonsog@ut.ee

Data mining approaches can uncover underlying patterns in chemical and pharmacological property space decisive for drug discovery and development. Two of the most common approaches are visualization and machine learning methods. Visualization methods use dimensionality reduction techniques in order to reduce multi-dimension data into 2D or 3D representations with a minimal loss of information. Machine learning attempts to find correlations between specific activities or classifications for a set of compounds and their features by means of recurring mathematical models. Both models take advantage of the different and deep relationships that can exist between features of compounds, and helpfully provide classification of compounds based on such features or in case of visualization methods uncover underlying patterns in the feature space. Drug-likeness has been studied from several viewpoints, but here we provide the first implementation in chemoinformatics of the t-Distributed Stochastic Neighbor Embedding (t-SNE) method for the visualization and the representation of chemical space, and the use of different machine learning methods separately and together to form a new ensemble learning method called AL Boost. The models obtained from AL Boost synergistically combine decision tree, random forests (RF), support vector machine (SVM), artificial neural network (ANN), *k* nearest neighbors (kNN), and logistic regression models. In this work, we show that together they form a predictive model that not only improves the predictive force but also decreases bias. This resulted in a corrected classification rate of over 0.81, as well as higher sensitivity and specificity rates for the models. In addition, separation and good models were also achieved for disease categories such as antineoplastic compounds and nervous system diseases, among others. Such models can be used to guide decision on the feature landscape of compounds and their likeness to either drugs or other characteristics, such as specific or multiple disease-category(ies) or organ(s) of action of a molecule.

Keywords: machine-learning, drug, data-mining, logistic, organ, drug design, multi-target

INTRODUCTION

An important task in drug design is to guide the synthesis, purchase, and testing of compounds based on their predicted properties. Proper prediction of properties can save time and resources, but also generate compounds not available beforehand. There are several methods to compare a real or virtual compound to known collection of compounds, from topological similarity, fingerprints, molecular features, among others (Ivanenkov et al., 2009; Akella and DeCaprio, 2010; García-Sosa et al., 2010, 2012a,b; Dhanda et al., 2013).

Machine learning allows observing hidden patterns in data, and modifying algorithms in order to better discern the patterns and improve robustness (Schneider, 2017; Gómez-Bombarelli et al., 2018). This includes several layers of data (deepness) and optimization of a function in order to better adopt the features of the (chemical) data (Schneider, 2017; Gómez-Bombarelli et al., 2018). Feedback loops can improve the learning process. The use of artificial intelligence and machine learning can enable the automated design of compounds according to several properties to be optimized (Schneider, 2017; Gómez-Bombarelli et al., 2018).

Visualization of high dimensional data is an important problem in many different domains and especially in drug design. Visualization of chemical data and a good representation of the chemical space are useful in many chemoinformatics and drug design applications including the selection of compounds for synthesis, the selection of compounds for biological evaluation, and the selection of subsets for the design of information-rich compound libraries (Ivanenkov et al., 2009; Akella and DeCaprio, 2010). The main problem of visualization of high dimensional data concerns the data representation in 2D or 3D with minimal loss of information. The dimensionality reduction aim is to preserve as much of the significant structure of the high-dimensional data as possible in the low-dimensional map.

The traditional approach for dimensionality reduction is principal component analysis (PCA) (Jolliffe, 2002), which assumes linear correlation between the dimensions and therefore, cannot adequately handle complex nonlinear data. In the last decade, a number of nonlinear techniques for dimensionality reduction have been proposed and implemented in chemoinformatics, such as self-organized map (SOM) (Zupan and Gasteiger, 1999) and generative topographic map (GTM) (Kireeva et al., 2012), to name but a few. In contrast to traditional linear techniques, nonlinear techniques have the ability to deal with complex nonlinear data, which is pervasive in drug design.

An important factor to consider in machine learning and artificial intelligence, as with any modeling work, is to properly account for the underlying data. The initial and sequential datasets must be well curated, to guarantee that the features and numbers are not biased and that they represent an important classification, optimization, or design task (Schneider, 2017).

Drug design requires an extremely high degree of selectivity. This implies a specific profile of interaction of a compound (or several compounds) with several targets, such as is the case seen in clinic-approved kinase inhibitors, while at the same time avoiding off- or anti-targets that may be responsible for side-effects (Campillos et al., 2008). Disease or organ classification is also important given that the same targets can be present in different tissues and therapeutic compounds need to have an efficient concentration at a specific place for effective action in an organism. These challenges have been approached using probability density functions (García-Sosa et al., 2012a), multivariate logistic regressions (García-Sosa et al., 2012b), PCA (García-Sosa et al., 2012c), and Bayesian naïve classifiers (García-Sosa and Maran, 2013), among others.

In the present work, the t-Distributed Stochastic Neighbor Embedding (t-SNE) method for the visualization and the representation of chemical space is implemented for the first time, and the use of different machine learning methods from decision tree, random forests (RF), support vector machine (SVM), artificial neural network (ANN), k-nearest neighbors (k-NN), and logistic regression models, separately and together, to form a new ensemble learning method called AL Boost for separation of drugs and nondrugs. Good models can also be achieved for disease categories such as antineoplastic compounds, cardiovascular system drugs, and nervous system diseases.

METHODS

Data Set

The full data set contains 762 compounds; compounds were classified into two classes: drug (366 compounds) and non-drug (396 compounds). The compounds were obtained from previous work (García-Sosa et al., 2010, 2012b), where the DrugBank (Wishart et al., 2006) was used to ascertain approved-drug status. Curation included that structure files were checked for consistency (chemical structure corresponds to chemical name) and cleaned, such as removing salts, counterions, etc. All compounds and features are provided in Table S1 on the Supporting Information.

Properties Calculation

Thirty five molecular properties were chosen and calculated for each compound, using ChemAxon[1] and XLogP (Wang et al., 2000) software, the same properties as in previous publications (see more details on the selection of properties in García-Sosa et al., 2012b; García-Sosa and Maran, 2013).

These physicochemical features were: the binding free energy to their target, ΔG_{bind}; log$P$; exact mass; Number of Carbons (NoC); Wiener index; molecular surface area (MSA); polar surface area (PSA); apolar surface area (apolarSA); hydrogen bond donor count; hydrogen bond acceptor count; rotatable bond count; atom count; hydrogen count; number of heavy atoms (NHA); molecular polarizability; aliphatic ring count; aromatic ring count; aromatic atom count; Balaban index; Harary index; bond count; hyperWiener index; Platt index; Randic index; ring count; Szeged index; Wiener polarity; and the ligand efficiencies (Kuntz et al., 1999) ΔG_{bind}_NHA; ΔG_{bind}_MW; ΔG_{bind}_PSA; ΔG_{bind}_MSA; ΔG_{bind}_apolarSA; ΔG_{bind}_Wiener; ΔG_{bind}_P; ΔG_{bind}_NoC. Free energies of binding were calculated using inhibition or dissociation constants from the SCORPIO (Ababou and Ladbury, 2007), KiBank (Zhang et al., 2004), and PDBbind (Wang et al., 2004) databases. Non-drugs had their nonexistence as drugs verified in the DrugBank (Wishart et al., 2006). Together, they composed a balanced set of drugs and nondrugs, which is important in order not to bias or skew the feature patterns toward one group

[1](v4.8.1, M., In; 2007)

of compounds against the other. Important features of the sets are that their distribution of binding energies and the number of compounds is similar for both drugs and non-drugs, and that the drugs include all administration routes, not only oral. This introduces a challenge to distinguish drugs from active, non-therapeutic compounds (non-drugs) because the differences between drugs and non-drugs are not judged by their binding energy (i.e., not only potency determines drug likeness), since other features then become more important to distinguish these groups of compounds.

In order to make a comparison to previous studies, no properties selection has been done, although to initially evaluate these properties, an information gain procedure has been implemented. Briefly, the information gain (Mitchell, 1997) of a property reflects the "degree of purity" of the partition obtained by splitting the parent data set using this property. The degree of purity is determined according to Shannon's entropy measure. This method has been widely used in chemoinformatics and bioinformatics and in a recent comparative study it was found to be highly effective for properties selection prior to model generation (Liu, 2004; Saeys et al., 2007). The information gain results indicated information gain (greater than 0) for 30 properties and no information gain (equal to zero) for five properties namely: hydrogen count; Platt index; ring count; Balaban index, and ΔG_{bind}_NoC.

The models and visualization use normalization of the features as a standard procedure.

Data Mining Workflow

The data mining procedure is derived using a workflow consisting of two main stages as follows: (1) Data visualization using the t-SNE method; (2) Classification models, which starts by dividing the data into training and test sets, followed by model generation with seven classification methods and model validation.

Data Visualization

The t-Distributed Stochastic Neighbor Embedding (t-SNE) (Maaten and Hinton, 2008) method is a non-linear dimensionality reduction algorithm that is especially designed for embedding high-dimensional data into a space of 2D or 3D. The t-SNE is capable of capturing much of the local information of the high-dimensional data, while also revealing global information such as clusters in the low dimensional representation. The basic idea of t-SNE is that similar objects are modeled by nearby points and dissimilar objects are modeled by distant points in the low dimensional embedding. The t-SNE algorithm consists of three main stages:

(1) Collection of the pairwise Euclidean distances between all high dimensional objects and convert them into conditional probabilities and then into joint probabilities, where similar objects get high probability and dissimilar ones get small probability
(2) Creation of an initial set of low-dimensional objects
(3) Iteratively update the low-dimensional objects to minimize a fitness function (the Kullback-Leibler (KL) divergence, i.e., how one probability distribution diverges from a second expected probability distribution) between a Gaussian distribution in the high-dimensional space and a t distribution in the low-dimensional space.

In order to evaluate the ability of the low dimensional representation to preserve the high-dimensional data and structure, we used the trust measure (Venna and Kaski, 2006). The trust measure defines the millieu of compounds, so that the neighborhood in the low dimensional representation is similar to the high dimension, and is given by Equation (1):

$$Trust = \frac{1}{n} * \frac{1}{k} \sum_{i=1}^{n} \sum_{j=1}^{k} \delta_j(s_{i,j}, \overline{x_i}) \tag{1}$$

where n represents the number of compounds, k the number of nearest neighbors, $s_{i,j}$ represents neighbor j for compound i in the low dimension representation, and $\overline{x_i}$ is the vector of compound i neighbors in the high dimension. δ_j is defined to be 1 if $s_{i,j}$ is found in $\overline{x_i}$ or 0 if not.

In this work, the neighborhood is defined as the 10 nearest neighbors, and we used the t-SNE algorithm as implemented in the MATLAB version R2017b.

Classification Models-Selection of Training Set and Test Set

In order to validate the classification model, compounds were divided into a training set (80%, 610 compounds), and a test set (20%, 152 compounds). Similar proportions (20%) of drug (73 compounds) and non-drug (79 compounds) compounds were selected for the test sets by applying independent selection procedures of a representativeness function (Yosipof and Senderowitz, 2014) to the two activity categories. Briefly, this method uses a simulated annealing optimization to select a subset of objects (e.g., compounds) which best represents the parent database from which it was selected. The models were built on the training set by using 10-fold cross-validation and seven methods and then tested on the test set.

Classification Methods

Six different algorithms, namely, decision tree, random forests (RF), support vector machine (SVM), artificial neural network (ANN), k-nearest neighbors (k-NN) and logistic regression (LR), and one newly boosting method named AL Boost, were used to build the classification models. In each case, a classification model was built using the training set and subsequently used to predict the activities (drug status) of the test set compounds for validation. The six models were generated with algorithms implemented in the WEKA version 3.9.1 (Hall et al., 2009) software using default parameters unless otherwise noted and the newly boosting method was self-coded.

The decision tree algorithm (Quinlan, 1986) operates by iteratively splitting a dataset characterized by activity data and features into smaller subsets. At each step, all features are considered in the search for one that, upon splitting a parent node, would produce the most uniform (activity-wise) child nodes. This procedure is repeated until no more splits are warranted, since either all compounds within all (terminal) nodes have identical activities, or since the gain in uniformity upon additional splits is not statistically significant. In the present study, we used the J4.8, a C4 variant algorithm.

Random forests (RF) (Breiman, 2001), as developed in 2001, with Breiman introducing the principle of random forests as an extension to the decision tree algorithm. In RF, multiple trees (rather than a single tree) are generated using randomly selected feature sets. Activity predictions are made by all trees and combined using a majority vote rule. In the present study, the number of trees was set to the default value of 100.

Support vector machine (SVM) (Vapnik, 1995) is an algorithm which has proven useful for noisy data. Under this paradigm, models are built by identifying a rigid decision hyperplane which leads to the greatest possible margins between activity classes. Nonlinear data could be handled by transposing the original feature space to higher dimensionalities using kernels. In this study, we have chosen to use the polynomial kernel function.

Artificial neural network (ANN) (Hassoun, 1995) is a non-linear classification method inspired by the behavior of biological networks of neurons. Within this approach, objects (i.e., compounds) are represented by vectors containing their features. Each feature is passed to one of the input neurons to which a weight is assigned. Based on these weights, input is passed to the output layer over a number of (optional) hidden layers. The output layer combines these signals to produce a result (e.g., activity or class prediction). Initially, weights are set to random values. As the network is repeatedly presented with input data, these weights are adjusted so that the total output of the network approximates the observed endpoint values associated with the compounds. In the present study we used multilayer perceptrons (MLP) with 19 hidden layers and 19 nodes.

k-Nearest Neighbor (*k*-NN) (Mitchell, 1997) is a *lazy learning* classification method, which assigns new compounds to the most common class of known compounds in their immediate neighborhood. Closest neighbors are identified by calculating Euclidian distances in a pre-defined feature space. In this present study, we used $k = 5$ neighbors.

The logistic regression (LR) (Mitchell, 1997) is a type of regression analysis where the dependent variable is binary (or binomial). The model is simply a non-linear transformation of the linear regression. The result is an equation which includes the impact of each variable on the odds ratio of the observed event of interest.

AL Boost: is a new chemoinformatics ensemble learning classification method which combines all the models obtained in this work (i.e., J4.8, RF, SVM, ANN, *k*-NN, and LR) together into one predictive model in order to improve the predictive force and decrease the bias. This method takes the predictions of each classification (learners) and combines them using a weighted majority voting function to determine the prediction of each compound. Each learner is assigned a weight according to its corrected classification rate error, given that poor learners get lower weights. For each compound, two functions are calculated as follows:

$$f\,(active) = \sum_{i=1}^{n} \frac{1}{w_i} * \delta_i \tag{2}$$

$$f\,(inactive) = \sum_{i=1}^{n} \frac{1}{w_i} * \delta_i \tag{3}$$

where i are the learner methods, w_i is the corrected classification rate error (CCR error, Equation 4) of learner i, and δ_i is 1 if the learner is predicted as active class (e.g., drug), or 0 if predicted as inactive class (e.g., non-drug), for Equation (2).

For Equation (3), δ_i is 1 if the learner is predicted as inactive class (e.g., non-drug) or 0 if it is predicted as active class (e.g., drug).

The majority vote between Equations (2) and (3) determines the prediction for the compound.

The last classification method detailed in this paper is Naïve Bayesian classifiers. This method was used in a previous publication (García-Sosa and Maran, 2013), thus it was not used for model building in this study, rather for comparison to the results obtained in García-Sosa and Maran (García-Sosa and Maran, 2013). The Naïve Bayesian classifiers use the distributions of features for different classes, and construct Gaussians for describing these distributions with characteristics being the mean and standard deviation. The probabilities (P) of a compound with certain features belonging to either class are computed, and that compound is assigned to the class for which the highest P is obtained.

Classification Models-Prediction Statistics

In all cases, classification predictions were evaluated using the corrected classification rate (CCR, also called "balanced accuracy"), accuracy, Matthews correlation coefficient (MCC), sensitivity, specificity, and the variance between the sensitivity and the specificity (Equations 5–10), where sensitivity is the percentage of truly active (e.g., drug) compounds being predicted from the model (Equation 8), and specificity is the percentage of truly inactive (e.g., non-drug) compounds being predicted from the model (Equation 9).

$$CCR\ \text{error} = 1 - \frac{1}{2}\left(\frac{T_N}{N_N} + \frac{T_P}{N_P}\right) \tag{4}$$

$$CCR = \frac{1}{2}\left(\frac{T_N}{N_N} + \frac{T_P}{N_P}\right) \tag{5}$$

$$Accuracy = \frac{T_N + T_P}{N_N + N_P} \tag{6}$$

$$MCC = \frac{T_N T_P - F_N F_P}{\sqrt{(T_P + F_P)\,(T_P + F_N)\,(T_N + F_P)\,(T_N + F_N)}} \tag{7}$$

$$Sensitivity = \frac{T_P}{T_P + F_N} \tag{8}$$

$$Specificity = \frac{T_N}{T_N + F_P} \tag{9}$$

$$Variance = \frac{1}{2}*(Sensitivity - \mu)^2 + \frac{1}{2}*(Specificity - \mu)^2 \quad (10)$$

where T_N and T_P represent the number of true negative (e.g., non-drug) and true positive (e.g., drug) predictions, respectively. N_N and N_P represent the total number of the two activity classes, and F_N and F_P represent the number of false negative and false positive predictions, respectively. μ represents the mean of the sensitivity and specificity.

Disease Categories

Further in the analysis of the drug/non-drug database, the drugs in the data set were characterized into their different anatomic therapeutical classifications, also called disease or organ category (DC). Here the comparison was not drugs *vs.* non-drugs, but drugs of one DC against another DC. In this work, we focus on the three largest DCs, namely cardiovascular, anti-neoplastic, and nervous systems. These three groups were evaluated against each other preforming three sub data sets Cardiovascular drugs vs. Anti-neoplastic agents, Cardiovascular drugs vs. Nervous system, and Anti-neoplastic agents vs. Nervous system. The same data mining workflow as before was applied. The number of compounds and the number of training and test sets (similar procedure and proportions as in the drug/non-drug database) for each DC are presented in **Table 1**.

RESULTS AND DISCUSSION

The properties of the compounds include widely used metrics such as size, weight, polarity, as well as topological indices, and ligand efficiencies. An important consideration for the data set construction was the curation of binding free energies of similar magnitude between drugs and non-drugs (bioactive compounds). Ligand efficiencies can normalize the binding energy of a compound according to other properties of a compound, such as size, lipophilicity, etc., and have a pragmatic use in developing series of compounds in order to improve or maintain binding strength while also improving their profile in other dimensions.

The first step of the data mining workflow is data visualization; the resulting 35 dimensional data of the drug/non-drug database was reduced into a 3D representation using t-SNE. The resulting trust measure of the low dimensional embedding was found to be 63%. A comparison to the common dimension reduction technique PCA, found that for a 3D representation using PCA, a trust measure of only 42% was obtained. This result indicates a good preservation of the structure and of the local information of the high dimensional data in the low embedding for the t-SNE.

TABLE 1 | The number of compounds, training, and test sets for the three different disease/organ category.

Disease/organ category	Compounds	Training set	Test set
Cardiovascular drugs	56	44	12
Anti-neoplastic agents	20	16	4
Nervous system	111	89	22

The distribution and the chemical space of the drug/non-drug compounds in the resulting t-SNE 3D space are presented in **Figure 1**.

From **Figure 1**, it can be broadly seen that drug compounds occupy mostly the central area (shown in the black square in **Figure 1**) of the plot in this perspective plane, and non-drugs are among the edges. The second step of the data mining workflow is the building and validation of the classification models. In order to build the classification models, we used six different classification methods, as well as the boosting method (AL Boost), the results obtained are shown in **Table 2**.

These results show that the separation between classes is good, and comparable to those found in other studies (García-Sosa and Maran, 2013). The AL Boost method performed as well as the best of the individual methods. The overall performances of the different models for the training set were evaluated by the CCR and are between 0.67 and 0.76. The best classification models based on this criterion are the AL Boost, the RF, and the LR (with CCR = 0.76) followed by the ANN (CCR = 0.75), SVM and k-NN (with CCR = 0.73), while the decision tree (with CCR = 0.67) lags behind. The overall performances of the different models for the test set largely mirror the results from the training set. However, some methods performed better, and the AL Boost method gave a good CCR of 0.81, while random forest had the highest CCR value of 0.82. On average, the CCR of the six other methods is 0.73 and 0.77 for the training set and test set, respectively, which is lower than the CCR results for AL Boost, but not statistically significant.

In order to evaluate the new AL Boost method, the variance between the specificity and the sensitivity was calculated as well. The variance represents the model balance between the two classes or the bias of the model toward one class. Lower variance values represent low bias and balanced models while higher variance values represent high bias and unbalanced models. The results for the training set and test set for the AL Boost method represent very similar results of specificity and sensitivity (training set 0.76 and 0.77 and test set 0.80 and 0.81 for the specificity and sensitivity, respectively). These results show a low bias and a well-balanced model with a variance of 0.01%^{2} and 0.22%^{2} for the training and test set, respectively, while on average, the variance of the six other methods is 0.93%^{2} and 7.22%^{2} for the training and test set, respectively. In addition, comparing the AL Boost to our previous publication (García-Sosa and Maran, 2013) using the naïve Bayesian method shows that the accuracy of AL Boost (0.81) is higher on the test set than the Bayesian classifier (0.70).

To evaluate the features used in this research, **Table 3** represents the most frequent features selected by the classifiers for the final model. In this case, the most frequent features are those that were both selected by the decision tree model and by the logistic regression models, while the other methods used all the features or combination of them for the final model. A comparison to previous publications reveals that there is common ground: the features of Acceptor Count, Donor Count, PSA, Log*P*, ΔG_{bind}_MSA, and Balaban Index were found to be features that separated drug and nondrug in REF (García-Sosa and Maran, 2013) and in REF (García-Sosa et al., 2012b). In addition, the Balaban Index was found to have an information gain of zero in the initial evaluation of the features (see Methods section), but here it was selected as one of the features that can separate drug and nondrug. Furthermore, it is interesting to note that most of the properties that correspond to the ones in Lipinski's rule of five (Lipinski et al., 2001) were found to have the ability to split the data set into drugs and non-drugs classes.

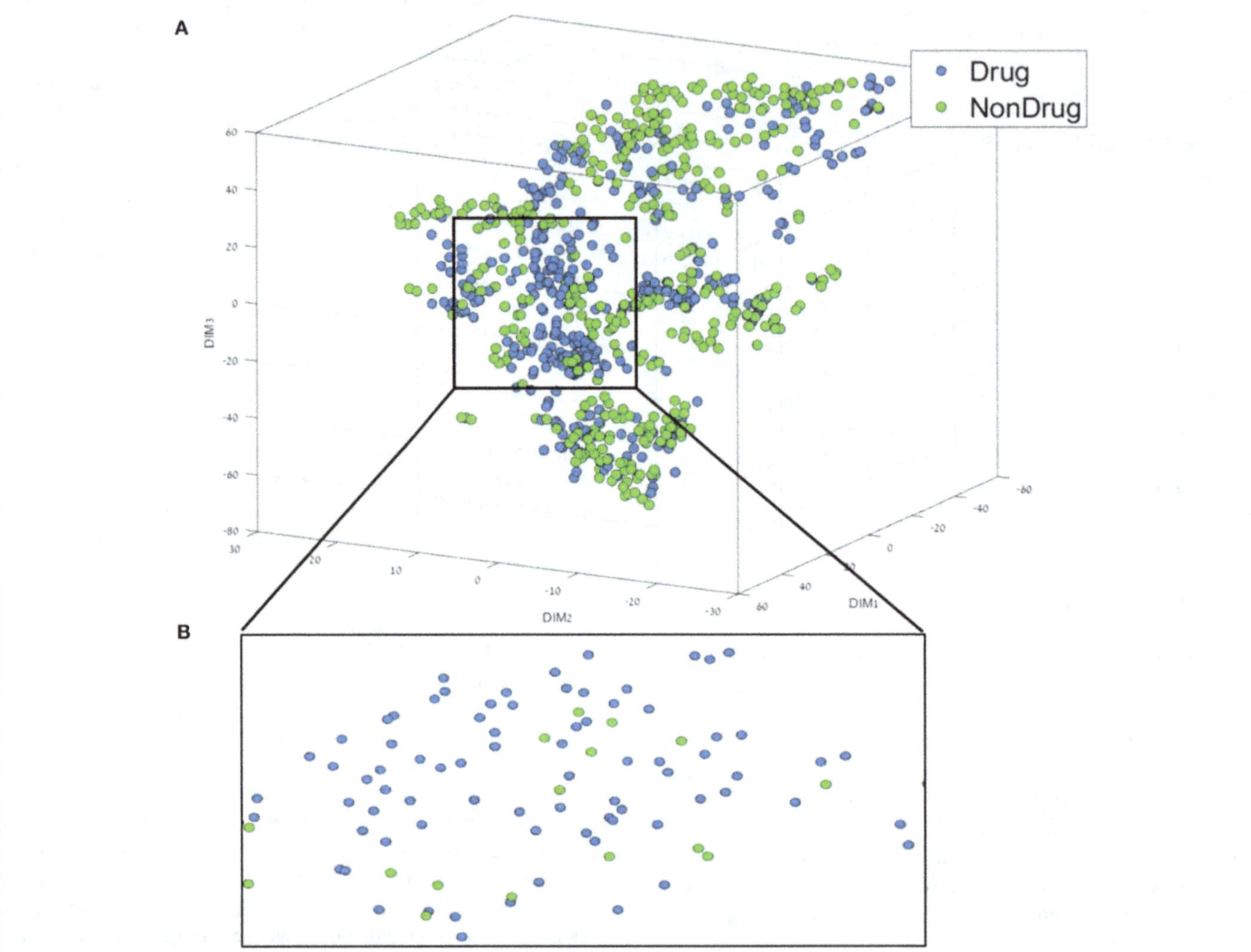

FIGURE 1 | (A) 3D representation of the Drug/Non-drug feature space using the t-SNE algorithm for dimension reduction. **(B)** A zoom into the drug area from the black square in **(A)**.

TABLE 2 | Drug/non-drug classification results.

	Training set						Test set					
Model	**Specificity**	**Sensitivity**	**CCR**	**Accuracy**	**Variance**	**MCC**	**Specificity**	**Sensitivity**	**CCR**	**Accuracy**	**Variance**	**MCC**
J4.8	0.67	0.67	0.67	0.67	0.01	0.35	0.72	0.81	0.75	0.76	18.90	0.52
RF	0.76	0.76	0.76	0.76	0.00	0.52	0.80	0.86	0.82	0.82	10.21	0.65
k-NN	0.73	0.73	0.73	0.73	0.06	0.46	0.75	0.78	0.76	0.76	1.34	0.53
SVM	0.73	0.74	0.73	0.73	0.25	0.47	0.74	0.73	0.74	0.74	0.17	0.47
ANN	0.77	0.72	0.75	0.75	5.25	0.50	0.81	0.81	0.81	0.81	0.12	0.62
LR	0.76	0.76	0.76	0.76	0.01	0.52	0.77	0.70	0.74	0.74	12.58	0.48
AL Boost	0.76	0.77	0.76	0.76	0.01	0.53	0.80	0.81	0.81	0.81	0.22	0.62
Naïve Bayesian*	0.74	0.89	–	0.82	–	0.64	0.50	0.92	–	0.70	–	0.46

**Naïve Bayesian results were taken from García-Sosa and Maran (2013).*

Having separated drugs and non-drugs, the next step was to consider separation of drugs into their different disease or organ category (DC). First, we visualize the feature space using t-SNE for each sub dataset. The resulting 3D representation of Anti-Neoplastic-Nervous system, Anti-Neoplastic-Cardiovascular, and Cardiovascular-Nervous system can be seen in **Figures 2–4**, respectively. The trust measure results can be seen in **Table 4**; these results clearly show the ability of the t-SNE methods to preserve the high-dimensional data and structure, with a trust between 70 and 74% for the three datasets. As before, a comparison to PCA was done, and again the t-SNE trust results were found to overcome the PCA. Although the trust results were found to be higher for the t-SNE than the PCA for each data set, no statistically significant difference was found between them.

Figure 2 presents the Anti-Neoplastic-Nervous system 3D representation. In this 3D representation a clear separation between the two DCs can be seen, with nervous system drugs in the center, and cancer drugs mostly on the edges, or not as well defined as nervous system. If one considers their place or target of action, nervous system drugs require locating in the brain and CNS, which requires the passing of specific membranes such as the blood-brain barrier that imposes a feature profile in the compounds. Two Anti-Neoplastic compounds (**Figure 2**, two blue dots in the black square, DR109.mol2, DR211.mol2) are markedly different from the rest of the Anti-neoplastic bulk. They correspond to compounds fluorouracil (5-FU), an atypically small compound – one ring –, and to pentostatin, also a small, polar compound; both of them acting as nucleoside analogs.

TABLE 3 | Most frequent model selected features.

Features		
Acceptor count	ΔG_{bind}	ΔG_{bind}_PSA
Donor count	Rotatable bond count	ΔG_{bind}_MSA
PSA	Hydrogen count	ΔG_{bind}_P
LogP	Aliphatic ring count	Number of carbons
Aromatic ring count	Balaban index	

Cardiovascular drugs were also majorly separated from cancer drugs (**Figure 3**), located mostly in the center as opposed to mostly on the edges for cancer drugs. Cancer affects all organs, so these system drugs tend to be not very located, which is also a major problem with cancer treatment, as side-effects are very common.

This separation between groups was not the case for the Cardiovascular vs. Nervous system drug plots, since both groups are very similar, perhaps only a cluster of cardiovascular drugs can be seen on the middle right.

Having visualized the data, the next step is to build classification models using the six classification methods and the ensemble learning AL Boost. The results for the Anti-Neoplastic vs. Nervous system, Anti-neoplastic vs. Cardiovascular, and Cardiovascular vs. Nervous System are presented in **Tables 5–7**, respectively.

The results in **Table 5** for the anti-Neoplastic vs. Nervous system classification models show good results for the training set with CCR $\geq$ 0.65, as well as for the test set with CCR $\geq$ 0.85. The ensemble learning model AL Boost provided a CCR of 0.74 and 0.88 on the training and test set, respectively, with the lowest variance of 1.93%^{2} and 4.73%^{2} on the training and test set, respectively. The accuracy for the AL Boost method was high, 0.91 for the training set, and 0.96 for the test set. These

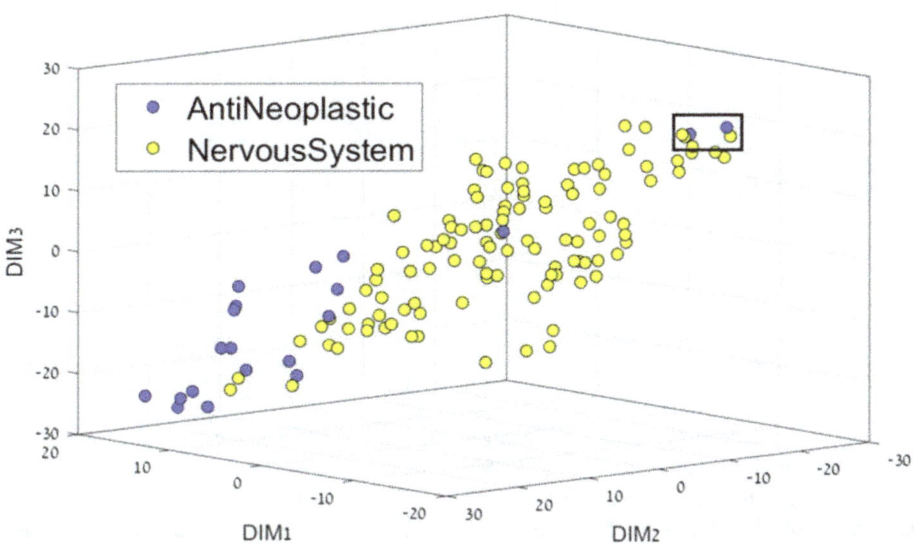

FIGURE 2 | 3D representation of the Anti-Neoplastic-Nervous system feature space using the t-SNE algorithm for dimension reduction. Two Anti-Neoplastic compounds (two blue dots in the black square) are markedly different from the rest of the Anti-neoplastic bulk. They correspond to compounds fluorouracil (5-FU), an atypically small compound – one ring –, and to pentostatin, also a small, polar compound; both of them acting as nucleoside analogs.

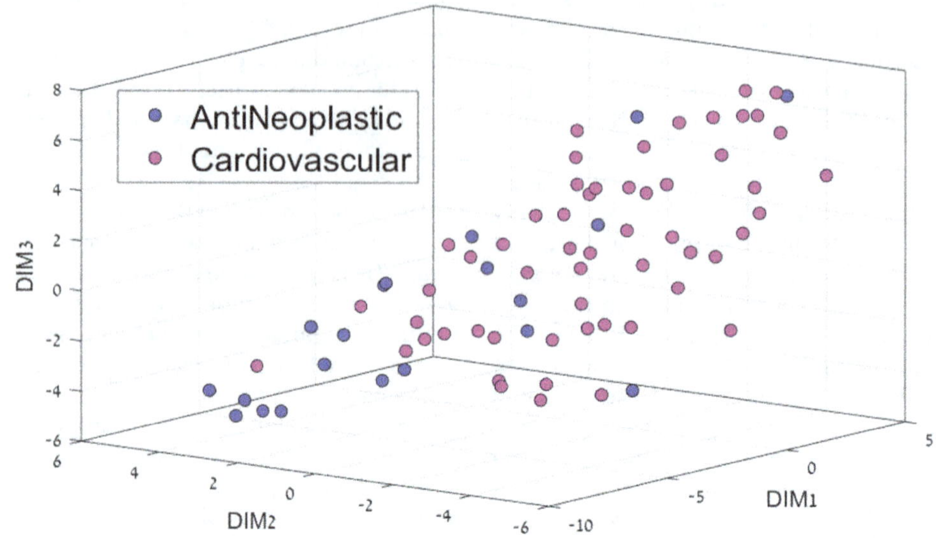

FIGURE 3 | 3D representation of the Anti-Neoplastic-Cardiovascular feature space using the t-SNE algorithm for dimension reduction.

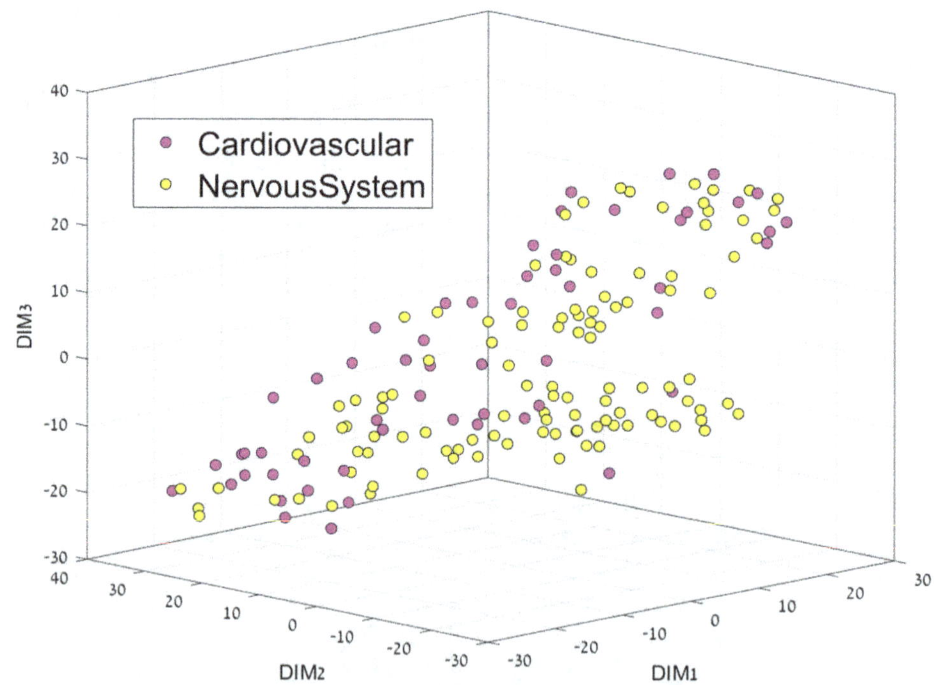

FIGURE 4 | 3D representation of the Cardiovascular-Nervous System feature space using the t-SNE algorithm for dimension reduction.

values are better when compared to those obtained previously using naïve Bayesian classifiers for the same data sets, 0.88 for training set, and 0.90 for the test set (García-Sosa and Maran, 2013). The sensitivity for the AL Boost method was much higher than using Bayesian classifiers, of 0.89 and 1.00 for training and test set for the former, vs. 0.50 and 0.60, respectively, for the latter. The values obtained for specificity are comparable for both methods, 0.97 and 0.96% for training and test sets for Bayesians, vs. 0.92 and 0.86, respectively, for AL Boost.

For the differences between cardiovascular drugs and cancer drugs (**Table 6**), good results were obtained for the AL Boost with CCR of 0.76 and 0.88 for the training set and test set, respectively, while on average, the CCR of the six other methods is 0.65 and 0.83 for the training set and test set, respectively. In addition, the accuracy for AL Boost is comparable for training set and higher for test set, with 0.85 and 0.94, respectively, vs. 0.88 and 0.90, respectively, for the Bayesian classifiers in previous work (García-Sosa and Maran, 2013). The sensitivity for the AL Boost method was comparable to Bayesian classifiers, with 0.82 and 1.00 for training and test set for the former, vs. 0.83 and 1.00, respectively, for the latter. The values for specificity are much higher for the AL Boost method than for Bayesians, with 0.27 and 0.43 for training and test sets for Bayesians, vs. 0.86 and 0.92, respectively, for AL Boost.

Another advantage of the AL Boost method, is that it could find a good distinction between cardiovascular and nervous system drugs with CCR of 0.68 and 0.72 for the training set and test set, respectively (shown in **Table 7**), which was not the case with naïve Bayesian classifiers, the latter being based on simple relationships between descriptors.

Summary of the classification results for the four databases presented here (drug/nondrug, anti-neoplastic vs. nervous system drugs, anti-neoplastic vs. cardiovascular drugs and cardiovascular drugs vs. nervous system drugs): a total of 24 results obtained for the individual classification models (e.g., J4.8, RF, *k*-NN, SVM, ANN, and LR) with an average CCR of 0.69 and 0.80 for the training set and test set, respectively. While the average CCR results for the four models of the AL Boost are 0.74 and 0.82 for the training set and test set, respectively. An independent sample *t*-test was performed among the individual CCR models results and the AL Boost CCR results which found no statically significant difference for the training set and not for the test set results. In summary, the average results for the AL Boost were found to overcome the average results for the individual classification models but weren't found to be significantly higher.

This research has several possible limitations including the data set, the classification method, and the visualization methods. One limitation is the number of compounds per disease category/organ classification. It would be good to have larger datasets for some disease groups, but we used the drugs that are

TABLE 4 | The trust results for the low-dimensional embedding (3D representation) using t-SNE and PCA.

System	t-SNE (%)	PCA (%)
Anti-neoplastic vs. nervous	72	66
Anti-neoplastic vs. cardiovascular	74	72
Cardiovascular vs. nervous	70	62

TABLE 5 | Classification results of anti-neoplastic vs. nervous system drugs, where specificity represents the nervous system and sensitivity represents the anti-neoplastic.

	Training set						Test set					
Model	**Specificity**	**Sensitivity**	**CCR**	**Accuracy**	**Variance**	**MCC**	**Specificity**	**Sensitivity**	**CCR**	**Accuracy**	**Variance**	**MCC**
J4.8	0.90	0.64	0.70	0.88	179.41	0.46	1.00	0.67	0.95	0.92	277.78	0.78
RF	0.93	0.82	0.77	0.91	28.81	0.63	0.96	1.00	0.88	0.96	4.73	0.85
k-NN	0.89	0.83	0.65	0.89	7.72	0.47	0.95	0.75	0.85	0.92	104.60	0.70
SVM	0.92	1.00	0.75	0.92	17.00	0.68	0.95	0.75	0.85	0.92	104.60	0.70
ANN	0.93	0.71	0.79	0.90	120.76	0.61	0.96	1.00	0.88	0.96	4.73	0.85
LR	0.92	0.89	0.74	0.91	1.93	0.63	0.96	1.00	0.88	0.96	4.73	0.85
AL Boost	0.92	0.89	0.74	0.91	1.93	0.63	0.96	1.00	0.88	0.96	4.73	0.85
Naïve Bayesian*	–	–	–	0.88	–	0.57	–	–	–	0.90	–	0.62

**Naïve Bayesian results were taken from García-Sosa and Maran (2013)*

TABLE 6 | Classification results of anti-neoplastic vs. cardiovascular drugs, where specificity represents the cardiovascular drugs and sensitivity represents the anti-neoplastic.

	Training set						Test set					
Model	**Specificity**	**Sensitivity**	**CCR**	**Accuracy**	**Variance**	**MCC**	**Specificity**	**Sensitivity**	**CCR**	**Accuracy**	**Variance**	**MCC**
J4.8	0.81	0.54	0.65	0.75	182.32	0.32	0.92	1.00	0.88	0.94	14.79	0.83
RF	0.83	0.62	0.69	0.78	114.92	0.41	0.92	1.00	0.88	0.94	14.79	0.83
k-NN	0.78	0.80	0.61	0.78	0.83	0.36	0.92	1.00	0.88	0.94	14.79	0.83
SVM	0.78	0.80	0.61	0.78	0.83	0.36	0.86	1.00	0.75	0.88	51.02	0.65
ANN	0.84	0.60	0.71	0.78	149.38	0.44	0.92	1.00	0.88	0.94	14.79	0.83
LR	0.80	0.55	0.63	0.75	156.83	0.30	0.86	1.00	0.75	0.88	51.02	0.65
AL Boost	0.86	0.82	0.76	0.85	3.79	0.59	0.92	1.00	0.88	0.94	14.79	0.83
Naïve Bayesian*	–	–	–	0.79	–	0.40	–	–	–	0.79	–	0.55

**Naïve Bayesian results were taken from García-Sosa and Maran (2013).*

TABLE 7 | Classification results of cardiovascular drugs vs. nervous system drugs, where specificity represents the nervous system and sensitivity represents the cardiovascular drugs.

	Training set						Test set					
Model	**Specificity**	**Sensitivity**	**CCR**	**Accuracy**	**Variance**	**MCC**	**Specificity**	**Sensitivity**	**CCR**	**Accuracy**	**Variance**	**MCC**
J4.8	0.76	0.55	0.64	0.70	105.33	0.30	0.74	0.55	0.64	0.68	93.78	0.28
RF	0.78	0.72	0.69	0.77	7.48	0.44	0.83	0.80	0.79	0.82	2.78	0.60
k-NN	0.71	0.57	0.59	0.69	51.02	0.22	0.70	0.57	0.60	0.68	43.74	0.23
SVM	0.77	0.82	0.68	0.77	6.87	0.46	0.75	0.83	0.69	0.76	17.36	0.47
ANN	0.78	0.56	0.67	0.71	120.60	0.33	0.83	0.73	0.77	0.79	24.41	0.54
LR	0.76	0.63	0.66	0.73	47.18	0.35	0.76	0.67	0.68	0.74	21.78	0.39
AL boost	0.77	0.73	0.68	0.76	3.17	0.42	0.79	0.70	0.72	0.76	21.01	0.47

available. New drugs are definitely needed in several categories, including cardiovascular, nervous system, and antineoplastic agents. Other limitations include the features selected by the models. Some of the classification methods employ all of the features in the data set, as well as combinations of different features in the final step. This makes the extraction of individual features harder.

A possible limitation for the t-SNE algorithm is the lack of an explicit mapping function. This limitation does not allow one to place any new data on an already existing map. In that case, a new map must be rebuilt from scratch and therefore, this method cannot be used as a supervised learning method (e.g., classification) for prediction.

CONCLUSIONS

To the best of our knowledge, this is the first example of the usage of t-SNE for the visualization and representation of the chemical space and the use of different machine learning methods separately and together to form a new ensemble learning method called AL Boost. Clear and good separations were obtained with the dimension reduction and machine learning approaches to distinguish drugs and non-drugs, as well as three major classes of drug compounds. The ability to use such tools for the identification of interesting trends, opens up new opportunities for understanding the factors affecting drugs performances and for designing new drugs. Considerations such as drug likeness and drug target, organ, and/or system class are thus made possible, providing another route for designing specificity into ligands and drugs. Clearly, this research should be conducted in close collaboration with experts in the medicinal/pharmaceutical chemistry field to both provide a chemistry-based explanation to the observed trends, as well as to capitalize on the results. We expect that the tools and methods implemented in this work will further be used in medicinal chemistry and drug design research.

AUTHOR CONTRIBUTIONS

AY applied the t-SNE and models and AL Boost algorithms, analyzed results, and wrote the manuscript. RG revised the manuscript. AG-S designed the research project, collected and curated the data, analyzed the results, and wrote the manuscript.

ACKNOWLEDGMENTS

Research work was supported by the Estonian Ministry for Education and Research (Grant IUT34-14) and the Portuguese Science Foundation (UID/DTP/04138/2013, SAICTPAC/0019/2015 and PTDC/QEQ-MED/7042/2014). Travel and open-access publication costs from the EU COST Action CA15135 Multi-target paradigm for innovative ligand identification in the drug discovery process (MuTaLig).

REFERENCES

Ababou, A., and Ladbury, J. E. (2007). Survey of the year: literature on applications of isothermal titration calorimetry. *J. Mol. Recognit.* 20, 4–14. doi: 10.1002/jmr.803

Akella, L. B., and DeCaprio, D. (2010). Cheminformatics approaches to analyze diversity in compound screening libraries. *Curr. Opin. Chem. Biol.* 14, 325–330. doi: 10.1016/j.cbpa.2010.03.017

Breiman, L. (2001). Random forests. *Mach. Learn.* 45, 5–32. doi: 10.1023/A:1010933404324

Campillos, M., Kuhn, M., Gavin, A. C., Jensen, L. J., and Bork, P. (2008). Drug target identification using side-effect similarity. *Science* 321, 263–266. doi: 10.1126/science.1158140

Dhanda, S. K., Singla, D., Mondal, A. K., and Raghava, G. P. S. (2013). DrugMint: a webserver for predicting and designing of drug-like molecules. *Biol. Direct.* 8:12. doi: 10.1186/1745-6150-8-28

García-Sosa, A. T., Hetenyi, C., and Maran, U. (2010). Drug efficiency indices for improvement of molecular docking scoring functions. *J. Comput. Chem.* 31, 174–184. doi: 10.1002/jcc.21306

García-Sosa, A. T., and Maran, U. (2013). Drugs, non-drugs, and disease category specificity: organ effects by ligand pharmacology. *SAR QSAR Environ. Res.* 24, 585–597. doi: 10.1080/1062936X.2013.773373

García-Sosa, A. T., Maran, U., and Hetenyi, C. (2012a). Molecular property filters describing pharmacokinetics and drug binding. *Curr. Med. Chem.* 19, 1646–1662. doi: 10.2174/092986712799945021

García-Sosa, A. T., Oja, M., Hetenyi, C., and Maran, U. (2012b). DrugLogit: logistic discrimination between drugs and nondrugs including disease-specificity by assigning probabilities based on molecular properties. *J. Chem. Inf. Model.* 52, 2165–2180. doi: 10.1021/ci200587h

García-Sosa, A. T., Oja, M., Hetenyi, C., and Maran, U. (2012c). Disease-specific differentiation between drugs and non-drugs using principal component analysis of their molecular descriptor space. *Mol. Inform.* 31, 369–383. doi: 10.1002/minf.201100094

Gómez-Bombarelli, R., Wei, J. N., Duvenaud, D., Hernández-Lobato, J. M., Sánchez-Lengeling, B., Sheberla, D., et al. (2018). Automatic chemical design using a data-driven continuous representation of molecules. *ACS Central Sci.* 4, 268–276. doi: 10.1021/acscentsci.7b00572

Hall, M., Frank, E., Holmes, G., Pfahringer, B., Reutemann, P., and Witten, I. H. (2009). The WEKA data mining software: an update. *ACM SIGKDD Explor. Newslett.* 11, 10–18. doi: 10.1145/1656274.1656278

Hassoun, M. H. (1995). *Fundamentals of Artificial Neural Networks*. Cambridge, MA: MIT Press.

Ivanenkov, Y. A., Savchuk, N. P., Ekins, S., and Balakin, K. V. (2009). Computational mapping tools for drug discovery. *Drug Discov. Today* 14, 767–775. doi: 10.1016/j.drudis.2009.05.016

Jolliffe, I. T. (2002). "Principal component analysis and factor analysis," in *Principal Component Analysis*, ed P. Bickel (New York, NY: Springer), 1–457.

Kireeva, N., Baskin, I. I., Gaspar, H. A., Horvath, D., Marcou, G., and Varnek, A. (2012). Generative topographic mapping (GTM): universal tool for data visualization, structure-activity modeling and dataset comparison. *Mol. Inform.* 31, 301–312. doi: 10.1002/minf.201100163

Kuntz, I. D., Chen, K., Sharp, K. A., and Kollman, P. A. (1999). The maximal affinity of ligands. *Proc. Natl. Acad. Sci. U.S.A.* 96, 9997–10002. doi: 10.1073/pnas.96.18.9997

Lipinski, C. A., Lombardo, F., Dominy, B. W., and Feeney, P. J. (2001). Experimental and computational approaches to estimate solubility and permeability in drug discovery and development. *Adv. Drug Deliv. Rev.* 46, 3–26. doi: 10.1016/S0169-409X(00)00129-0

Liu, Y. (2004). A comparative study on feature selection methods for drug discovery. *J. Chem. Inf. Comput. Sci.* 44, 1823–1828. doi: 10.1021/ci049875d

Maaten, L. V. D., and Hinton, G. (2008). Visualizing data using t-SNE. *J. Mach. Learn. Res.* 9, 2579–2605.

Mitchell, T. M. (1997). *Machine Learning*. New York, NY: McGraw-Hill.

Quinlan, J. R. (1986). Induction of decision trees. *Mach. Learn.* 1, 81–106. doi: 10.1007/BF00116251

Saeys, Y., Inza, I., and Larrañaga, P. (2007). A review of feature selection techniques in bioinformatics. *Bioinformatics* 23, 2507–2517. doi: 10.1093/bioinformatics/btm344

Schneider, G. (2017). Automating drug discovery. *Nat. Rev. Drug Discov.* 17:97. doi: 10.1038/nrd.2017.232

Vapnik, V. N. (1995). *The Nature of Statistical Learning Theory*. New York, NY: Springer-Verlag. doi: 10.1007/978-1-4757-2440-0

Venna, J., and Kaski, S. (2006). "Visualizing gene interaction graphs with local multidimensional scaling," in *ESANN*, vol. 6, (Bruges: European Symposium on Artificial Neural Networks), 557–562.

Wang, R. X., Fang, X. L., Lu, Y. P., and Wang, S. M. (2004). The PDBbind database: Collection of binding affinities for protein-ligand complexes with known three-dimensional structures. *J. Med. Chem.* 47, 2977–2980. doi: 10.1021/jm030580l

Wang, R. X., Gao, Y., and Lai, L. H. (2000). Calculating partition coefficient by atom-additive method. *Perspect. Drug Discov. Design* 19, 47–66. doi: 10.1023/A:1008763405023

Wishart, D. S., Knox, C., Guo, A. C., Shrivastava, S., Hassanali, M., Stothard, P., et al. (2006). DrugBank: a comprehensive resource for *in silico* drug discovery and exploration. *Nucleic Acids Res.* 34, D668–D672. doi: 10.1093/nar/gkj067

Yosipof, A., and Senderowitz, H. (2014). Optimization of molecular representativeness. *J. Chem. Inf. Model.* 54, 1567–1577. doi: 10.1021/ci40 0715n

Zhang, J. W., Aizawa, M., Amari, S., Iwasawa, Y., Nakano, T., and Nakata, K. (2004). Development of KiBank, a database supporting structure-based drug design. *Comput. Biol. Chem.* 28, 401–407. doi: 10.1016/j.compbiolchem.2004.09.003

Zupan, J., and Gasteiger, J. (1999). *Neural Networks in Chemistry and Drug Design*. Weinheim: John Wiley & Sons, Inc.

18

Application of Pharmacokinetic-Pharmacodynamic Modeling in Drug Delivery: Development and Challenges

*Huixi Zou, Parikshit Banerjee, Sharon Shui Yee Leung and Xiaoyu Yan**

School of Pharmacy, Faculty of Medicine, The Chinese University of Hong Kong, Hong Kong, Hong Kong

Correspondence:
Xiaoyu Yan
xiaoyuyan@cuhk.edu.hk

With the advancement of technology, drug delivery systems and molecules with more complex architecture are developed. As a result, the drug absorption and disposition processes after administration of these drug delivery systems and engineered molecules become exceedingly complex. As the pharmacokinetic and pharmacodynamic (PK-PD) modeling allows for the separation of the drug-, carrier- and pharmacological system-specific parameters, it has been widely used to improve understanding of the *in vivo* behavior of these complex delivery systems and help their development. In this review, we summarized the basic PK-PD modeling theory in drug delivery and demonstrated how it had been applied to help the development of new delivery systems and modified large molecules. The linkage between PK and PD was highlighted. In particular, we exemplified the application of PK-PD modeling in the development of extended-release formulations, liposomal drugs, modified proteins, and antibody-drug conjugates. Furthermore, the model-based simulation using primary PD models for direct and indirect PD responses was conducted to explain the assertion of hypothetical minimal effective concentration or threshold in the exposure-response relationship of many drugs and its misconception. The limitations and challenges of the mechanism-based PK-PD model were also discussed.

Keywords: drug delivery, modified protein, pharmacokinetic modeling, pharmacodynamic modeling, mechanism-based PK-PD modeling, the minimal effective concentration

INTRODUCTION

The research field of drug delivery focuses on the development of new techniques to manipulate drug absorption and disposition to achieve a desirable effect (Anselmo and Mitragotri, 2014; Asiri and Mohammad, 2018). With the advancement of technology, drug delivery systems with more complex architectures are developed. As a result, the drug absorption and disposition processes after administration of these drug delivery systems become exceedingly complex. The lack of understanding of the *in vivo* behavior of these delivery systems may limit their successful translation into clinics. Mechanism-based pharmacokinetic-pharmacodynamic (PK-PD) modeling could be used to untangle these complexities and improve the understanding of the *in vivo* behavior of these drug delivery systems, consequently informing their preclinical-to-clinical translation and clinical development.

PK-PD modeling, an indispensable component of drug discovery and development, is a mathematical approach to study pharmacokinetics (PK), pharmacodynamics (PD), and their relationship (Peck et al., 1992; Danhof et al., 2005). As **Figure 1** shows, the mechanism-based PK-PD model can be incorporated into multiple stages in drug development. Explicitly, PK modeling quantitatively describes the process of absorption and disposition of drug in the body. PD modeling evaluates the time course of the pharmacological effects of drugs, with the consideration of the mechanism of drug action and major rate-limiting steps in the biology of the system (Mager et al., 2003). The PK and PD modeling can quantify the relationship of drug exposure and response, and further characterize the influences of drug-specific, delivery system-specific, physiological and pathological system-specific parameters on this relationship (Agoram et al., 2007; Danhof et al., 2007). Drug-specific parameters (e.g., drug clearance and receptor binding affinity) illustrate the interaction between the drug and the biological system. The drug delivery system-specific parameters represent the properties of carriers, such as the clearance, release rate, and the internalization rate of the carrier. The physiological system-specific parameters represent physiological values such as blood flow, life-span of cells, expression of enzymes, and transporters (Danhof et al., 2005; Danhof et al., 2007; Sager et al., 2015).

Through the separation of drug-specific and system-specific parameters in PK-PD modeling, the influences of various properties of the delivery system on the *in vivo* drug effect would be evaluated and facilitate its development. As shown in the bottom panel of **Figure 1**, the mechanism-based PK-PD models, developed based on the PK-PD data from preclinical studies, can be used to optimize the drug delivery system and predict the dosing regimen in humans. Once the clinical PK-PD data is available, they can be incorporated into the PK-PD models to further optimize their design. The PK-PD modeling can also evolve together with the clinical development to support the final approval.

Currently, modeling technique is commonly applied in the drug delivery system and modified large molecules. In the classic drug delivery system, modeling has been widely utilized in aiding the formulation design based on preclinical studies, such as liposome, nanoparticle, and nanoemulsion (Soininen et al., 2016; Benchimol et al., 2019; Kadakia et al., 2019). As for the modification of large molecules related to drug delivery, such as PEGylated protein, Fc-modified mAbs and antibody-drug conjugate (ADC), modeling technique has been widely used in both preclinical studies and clinical trials, providing valuable information for the animal-to-human translation and dose regimen selection in clinical trials (Mager et al., 2005; Zheng et al., 2011; Krzyzanski et al., 2013; Ait-Oudhia et al., 2017; McSweeney et al., 2018). There are also many review papers and book chapters on the recent advancement of modeling in drug delivery, while those publications focused more on pharmacokinetics (Yamashita and Hashida, 2013; Ait-Oudhia et al., 2014; Diao and Meibohm, 2015; Singh et al., 2015; Hedrich et al., 2018; Rodallec et al., 2018; Singh and Shah, 2018; Glassman and Muzykantov, 2019; He et al., 2019; Park, 2019). On the contrary, in this review, the linkage between PK and PD is highlighted. We introduce the basic theory of PK-PD modeling and its application relevant to drug delivery. The theory of PK focuses on the modeling of absorption and deconvolution, which is a technique used to identify an appropriate model structure for describing complex absorption. We further discuss the basic PD theory that links drug concentration and therapeutic effect. A few case studies, including the classic drug delivery system and modified large molecules, are presented to exemplify the application of this theoretical framework in practice. A model-based simulation is conducted to explain the

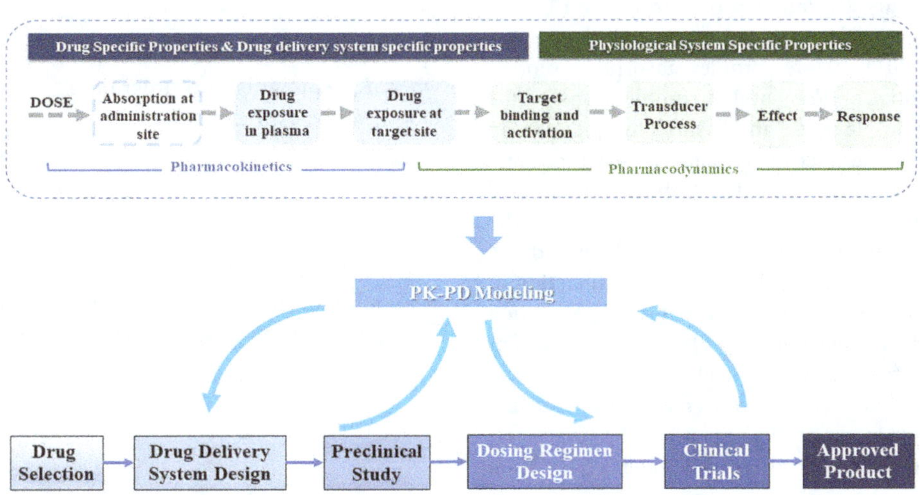

FIGURE 1 | Schematic of PK-PD modeling in the drug delivery system development. In the development of the drug delivery system, PK-PD modeling could guide the formulation design and dosing regimen selection based on the preclinical and clinical data. This technique connects the drug dose to the physiological response, related to the properties of the drug delivery system and physiological system. A chain of events illustrates the flow from the administration, drug exposure (plasma and target site), receptor binding and activation, transduction to effect, and the effect on physiological response.

assertion and misconception of a hypothetical minimal effective concentration or threshold, which has been used to guide the development of many drugs. Furthermore, the limitations and challenges of the mechanism-based PK-PD model are discussed.

BASIC THEORY

Pharmacokinetic Modeling

PK modeling is critical to understand the time courses of drug concentration following administration of various formulations and quantify the dose-concentration relationship. The method of compartmental modeling is commonly used to characterize PK (Jones and Rowland-Yeo, 2013). After the drug enters the central compartment (blood) *via* intravenous (IV) administration, distribution, and elimination occur. A one-compartment model is often used to describe the PK showing a monoexponential decline. It assumes the entire body (including blood, organs, and tissues) acts like a single, uniform compartment (Shargel et al., 1999). A two- or three-compartment model describes the PK curve that shows multi-exponential decay. Blood and well-perfused organs are usually lumped together and considered as a central compartment, while tissues with relatively slow but similar distribution rate are grouped together as one or more peripheral compartments (Ahmed, 2015). For drug administered *via* extravascular routes, its absorption to the central compartment is usually described by a first-order or zero-order process.

New drug delivery systems often significantly influence the PK by modifying the *in vivo* drug release and absorption process. By tuning the drug release profile, the apparent half-life of the drug could be prolonged, and drug accumulation at the target site may be enhanced (Shargel et al., 1999). Complex absorption can involve multiple pathways that occur simultaneously or sequentially, which could be challenging to model. Thus, modelers often use a numerical deconvolution technique to recover the complex drug absorption profile from the PK data so that an appropriate model structure can be used accordingly (Bonate and Steimer, 2011). More complex absorption models may consist of sequential and/or parallel combinations of the simple ones. Here, the simple model and basic techniques used in the absorption modeling are discussed, including first-order and zero-order absorption kinetics, flip-flop kinetics, and deconvolution. While other PK techniques, such as the population PK modeling and the physiologically based PK (PBPK) modeling, are also commonly used in the modeling of drug delivery system, basic concepts and principles of population PK and PBPK modeling are beyond the scope of this report. For readers who are interested with those two topics, several papers in the literature provided recent advancement and excellent review of these fields (Moss and Siccardi, 2014; Lestner et al., 2016; Li et al., 2017; Chetty et al., 2018; Nikanjam et al., 2018; Siccardi et al., 2018).

First-Order Absorption

The most common method to describe drug absorption after extravascular administration assumes a first-order absorption. **Figure 2** shows a one-compartment model with first-order absorption and first-order elimination. The model equations are as follows:

$$\frac{dA_1}{dt} = -k_a \cdot A_1 \tag{1}$$

$$\frac{dA_2}{dt} = k_a \cdot A_1 - \left(\frac{CL}{V}\right) \cdot A_2 \tag{2}$$

$$C_p = \frac{A_2}{V} \tag{3}$$

where A_1 denotes the mass of drug at the administration site, k_a is the absorption rate, A_2 denotes the mass of drug in the body, CL represents the clearance, V represents the volume of distribution, and C_p denotes the plasma drug concentration. The initial conditions for Eqs. 1 and 2 are:

$$A_{1_0} = Dose \cdot F \tag{4}$$

$$A_{2_0} = 0 \tag{5}$$

where *Dose* denotes the amount of drug administered, and F represents the bioavailability. By solving the above differentiation equations, the drug concentration, C_p, can be expressed as:

$$C_p = \frac{F \cdot k_a \cdot Dose}{V(k_a - \frac{CL}{V})} \cdot (e^{-\frac{CL}{V} \cdot t} - e^{-k_a \cdot t}) \tag{6}$$

Zero-Order Absorption

Zero-order processes have also been used to describe the absorption after extravascular drug administration, where the drug is absorbed at a constant rate. The equations (Eqs.7 and 8) for the one-compartment model with zero-order absorption and linear elimination are:

$$\frac{dA_2}{dt} = K_0 - \left(\frac{CL}{V}\right) \cdot A_2 \tag{7}$$

where K_0 represents zero-order input. The drug concentration in blood can be expressed as:

$$C_p = \frac{K_0}{CL} \cdot \left(1 - e^{-\frac{CL}{V} \cdot t}\right) \tag{8}$$

Flip-Flop Kinetics

A popular formulation approach is to extend the release of drug from the delivery system to reduce the dosing frequency and

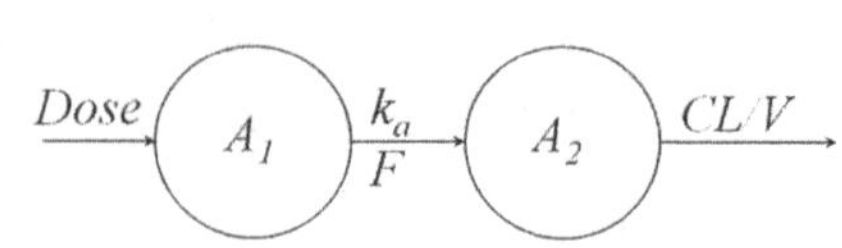

FIGURE 2 | One compartment model with first-order absorption and first-order elimination.

improve patient compliance (Stege et al., 1996; Jadhav et al., 2006). When the absorption process is much slower than the elimination process, the apparent half-life significantly increases due to the slow absorption step, resulting in flip-flop kinetics (Davis, 2018). For instance, in a one-compartment model with first-order absorption and elimination (**Figure 2**), when absorption rate k_a is much smaller than the elimination rate k_{el} (derived by CL/V), resulting in the flip-flop phenomenon. A schematic of flip-flop kinetics in **Figure 3** shows the simulated PK profile of a drug upon IV and extravascular administration. With a rapid absorption ($k_a > k_{el}$), the terminal slope of the concentration-time profile is similar to that after IV administration route, reflecting the k_{el}. However, when drug absorption is slower than the elimination ($k_a < k_{el}$), the absorption process becomes the rate-limiting step. The downward concentration-time curve is less steep and reflects the k_a, while the upward curve reflects the elimination process, k_{el}.

Flip-flop kinetics is commonly observed in the sustained- and controlled-release formulations (Idkaidek et al., 1998; Stepensky et al., 2001). However, the unawareness of flip-flop kinetics can lead to the incorrect characterization of the absorption process. In particular, the terminal phase of the PK profile might be controlled by drug absorption instead of the elimination, which cannot be distinguished with only PK data after extravascular administration. Therefore, the IV data is indispensable to recognize the flip-flop phenomenon and to accurately estimate the PK parameters associated with the drug absorption (Reed et al., 2017).

Deconvolution

Deconvolution has been widely used in PK modeling of drug absorption. It generates an input profile that can be used to guide the selection of the model structure for absorption (Deslandes et al., 1992). By deconvolution, one can estimate the rate and extent of absorption of various formulations *via* extravascular routes, such as subcutaneous, oral, intranasal, rectal, and transdermal (Larsen et al., 1991; Fiset et al., 1995; Björkman et al., 1997; Duquesnoy et al., 1998).

Deconvolution is achieved by the inverse operation of convolution, which is an approach to create a new function by combining two mathematical functions (Yanez et al., 2011). For example, the time courses of drug concentration in plasma after extravascular administration (Eq. 9) can be considered as a convolution of absorption and disposition functions and expressed as:

$$F(t) = In(t) * D(t) \tag{9}$$

where $F(t)$ represents the function describing the drug concentration-time profile, and $In(t)$ and $D(t)$ denote the input/absorption function and output/disposition function, respectively. The symbol "*" represents the convolution operation. The disposition function $D(t)$ can be obtained from the PK profile after IV administration. As long as PK profiles after IV and extravascular administrations are known, the profile for absorption function $In(t)$ can be derived by numerical deconvolution algorithms in software. Currently, deconvolution algorithms are readily available in commercial software such as Phoenix WinNonlin 8.1 (Pharsight Corporation, Cary, North Carolina), Kinetica (Thermo Scientific), and GastroPlus (Simulations Plus, Lancaster, CA) (da Silva Honório et al., 2013; Balakrishnan, 2014).

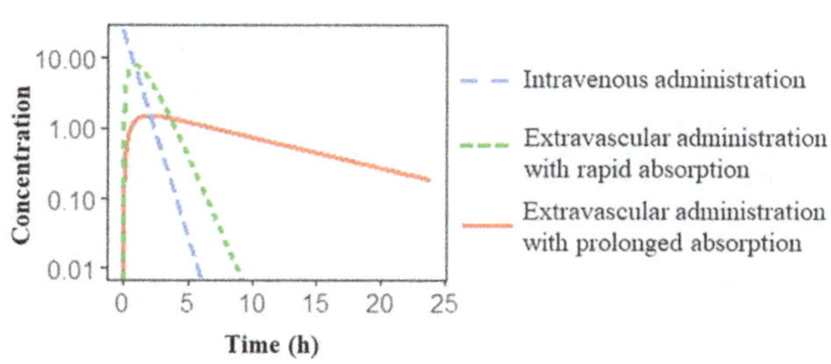

FIGURE 3 | Schematic of extravascular administration with flip-flop kinetics. Simulated PK profile of the same drug to illustrate the effect of differences in the absorption rate. The slow absorption process results in a prolonged half-life.

Pharmacodynamic Modeling

PD models quantify the relationship between drug concentration and therapeutic effect. In this section, the PD models that capture the main mechanisms of drug action are presented, including direct effect, biophase, and indirect response models. Similar to PK, PD is usually described by the compartmental models, and complex PD models are created by combining the simple model.

Direct Effect Models

At the beginning of the research field of pharmacodynamics, it is recognized that the pharmacological effect is linearly related to drug concentration or logarithm of drug concentration (Levy, 1964). It was supported by the clinical data of tubocurarine (Levy, 1966). The plasma drug concentration decreased exponentially after intramuscular injection, and the degree of muscle relaxation decreased linearly with time. However, the relationship between the effect and tubocurarine concentration is linear only if the effect is either less than 20% (linear) or within 20 to 80% of the maximum (log-linear) effect (E_{max}) (Mager et al., 2003). Due to the limitation, the nonlinear E_{max} model was introduced (Wagner, 1968). The rationale for the E_{max} model is based on the classic receptor occupancy theory, and it assumes the drug effect (E) is directly proportional to the fraction of occupied receptors:

$$E = \gamma \cdot RC \tag{10}$$

where RC represents the concentration of drug-receptors complex, and γ is the proportional factor. The drug-receptor complex equilibrium function is described as below:

$$RC = \frac{R_0 \cdot C_p}{K_D + C_p} \tag{11}$$

where R_0 is the total receptor concentration in the tissue, and K_D is the dissociation constant for the drug-receptor complex. By combining Eq. 10 to 11, the E_{max} model equation could be derived:

$$E = \frac{E_{max} \cdot C_p}{EC_{50} + C_p} \tag{12}$$

where E_{max} is the maximum possible effect and equal to γRC, and EC_{50} is a sensitivity parameter representing the drug concentration producing the half-maximal effect. The E_{max} model is frequently used to describe the *in vivo* exposure-effect relationship of many central system drugs and cardiovascular agents (Minematsu et al., 2001; Friberg et al., 2005), where a rapid onset of drug effect is induced. For instance, the E_{max} model has been used to describe the relationship between cocaine concentration and cardiovascular effect, including systolic and diastolic blood pressures as well as the heart rate (Laizure and Parker, 2009).

In addition to the linear relationship between the effect and the drug-receptor complex, a nonlinear relationship has also been proposed as the operational model of agonism (Black and Leff, 1983). The model is expressed as:

$$E = \frac{E_{max} \cdot RC}{K_E + RC} \quad (13)$$

where K_E is the concentration of the drug-receptor complex that triggers a half-maximum effect. By combining Eq.11 and Eq.13, the relationship between the drug effect and the concentration of agonist (A) can be derived as below:

$$E = \frac{E_{max} \cdot \tau \cdot A}{K_D + (\tau + 1) \cdot A} \quad (14)$$

where τ represents the operational efficacy of agonist and is defined by the total concentration of receptor (R_O) divided by K_E. It should be noted that the concentration of drug achieving maximum effect is no longer EC_{50} as defined in Eq.12. As the concentration of drug (A) goes to infinity, the maximal effect is described by the asymptote parameter (α) of Eq.15:

$$\alpha = \frac{E_{max} \cdot \tau}{1 + \tau} \quad (15)$$

The concentration of agonist producing the half-maximal effect (A_{50}) could be derived and shown in Eq. 16:

$$A_{50} = \frac{K_D}{1 + \tau} \quad (16)$$

In Eq.15, when τ is large ($\frac{\tau}{1+\tau}$ approaches to 1), α approaches to E_{max}, and A_{50} is much smaller than K_D, suggesting the drug is a full agonist. However, when τ is small ($\frac{\tau}{1+\tau}$ approaches to 0), α is smaller than E_{max}, and A_{50} approaches to K_D, indicating a partial agonism. The operational model of agonism suggested that the drug triggering effect is a two-step process, where the first step is the receptor binding process, and the second step is the signal-transduction process. Therefore, it can simultaneously analyze concentration-response data of compounds with different binding affinities (K_D) and efficacy (τ), such as full and partial receptor agonists (Danhof et al., 2007). It has been applied in μ opioid (MOP) receptor agonists with varying affinities of receptor and intrinsic efficacies (Scott et al., 1991; Cox et al., 1999).

The models mentioned above (the E_{max} model and the operational model of agonism) describe the direct effect of drugs, when there is no time delay between plasma concentration and response. However, the lag between therapeutic effect and plasma concentration is commonly observed. Depending on the mechanism of the delay, this phenomenon can often be explained by either the biophase model or the indirect response model.

Biophase Distribution Model

The biophase model attributes the delay between the drug concentration and therapeutic effect to the time that it takes for the drug in the plasma to distribute to the target site (Sheiner et al., 1979; Danhof et al., 2007). A biophase compartment was proposed to represents the drug at the target site. In **Figure 4**, a biophase model has been utilized to explain the delayed effect in relation to the plasma drug concentration of d-tubocurarine (Sheiner et al., 1979), where the plasma concentration is linked to biophase concentration with the following differential equation:

$$\frac{dC_e}{dt} = k_{eo} \cdot C_p - k_{eo} \cdot C_e \quad (17)$$

where C_e and C_p represent the concentrations in the biophase and plasma, respectively, and k_{eo} represents the first-order distribution rate constant. As the delay in response due to the distribution process, it could be affected by the physicochemical properties of the drug (e.g., molecule size), binding to plasma protein, and transporter expression (Danhof et al., 2007).

Indirect Response Models

Indirect response (IDR) models are widely used to describe the delayed response generated by the indirect mechanism. Specifically, the drug could stimulate or inhibit either the production or the dissipation of drug response, causing the delay. Jusko and his group formalized four basic indirect response models to describe diverse clinical pharmacodynamic data (Dayneka et al., 1993; Jusko and Ko, 1994). As shown in **Figure 5**, Model I and Model II show the inhibitory effect on the input or loss of response, and Model III and Model IV show the stimulatory effect. The models are expressed as:

$$\frac{dR}{dt} = k_{in}\left(1 - \frac{I_{max} \cdot C_p}{IC_{50} + C_p}\right) - k_{out} \cdot R \quad Model\ I \quad (18)$$

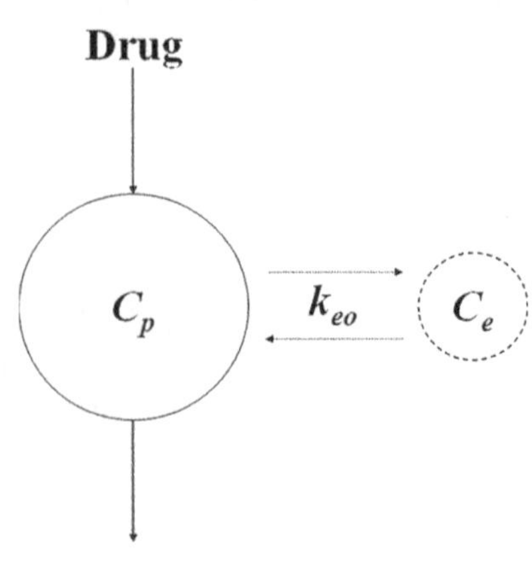

FIGURE 4 | Schematic of biophase model. C_e and C_p represent the concentration at the biophase and plasma, respectively. k_{eo} represents the first-order distribution rate constant.

FIGURE 5 | Indirect response model structure. k_{in} and k_{out} represent the first-order production constant and the first-order dissipation rate constant of the response, respectively. The open and solid box represents the inhibitory and stimulatory effect, respectively.

$$\frac{dR}{dt} = k_{in} - k_{out} \left(1 - \frac{I_{max} \cdot C_p}{IC_{50} + C_p}\right) \cdot R \quad \textit{Model II} \tag{19}$$

$$\frac{dR}{dt} = k_{in} \left(1 + \frac{S_{max} \cdot C_p}{SC_{50} + C_p}\right) - k_{out} \cdot R \quad \textit{Model III} \tag{20}$$

$$\frac{dR}{dt} = k_{in} - k_{out} \left(1 + \frac{S_{max} \cdot C_p}{SC_{50} + C_p}\right) \cdot R \quad \textit{Model IV} \tag{21}$$

where R represents the response; $I_{\max}$ and $S_{\max}$ are defined as the maximal effect of inhabitation or stimulation, respectively; IC_{50} and SC_{50} are the concentration trigger the half-maximal effect of inhibition or stimulation, respectively. The IDR model I has been applied to describe the PK-PD relationship of Warfarin, a vitamin K epoxide reductase inhibitor. Warfarin takes effect by inhibiting the production of prothrombin and cause a delayed anticoagulant effect (Nagashima et al., 1969). A number of papers have reviewed the applications of IDR models (Sharma and Jusko, 1998; Mager et al., 2003; Danhof et al., 2007). The IDR models can be extended to characterize more complex dynamics. A life-span based IDR model has been developed for therapeutic growth factors that alter the production of natural cells (Krzyzanski et al., 1999). A precursor-dependent IDR model has been used to describe the drug effect on the production of endogenous mediators from a specific precursor (Sharma et al., 1998).

Furthermore, integration of IDR model I with the operational model (Eq.22) has been applied in A_1 adenosine receptor agonists with different binding affinities, to describe the relationship between their plasma concentrations and antilipolytic effects (Van der Graaf et al., 1997; Van der Graaf et al., 1999):

$$\frac{dR}{dt} = k_{in} \cdot \left(1 - \frac{E_{max} \cdot \tau \cdot A}{K_A + (\tau + 1) \cdot A}\right) - k_{out} \cdot R \tag{22}$$

The operational model with IDR model I (Eq. 22) might be preferred than the original IDR model I (Eq.18), because it assumes the nonlinear transduction between the drug-receptor complex and the effect of stimulation of k_{in}. However, this model requires PK-PD data from both full and partial agonists to resolve the model parameters. Given such data are often not available, the original IDR model is more commonly applied to characterize the PK-PD relationship of a single compound.

Application of PK-PD Modeling

In this section, we will discuss the application of PK-PD modeling in the development of four different types of drug delivery systems, including extended-release formulation, modified protein, liposome, and antibody-drug conjugates. Furthermore, a model-based simulation using a spectrum of basic PD models was conducted to illustrate the hypothetical minimum effective concentration (MEC).

Complex PK-PD models, as shown in **Figures 6–9**, are often constructed by assembling basic PK and PD model components that have been discussed in previous sections. **Table 1** summarizes the building blocks of PK and PD models that are used to characterize the activity of the compounds in the case studies. For example, the PK-PD model for rHuEPO in **Figure 8** is a combination of the first-order absorption model, target-mediated drug disposition (TMDD) model (Mager and Jusko, 2001a), operational model of agonism (Black and Leff, 1983), precursor-pool dependent IDR model (Sharma et al., 1998), and transit compartment model for transduction process (Mager and Jusko, 2001b).

Application to Paliperidone Palmitate

The development of a 3-month extended-release (ER) formulation of paliperidone palmitate (PP3M), demonstrates how the PK-PD modeling can contribute to the development of new ER formulation. Paliperidone (9-hydroxy-risperidone) is an antipsychotic agent for the acute and maintenance treatment of schizophrenia (Samtani et al., 2009). PP3M is a long-acting injectable formulation of paliperidone palmitate, which is the insoluble ester prodrug of paliperidone (Cleton et al., 2014; Gopal et al., 2015). After intramuscular injection, paliperidone palmitate particles slowly dissolve into the local fluids at the injection site. Due to the poor aqueous solubility, the drug release from the formulation is a dissolution-driven process and becomes the rate-

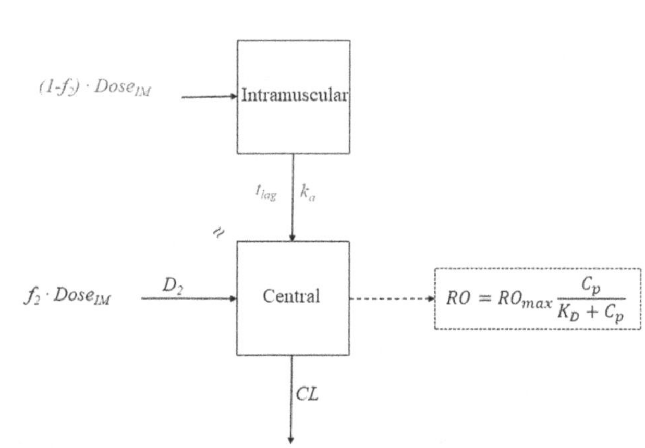

FIGURE 6 | The PK-PD model of paliperidone palmitate. The absorption model was divided into two components: f_2 and *(1- f_2)*. f_2 denotes the fraction that enters the central compartment *via* a zero-order process, and *(1-f_2)* denotes the fraction that enters the central compartment *via* a first-order process. t_{lag} is the lag time, k_a is the absorption rate, D_2 is the duration of f_2 for zero-process and equal to t_{lag}, *CL* represents clearance, *RO* represents receptor occupancy, RO_{max} represents the maximal occupancy can be achieved, C_p represents the plasma concentration, and K_D is the equilibrium dissociation constant.

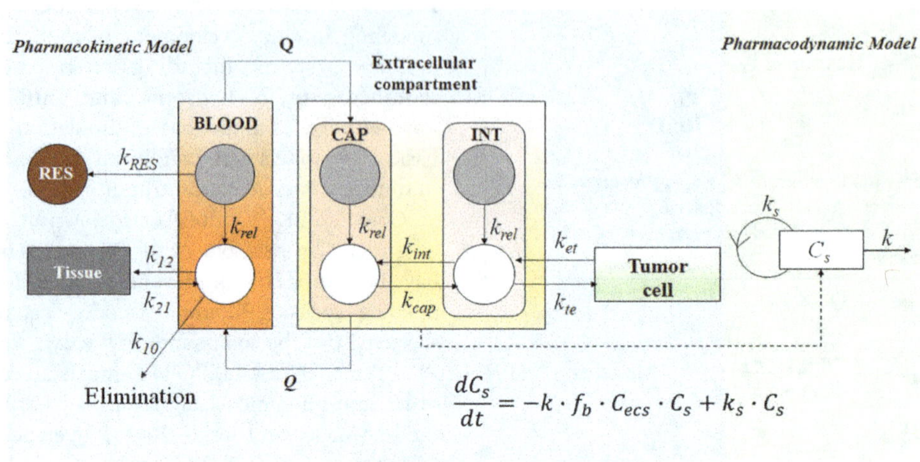

FIGURE 7 | The PK-PD model of the free doxorubicin and liposomal doxorubicin. Free doxorubicin and liposomal doxorubicin are represented by white and grey circles, respectively; the disposition of free doxorubicin and liposomal doxorubicin was described by a two-compartment and a one-compartment model, respectively. The intra-tumor disposition is described by a physiological model linked with tumor blood flow rate (*Q*). Tumor tissue was divided into three compartments: capillary (CAP), interstitial (INT), and tumor cell. The former two are considered in the extracellular compartment (ESC). k_{RES} represents reticuloendothelial system (RES) mediated elimination rate constant of liposomal doxorubicin; liposomal doxorubicin was unidirectionally transported from CAP into INT (k_{tu}); k_{rel} represents the first-order release rate constant of free doxorubicin from liposomes in blood, CAP and INT; distribution of free doxorubicin to tumor cells was described using k_{te} and k_{et}; k_{21}, k_{12}, and k_{10} represent the micro-pharmacokinetic constants for free doxorubicin. For the pharmacodynamic model, a cell-kill kinetic model was linked with the PK model. The mass balance equation describes the change rate of cell number, where C_s represents cell number, $f_b \cdot C_{ecs}$ represents the unbound drug concentration in ESC, k_s is the cell proliferation rate constant, and k is the drug-induced irreversible cell-death rate constant.

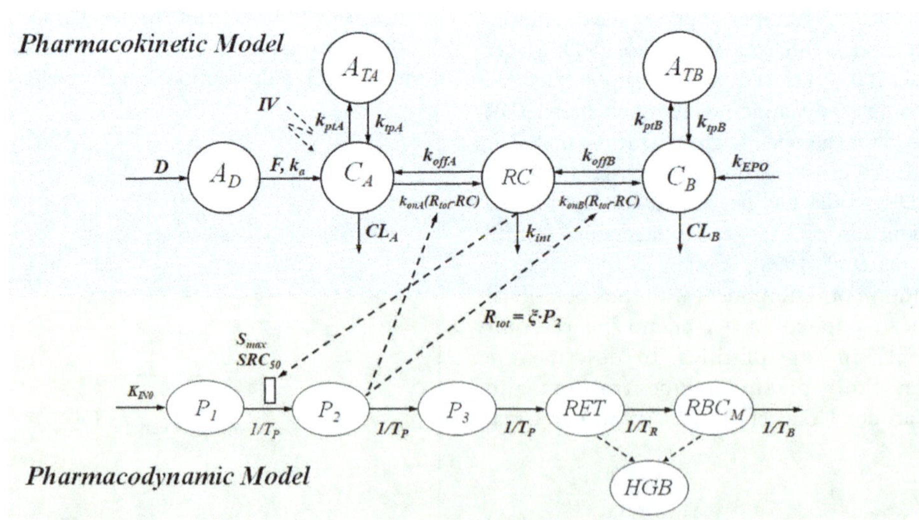

FIGURE 8 | Mechanism-based PK-PD model of ESAs. The upper panel of the flow schematic is based on the TMDD model to describe the PK process. *D* and A_D represent the duration of the zero-order input and absorption compartment for the SC route, respectively. *F* is the bioavailability, and k_a is the first-order absorption rate constant. C_A, C_B, and RC represent the concentration of free ESAs, endogenous EPO (eEPO), and the EPO-receptor complex, respectively. A_{TA} and A_{TB} are tissue compartments, k_{tpA}, k_{tpB}, k_{ptA}, and k_{ptB} are tissue distribution rate constants; k_{onA}, k_{onB}, k_{offA}, and k_{offB} represents second-order rate constants for forming RC and first-order dissociation rate constants of ESAs and eEPO; R_{tot} represents total receptor concentration; CL_A and CL_B are the first-order elimination rate constants; k_{int} is the first-order internalization and degradation rate constant; k_{EPO} represents the synthesis rate of eEPO. The PD model contains delay parameters, indicating the life span of various erythropoietic cells. P_1, P_2, and P_3 represent three different maturation-level erythroid precursor cell compartments; *RET* is reticulocytes, and *RBCM* is mature red blood cell; HGB represents hemoglobin. K_{IN0} represents production process for P_1 cells, S_{max} represents the maximal effect of RC on the proliferation of precursor cells, and SRC_{50} is the concentration of drug-receptor complex to induce half of S_{max}; T_P, T_R, T_B, mean residence time for precursor cell, reticulocytes, and mature red blood cell. PD effect of the expansion of precursor cell on R_{tot} mediates the PK process in return, and ξ is the factor of proportionality.

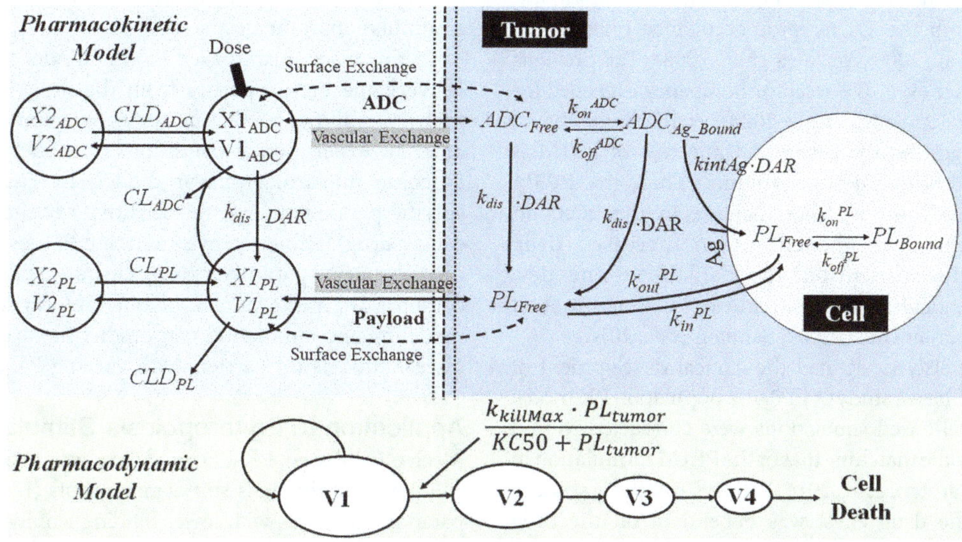

FIGURE 9 | The multiscale PK-PD model of brentuximab-vedotin. The PK model is an integration of a modified two-compartment model in tumor to simultaneously characterize the plasma and intracellular PK of ADC and the payload. After the IV administration of ADC, partial ADC dissociates and releases payloads. ADC and the free drug in the central compartment can be eliminated, distribute to the peripheral compartment, or distribute to the tumor compartment. In the tumor tissue, the free drug could enter the cell by passive diffusion and bind to the target or go back into the extracellular environment. ADC in the tumor environment interacts with the antigen on the tumor cell membrane, and is internalized into the tumor cell. Subsequently, ADC is degraded in lysosomes to release the free drug intracellularly. The intracellular concentration is considered as the concentration in the biophase compartment. $X1_{ADC}$, $X2_{ADC}$, $X1_{PL}$, and $X2_{PL}$, the amount of ADC or payload in the central or peripheral compartment; $V1_{ADC}$, $V2_{ADC}$, $V1_{PL}$, and $V2_{PL}$, volume of distribution of ADC or payload in the central or peripheral compartment; CL_{ADC}, plasma clearance of ADC; CLD_{ADC}, distribution clearance of ADC; ADC_{Free} and ADC_{Bound}, free and bound ADC concentration in tumor tissue; Ag: total antigen; PL_{Free} and PL_{Bound}, free and bound payload concentration in cancer cell; DAR, average drug antibody ratio; k_{dis}, dissociation rate of payload from antibody-drug conjugate; k_{int}^{Ag}, internalization rate of antigen inside the cell; k_{on}^{ADC} and k_{off}^{ADC}, association and dissociation rate constants between antibody-drug conjugate and antigen; k_{on}^{PL} and k_{off}^{PL}, association and dissociation rate constants between drug and intracellular drug target; k_{in}^{PL}, drug nonspecific uptake rate in cancer cell; k_{out}^{PL}, efflux rate of payload from the cancer cell; V1, V2, V3, and V4, tumor volume in the growth.

TABLE 1 | PK-PD model components and related mechanisms of action of drugs.

Drug	PK model components	PD model components	Contribution of PK-PD modeling
Paliperidone palmitate	One-compartment model with First-order elimination First-order absorption Zero-order absorption Flip-flop kinetics	Dopamine D_2 receptor occupancy regulation (Kapur et al., 2000)	Optimized formulation and dose regimen Accelerated the clinical trial
Liposomal doxorubicin	Two-compartment model for doxorubicin One-compartment model for liposome Flip-flop kinetics	Biophase model (Sheiner et al., 1979) Cell-killing kinetic model (Jusko, 1973)	Evaluated the influence of drug-, carrier-, and system-specific parameter on anti-tumor efficacy
Erythropoiesis stimulating agents	Two-compartment model First-order absorption Flip-flop kinetics TMDD model (Mager and Jusko, 2001a)	The operational model of agonism (Black and Leff, 1983) Precursor-Pool dependent indirect response model (Sharma et al., 1998) Transit compartment model (Mager and Jusko, 2001b)	Quantified minimal-effect concentration Explained the relationship between *in vivo* binding affinity and effect
Brentuximab-vedotin	Two-compartment model with first-order elimination	E_{max} model (Wagner, 1968) Biophase model (Sheiner et al., 1979) Transit compartment model (Mager and Jusko, 2001b)	Predicted the clinical response by preclinical data

limiting step of absorption. Ultimately, the slow absorption resulted in flip-flop kinetics and prolonged apparent half-life.

The formulation of PP3M was developed from a 1-month formulation (PP1M) based on the knowledge gained from PK-PD modeling, which identified the injection volume as a significant factor affecting the release rate (Samtani et al., 2009). The PK-PD model of paliperidone palmitate is shown in **Figure 6**. For the PK modeling in PP1M, the deconvolution technique was utilized to identify the appropriate absorption model. A fraction of the dose was initially absorbed *via* a zero-order process, and the remaining fraction entered the central compartment *via* a first-order process after a delay. Since paliperidone is a dopamine receptor D_2 antagonist, the clinical response is linked with the D_2 receptor occupancy (Nordström et al., 1993; Kapur et al., 2000; Arakawa et al., 2008). The previous study has indicated that over 70% receptor occupancy is needed for the therapeutic effect (Arakawa et al., 2008). A PK model-based covariate analysis suggested the absorption rate (k_a) of PP1M is negatively associated with injection volume. Thus, the PP3M formulation was developed with an increase in the injection volume. Together with the benefit of an increased drug concentration in the suspension, the half-life of the new formulation is long enough to maintain an effective concentration over three months (Samtani et al., 2009; Samtani et al., 2016).

PK-PD modeling also accelerated the clinical development of PP3M. Based on the Phase I study of PP3M, a population PK model was developed. Model-based simulations were conducted to find the dose with a PK profile matching that of the PP1M formulation in the Phase III study (Samtani et al., 2016). The PK matching strategy hypothesized that the drug effect was dependent on the drug concentration in plasma above a targeting concentration supported by the PP1M PK/PD studies. Eventually, based on the PK-PD study of PP1M and limited single-dose Phase I data of PP3M, a prospective dose in Phase III was selected without conducting any Phase II dose-finding study. The Phase III study in the end achieved predicted PK and efficacy. The development of the PP3M formulation is a successful case, demonstrating that PK-PD modeling can significantly accelerate the clinical development of a drug delivery system and reduce the cost.

Application to Long-Circulating Liposomal Doxorubicin

The PK-PD model in **Figure 7** described the disposition of liposomal doxorubicin and free doxorubicin, and quantitatively evaluated the relationship between drug exposure and anti-tumor effect by separating the carrier specific-, drug-specific- and system-specific parameters (Harashima et al., 1999). The model was developed based on reported and experimentally obtained preclinical data. The PK profile of liposomal doxorubicin and free doxorubicin in the blood were described by one- and two-compartment models, respectively. Extracellular (ESC) compartment at the tumor site is considered as the biophase compartment, where the concentration has been linked with a cell-killing function. A sensitivity analysis suggested that the rates of liposome clearance (k_{RES}) and drug release (k_{rel}) play critical roles in drug delivery. Lower k_{RES} could mitigate the loss of liposomal doxorubicin in blood to maintain a longer blood circulation period of liposomes. Subsequently, the accumulation of liposomes in the tumor site (ESC) would increase, resulting in a better tumor-killing effect. Furthermore, the simulation results suggested that a medium release rate (k_{rel} at 0.06 h^{-1}) was optimal to achieve higher efficiency in rodents. Compared with the rapid-release formulations, a slower release rate could increase the free drug accumulation in the ESC compartment, instead of being cleared in blood. However, if the release rate was too low (k_{rel} at 0.006 h^{-1}), the formulation failed to achieve the critical drug concentration to inhibit tumor proliferation (Harashima et al., 1999). Therefore, the optimal medium release rate suggested by the model was a balance between the drug elimination from blood and the drug accumulation in the tumor site.

In this mechanism-based PK-PD model, the separation of the delivery-specific properties from the drug- and system-specific properties allows predicting the *in vivo* anti-tumor effect under different experimental conditions. One can predict the *in vivo* outcome in various tumor models by changing the system-specific parameter (e.g., the sensitivity of the tumor to the anti-cancer drug). Similarly, by simulating PD associated with various carrier-specific parameters (e.g., clearance of the carrier), one can compare the performance of different carriers. Hence, PK-PD modeling and simulation can predict the drug effect in different disease models for carriers with varying PK properties.

Application to Erythropoiesis-Stimulating Agents

Mechanism-based PK-PD modeling was applied to quantify the MEC of erythropoiesis-stimulating agents (ESAs), and explain the paradox that ESAs with lower binding affinity has a higher *in vivo* activity (Yan and Krzyzanski, 2013). By binding to the erythropoietin receptor (EPOR) on the membrane of erythroid precursor cells, ESAs stimulate the proliferation and differentiation of erythroid precursor cells (Elliott et al., 2008). Current ESAs include epoetin alfa, darbepoetin alfa, and continuous erythropoietin receptor activator (CERA) (Locatelli and Del Vecchio, 2011). Epoetin, the first recombinant human erythropoietin (rHuEPO), has a half-life between 5 and 12 hours and requires thrice-weekly dosing. Darbepoetin, a hyperglycosylated analog of rHuEPO, has 3- to 4-fold longer half-life than epoetin. However, the receptor binding affinity of darbepoetin is 4.3-times lower than that of epoetin, yet it has higher *in vivo* efficacy (Egrie and Browne, 2001). CERA was developed by incorporating a 30 kDa methoxy polyethylene glycol polymer chain to rHuEPO (Macdougall, 2005). It has a longer half-life, but its receptor binding affinity is much lower (50–100 times) than that of epoetin.

It was hypothesized that the effect of ESAs is not dependent on the peak concentration but on the duration of drug concentration above a 'critical concentration', also known as the MEC (Kiss et al., 2010). ESAs with a lower receptor-binding affinity are considered to have a higher MEC level to ensure sufficient receptor binding. Given MEC varies among various ESAs with different receptor binding affinity, the dosing of darbepoetin and CERA cannot be directly derived by PK matching with their predecessor, epoetin. Without the quantitative definition of MEC, a large number of clinical trials had been conducted to optimize the dosing regimen of darbepoetin (Glaspy et al., 2001; Glaspy et al., 2002; Vansteenkiste et al., 2002).

It was believed that establishing a relationship between the MEC and receptor binding affinity may help to find the optimal regimen for various ESAs. A mechanism-based PK-PD model was, therefore, developed to quantify the MEC of various ESAs based on the clinical PK-PD data of rHuEPO (Yan et al., 2012; Yan and Krzyzanski, 2013). The model structure is provided in **Figure 8**. This model incorporated the operational model of agonism into the PK-PD modeling, which helped to dissect the influence of receptor binding affinity on the drug effect. Furthermore, the binding between ESAs and EPOR results in receptor-mediated drug elimination (Yan and Krzyzanski, 2013). A model-based simulation was conducted to simulate the PK-PD profile of epoetin and darbepoetin under a thricely weekly IV bolus regimen. The PK profiles were overplayed with the C_{50} (Eq. 23) and showed that C_{50} could be considered as the MEC:

$$C_{50} = \frac{K_D}{1+\tau} \tag{23}$$

where C_{50} is the ESA concentration that triggers the half-maximal effect, τ is the efficacy parameter in the operational model of agonism, and K_D is the dissociation equilibrium constant of ESAs. Consistent with the MEC hypothesis, darbepoetin has with a lower binding affinity (higher K_D), but a higher C_{50} value compared to epoetin. However, the simulation also demonstrated that lower binding affinity of darbepoetin leads to lower receptor-mediated drug elimination and hence a slower clearance of the drug compared to epoetin. Therefore, the duration of darbepoetin concentration maintained above C_{50} is longer than that of epoetin, leading to a higher *in vivo* activity (Yan and Krzyzanski, 2013). In other words, the higher concentration and prolonged duration above MEC will eventually compensate for the counteracting effects of lower receptor binding affinity, thereby increasing their *in vivo* activities. Model-based simulations further successfully predicted that CERA had the highest *in vivo* potency among the three ESAs when administered with the same molar dose at any of the approved dosing regimens (i.e., thrice weekly, once weekly, and once every 2 weeks). The model also predicted that if the receptor binding affinity was too low, the benefit (i.e., longer half-life) of lower receptor binding affinity dissipated and eventually led to a lower *in vivo* activity.

Application to Brentuximab-Vedotin

PK-PD modeling is applied to improve the understanding of the complex PK-PD relationship of ADC. ADC consists of a monoclonal antibody (mAb), a cytotoxic payload, and a linker (Tsuchikama and An, 2018). After binding to the antigen expressed on the surface of a tumor cell, ADC is internalized and transported to lysosomes. Once inside of lysosomes, the linker is cleaved to release the cytotoxic payload. It can enhance the selective delivery of the payload to the tumor cell and reduce the systemic toxicity. Brentuximab-vedotin is an anti-CD30 based ADC (Shah et al., 2012). A multiscale PK-PD model (**Figure 9**) was developed to simultaneously captures the disposition of brentuximab-vedotin and its payload, at the cellular and physiological (plasma and tumor tissue) level. The detailed description of the model is provided in the legend of **Figure 9**. A cellular PK model was developed based on *in vitro* experiments, to mimic the intracellular and extracellular (tumor) PK activities of the payload and the ADC. Then, based on the preclinical and clinical *in vivo* data, the PK model of ADC and payload in plasma and tumor was developed. In terms of the PD model, the E_{max} model was used to describe the nonlinear relationship between the intracellular concentration and the tumor-killing rate. The PD parameters were estimated based on the preclinical tumor growth inhibition data in mice. By integration of the multiscale PK-PD model and PK data of brentuximab-vedotin in patients, clinical responses were predicted. A retrospective comparison suggested that model-predicted progression-free survival and complete response rates were comparable to those observed in clinical trials (Bartlett et al., 2009; Younes et al., 2010; Fanale et al., 2012). This example shows that the PK-PD model could integrate the *in vitro* and *in vivo* preclinical information to predict the ultimate clinical response.

Furthermore, this ADC disposition model offers a conceptual framework for the design of ADC and facilitates the preclinical-to-clinical translation. The PK model described above has been applied in auristatin-based anti-5T4 antibody-drug conjugates (Shah et al., 2014). It was discovered that the stability of the payload on the ADC and tumor size are the two most influential factors to the payload exposure in plasma. The linker controls the stability of payload and its dissociation from the antibody. The occurrence of extracellular dissociation increases the systemic exposure of toxic payload and results in a severe adverse effect. Therefore, it offered a rationale to modify the linker to increase the stability of the payload on ADC. Also, the sensitivity analysis suggested an increase in tumor size may lead to a rise in payload exposure in plasma. When tumors are small and avascular, ADC could only diffuse from the tumor periphery to the tumor. However, as a tumor grows and becomes vascularized, ADC can quickly enter the tumor by diffusion from the vasculature. Subsequently, the payload released from ADC inside of the tumor would also increase and diffuse to the systemic circulation. The author suggested that the difference in tumor size between animals and patients should be considered during the preclinical-to-clinical translation.

Model-Based Simulation to Illustrate the Hypothetical MEC

During the development of delivery system, maintaining drug concentration at a threshold concentration (e.g., IC_{50} and EC_{50}) in blood or target site has often been used as a simple method to evaluate the performance of diverse formulation (Mishra et al., 2011). For example, drug release from nanocarriers is often deliberately controlled to maintain the plasma drug level within the therapeutic window between the MEC and the minimum toxic concentration (Siegel and Rathbone, 2012). The presented case studies also implied the presence of MEC and the importance of maintaining drug concentration above a MEC.

In this section, we use PK-PD modeling and simulation to illustrate the assertion and misconception of MEC. Simple direct response model (Eq. 12), indirect response model III (Eq. 20), and indirect model III with the operational model of agonism (Eqs. 15 and 20) are used in PD simulations to accommodate major mechanisms of drug action. A one-compartment model with first-order absorption and first-order elimination is used to simulate PK. The duration of drug concentration above a threshold was manipulated by changing the value of the absorption rate (k_a), mimicking the different release rates of various drug delivery systems. EC_{50} and A_{50} are used as the concentration threshold in the simulation. The relationship between duration of drug concentration above a threshold, and the response was investigated. All the simulations were performed using mrgsolve, an open-source R package (Elmokadem et al., 2019). Parameter values are provided in the legend of **Figure 10**.

Figure 10 shows the simulated PK, PD, and the area under the effect versus time curve (AUEC) for each model with different absorption rates (k_a), which controls the duration of concentration

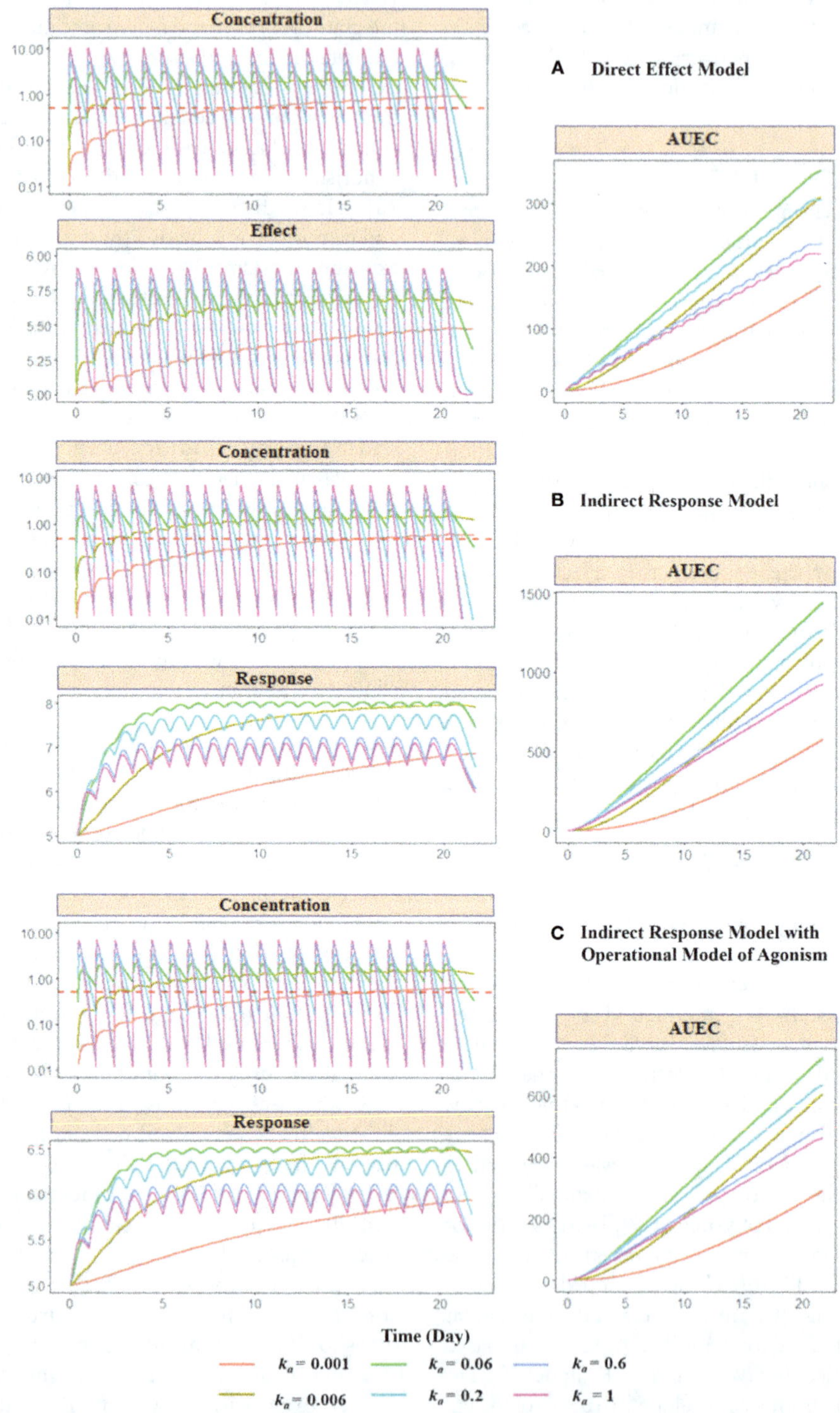

FIGURE 10 | Model-based simulations with different absorption rates. Drug concentration, response (effect), and area under response (AUEC) versus time profiles have been simulated with different PD models: **(A)** direct response model, **(B)** indirect model, and **(C)** indirect response model with operational model of agonism. The dose is 1000 mg. The absorption rate varies from 0.001 to 1 h^{-1}. The red dashed line shows the EC_{50} values or the A_{50} values, which are equal to 1 mg/L. Clearance (*CL*) is 27 L/h, the volume of distribution (*V*) is 90 L (k_{el} = 0.3 h^{-1}), concentration of receptor complex that triggers the half-maximum effect (K_E) is 5 mg/L, E_{max} is 1, response production rate constant (k_{in}) is 0.1 h^{-1}, response elimination rate constant (k_{out}) is 0.02 h^{-1}, equilibrium dissociate rate (K_D) is 2, target production (k_{syn}) are 1 h^{-1}, and degradation (k_{deg}) rate are 0.2 h^{-1}.

above EC_{50} or A_{50}. After the last dose treatment on day 21, the order of the AUEC under varying k_a values are $k_a = 0.06 > k_a = 0.2 > k_a = 0.006 > k_a = 0.6 > k_a = 1 > k_a = 0.001$, which is consistent with the order of duration of drug concentration maintained above the threshold (red dashed line) in the PK profiles. The medium value of absorption $k_a = 0.06$ triggers the highest effect in all three models. Compared with $k_a = 0.06$ group, a larger k_a value ($k_a = 0.2, 0.6$, and 1) results in faster absorption and subsequent elimination, and a shorter duration of concentration above the threshold. On the other hand, when k_a is smaller ($k_a = 0.006$ and 0.001), the absorption is too slow to achieve the threshold concentration during the dosing period. These simulations demonstrate that the duration of drug concentration above a threshold is the determining factor for the therapeutic effect. Therefore, many formulations have focused on optimizing the drug release rate for maintaining drug concentration above MEC.

Although EC_{50} and A_{50} are used as the threshold in the present simulation, it should be noted that the threshold is a hypothetical concept and arbitrarily selected. The concentration-effect relationship (as expressed as E_{max} model or the operational model) is a continuous function without such a threshold. It means maintaining concentration above a specific threshold may not be appropriate for formulation selection, unless the concentration and response relationship is known, and the response associated with this threshold concentration is desired. Therefore, simulation based on the PK-PD relationship is preferred than a single threshold to select the formulation and dosing regimens.

CHALLENGE AND STRATEGY

Although PK-PD modeling has facilitated drug development, several challenges are associated with its application. First, assumptions that are used to simplify the drug delivery process in PK-PD modeling might not always be appropriate. A reliable assumption requires a detailed understanding of both the physiological system and a drug delivery system. Due to the lack of relevant information, it's challenging to validate these assumptions (Suryawanshi et al., 2010). For instance, the PK-PD model of ADC we discussed previously assumed the drug concentration in tumor cells was related to the cell-killing effect (Shah et al., 2012). However, without actual measurement in the distribution cascade, the validity of this assumption is uncertain.

Furthermore, extrapolation from animals to humans based on the PK-PD modeling is also challenging. For instance, in the case study of liposomal doxorubicin, the author suggested that the optimal rate of drug release in rodents was different from that in humans (Harashima et al., 1999). Although there is no universal solution, some methods could be considered to minimize the error of scaling. First, we should always select the appropriate animal species for scalling to humans (Tibbitts et al., 2010). For instance, it is known that dog is the most relevant species to human for preclinical cardiacsafety assessment (Gralinski, 2003; Dubois et al., 2017). Second, allometric scaling using multiple species has been applied to minimize the error and increase the accuracy of prediction (Huh et al., 2011). This method is commonly used to predict human PK (Amantana et al., 2013; Di Martino et al., 2019). Third, for some pharmacological systems, such as the erythropoietic system, the method of scaling from animal to human has already been established (Mager et al., 2009). Thus, given the available prior information, it is relatively more acceptable to scale from animal to human. Fourth, PK-PD modeling based on data collected from tumor xenograft mice model has been extensively used in oncology. This is supported by that the predicted threshold concentration derived from xenograft experiments correlates with the active dose in humans for several marketed chemotherapy drug (Rocchetti et al., 2007). Such a correlation can also be observed in targeted therapies, including both small and large molecules (Yamazaki, 2013; Lindauer et al., 2017). Therefore, the effective concentration in preclinical species could serve as a minimum target concentration that needs to be achieved in humans.

It should be pointed out that modeling assumptions are usually based on prior experience and knowledge and are not equal to random guessing (even they are often not be provided by modelers). They contribute to the power of modeling. Having assumptions helps us to fill the missing pieces among existing information and simplify the understanding of a complex system. However, modelers should be mindful of and acknowledge explicitly the assumptions and limitations of the model, and develop models that are fit for their purpose (Zhang et al., 2008). Methods like sensitivity analysis and external validation can check model's dependency on assumptions, and allows to identify alternative assumption and the information that is needed to in future experiments. An optimal study design can be achieved by simulation and re-estimation, to ensure that the information collected in future experiments is informative on the new assumption (Suryawanshi et al., 2010). Once the new data become available to validate the predicted outcome, the assumption can be further refined and updated. Such a process can be repeated until the final goal of modeling is achieved.

SUMMARY

In this review, we have presented the basic theory and techniques of PK-PD modeling and highlighted its application in the development of different drug delivery systems and modified large molecules. PK-PD modeling and simulation are used to illustrate the misconception of the concentration threshold. The development of new technology can improve the understanding of the physicochemical properties of the delivery system and their interactions with the physiological system. Thus, the predictive ability of PK-PD modeling can be enhanced to guide the development of new drug delivery systems.

AUTHOR CONTRIBUTIONS

HZ performed the model simulation and wrote the manuscript. XY supervised and contributed to the simulation and editing of the review. SL and PB contributed to the revision of the review.

FUNDING

This work was supported by the start-up grant from School of Pharmacy, The Chinese University of Hong Kong.

REFERENCES

Agoram, B. M., Martin, S. W., and van der Graaf, P. H. (2007). The role of mechanism-based pharmacokinetic-pharmacodynamic (PK-PD) modelling in translational research of biologics. *Drug Discovery Today* 12 (23-24), 1018–1024. doi: 10.1016/j.drudis.2007.10.002

Ahmed, T. (2015). "Pharmacokinetics of drugs following IV Bolus, IV infusion, and oral administration," in *Basic Pharmacokinetic Concepts and Some Clinical Applications*. Ed. T. A. Ahmed (Rijeka: IntechOpen), 53–98. doi: 10.5772/61573

Ait-Oudhia, S., Mager, D. E., and Straubinger, R. M. (2014). Application of pharmacokinetic and pharmacodynamic analysis to the development of liposomal formulations for oncology. *Pharmaceutics* 6 (1), 137–174. doi: 10.3390/pharmaceutics6010137

Ait-Oudhia, S., Zhang, W., and Mager, D. E. (2017). A mechanism-based PK/PD model for hematological toxicities induced by antibody-drug conjugates. *AAPS J.* 19 (5), 1436–1448. doi: 10.1208/s12248-017-0113-5

Amantana, A., Chen, Y., Tyavanagimatt, S. R., Jones, K. F., Jordan, R., Chinsangaram, J., et al. (2013). Pharmacokinetics and interspecies allometric scaling of ST-246, an oral antiviral therapeutic for treatment of orthopoxvirus infection. *PloS One* 8 (4), e61514. doi: 10.1371/journal.pone.0061514

Anselmo, A. C., and Mitragotri, S. (2014). An overview of clinical and commercial impact of drug delivery systems. *J. Controlled Release* 190, 15–28. doi: 10.1016/j.jconrel.2014.03.053

Arakawa, R., Ito, H., Takano, A., Takahashi, H., Morimoto, T., Sassa, T., et al. (2008). Dose-finding study of paliperidone ER based on striatal and extrastriatal dopamine D 2 receptor occupancy in patients with schizophrenia. *Psychopharmacology* 197 (2), 229–235. doi: 10.1007/s00213-007-1029-z

Asiri, A. M., and Mohammad, A. (2018). *Applications of nanocomposite materials in drug delivery* (Cambridge: Woodhead Publishing).

Balakrishnan, N. (2014). *Methods and applications of statistics in clinical trials, volume 2: Planning, analysis, and inferential methods* (New Jersey: John Wiley & Sons).

Bartlett, N., Forero-Torres, A., Rosenblatt, J., Fanale, M., Horning, S., and Thompson, S. (2009). Complete remissions with SGN-35 weekly dosing: a phase I dose-escalation study in relapsed/refractory Hodgkin lymphoma or systemic ALCL patients. *J. Clin. Oncol.* 17, 8500. doi: 10.1200/jco.2009.27.15_suppl.8500

Benchimol, M. J., Bourne, D., Moghimi, S. M., and Simberg, D. (2019). Pharmacokinetic analysis reveals limitations and opportunities for nanomedicine targeting of endothelial and extravascular compartments of tumours. *J. Drug Target* 27 (5-6), 690–698. doi: 10.1080/1061186X.2019.1566339

Björkman, S., Rigemar, G., and Idvall, J. (1997). Pharmacokinetics of midazolam given as an intranasal spray to adult surgical patients. *Br. J. Anaesth.* 79 (5), 575–580. doi: 10.1093/bja/79.5.575

Black, J. W., and Leff, P. (1983). Operational models of pharmacological agonism. *Proc. R. Soc. London Ser. B: Biol. Sci.* 220 (1219), 141–162. doi: 10.1098/rspb.1983.0093

Bonate, P. L., and Steimer, J.-L. (2011). *Pharmacokinetic-pharmacodynamic modeling and simulation* (New York: Springer).

Chetty, M., Johnson, T. N., Polak, S., Salem, F., Doki, K., and Rostami-Hodjegan, A. (2018). Physiologically based pharmacokinetic modelling to guide drug delivery in older people. *Adv. Drug Delivery Rev.* 135, 85–96. doi: 10.1016/j.addr.2018.08.013

Cleton, A., Rossenu, S., Crauwels, H., Berwaerts, J., Hough, D., Gopal, S., et al. (2014). A single-dose, open-label, parallel, randomized, dose-proportionality study of paliperidone after intramuscular injections of paliperidone palmitate in the deltoid or gluteal muscle in patients with schizophrenia. *J. Clin. Pharmacol.* 54 (9), 1048–1057. doi: 10.1002/jcph.295

Cox, E. H., Langemeijer, M. W., Gubbens-Stibbe, J. M., Muir, K. T., and Danhof, M. (1999). The comparative pharmacodynamics of remifentanil and its metabolite, GR90291, in a rat electroencephalographic model. *Anesthesiol.: J. Am. Soc. Anesthesiol.* 90 (2), 535–544. doi: 10.1097/00000542-199902000-00030

da Silva Honório, T., Pinto, E. C., Rocha, H. V. A., Esteves, V. S. A. D., dos Santos, T. C., Castro, H. C. R., et al. (2013). In vitro–in vivo correlation of efavirenz tablets using GastroPlus®. *AAPS Pharm. Sci. Tech.* 14 (3), 1244–1254. doi: 10.1208/s12249-013-0016-4

Danhof, M., Alvan, G., Dahl, S. G., Kuhlmann, J., and Paintaud, G. (2005). Mechanism-based pharmacokinetic-pharmacodynamic modeling-a new classification of biomarkers. *Pharm. Res.* 22 (9), 1432–1437. doi: 10.1007/s11095-005-5882-3

Danhof, M., de Jongh, J., De Lange, E. C., Della Pasqua, O., Ploeger, B. A., and Voskuyl, R. A. (2007). Mechanism-based pharmacokinetic-pharmacodynamic modeling: biophase distribution, receptor theory, and dynamical systems analysis. *Annu. Rev. Pharmacol. Toxicol.* 47, 357–400. doi: 10.1146/annurev.pharmtox.47.120505.105154

Davis, J. L. (2018). "Pharmacologic Principles," in *Equine Internal Medicine* (Philadelphia: W.B. Saunders), vol. 79–137.

Dayneka, N. L., Garg, V., and Jusko, W. J. (1993). Comparison of four basic models of indirect pharmacodynamic responses. *J. Pharmacokinet. Pharmacodyn.* 21 (4), 457–478. doi: 10.1007/bf01061691

Deslandes, A., Westphal, J. F., Trouvin, J. H., and Farinotti, R. (1992). Adaptive computer program for determination of absorption profiles by numerical deconvolution: application to amoxicillin absorption. *J. Pharm. Sci.* 81 (8), 802–807. doi: 10.1002/jps.2600810816

Di Martino, M. T., Arbitrio, M., Fonsi, M., Erratico, C. A., Scionti, F., Caracciolo, D., et al. (2019). Allometric Scaling Approaches for Predicting Human Pharmacokinetic of a Locked Nucleic Acid Oligonucleotide Targeting Cancer-Associated miR-221. *Cancers (Basel)* 12 (1), 27. doi: 10.3390/cancers12010027

Diao, L., and Meibohm, B. (2015). Tools for predicting the PK/PD of therapeutic proteins. *Expert Opin. Drug Metab. Toxicol.* 11 (7), 1115–1125. doi: 10.1517/17425255.2015.1041917

Dubois, V. F., Smania, G., Yu, H., Graf, R., Chain, A. S., Danhof, M., et al. (2017). Translating QT interval prolongation from conscious dogs to humans. *Br. J. Clin. Pharmacol.* 83 (2), 349–362. doi: 10.1111/bcp.13123

Duquesnoy, C., Mamet, J., Sumner, D., and Fuseau, E. (1998). Comparative clinical pharmacokinetics of single doses of sumatriptan following subcutaneous, oral, rectal and intranasal administration. *Eur. J. Pharm. Sci.* 6 (2), 99–104. doi: 10.1016/S0928-0987(97)00073-0

Egrie, J. C., and Browne, J. K. (2001). Development and characterization of novel erythropoiesis stimulating protein (NESP). *Br. J. Cancer* 84 (1), 3–10. doi: 10.1054/bjoc.2001.1746

Elliott, S., Pham, E., and Macdougall, I. C. (2008). Erythropoietins: a common mechanism of action. *Exp. Hematol.* 36 (12), 1573–1584. doi: 10.1016/j.exphem.2008.08.003

Elmokadem, A., Riggs, M. M., and Baron, K. T. (2019). Quantitative Systems Pharmacology and Physiologically-Based Pharmacokinetic Modeling With mrgsolve: A Hands-On Tutorial. *CPT: Pharmacometrics Syst. Pharmacol.* 8 (12), 883–893. doi: 10.1002/psp4.12467

Fanale, M. A., Forero-Torres, A., Rosenblatt, J. D., Advani, R. H., Franklin, A. R., Kennedy, D. A., et al. (2012). A phase I weekly dosing study of brentuximab vedotin in patients with relapsed/refractory CD30-positive hematologic malignancies. *Clin. Cancer Res.* 18 (1), 248–255. doi: 10.1158/1078-0432.CCR-11-1425

Fiset, P., Cohane, C., Browne, S., Brand, S. C., and Shafer, S. L. (1995). Biopharmaceutics of a new transdermal fentanyl device. *Anesthesiology* 83 (3), 459–469. doi: 10.1097/00000542-199509000-00004

Friberg, L. E., Isbister, G. K., Hackett, L. P., and Duffull, S. B. (2005). The population pharmacokinetics of citalopram after deliberate self-poisoning: A Bayesian approach. *J. Pharmacokinet. Phar.* 32 (3-4), 571–605. doi: 10.1007/s10928-005-0022-6

Glaspy, J., Jadeja, J. S., Justice, G., Kessler, J., Richards, D., Schwartzberg, L., et al. (2001). A dose-finding and safety study of novel erythropoiesis stimulating protein (NESP) for the treatment of anaemia in patients receiving multicycle chemotherapy. *Br. J. Cancer* 84 (1), 17–23. doi: 10.1054/bjoc.2001.1748

Glaspy, J., Jadeja, J., Justice, G., Kessler, J., Richards, D., Schwartzberg, L., et al. (2002). Darbepoetin alfa given every 1 or 2 weeks alleviates anaemia associated with cancer chemotherapy. *Br. J. Cancer* 87 (3), 268–276. doi: 10.1038/sj.bjc.6600465

Glassman, P. M., and Muzykantov, V. R. (2019). Pharmacokinetic and Pharmacodynamic Properties of Drug Delivery Systems. *J. Pharmacol. Exp. Ther.* 370 (3), 570–580. doi: 10.1124/jpet.119.257113

Gopal, S., Vermeulen, A., Nandy, P., Ravenstijn, P., Nuamah, I., Buron Vidal, J. A., et al. (2015). Practical guidance for dosing and switching from paliperidone palmitate 1 monthly to 3 monthly formulation in schizophrenia. *Curr. Med. Res. Opin.* 31 (11), 2043–2054. doi: 10.1185/03007995.2015.1085849

Gralinski, M. R. (2003). The dog's role in the preclinical assessment of QT interval prolongation. *Toxicol. Pathol.* 31 (1_suppl), 11–16. doi: 10.1080/01926230390174887

Harashima, H., Tsuchihashi, M., Iida, S., Doi, H., and Kiwada, H. (1999). Pharmacokinetic/pharmacodynamic modeling of antitumor agents encapsulated into liposomes. *Adv. Drug Deliv. Rev.* 40 (1-2), 39–61. doi: 10.1016/S0169-409x(99)00039-3

He, H., Yuan, D., Wu, Y., and Cao, Y. (2019). Pharmacokinetics and Pharmacodynamics Modeling and Simulation Systems to Support the Development and Regulation of Liposomal Drugs. *Pharmaceutics* 11 (3), 110. doi: 10.3390/pharmaceutics11030110

Hedrich, W. D., Fandy, T. E., Ashour, H. M., Wang, H., and Hassan, H. E. (2018). Antibody-Drug Conjugates: Pharmacokinetic/Pharmacodynamic Modeling, Preclinical Characterization, Clinical Studies, and Lessons Learned. *Clin. Pharmacokinet.* 57 (6), 687–703. doi: 10.1007/s40262-017-0619-0

Huh, Y., Smith, D. E., and Feng, M. R. (2011). Interspecies scaling and prediction of human clearance: comparison of small- and macro-molecule drugs. *Xenobiotica* 41 (11), 972–987. doi: 10.3109/00498254.2011.598582

Idkaidek, N. M., Amidon, G. L., Smith, D. E., Najib, N. M., and Hassan, M. M. (1998). Determination of the population pharmacokinetic parameters of sustained-release and enteric-coated oral formulations, and the suppository formulation of diclofenac sodium by simultaneous data fitting using NONMEM. *Biopharm. Drug Dispos.* 19 (3), 169–174. doi: 10.1002/(SICI)1099-081X(199804)19:3<169::AID-BDD83>3.0.CO;2-C

Jadhav, P. R., Agersø, H., Tornøe, C. W., and Gobburu, J. V. (2006). Semi-mechanistic pharmacodynamic modeling for degarelix, a novel gonadotropin releasing hormone (GnRH) blocker. *J. Pharmacokinetics Pharmacodyn.* 33 (5), 609–634. doi: 10.1007/s10928-006-9025-1

Jones, H., and Rowland-Yeo, K. (2013). Basic concepts in physiologically based pharmacokinetic modeling in drug discovery and development. *CPT Pharmacometrics Syst. Pharmacol.* 2, e63. doi: 10.1038/psp.2013.41

Jusko, W. J., and Ko, H. C. (1994). Physiologic indirect response models characterize diverse types of pharmacodynamic effects. *Clin. Pharmacol. Ther.* 56 (4), 406–419. doi: 10.1038/clpt.1994.155

Jusko, W. J. (1973). A pharmacodynamic model for cell-cycle-specific chemotherapeutic agents. *J. Pharmacokinetics Biopharm.* 1 (3), 175–200. doi: 10.1007/BF01062346

Kadakia, E., Bottino, D., and Amiji, M. (2019). Mathematical Modeling and Simulation to Investigate the CNS Transport Characteristics of Nanoemulsion-Based Drug Delivery Following Intranasal Administration. *Pharm. Res.* 36 (5), 75. doi: 10.1007/s11095-019-2610-y

Kapur, S., Zipursky, R., Jones, C., Remington, G., and Houle, S. (2000). Relationship between dopamine D2 occupancy, clinical response, and side effects: a double-blind PET study of first-episode schizophrenia. *Am. J. Psychiatry* 157 (4), 514–520. doi: 10.1176/appi.ajp.157.4.514

Kiss, Z., Elliott, S., Jedynasty, K., Tesar, V., and Szegedi, J. (2010). Discovery and basic pharmacology of erythropoiesis-stimulating agents (ESAs), including the hyperglycosylated ESA, darbepoetin alfa: an update of the rationale and clinical impact. *Eur. J. Clin. Pharmacol.* 66 (4), 331–340. doi: 10.1007/s00228-009-0780-y

Krzyzanski, W., Ramakrishnan, R., and Jusko, W. J. (1999). Basic pharmacodynamic models for agents that alter production of natural cells. *J. Pharmacokinetics Biopharm.* 27 (5), 467–489. doi: 10.1023/A:1023249813106

Krzyzanski, W., Sutjandra, L., Perez-Ruixo, J. J., Sloey, B., Chow, A. T., and Wang, Y.-M. (2013). Pharmacokinetic and pharmacodynamic modeling of romiplostim in animals. *Pharm. Res.* 30 (3), 655–669. doi: 10.1007/s11095-012-0894-2

Laizure, S. C., and Parker, R. B. (2009). Pharmacodynamic Evaluation of the Cardiovascular Effects after the Coadministration of Cocaine and Ethanol. *Drug Metab. Dispos.* 37 (2), 310–314. doi: 10.1124/dmd.108.023531

Larsen, F., Clausen, T., Wolff, J., Hansen, P., and Rasmussen, S. (1991). Absorption profiles of rectally administered midazolam estimated by deconvolution. *Eur. J. Drug Metab. Pharmacokinetics* 291–296.

Lestner, J. M., Groll, A. H., Aljayyoussi, G., Seibel, N. L., Shad, A., Gonzalez, C., et al. (2016). Population pharmacokinetics of liposomal amphotericin B in immunocompromised children. *Antimicrob. Agents Chemother.* 60 (12), 7340–7346. doi: 10.1128/AAC.01427-16

Levy, G. (1964). Relationship between elimination rate of drugs and rate of decline of their pharmacologic effects. *J. Pharm. Sci.* 53 (3), 342–343. doi: 10.1002/jps.2600530325

Levy, G. (1966). Kinetics of pharmacologic effects. *Clin. Pharmacol. Ther.* 7 (3), 362–372. doi: 10.1002/cpt196673362

Li, M., Zou, P., Tyner, K., and Lee, S. (2017). Physiologically Based Pharmacokinetic (PBPK) Modeling of Pharmaceutical Nanoparticles. *AAPS J.* 19 (1), 26–42. doi: 10.1208/s12248-016-0010-3

Lindauer, A., Valiathan, C. R., Mehta, K., Sriram, V., de Greef, R., Elassaiss-Schaap, J., et al. (2017). Translational Pharmacokinetic/Pharmacodynamic Modeling of Tumor Growth Inhibition Supports Dose-Range Selection of the Anti-PD-1 Antibody Pembrolizumab. *CPT Pharmacometrics Syst. Pharmacol.* 6 (1), 11–20. doi: 10.1002/psp4.12130

Locatelli, F., and Del Vecchio, L. (2011). Erythropoiesis-stimulating agents in renal medicine. *Oncologist* 16, 19–24. doi: 10.1634/theoncologist.2011-S3-19

Macdougall, I. (2005). CERA (Continuous Erythropoietin Receptor Activator): a new erythropoiesis-stimulating agent for the treatment of anemia. *Curr. Hematol. Rep.* 4 (6), 436–440.

Mager, D. E., and Jusko, W. J. (2001a). General pharmacokinetic model for drugs exhibiting target-mediated drug disposition. *J. Pharmacokinet. Pharmacodyn.* 28 (6), 507–532. doi: 10.1023/a:1014414520282

Mager, D. E., and Jusko, W. J. (2001b). Pharmacodynamic modeling of time-dependent transduction systems. *Clin. Pharmacol. Ther.* 70 (3), 210–216. doi: 10.1067/mcp.2001.118244

Mager, D. E., Wyska, E., and Jusko, W. J. (2003). Diversity of mechanism-based pharmacodynamic models. *Drug Metab. Dispos.* 31 (5), 510–518. doi: 10.1124/dmd.31.5.510

Mager, D. E., Neuteboom, B., and Jusko, W. J. (2005). Pharmacokinetics and pharmacodynamics of PEGylated IFN-β 1a following subcutaneous administration in monkeys. *Pharm. Res.* 22 (1), 58–61. doi: 10.1007/s11095-004-9009-z

Mager, D. E., Woo, S., and Jusko, W. J. (2009). Scaling pharmacodynamics from in vitro and preclinical animal studies to humans. *Drug Metab. Pharmacokinet.* 24 (1), 16–24. doi: 10.2133/dmpk.24.16

McSweeney, M., Wessler, T., Price, L., Ciociola, E., Herity, L., Piscitelli, J., et al. (2018). A minimal physiologically based pharmacokinetic model that predicts anti-PEG IgG-mediated clearance of PEGylated drugs in human and mouse. *J. Controlled Release* 284, 171–178. doi: 10.1016/j.jconrel.2018.06.002

Minematsu, T., Ohtani, H., Yamada, Y., Sawada, Y., Sato, H., and Iga, T. (2001). Quantitative relationship between myocardial concentration of tacrolimus and QT prolongation in guinea pigs: Pharmacokinetic/pharmacodynamic model incorporating a site of adverse effect. *J. Pharmacokinet. Phar.* 28 (6), 533–554. doi: 10.1023/A:1014460404352

Mishra, G. P., Bagui, M., Tamboli, V., and Mitra, A. K. (2011). Recent applications of liposomes in ophthalmic drug delivery. *J. Drug Deliv.* 2011, 1–14. doi: 10.1155/2011/863734

Moss, D. M., and Siccardi, M. (2014). Optimizing nanomedicine pharmacokinetics using physiologically based pharmacokinetics modelling. *Br. J. Pharmacol.* 171 (17), 3963–3979. doi: 10.1111/bph.12604

Nagashima, R., O'reilly, R., and Levy, G. (1969). Kinetics of pharmacologic effects in man: the anticoagulant action of warfarin. *Clin. Pharmacol. Ther.* 10 (1), 22–35. doi: 10.1002/cpt196910122

Nikanjam, M., Capparelli, E. V., Lancet, J. E., Louie, A., and Schiller, G. (2018). Persistent cytarabine and daunorubicin exposure after administration of novel liposomal formulation CPX-351: population pharmacokinetic assessment. *Cancer Chemother. Pharmacol.* 81 (1), 171–178. doi: 10.1007/s00280-017-3484-5

Nordström, A.-L., Farde, L., Wiesel, F.-A., Forslund, K., Pauli, S., Halldin, C., et al. (1993). Central D2-dopamine receptor occupancy in relation to antipsychotic drug effects: a double-blind PET study of schizophrenic patients. *Biol. Psychiatry* 33 (4), 227–235. doi: 10.1016/0006-3223(93)90288-O

Park, K. (2019). PK/PD model for liposomal chemophototherapy. *J. Control Release* 297, 102. doi: 10.1016/j.jconrel.2019.02.022

Peck, C. C., Barr, W. H., Benet, L. Z., Collins, J., Desjardins, R. E., Furst, D. E., et al. (1992). Opportunities for integration of pharmacokinetics, pharmacodynamics, and toxicokinetics in rational drug development. *Clin. Pharmacol. Ther.* 51 (4), 465–473. doi: 10.1038/clpt.1992.47

Reed, S. M., Bayly, W. M., and Sellon, D. C. (2017). *Equine Internal Medicine-E-Book* (New York: Elsevier Health Sciences).

Rocchetti, M., Simeoni, M., Pesenti, E., De Nicolao, G., and Poggesi, I. (2007). Predicting the active doses in humans from animal studies: a novel approach in oncology. *Eur. J. Cancer* 43 (12), 1862–1868. doi: 10.1016/j.ejca.2007.05.011

Rodallec, A., Fanciullino, R., Lacarelle, B., and Ciccolini, J. (2018). Seek and destroy: improving PK/PD profiles of anticancer agents with nanoparticles. *Expert Rev. Clin. Pharmacol.* 11 (6), 599–610. doi: 10.1080/17512433.2018.1477586

Sager, J. E., Yu, J., Ragueneau-Majlessi, I., and Isoherranen, N. (2015). Physiologically based pharmacokinetic (PBPK) modeling and simulation approaches: a systematic review of published models, applications, and model verification. *Drug Metab. Dispos.* 43 (11), 1823–1837. doi: 10.1124/dmd.115.065920

Samtani, M. N., Vermeulen, A., and Stuyckens, K. (2009). Population pharmacokinetics of intramuscular paliperidone palmitate in patients with schizophrenia: a novel once-monthly, long-acting formulation of an atypical antipsychotic. *Clin. Pharmacokinet.* 48 (9), 585–600. doi: 10.2165/11316870-000000000-00000

Samtani, M. N., Nandy, P., Ravenstijn, P., Remmerie, B., Vermeulen, A., Russu, A., et al. (2016). Prospective dose selection and acceleration of paliperidone palmitate 3-month formulation development using a pharmacometric bridging strategy. *Br. J. Clin. Pharmacol.* 82 (5), 1364–1370. doi: 10.1111/bcp.13050

Scott, J. C., Cooke, J. E., and Stanski, D. R. (1991). Electroencephalographic quantitation of opioid effect: comparative pharmacodynamics of fentanyl and sufentanil. *Anesthesiology* 74 (1), 34–42. doi: 10.1097/00000542-199101000-00007

Shah, D. K., Haddish-Berhane, N., and Betts, A. (2012). Bench to bedside translation of antibody drug conjugates using a multiscale mechanistic PK/PD model: a case study with brentuximab-vedotin. *J. Pharmacokinet. Pharmacodyn.* 39 (6), 643–659. doi: 10.1007/s10928-012-9276-y

Shah, D. K., King, L. E., Han, X. G., Wentland, J. A., Zhang, Y. H., Lucas, J., et al. (2014). A Priori Prediction of Tumor Payload Concentrations: Preclinical Case Study with an Auristatin-Based Anti-5T4 Antibody-Drug Conjugate. *AAPS J.* 16 (3), 452–463. doi: 10.1208/s12248-014-9576-9

Shargel, L., Andrew, B., and Wu-Pong, S. (1999). *Applied biopharmaceutics and pharmacokinetics* (New York: Appleton & Lange Stamford).

Sharma, A., and Jusko, W. J. (1998). Characteristics of indirect pharmacodynamic models and applications to clinical drug responses. *Br. J. Clin. Pharmacol.* 45 (3), 229–239. doi: 10.1046/j.1365-2125.1998.00676.x

Sharma, A., Ebling, W. F., and Jusko, W. J. (1998). Precursor-dependent indirect pharmacodynamic response model for tolerance and rebound phenomena. *J. Pharm. Sci.* 87 (12), 1577–1584. doi: 10.1021/js980171q

Sheiner, L. B., Stanski, D. R., Vozeh, S., Miller, R. D., and Ham, J. (1979). Simultaneous modeling of pharmacokinetics and pharmacodynamics: application to d-tubocurarine. *Clin. Pharmacol. Ther.* 25 (3), 358–371. doi: 10.1002/cpt1979253358

Siccardi, M., Rannard, S., and Owen, A. (2018). The emerging role of physiologically based pharmacokinetic modelling in solid drug nanoparticle translation. *Adv. Drug Deliv. Rev.* 131, 116–121. doi: 10.1016/j.addr.2018.06.016

Siegel, R. A., and Rathbone, M. J. (2012). "Overview of controlled release mechanisms," in *Fundamentals and applications of controlled release drug delivery* (New York: Springer), 19–43.

Singh, A. P., and Shah, D. K. (2018). Utility of PK-PD Modeling and Simulation to Improve Decision Making for Antibody-Drug Conjugate Development. *Innovations Next-Gener. Antibody-Drug Conjugates* 73–97. doi: 10.1007/978-3-319-78154-9

Singh, A. P., Shin, Y. G., and Shah, D. K. (2015). Application of Pharmacokinetic-Pharmacodynamic Modeling and Simulation for Antibody-Drug Conjugate Development. *Pharm. Res.* 32 (11), 3508–3525. doi: 10.1007/s11095-015-1626-1

Soininen, S. K., Vellonen, K. S., Heikkinen, A. T., Auriola, S., Ranta, V. P., Urtti, A., et al. (2016). Intracellular PK/PD Relationships of Free and Liposomal Doxorubicin: Quantitative Analyses and PK/PD Modeling. *Mol. Pharm.* 13 (4), 1358–1365. doi: 10.1021/acs.molpharmaceut.6b00008

Stege, R., Gunnarsson, P. O., Johansson, C. J., Olsson, P., Pousette, Å., and Carlström, K. (1996). Pharmacokinetics and testosterone suppression of a single dose of polyestradiol phosphate (Estradurin®) in prostatic cancer patients. *Prostate* 28 (5), 307–310. doi: 10.1002/(SICI)1097-0045(199605)28:5<307::AID-PROS6>3.0.CO;2-8

Stepensky, D., Friedman, M., Srour, W., Raz, I., and Hoffman, A. (2001). Preclinical evaluation of pharmacokinetic–pharmacodynamic rationale for oral CR metformin formulation. *J. Controlled Rel.* 71 (1), 107–115. doi: 10.1016/S0168-3659(00)00374-6

Suryawanshi, S., Zhang, L., Pfister, M., and Meibohm, B. (2010). The current role of model-based drug development. *Expert Opin. Drug Discovery* 5 (4), 311–321. doi: 10.1517/17460441003713470

Tibbitts, J., Cavagnaro, J. A., Haller, C. A., Marafino, B., Andrews, P. A., and Sullivan, J. T. (2010). Practical approaches to dose selection for first-in-human clinical trials with novel biopharmaceuticals. *Regul. Toxicol. Pharmacol.* 58 (2), 243–251. doi: 10.1016/j.yrtph.2010.06.007

Tsuchikama, K., and An, Z. (2018). Antibody-drug conjugates: recent advances in conjugation and linker chemistries. *Protein Cell* 9 (1), 33–46. doi: 10.1007/s13238-016-0323-0

Van der Graaf, P., Van Schaick, E., Mathot, R., Ijzerman, A., and Danhof, M. (1997). Mechanism-based pharmacokinetic-pharmacodynamic modeling of the effects of N6-cyclopentyladenosine analogs on heart rate in rat: estimation of in vivo operational affinity and efficacy at adenosine A1 receptors. *J. Pharmacol. Exp. Ther.* 283 (2), 809–816.

Van der Graaf, P. H., Van Schaick, E. A., Visser, S. A. G., De Greef, H. J. M. M., Ijzerman, A. P., and Danhof, M. (1999). Mechanism-based pharmacokinetic-pharmacodynamic modeling of antilipolytic effects of adenosine A(1) receptor agonists in rats: Prediction of tissue-dependent efficacy in vivo. *J. Pharmacol. Exp. Ther.* 290 (2), 702–709.

Vansteenkiste, J., Pirker, R., Massuti, B., Barata, F., Font, A., Fiegl, M., et al. (2002). Double-blind, placebo-controlled, randomized phase III trial of darbepoetin alfa in lung cancer patients receiving chemotherapy. *J. Natl. Cancer Inst.* 94 (16), 1211–1220. doi: 10.1093/jnci/94.16.1211

Wagner, J. (1968). Kinetics of pharmacologic response I. Proposed relationships between response and drug concentration in the intact animal and man. *J. Theor. Biol.* 20 (2), 173–201. doi: 10.1016/0022-5193(68)90188-4

Yamashita, F., and Hashida, M. (2013). Pharmacokinetic considerations for targeted drug delivery. *Adv. Drug Delivery Rev.* 65 (1), 139–147. doi: 10.1016/j.addr.2012.11.006

Yamazaki, S. (2013). Translational pharmacokinetic-pharmacodynamic modeling from nonclinical to clinical development: a case study of anticancer drug, crizotinib. *AAPS J.* 15 (2), 354–366. doi: 10.1208/s12248-012-9436-4

Yan, X., and Krzyzanski, W. (2013). Quantitative assessment of minimal effective concentration of erythropoiesis-stimulating agents. *Cpt-Pharmacometrics Syst. Pharmacol.* 2 (8), 1–10. doi: 10.1038/psp.2013.39

Yan, X., Lowe, P. J., Fink, M., Berghout, A., Balser, S., and Krzyzanski, W. (2012). Population pharmacokinetic and pharmacodynamic model-based comparability assessment of a recombinant human Epoetin Alfa and the Biosimilar HX575. *J. Clin. Pharmacol.* 52 (11), 1624–1644. doi: 10.1177/0091270011421911

Yanez, J. A., Remsberg, C. M., Sayre, C. L., Forrest, M. L., and Davies, N. M. (2011). Flip-flop pharmacokinetics–delivering a reversal of disposition: challenges and opportunities during drug development. *Ther. Delivery* 2 (5), 643–672. doi: 10.4155/tde.11.19

Younes, A., Bartlett, N. L., Leonard, J. P., Kennedy, D. A., Lynch, C. M., Sievers, E. L., et al. (2010). Brentuximab vedotin (SGN-35) for relapsed CD30-positive lymphomas. *New Engl. J. Med.* 363 (19), 1812–1821. doi: 10.1056/NEJMoa1002965

Zhang, L., Pfister, M., and Meibohm, B. (2008). Concepts and Challenges in Quantitative Pharmacology and Model-Based Drug Development. *AAPS J.* 10 (4), 552–559. doi: 10.1208/s12248-008-9062-3

Zheng, Y., Scheerens, H., Davis, J. C.Jr., Deng, R., Fischer, S. K., Woods, C., et al. (2011). Translational pharmacokinetics and pharmacodynamics of an FcRn-variant anti-CD4 monoclonal antibody from preclinical model to phase I study. *Clin. Pharmacol. Ther.* 89 (2), 283–290. doi: 10.1038/clpt.2010.311

Permissions

All chapters in this book were first published by Frontiers; hereby published with permission under the Creative Commons Attribution License or equivalent. Every chapter published in this book has been scrutinized by our experts. Their significance has been extensively debated. The topics covered herein carry significant findings which will fuel the growth of the discipline. They may even be implemented as practical applications or may be referred to as a beginning point for another development.

The contributors of this book come from diverse backgrounds, making this book a truly international effort. This book will bring forth new frontiers with its revolutionizing research information and detailed analysis of the nascent developments around the world.

We would like to thank all the contributing authors for lending their expertise to make the book truly unique. They have played a crucial role in the development of this book. Without their invaluable contributions this book wouldn't have been possible. They have made vital efforts to compile up to date information on the varied aspects of this subject to make this book a valuable addition to the collection of many professionals and students.

This book was conceptualized with the vision of imparting up-to-date information and advanced data in this field. To ensure the same, a matchless editorial board was set up. Every individual on the board went through rigorous rounds of assessment to prove their worth. After which they invested a large part of their time researching and compiling the most relevant data for our readers.

The editorial board has been involved in producing this book since its inception. They have spent rigorous hours researching and exploring the diverse topics which have resulted in the successful publishing of this book. They have passed on their knowledge of decades through this book. To expedite this challenging task, the publisher supported the team at every step. A small team of assistant editors was also appointed to further simplify the editing procedure and attain best results for the readers.

Apart from the editorial board, the designing team has also invested a significant amount of their time in understanding the subject and creating the most relevant covers. They scrutinized every image to scout for the most suitable representation of the subject and create an appropriate cover for the book.

The publishing team has been an ardent support to the editorial, designing and production team. Their endless efforts to recruit the best for this project, has resulted in the accomplishment of this book. They are a veteran in the field of academics and their pool of knowledge is as vast as their experience in printing. Their expertise and guidance has proved useful at every step. Their uncompromising quality standards have made this book an exceptional effort. Their encouragement from time to time has been an inspiration for everyone.

The publisher and the editorial board hope that this book will prove to be a valuable piece of knowledge for researchers, students, practitioners and scholars across the globe.

List of Contributors

Mariana González-Medina, Mario Figueroa and José L. Medina-Franco
Departamento de Farmacia, Facultad de Química, Universidad Nacional Autónoma de México, México

John R. Owen
High-Performance Computing Research Group, ECIT Institute, Northern Ireland Science Park, Belfast, UK

Tamam El-Elimat
Department of Medicinal Chemistry and Pharmacognosy, Faculty of Pharmacy, Jordan University of Science and Technology, Irbid, Jordan

Cedric J. Pearce
Mycosynthetix, Inc., Hillsborough, NC, USA

Nicholas H. Oberlies
Department of Chemistry and Biochemistry, University of North Carolina at Greensboro, Greensboro, NC, USA

Marilia N. N. Lima, Cleber C. Melo-Filho, Vinicius M. Alves and Rodolpho C. Braga
LabMol - Laboratory for Molecular Modeling and Drug Design, Faculty of Pharmacy, Federal University of Goiás, Goiânia, Brazil

Gustavo C. Cassiano and Fabio T. M. Costa
Laboratory of Tropical Diseases - Prof. Dr. Luiz Jacintho da Silva, Department of Genetics, Evolution, Microbiology and Immunology, Institute of Biology, UNICAMP, Campinas, Brazil

Bruno J. Neves
LabMol - Laboratory for Molecular Modeling and Drug Design, Faculty of Pharmacy, Federal University of Goiás, Goiânia, Brazil
Laboratory of Cheminformatics, PPG-SOMA, University Center of Anápolis/UniEVANGELICA, Anápolis, Brazil

Pedro V. L. Cravo
Global Health and Tropical Medicine Centre, Unidade de Parasitologia Médica, Instituto de Higiene e Medicina Tropical, Universidade Nova de Lisboa, Lisbon, Portugal

Alexey A. Lagunin and Sergey M. Ivanov
Department of Bioinformatics, Institute of Biomedical Chemistry, Moscow, Russia
Department of Bioinformatics, Pirogov Russian National Research Medical University, Moscow, Russia

Eugene N. Muratov
Laboratory for Molecular Modeling, Division of Chemical Biology and Medicinal Chemistry, Eshelman School of Pharmacy, University of North Carolina at Chapel Hill, Chapel Hill, NC, United States
Department of Chemical Technology, Odessa National Polytechnic University, Odessa, Ukraine

Juliana Calit and Daniel Y. Bargieri
Department of Parasitology, Institute of Biomedical Sciences, University of São Paulo, São Paulo, Brazil

Carolina H. Andrade
LabMol - Laboratory for Molecular Modeling and Drug Design, Faculty of Pharmacy, Federal University of Goiás, Goiânia, Brazil
Laboratory of Tropical Diseases - Prof. Dr. Luiz Jacintho da Silva, Department of Genetics, Evolution, Microbiology and Immunology, Institute of Biology, UNICAMP, Campinas, Brazil

Chun Xie, Ying Li, Xing-Xing Fan, Yu-Wei Wang, Chun-Li Wei, Liang Liu and Elaine Lai-Han Leung
State Key Laboratory of Quality Research in Chinese Medicine, Macau Institute for Applied Research in Medicine and Health, Macau University of Science and Technology, Macau, China

Lan-Lan Li
State Key Laboratory of Applied Organic Chemistry and Department of Chemistry, Lanzhou University, Lanzhou, China

Xiao-Jun Yao
State Key Laboratory of Quality Research in Chinese Medicine, Macau Institute for Applied Research in Medicine and Health, Macau University of Science and Technology, Macau, China
State Key Laboratory of Applied Organic Chemistry and Department of Chemistry, Lanzhou University, Lanzhou, China

Maria A. Romanova, Anton D. Zadorozhny, Natalia S. Kurilenko and Boris V. Shilov
Department of Bioinformatics, Pirogov Russian National Research Medical University, Moscow, Russia

Pavel V. Pogodin, Dmitry A. Filimonov and Vladimir V. Poroikov
Department of Bioinformatics, Institute of Biomedical Chemistry, Moscow, Russia

Rodolfo S. Simões and Patricia R. Oliveira
School of Arts, Sciences and Humanities, University of São Paulo, São Paulo, Brazil

Vinicius G. Maltarollo
Department of Pharmaceutical Products, Faculty of Pharmacy, Federal University of Minas Gerais, Belo Horizonte, Brazil

Kathia M. Honorio
School of Arts, Sciences and Humanities, University of São Paulo, São Paulo, Brazil
Center for Natural and Human Sciences, Federal University of ABC, Santo André, Brazil

Patric Schyman, Ruifeng Liu, Valmik Desai and Anders Wallqvist
DoD Biotechnology High Performance Computing Software Applications Institute, Telemedicine and Advanced Technology Research Center, U.S. Army Medical Research and Materiel Command, Fort Detrick, MD, United States

Lewis H. Mervin, Avid M. Afzal and Andreas Bender
Centre for Molecular Informatics, Department of Chemistry, University of Cambridge, Cambridge, United Kingdom

Lars Brive
Cygnal Bioscience, Pixbo, Sweden

Ola Engkvist
Hit Discovery, Discovery Sciences, IMED Biotech Unit, AstraZeneca, Gothenburg, Sweden

Manon Réau, Florent Langenfeld, Jean-François Zagury, Nathalie Lagarde and Matthieu Montes
Laboratoire GBA, EA4627, Conservatoire National des Arts et Métiers, Paris, France

Péter Bencsik, Anikó Görbe and Éva Kenyeres
Cardiovascular Research Group, Department of Biochemistry, Faculty of Medicine, University of Szeged, Szeged, Hungary
Pharmahungary Group, Szeged, Hungary

Krisztina Kupai, Renáta Gáspár, Tamás Csont and Csaba Csonka
Department of Biochemistry, Faculty of Medicine, University of Szeged, Szeged, Hungary

Zoltán V. Varga and János Pálóczi
Department of Pharmacology and Pharmacotherapy, Faculty of Medicine, Semmelweis University, Budapest, Hungary

László Kovács and Ferenc Takács
Infarmatik, Budapest, Hungary

Lutz Weber
OntoChem GmbH, Halle (Saale), Germany

István Hajdú
OntoChem GmbH, Halle (Saale), Germany
Research Centre for Natural Sciences, Institute of Enzymology, Hungarian Academy of Sciences, Budapest, Hungary

Gabriella Fabó, Sándor Cseh and György Dormán
Targetex Biosciences, Dunakeszi, Hungary

László Barna
Research Centre for Natural Sciences, Institute of Enzymology, Hungarian Academy of Sciences, Budapest, Hungary
Microscopy Center at IEM HAS, Institute of Experimental Medicine, Hungarian Academy of Sciences, Budapest, Hungary

Péter Ferdinandy
Pharmahungary Group, Szeged, Hungary
Department of Pharmacology and Pharmacotherapy, Faculty of Medicine, Semmelweis University, Budapest, Hungary

Yin-Hua Deng, Ning-Ning Wang and Kang-Ping Xu
Xiangya School of Pharmaceutical Sciences, Central South University, Changsha, China

Zhen-Xing Zou and Gui-Shan Tan
Xiangya School of Pharmaceutical Sciences, Central South University, Changsha, China
Pharmacy Department, Xiangya Hospital, Central South University, Changsha, China

Lin Zhang
College of Food Science and Technology, Central South University of Forestry and Technology, Changsha, China

Alex F. Chen and Dong-Sheng Cao
Xiangya School of Pharmaceutical Sciences, Central South University, Changsha, China
Center for Vascular Disease and Translational Medicine, Third Xiangya Hospital, Central South University, Changsha, China

Shan Wang, Yu Tian, Gui-bo Sun and Xiao-bo Sun
Beijing Key Laboratory of Innovative Drug Discovery of Traditional Chinese Medicine (Natural Medicine) and Translational Medicine, Institute of Medicinal Plant Development, Chinese Academy of Medical Sciences and Peking Union Medical College, Beijing, China

Min Wang
Life and Environmental Science Research Center, Harbin University of Commerce, Harbin, China
Beijing Key Laboratory of Innovative Drug Discovery of Traditional Chinese Medicine (Natural Medicine) and Translational Medicine, Institute of Medicinal Plant Development, Chinese Academy of Medical Sciences and Peking Union Medical College, Beijing, China

Shaherin Basith, Minghua Cui, Stephani J. Y. Macalino, Jongmi Park, Nina A. B. Clavio, Soosung Kang and Sun Choi
College of Pharmacy and Graduate School of Pharmaceutical Sciences, Ewha Womans University, Seoul, South Korea

Fang-Yu Lin
Graduate Institute of Biomedical Electronics and Bioinformatics, National Taiwan University, Taipei, Taiwan

Emilio Xavier Esposito
exeResearch, LLC, East Lansing, MI, United States

Yufeng J. Tseng
Department of Computer Science and Information Engineering, National Taiwan University, Taipei, Taiwan

Yuqing Cui, Shaohua Liu, Xiaojuan Zhang, Xianfei Ding, Xiaoguang Duan, Huoyan Liang, Dong Wang and Tongwen Sun
General ICU, The First Affiliated Hospital of Zhengzhou University, Henan Key Laboratory of Critical Care Medicine, Zhengzhou Key Laboratory of Sepsis, Zhengzhou, China

Zijia Zhu and Ji Zhang
Department of Pharmacy, The First Affiliated Hospital of Zhengzhou University, Zhengzhou, China

Guojun Zhang
Department of Respiratory, The First Affiliated Hospital of Zhengzhou University, Zhengzhou, China

Zujiang Yu
Department of Infectious Diseases, The First Affiliated Hospital of Zhengzhou University, Zhengzhou, China

Jianjun Yang
Department of Anesthesiology, The First Affiliated Hospital of Zhengzhou University, Zhengzhou, China

Aman Chandra Kaushik and Xiaofeng Dai
Wuxi School of Medicine, Jiangnan University, Wuxi, China

Aamir Mehmood and Dong-Qing Wei
School of Life Sciences and Biotechnology, Shanghai Jiao Tong University, Shanghai, China
Peng Cheng Laboratory, Vanke Cloud City Phase I, Guangdong, China

Francesco Ortuso, Donatella Bagetta, Annalisa Maruca, Carmine Talarico and Stefano Alcaro
Department of Health Sciences, Magna Græcia University of Catanzaro, Catanzaro, Italy

Maria L. Bolognesi
Department of Pharmacy and Biotechnology, Università di Bologna, Bologna, Italy

Norbert Haider and Thierry Langer
Department of Pharmaceutical Chemistry, Faculty of Life Sciences, University of Vienna, Vienna, Austria

Fernanda Borges
Department of Chemistry and Biochemistry, Faculty of Sciences, CIQUP, Universidade do Porto, Porto, Portugal

Sharon Bryant
Inte:Ligand GmbH, Vienna, Austria

Hanoch Senderowitz
Department of Chemistry, Bar-Ilan University, Ramat Gan, Israel

Abraham Yosipof
Department of Information Systems and Department of Business Administration, College of Law & Business, Ramat-Gan, Israel

Rita C. Guedes
Department of Medicinal Chemistry, Faculty of Pharmacy, Research Institute for Medicines (iMed. ULisboa), Universidade de Lisboa, Lisbon, Portugal

Alfonso T. García-Sosa
Department of Molecular Technology, Institute of Chemistry, University of Tartu, Tartu, Estonia

Huixi Zou, Parikshit Banerjee, Sharon Shui Yee Leung and Xiaoyu Yan
School of Pharmacy, Faculty of Medicine, The Chinese University of Hong Kong, Hong Kong

Index

www.ingramcontent.com/pod-product-compliance
Lightning Source LLC
Chambersburg PA
CBHW080303300426
44173CB00005B/27